Comprehensive Periodontics for the Dental Hygienist

Mea A. Weinberg, D.M.D., M.S.D., R.Ph.
Clinical Associate Professor
Director of Second Year Periodontics
Department of Periodontics
Division of Diagnostics, Infectious Diseases and Health Promotion
New York University College of Dentistry
New York, New York

Cheryl Westphal, R.D.H., M.S.
Clinical Associate Professor
Assistant Dean for Allied Health Programs
Director, Dental Hygiene Program
New York University College of Dentistry
New York, New York

Milton Palat, D.D.S., J.D.
Associate Professor
Director of Undergraduate Periodontics
Department of Periodontics
Division of Diagnostics, Infectious Disease and Health Promotion
New York University College of Dentistry
New York, New York

Stuart J. Froum, D.D.S.
Clinical Professor
Director of Research, Department of Implantology
Department of Periodontics
Division of Diagnostics, Infectious Disease and Health Promotion
New York University College of Dentistry
New York, New York

Prentice
Hall

Upper Saddle River, New Jersey, 07458

Library of Congress Cataloging-in-Publication Data

Comprehensive periodontics for the dental hygienist / [edited by] Mea A. Weinberg ...
[et al.].
    p. cm.
  Includes bibliographical references and index.
  ISBN 0-8385-1554-1
    1. Periodontics. 2. Dental hygienists. I. Weinberg, Mea A.
  RK361 .C58 2001
  617.6'32—dc21

                        00-063717

Publisher: Julie Alexander
Executive Editor: Greg Vis
Acquisitions Editor: Mark Cohen
Editorial Assistant: Melissa Kerian
Director of Manufacturing and Production: Bruce Johnson
Managing Editor: Patrick Walsh
Production Editor: Carlisle Publishers Services
Production Liaison: Cathy O'Connell
Manufacturing Manager: Ilene Sanford
Director of Marketing: Leslie Cavaliere
Marketing Manager: Kristin Walton
Marketing Coordinator: Cindy Frederick
Creative Director: Marianne Frasco
Cover Design: Dennis Moller
Composition and Interior Design: Carlisle Communications
Printing and Binding: Courier Stoughton

Notice: The authors and the publisher of this volume have taken care that the information and technical recommendations contained herein are based on research and expert consultation, and are accurate and compatible with the standards generally accepted at the time of publication. Nevertheless, as new information becomes available, changes in clinical and technical practices become necessary. The reader is advised to carefully consult manufacturers' instructions and information material for all supplies and equipment before use, and to consult with a health care professional as necessary. This advice is especially important when using new supplies or equipment for clinical purposes. The authors and publisher disclaim all responsibility for any liability, loss, injury, or damage incurred as a consequence, directly or indirectly, of the use and application of any of the contents of this volume.

Prentice-Hall International (UK) Limited, *London*
Prentice-Hall of Australia Pty. Limited, *Sydney*
Prentice-Hall Canada Inc., *Toronto*
Prentice-Hall Hispanoamericana, S.A., *Mexico*
Prentice-Hall of India Private Limited, *New Delhi*
Prentice-Hall of Japan, Inc., *Tokyo*
Prentice-Hall Singapore Pte. Ltd.
Editoria Prentice-Hall do Brasil, Ltda., *Rio de Janeiro*

10 9 8 7 6 5 4 3
ISBN 0-8385-1554-1

Contents

Fall 2003 Midterm + Final SDHS

In the increasingly complicated world of periodontics, it is important that the fundamental principles of therapy and pathogenesis remain the unifying theme of any text on the subject. This text, anchored in evidence-based learning, offers these fundamental principles with concise definitions, precise objectives, and helpful lists not only of key words but also of key points. It simplifies many of the complexities of the disease process without confusing them and provides clear links back to practical aspects of therapy.

Importantly, while basic biologic principles unify the text, timely discussions of implant care, medically compromised patients, and chemotherapeutics add a high degree of relevance. Indeed, at the dawn of the new millennium, it is critical to prepare clinicians for the inevitable advances in chemotherapy and diagnostics that will be the hallmark of clinical management of periodontal diseases in the future.

The reader is urged to take full advantage of the many learning tools incorporated into this text. These tools include frequent references, definitions, key words, key points, and self-quiz questions. When more details are required than are possible in a book of this type, the reader is urged to consult the references. Hopefully, on completion of this text the reader will fully understand the evidence-based nature of periodontal diseases and their many modes of treatment. Moreover, it is the purpose of this book to be both clear and concise, and it is expected that readers will be able to use similar clear explanations of therapy and etiology when discussing periodontal problems with both patients and colleagues. This clarity of thought will inspire readers to seek further illumination of the topics through the biomedical literature, consultation with learned faculty, and a zest for lifelong learning.

Dean Michael C. Alfano, D.M.D., Ph.D.
Professor and Dean, College of Dentistry
New York University
New York, New York

There is now a significant body of knowledge about the risk factors, pathogenesis and treatment, and prevention of periodontal diseases. Yet this knowledge is rarely applied as an evidence-based approach to the difficult problem of deciding when specific treatments or examination methods work. Thus, both classic and current references are included in each chapter.

This basic text has been written in an attempt to make our understanding of periodontal diseases accessible to the dental hygiene student and to the practicing dental hygienist and dentist needing to update basic knowledge or acquire a concise synopsis of clinical periodontics. This text is presented in three sections:

Section I deals with the anatomy of the periodontium, progression of periodontal diseases, risk factors (e.g., dental biofilms, smoking, and diabetes mellitus) for periodontal diseases, and periodontal disease as a risk factor for systemic conditions such as stroke, cardiovascular disease, emphysema, and premature low-birth-weight babies.

Section II deals with the clinical examination and treatment planning for the management of patients with periodontal diseases.

Section III comprises the remaining chapters, which discuss the nonsurgical and surgical therapy. Included in this section is an extensive review of drugs used in periodontal therapy including various controlled-release drug devices (e.g., PerioChip™, Atridox®, Actiste®) and enzyme suppression drugs (e.g., Periostat™) used as adjunctive treatment. The appendices include the steps needed for the prevention of infective endocarditis, periodontic informatics, how to critically review the periodontal literature, and periodontal issues pertaining to women. Extensive tables feature clinical applications of periodontal therapy.

At the 1999 International Workshop for a Classification of Periodontal Diseases and Conditions in Illinois, a new classification system was developed. This is reviewed in Appendix 5. It is the intentions of The Academy of Periodontology to integrate this new system into education as early as possible. Since this classification was published during the final stages of publication of this textbook, we attempted to incorporate the new terminology, at times referring to the older, out-of-date terms. However, the reader should refer to Chapter 4 for a more in-depth description of the new terminology.

We hope this book will serve as a helpful text for all dental practitioners.

Mea A. Weinberg, D.M.D., M.S.D., R.Ph.
Cheryl Westphal, R.D.H., M.S.
Milton Palat, D.D.S, J.D.
Stuart J. Froum, D.D.S.

Preface

Contributors

Mary Elizabeth Aichelmann-Reidy, D.D.S.
Assistant Professor
Department of Periodontics
University of Maryland
Baltimore, Maryland

Fadi I. Beydoun, D.D.S., M.S.
Clinical Assistant Professor
Department of Periodontics
Division of Diagnostics, Infectious Disease
    and Health Promotion
New York University College of Dentistry
New York, New York

Ulana K. Cirincione, R.D.H., M.S., M.P.H.
Clinical Associate Professor
Department of Periodontics
Northwestern University School of
    Dentistry
Chicago, Illinois

Denise Estafan, D.D.S, M.S.
Assistant Professor
Director of Clinical Esthetics
Division of Reconstructive and Compre-
    hensive Care
New York University College of Dentistry
New York, New York

Suzanne K. Farrar, B.S., R.D.H.
Clinical Instructor
Department of Periodontics
Louisiana State University School of
    Dentistry
New Orleans, Louisiana

Cynthia Fong, R.D.H., M.S.
Lecturer/Instructor in Periodontics
Pierce College
Department of Dental Hygiene
Tacoma, Washington

Herbert Frommer, D.D.S.
Professor
Director of Radiology
New York University College of Dentistry
New York, New York

Stuart J. Froum, D.D.S.
Clinical Professor, Director of Research
Department of Implantology
Department of Periodontics
Division of Diagnostics, Infectious Disease
    and Health Promotion
New York University College of Dentistry
New York, New York

Diana L. Mercado Galvis, R.D.H., M.S.
Former Clinical Associate Professor
Dental Hygiene Program
New York University College of Dentistry
New York, New York

Ann M. Goodwin, R.D.H., M.S.
Clinical Associate Professor
Dental Hygiene Program
New York University College of Dentistry
New York, New York

Rosemary DeRosa Hays, R.D.H., M.S.
Clinical Associate Professor
Dental Hygiene Program
New York University College of Dentistry
New York, New York

Cheng-Sheng Ho, D.D.S., M.S.
Department of Periodontics and Implant
    Dentistry
China Medicine College Hospital
China Medicine College Dental School
Taiwan

Judith Kreismann, R.D.H., B.S., M.S.
Clinical Associate Professor
Dental Hygiene Program
New York University College of Dentistry
New York, New York

Eva M. Lupovici, R.D.H., M.S.
Clinical Associate Professor
Dental Hygiene Program
New York University College of Dentistry
New York, New York

John D. Mason, B.A., D.D.S.
Assistant Professor
Department of Periodontics
Louisiana State University School of
  Dentistry
New Orleans, Louisiana

Trisha E. O'Hehir, R.D.H., B.S.
Editor of Perio Reports
Senior Consulting Editor, RHD Magazine
Vice President, Perio-Data™ Company
Assistant Visiting Professor, Northern
  Arizona University
Flagstaff, Arizona

Milton Palat, D.D.S., J.D.
Associate Professor
Director of Undergraduate Periodontics
Department of Periodontics; Division of
  Diagnostics, Infectious Disease and
  Health Promotion
New York University College of Dentistry
New York, New York

Jill Rethman, R.D.H., B.A.
Visiting Clinical Instructor
University of Pittsburgh
School of Dental Medicine, Department of
  Dental Hygiene
Pittsburgh, Pennsylvania

Michael P. Rethman, D.D.S., M.S.
Chief of Periodontics
Tripler Medical Center
Honolulu, Hawaii

Robert S. Schoor, D.D.S.
Associate Professor
Director of Postgraduate Periodontics
Department of Periodontics
Division of Diagnostics, Infectious Disease
  and Health Promotion
New York University College of Dentistry
New York, New York

Surendra Singh, D.D.S., M.S.
Professor
Department of Periodontics
University of Medicine and Dentistry of
  New Jersey School of Dentistry
Newark, New Jersey

Jeanne St. Germain, B.S., R.D.H.
Clinical Instructor
Department of Periodontics
Louisiana State University School of
  Dentistry
New Orleans, Louisiana

Mea A. Weinberg, D.M.D., M.S.D., R.Ph.
Clinical Associate Professor
Director of Second Year Periodontics
Department of Periodontics
Division of Diagnostics, Infectious Dis-
  eases and Health Promotion
New York University College of Dentistry
New York, New York

Theodore L. West, D.D.S., M.D.S.
Clinical Professor
Department of Periodontics
School of Dental and Oral Surgery
Columbia University
New York, New York

Cheryl Westphal, R.D.H., M.S.
Clinical Associate Professor
Assistant Dean for Allied Health Programs
Director, Dental Hygiene Program
New York University College of Dentistry
New York, New York

Raymond A. Yukna, D.M.D., M.S.
Professor, Coordinator Postgraduate
  Periodontics
Louisiana State University School of
  Dentistry
New Orleans, Louisiana

Reviewers

Deedee McClain Smith, C.D.A., R.D.H., M.S.
York Technical College
Rock Hill, South Carolina

Linda DeVore, R.D.H., M.A.
University of Maryland Dental School
Baltimore, Maryland

Carol Johnson, M.S.H.A.
Carroll Technical Institute
Douglasville, Georgia

C. Merry LeBlond, R.D.H., M.S.
Middlesex County College
Edison, New Jersey

Joan Otomo-Corgel, D.D.S., M.P.H.
VAMC Postdoctoral Periodontics Residency
Faculty and Chair of Research
Adjunct Assistant Professor in Residence
UCLA School of Dentistry
Department of Periodontics
Los Angeles, California

PERIODONTAL DISEASES: INTRODUCTION AND BACKGROUND

Section I

ANATOMY OF THE PERIODONTAL STRUCTURES: THE HEALTHY STATE

Mea A. Weinberg, D.M.D., M.S.D., R.Ph.

Outline:

Clinical Anatomy of the Gingival Unit
Microscopic Anatomy of the Gingival Unit
Attachment Apparatus
Physiology of the Periodontium
Changes with Aging
Summary
Key Points
References
Self-Quiz

Goal:

To provide the dental hygienist with knowledge of the structures and functions of the periodontium in health.

Educational Objectives:

Upon completion of this chapter, the reader should be able to:

Illustrate and discuss the clinical anatomy of the periodontium;

Illustrate and describe the microscopic anatomy of the periodontium;

List and describe the functions of the periodontium;

Discuss the importance of the dentogingival unit; and

Describe the blood supply to the gingiva and the attachment apparatus.

KEY WORDS
• periodontium
• attachment apparatus
• connective tissue attachment
• dentogingival unit
• biologic width

*T*he **periodontium,** translated in Latin to mean "around the tooth," consists of the gingiva, periodontal ligament, cementum, and alveolar and supporting bone which surrounds and supports the teeth (Fig. 1–1a ■). The **attachment apparatus** consists of periodontal tissues involved in the attachment and support of the root in the tooth socket, specifically the periodontal ligament, cementum, and alveolar and supporting bone (Hassell 1993). Although each component differs in function and character, they are all biologically dependent upon each other and are considered important in the functioning of the oral cavity. A working knowledge of the ultrastructural anatomy and biology of the periodontal tissues is an important prerequisite for practitioners to recognize and treat periodontal diseases.

In order to understand the different stages of diseases in the periodontium, it is necessary to recognize the structures and functions of the periodontium in health. This chapter describes the clinical and microscopic features of the periodontium in health and will be the foundation for ensuing discussions in this text.

CLINICAL ANATOMY OF THE GINGIVAL UNIT

The oral mucosa is divided into three types: (1) masticatory mucosa, which includes the gingiva and hard palate; (2) lining mucosa, which consists of the alveolar mucosa, soft palate, lining of lips, cheeks, and sublingual area; and (3) specialized mucosa, which is found on the dorsum of the tongue.

MASTICATORY MUCOSA (GINGIVA)

The gingiva forms a protective covering over the other components of the periodontium and is well adapted to protect against mechanical insults (e.g., toothbrushing and chewing). The gingiva encircles the cervical portion of the teeth and covers the alveolar process. Anatomically, the gingiva is subdivided into the free gingiva, attached gingiva, and interdental gingiva or papilla (Fig. 1–1b ■). The outer surface of the gingiva consists of stratified squamous epithelium. Underneath the epithelium is gingival connective tissue, which is termed the *lamina propria.*

Free gingiva (marginal gingiva)

The free gingiva or marginal gingiva surrounds the neck of the tooth. Its boundaries are coronally, the free gingival margin; apically, the free gingival groove; and laterally, the gingival crevice and the tooth (Fig. 1–1b). The free gingiva is approximately 1.5 mm wide and has a smooth surface. The free gingiva lies on and adapts to the enamel and can be separated from the tooth with a periodontal instrument (Schroeder and Listgarten 1997).

The free gingival margin is the edge or the most coronal part of the free gingiva and in a fully erupted tooth is located on the enamel approximately 0.5 to 2 mm coronal to the cementoenamel junction (CEJ). It is the entry into the gingival crevice. The free gingival margin has a scalloped outline following the contour of the cementoenamel junction (Fig. 1–1b). In the posterior region the architecture becomes less scalloped. Up to the completed eruption of permanent teeth in children, the free gingival margin usually remains located on the cervical bulge of

FIGURE 1-1

(a) Schematic drawing of a tooth with its periodontium: G = gingiva; PDL = periodontal ligament fibers; RC = root cementum; ABP = alveolar bone proper; AP = alveolar process. (b) Landmarks of the gingival unit. The gingiva is salmon pink, while the alveolar mucosa is thinner and redder in color. (Right side) Schematic drawing of a cross section of the periodontium: E = enamel; FGM = Free gingival margin; FG = free gingiva; AG = attached gingiva; MGJ = mucogingival junction; AM = alveolar mucosa; FN = frenum; AP = alveolar process; CEJ = cementoenamel junction. (Copyright © 1997 by J. Lindhe and T. Karring, Anatomy of the periodontium, in *Clinical periodontology and implant dentistry*, ed. J. Lindhe. Copenhagen: Munksgaard.)

(a)

(b)

the enamel. This is a normal situation and as the tooth erupts the free gingival margin will ultimately move apically.

Gingival Crevice   The gingival crevice is the space between the free gingiva and the tooth surface and is lined by nonkeratinized stratified squamous epithelium. In gingival health the gingival crevice is known as a *sulcus,* whereas in disease it is termed a *pocket*. The normal sulcular depth is approximately 1 to 3 mm when measured with a periodontal probe.

Gingival crevicular fluid (GCF) is the fluid that originates from blood vessels within the underlying connective tissue (lamina propria) and flows through the tissue into the gingival crevice. The rate of passage of this fluid is, apparently, dependent upon the absence or presence of inflammation in the connective tissue of the gingiva. The flow is minimal to absent in health, but increases due to the accumulation of plaque in the gingival crevice (Alfano 1974). Components of GCF resemble blood serum components and include elements such as calcium, sodium, potassium, and phosphorous, along with cells and bacteria. The role of GCF is both protective and harmful. While crevicular fluid flow cleanses the sulcus, it is also a source of nutrients for subgingival bacteria and supports subgingival calculus formation (Mukherjee 1985). Certain antibiotics including tetracyclines used in the treatment of periodontal diseases have been found to concentrate in higher levels locally in the GCF (pocket area) than in the serum (Gordon et al. 1981).

Free Gingival Groove   The free gingival groove, a shallow depression on the outer surface of the gingiva, is about 1 to 2 mm apical from the margin of the gingiva and corresponds approximately to the level of the cementoenamel junction. This groove separates the free gingiva from the attached gingiva. The free gingival groove is present in about 30 to 40% of adults and occurs most frequently in the mandibular premolar and incisor areas. It is more pronounced on the facial than on the lingual regions. Its absence or presence is not related to the health of the gingiva.

Attached gingiva

The attached gingiva is continuous with the free gingiva and is firmly attached to the underlying cementum and periosteum (connective tissue) covering the alveolar process. It extends apically from the free gingival groove to the mucogingival junction (MGJ) or mucogingival line. The mucogingival junction joins the attached gingiva to the alveolar mucosa (Fig. 1–1b). The scalloped mucogingival junction is not discernible on the palate because the attached gingiva runs into the palatal mucosa. The width of the free gingiva and the attached gingiva consists of the total width of gingiva.

Since attached gingiva is not movable and is firmly bound down to the tooth and bone, it is capable of withstanding forces from toothbrushing and chewing. The width of the attached gingiva varies in different areas of the mouth and between individuals (Fig. 1–2 ■). On the facial aspect, the attached gingiva is widest in the incisor region and narrowest in the first premolar area. On the lingual aspect, the attached gingiva is widest in the molar region and narrowest in the incisor region. The width of attached gingiva increases with age because teeth will slowly erupt continuously throughout life as a result of natural attrition or occlusal wear (Ainamo and Talari 1976).

The color of the gingiva is normally salmon pink with slight variations. The gingiva shows varying degrees of brownish color depending on ethnic variation (Fig. 1–3 ■). This is considered to be normal gingival pigmentation.

Stippling   Clinically, the outer surface of the attached gingiva has an appearance similar to an orange peel with shallow depressions between elevations referred to as being *stippled*. The free gingiva has a smooth surface and is not stippled (Fig. 1–4 ■). A histologic description of stippling is discussed in the following section.

FIGURE 1–2

Varying amounts of attached gingiva; the narrowest width is on the mandibular premolars and the widest is on the maxillary incisors.

FIGURE 1–3

Physiological gingival pigmentation in a 30-year-old patient from India.

FIGURE 1–4

Surface stippling of the attached gingiva and the interdental gingiva. Note the dimpling or depressions on the surface. The surface of the free gingiva is not stippled.

Stippling may be present in health or disease. The absence of stippling does not necessarily indicate the presence of disease. On the other hand, the presence of inflammation with the loss of stippling can be considered part of the disease process, assuming stippling was present initially.

Stippling is present in only about 40% of adults and varies in different individuals, ages, and sexes. Stippling of the attached gingiva is absent in children under 5 years of age and may be more evident in men than women. It is more prominent in the anterior than the posterior region and may even be absent in the molar areas. The facial gingiva shows more prominent stippling than the lingual.

Interdental gingiva (interdental papilla)

In health the interdental gingiva tightly fills the gingival embrasure, which is the space between the contact point and alveolar bone of two adjacent teeth. The margin and lateral borders of the interdental gingiva are an extension of the free gingiva, whereas the remaining parts are attached gingiva (Fig. 1–5a ■).

FIGURE 1–5

Features of the interdental gingiva. (a) In health the interdental gingiva fills the gingival embrasure (G). (b) The col is directly under the contact point of the teeth. (From P. F. Fedi, Jr., and A. R. Vernino. *The periodontic syllabus.* Copyright © 2000 by Williams & Wilkins.)

(a)

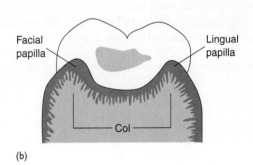

(b)

The size and shape of the papillae are determined by tooth-to-tooth contact, the curvature of the cementoenamel junction, and the width (faciolingually) of the interproximal tooth surfaces. When teeth are crowded, as often seen in mandibular incisors, the papillae may be slender and narrow. Anterior papillae are pyramidal in shape while posterior papillae are rounder and slightly flatter. An anterior papilla forms a single pyramidal structure because there is only one papilla. The papillae of posterior teeth (premolars and molars) are wedge shaped, with one vestibular (facial) and one oral (lingual) papilla connected by a concave area called the *col* (Fig. 1–5b ■). The col is directly apical to the contact point, representing the fusion of the interproximal junctional epithelia of two adjacent teeth. While an anterior papilla can form a col shape, it is more prominent in posterior papillae. When a diastema (loss of contact between two adjacent teeth) is present the interdental papilla is absent and there is no col. Since the shape of a col is concave it may predispose the interproximal area to the accumulation of dental plaque.

LINING MUCOSA

Alveolar mucosa

Although not actually part of the periodontium, the alveolar mucosa is an important periodontal structure and deserves discussion. The alveolar mucosa extends apically from the mucogingival junction to the mucous membrane of the cheek, lip, and floor of the mouth (Fig. 1–1b). In comparison to the attached gingiva, alveolar mucosa is thinner and redder in color, has a smooth surface, and is movable.

Frenum Attachments   Frenum (pleural: frena) attachments are folds of alveolar mucosa. They are not concentrations of muscle, having no more muscle fibers than alveolar mucosa. The function of a frenum is to attach lips and cheeks to the maxillary and mandibular mucosa and to limit the movement of the lips and cheeks. There are usually seven frena located in the canine/premolar area, between the central incisors and in the mandibular anterior lingual area. A frenum should originate and end in alveolar mucosa near the mucogingival junction.

SPECIALIZED MUCOSA

The mucosa of the dorsum of the tongue contains numerous papillae of three types: filiform, fungiform, and circumvallate. The circumvallate papillae are located along the V-shaped groove on the back of the tongue. Each papilla is surrounded by a circular groove. The taste buds are located mainly on the sides of these papillae. The filiform papillae are slender ones and the most abundant, covering the entire top or dorsal surface of the tongue. No taste buds are associated with these papillae; they respond only to heat and mechanical stimuli. The fungiform papillae, which are broad and flat, are found chiefly at the edges of the tongue and are provided with taste buds.

MICROSCOPIC ANATOMY OF THE GINGIVAL UNIT

GINGIVAL EPITHELIUM

The gingiva is covered by a layer of stratified squamous epithelium with an underlying core of connective tissue called the *lamina propria* (Fig. 1–6 ■). The gingival epithelium exists as structurally different forms specific to certain areas of the teeth. Thus, the gingival epithelium can be divided into (Fig. 1–7 ■):

- the oral epithelium (OE);
- the sulcular or crevicular epithelium (SE); and
- the junctional epithelium (JE).

The gingival epithelium is avascular and relies upon the underlying lamina propria for its blood supply and nutrients. The epithelium found in the oral cavity consists of several layers of cells (Fig. 1–7):

1. stratum basale or stratum germinativum (basal cell layer); deepest layer next to the lamina propria;

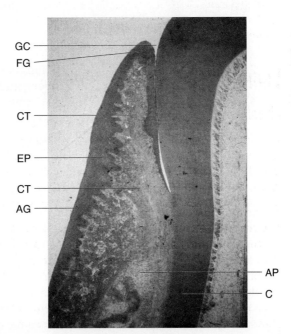

FIGURE 1–6

Photomicrograph of the gingival epithelium (EP) and the gingival connective tissue or lamina propria (CT). AG = attached gingiva; FG = free gingiva; GC = gingival crevice; C = cementum; AP = alveolar process. (Courtesy of Dr. Harvey Wishe, New York University College of Dentistry.)

Diagram of the layers of the gingival epithelium. Underlying the epithelium is the gingival connective tissue (lamina propria). OE = oral epithelium; SE = sulcular epithelium; JE = junctional epithelium; CT = gingival connective tissue or lamina propria; GF = gingival fibers; GS = gingival sulcus; E = enamel; D = dentin; C = cementum; AP = Alveolar process; BCL = basal cell layer; PCL = prickle cells layer; SL = superficial layer.

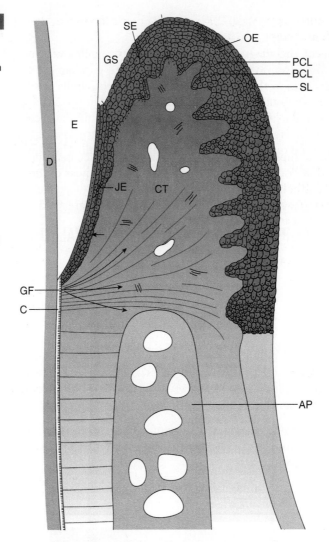

2. stratum spinosum (prickle or spinous cell layer);
3. stratum granulosum (granular layer); and
4. the stratum corneum (keratinized/cornified cell layer; also called the *superficial cell layer*); this outermost layer serves as a barrier membrane protecting the underlying periodontal tissues from invasion by foreign substances.

Cell renewal

Since the epithelium is subject to considerable insult, it must have a means of regular renewal. The epithelium achieves this renewal by producing a pool of cells that migrate from the basal layer to the oral environment. This process by which epithelial cells differentiate or mature is called *keratinization*. The type of differentiation reflects the functional demands or stimulus placed on the tissue. During keratinization, the entire thickness of the epithelium is replaced. The time it takes for this replacement or cell renewal is called the *turnover time.* This time differs with the various types of epithelium. Such differences become important during tissue healing after periodontal surgery or tissue damage.

The keratinization process occurs as follows (Moss-Salentijn and Hendricks-Klyvert 1990):

- basal cells in the basal cell layer divide and produce new cells;
- the "older" basal cells travel or move into the next layer, the spinous cell layer, on their way to the most outer epithelial cell layer;
- once in the spinous cell layer, the basal cells becomes keratinocytes. On their way to the outer surface, the keratinocytes synthesize or produce keratin;
- keratin is a protein that contributes to the mechanical toughness of the outer surface of the epithelium; and
- when the keratinocytes reach the outer epithelial surface, they are shed from the surface into the oral cavity.

Three grades of keratinization or maturation are identified according to the completeness of the transition of the keratinocyte from the basal cell layer to the outermost, superficial cell layer. Consequently, epithelium can be keratinized, parakeratinized, or nonkeratinized. Keratinized epithelium is composed of all four layers and is primarily seen in the skin. Fully keratinized cells form keratin and lose their nuclei by the time they migrate to the outer surface. Parakeratinized cells, which are found in the mouth in areas such as the gingival oral epithelium, retain their nuclei but show some signs of being keratinized. The stratum granulosum is usually difficult to recognize and a surface parakeratinized outer layer is present. Epithelial cells found in the junctional epithelium and alveolar mucosas are nonkeratinized and do not undergo keratinization.

Oral epithelium

The oral epithelium faces the oral cavity on the outer surface of the free and attached gingivae extending from the free gingival margin to the mucogingival junction. The gingiva is usually composed of parakeratinized stratified squamous epithelium.

The gingiva has an epithelial turnover time of approximately 10 days as demonstrated in an animal model (Schroeder and Listgarten 1997), while in the skin it is approximately 28 days.

Cells in the Oral Epithelium   The function of the oral epithelium is to protect the underlying structures and acts as a mechanical barrier. The oral epithelium contains cells:

- keratinocytes
- nonkeratinocytes (also called clear cells)
  - melanocytes
  - Langerhans cells
  - Merkel cells

Keratinocytes make up the majority of oral epithelial cells. Keratinocytes function to synthesize keratin which contributes to the mechanical toughness of the outer surface of the oral epithelium and relative impermeability to fluids and cells. It is also responsible for the salmon pink color of the gingiva.

Melanocytes located in the basal cell layer secrete melanin, which is responsible for the brownish pigmentation in the gingiva. Pigmentation is more prominent in darker-skinned individuals (Fig. 1–3). The amount of pigmentation is genetically predetermined according to the potential of the cells to produce melanin, rather than to the number of cells present.

Other cell types in the gingival epithelium are the Langerhans cells, which are located in the stratum spinosum and are involved in the early defense mechanism of the gingiva. Merkel cells are found in the basal cell layer and are associated with nerve endings acting as touch-sensory cells. White blood cells such as lymphocytes and neutrophils or polymorphonuclear leukocytes (PMNs) are transiently found in the epithelial layers in health but increase in numbers in periodontal disease, functioning to defend the body against bacteria and other invaders.

Sulcular epithelium

Overall, the sulcular epithelum is structurally similar to the oral epithelium except that it is less keratinized. The sulcular epithelium has epithelial ridges as does the oral epithelium. Sulcular or crevicular epithelium lines the gingival sulcus without being in contact with the tooth surface. It is generally nonkeratinized and thin but can become parakeratinized if given the appropriate stimulus. The sulcular epithelium exhibits two or three cell layers and a definitive and continuous cornified layer is absent. At the free gingival margin, it is continuous with, and structurally similar to, the oral epithelium. Apically it overlaps the coronal surface of the junctional epithelium and faces the tooth surface (Fig. 1–7).

Junctional epithelium

The junctional epithelium is the epithelial part of the free gingiva not visible from the outside. It provides the contact between the gingiva and the tooth. The junctional epithelium can be regarded as a downgrowth of the squamous epithelium of the gingiva and is continuous with the sulcular epithelium, extending from the bottom of the crevice to the cementoenamel junction. It forms a collar around the neck of the tooth on the cervical part of the enamel.

The junctional epithelium is composed of nonkeratinized stratified squamous epithelium. It is composed of only two epithelial layers, either an active basal cell layer and an inactive suprabasal cell layer or a basal cell and spinous cell layer (Hassell 1993; Schroeder and Listgarten 1997).

The junctional epithelium, through the epithelial attachment, contributes to the direct attachment of the gingiva to the tooth surface and thus serves a significant role in periodontal health and disease when this attachment to the tooth is lost.

At the coronal portion, the thickness of the junctional epithelium is about fifteen to thirty cells, while apically, near the cementoenamel junction, there may be only one to two cells (Fig. 1–7). Interproximally, the junctional epithelium of adjacent teeth fuses coronally to form the lining of the col area (Schroeder and Listgarten 1997).

Semipermeable Membrane The junctional epithelium is more permeable than the oral or sulcular epithelium. Thus, the junctional epithelium is referred to as a *semipermeable membrane* allowing the movement of fluid and cells of certain sizes (Kornman, Page, and Tonetti 1997). There are fewer intercellular junctions and thus wider spaces between the cells than in the oral or sulcular epithelium, and the cells are arranged in a parallel fashion. This allows for passage of cells and tissue fluid from the lamina propria into the sulcus and for passage of bacteria and its by-products from the gingival sulcus into the lamina propria. It is also more permeable because the cells do not keratinize. The coronal part of the junctional epithelium that is closest to the bottom of the sulcus is the most permeable part, while the apical part is where cell division for tissue renewal occurs.

Cells in the Junctional Epithelium   In addition to keratinocytes, the junctional epithelium may contain clear cells. In health, small numbers of PMNs are transiently seen in the junctional epithelium (Tonetti et al. 1995). They will usually pass through the junctional epithelium into the gingival sulcus, where they play a role in the defense of the host (body) against bacteria and other microorganisms.

Cellular Turnover   A unique characteristic of the junctional epithelium is its high rate of cellular turnover. As demonstrated in an animal model, the cells of the junctional epithelium undergo constant turnover every 4 to 7 days, whereby the basal cells migrate coronally out through the sulcus where the old cells are shed into the oral cavity.

ALVEOLAR MUCOSA

Alveolar mucosa is compressible and movable due to the presence of a submucosa between the thin lamina propria and the underlying tissue, usually muscle, the presence of elastic fibers, and an underlying loose connective tissue that is attached to the underlying periosteum of the alveolar process.

The epithelium of the alveolar mucosa has about the same thickness as that of the gingiva, but its structure is completely different (Schroeder 1991; Schroeder and Listgarten 1997). A granular layer is not present and the superficial layer does not stain, as does the surface of parakeratinized epithelium (Squier and Hill 1998). The epithelium contains melanocytes, Langerhans cells, Merkel cells, and small lymphocytes.

Epithelial ridges are either not present or if present they are indistinct because they are shorter and wider than in the gingiva, giving a smoother surface texture. The color is darker red than the gingiva because of its highly vascular underlying connective tissue. The point where there is a marked increase in elastic fibers within the underlying connective tissue demarcates the mucogingival junction.

GINGIVAL CONNECTIVE TISSUE

Underlying the stratified squamous epithelium and encircling the tooth is the gingival connective tissue or lamina propria.

Connective tissue/epithelium interface

The interface between the connective tissue and oral epithelium is not smooth, but rather the undersurface of the epithelium has connecting epithelial ridges that extend into the connective tissue (Fig. 1–8 ■). At the intersection of epithelial ridges are pits or depressions that contain connective tissue extensions called *connective tissue papillae.* Clinically these depressions evident on the surface of the gingiva represent stippling. Stippling is established at the areas of fusion between adjacent epithelial ridges. In periodontal health the epithelial ridges are absent from the junctional epithelium and are not well developed in the sulcular epithelium. The

FIGURE 1–8

A photomicrograph of the gingival oral epithelium (OE)/connective tissue (CT) interface. Note prominent epithelial ridges (ER). Intersections between the epithelial ridges under the epithelial surface correspond to depressions seen on the surface of the gingiva. Fingerlike projections termed *connective tissue papillae* (CP) extend into the depressions on the undersurface of the epithelium. This produces the characteristic stippled appearance of the attached gingiva. (Courtesy of Dr. Harvey Wishe, New York University College of Dentistry.)

main purposes of stippling is to aid in the increased strength between the epithelium and connective tissue and to enable the epithelium to obtain its blood supply from the connective tissue papillae in the shortest distance possible.

Gingival connective tissue

The main component of the gingival connective tissue, as well as all connective tissue in the body, is collagen fibers, which accounts for about 60% of the total volume. Collagen is a protein composed of amino acids. There are many different types of collagen, with Type I and III primarily found in most connective tissues. The lamina propria provides mechanical support and nutrients for the avascular epithelium. Type I collagen fibers give the gingiva its firmness and resiliency. The remainder of gingival connective tissue consists of ground substance, which is composed of proteins termed *proteoglycans,* in which the collagen fibers, cells, nerves, and blood vessels are embedded. Proteoglycans have a protein core with carbohydrate side chains (glycosaminoglycans) of chondroitin sulphate, heparin sulphate, and hyaluronic acid. The ground substance also allows for the transportation of water and nutrients through the tissue.

Gingival Fibers   The free and attached gingivae are attached to the tooth surface through a **connective tissue attachment.** Collagen fibers in the gingiva are arranged in such a way that they maintain the gingiva against the tooth and bone. The collagen fibers are organized in bundles or groups according to their origin and insertion (Schroeder and Listgarten 1997). The collagen fibers embedded on one end in the cementum are termed Sharpey's fibers (Goldman 1951). Collectively the gingival fiber bundles are called the *gingival fibers,* the *supracrestal fiber apparatus* (because they are located coronal to the crest of alveolar bone), or the *gingival connective tissue attachment.* These three terms will be used interchangeably throughout the text. Table 1–1 ■ reviews the primary collagen fiber

TABLE 1–1		
CLASSIFICATION OF THE GINGIVAL FIBERS		
NAME OF FIBER	**ORIGIN AND DISTRIBUTION**	**FUNCTION**
Circular	Encircles the tooth within the free gingiva	Provides support and contour to the free gingiva
Dentogingival	From the cementum at the base of the gingival sulcus, flares coronally into the free gingiva (group A), laterally into the attached gingiva (group B), and apically into the periosteum (group C); found on the facial, lingual, and interproximal surfaces	Contributes to the support of the gingiva
Dentoperiosteal	Extends from the cementum apically over the alveolar crest into the periosteum	Anchors the tooth to the bone
Alveologingival	Extends from the periosteum of the alveolar crestal bone coronally into the connective tissue	Attaches the gingiva to the alveolar bone
Transseptal	Runs from the cementum of one tooth interproximal to the cementum of the adjacent tooth	Keeps teeth in alignment and protects the interproximal bone from the inflammatory infiltrate; resistant to inflammation and will continuously reform when bone and fibers are destroyed

FIGURE 1–9

The major part of the connective tissue of the free and attached gingivae are composed of collagen fibers that are arranged in groups or bundles. The name indicates the origin and insertion of the fibers: CF = circular fibers; DGF = dentogingival fibers; DPF = dentoperiosteal fibers; TF = transseptal fibers. (Copyright © 1997 by J. Lindhe and T. Karring, Anatomy of the periodontium, in *Clinical periodontology and implant dentistry,* ed. J. Lindhe. Copenhagen: Munksgaard.)

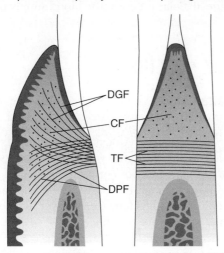

groups in the gingiva (Fig. 1–9 ■), including the circular, dentogingival, dentoperiosteal, alveologingival, and transseptal fibers. Secondary gingival fiber groups include periostogingival, interpapillary, transgingival, intercrevicular, semicircular, and intergingival fibers (Page et al. 1974; Goldman 1951). Their function is to support and give contour to the free and attached gingivae and firmly connect the attached gingiva to the underlying cementum and alveolar bone. The free gingiva is not actually free nor is it attached to the tooth, but rather it is held in close proximity to the tooth by the gingival fibers, which prevent the free gingiva from being deflected from the tooth during mastication.

Collagen organization

Collagen fibers are either densely or loosely organized. Dense connective tissue that is found in the lamina propria of the gingiva consists of heavy, tightly packed fibers that function to resist tension. Loose connective tissue, as exemplified by alveolar mucosa, is composed of the collagen fibers that are thin and delicate and do not have a mechanical protective function. Collagen is constantly being synthesized and degraded as part of the normal remodeling or turnover of gingival connective tissue.

Cellular and vascular elements

The cellular part of the lamina propria predominately consists of

- fibroblasts;
- macrophages;
- mast cells; and
- plasma cells, lymphocytes, and neutrophils.

Fibroblasts synthesize ground substance, collagen, and collagenase. Collagenase is an enzyme responsible for the breakdown of collagen during remodeling. Thus, fibroblasts play a chief role in the maintenance and remodeling of connective tissue. Other cells in the lamina propria include red blood cells, PMNs, macrophages, lymphocytes, and mast cells, which are involved in the defense of the host against toxins.

A rich vascular complex is found in the lamina propria. Since there is no submucosa, as is found in the alveolar mucosa, the blood supply passes directly to the lamina propria.

CELL-TO-CELL TISSUE JUNCTION

Epithelial cell-to-cell attachment

Electron microscopy has demonstrated that epithelial cells are held together by intercellular bridges or desmosomes. A desmosome consists of two adjacent attachment plaques, which are continuous with the innermost leaflet of the cell membrane (Fig. 1–10 ■). A space exists between adjacent desmosomes allowing passage of material and fluid through the tissue while holding together epithelial cells. Since junctional epithelium has four times fewer desmosomes than oral epithelium, the intercellular spaces are wider.

Epithelium-tooth surface/connective tissue interface

The junctional epithelium adheres to the tooth surface (e.g., enamel) through the epithelial attachment. The basal cells of the junctional epithelium do not contact the enamel or the connective tissue directly. Instead, between the junctional epithelium and the tooth and connective tissue is a basal lamina and hemidesmosomes (Stern 1965; also see Fig. 1–10). The basal lamina and the hemidesmosomes are referred to as the *epithelial attachment* and it provides the attachment of the junctional ep-

FIGURE 1–10

Schematic illustration showing the attachment of the junctional epithelium to the tooth surface and the underlying connective tissue and (E) enamel. The electron-dense zone (1) is a continuation of the lamina densa (LD); the electron-lucent zone (2) is a continuation of the lamina lucida (LL); anchoring fibrils (AF) radiate out into the lamina propria. The cell membrane of the epithelial cells harbor hemidesmosomes (HD) toward the enamel and the connective tissue. Adjacent epithelial cell membranes also harbor desmosomes (D) which hold epithelial cells together. GCT = gingival connective tissue attachment (Copyright © 1997 by J. Lindhe and T. Karring, Anatomy of the periodontium, in *Clinical periodontology and implant dentistry,* ed. J. Lindhe. Copenhagen: Munksgaard.)

ithelium to the tooth surface as seen under the electron microscope. Epithelial attachment is not synonymous with junctional epithelium, which refers to the entire epithelium. The basal lamina has an outer electron lucent (lighter) zone called the *lamina lucida* and an inner electron dense (darker) zone called the *lamina densa.* The basal lamina is continuous around the base of the junctional epithelium. These structures lie in a sandwich-like arrangement, one on top of each other.

A hemidesmosome consists of one attachment plaque continuous with the cell membrane and attaches the epithelial (basal) cell to the basal lamina. This in turn attaches to the enamel on one side and the underlying connective tissue on the other side (Fig. 1–10). Connective tissue fibers called *anchoring fibrils* attach the lamina densa to the underlying connective tissue. This same structural relationship also exists between the oral and sulcular epithelium, where a basal lamina separates the epithelium from the connective tissue.

DENTOGINGIVAL UNIT

The **dentogingival unit** collectively refers to the epithelial attachment and the gingival connective tissue attachment (gingival fibers) to the cementum, both of which are involved in the stabilization of the gingiva to the tooth. Of the two types of attachment, the gingival connective tissue (gingival fibers) forms a firmer one, supporting the epithelium and probably inhibiting movement of the epithelium apically.

The combined length of the dentogingival unit has been described in the literature as the **biologic width** (Fig. 1–11 ■). A study using human cadaver models

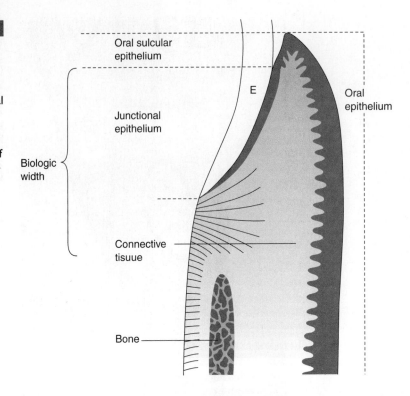

FIGURE I–II

Schematic illustration of the biologic width includes the length of the junctional epithelium (0.97 mm) and the gingival connective tissue attachment (1.07 mm). (Copyright © 1997 by J. Lindhe and T. Karring, Anatomy of the periodontium, in *Clinical periodontology and implant dentistry*, ed. J. Lindhe. Copenhagen: Munksgaard.)

determined that the components of the biologic width included the junctional epithelium with a mean length of 0.97 mm and gingival connective tissue attachment with a mean length of 1.07 mm (Gargiulo, Wentz, and Orban 1961). This soft-tissue dimension is essential to maintain gingival health. Biologic width or the length (coronal-apical dimension) of the soft tissue attachments becomes important during periodontal-prosthetic (restorative) treatment. The margin of a restoration should not disturb the biologic width. Thus, the margin of a restoration should not be closer than 2 mm to the alveolar bone crest.

Formation of the dentogingival unit

The formation of the dentogingival unit has important clinical considerations during the periodontal evaluation and in the healing of the gingiva after periodontal treatment. After completion of the enamel, the ameloblasts produce the primary enamel cuticle as their last function before they degenerate and become part of the reduced enamel epithelium. At the time of tooth eruption, the enamel is still covered with reduced enamel epithelium, which is connected to the enamel by the primary enamel cuticle. As tooth eruption occurs, the reduced enamel epithelium fuses with the oral epithelium at the base of the sulcus forming the junctional epithelium. The reduced enamel epithelium forms the lining of the gingival sulcus. The junctional epithelium produces another cuticle between itself and the enamel called the *secondary cuticle,* which holds the junctional epithelium in close proximity to the tooth. While the tooth erupts into occlusion, the junctional epithelium gradually moves apically down the crown exposing it. Several stages occur during this passive eruption process. Initially, the junctional epithelium ends at the cementoenamel junction. In periodontal

FIGURE 1-12

Photomicrograph of the attachment apparatus. D = dentin; C = cementum; PDL = periodontal ligament; AP = alveolar process; MS = marrow spaces; CM = cementicles. (Courtesy of Dr. Harvey Wishe, New York University College of Dentistry.)

disease, the junctional epithelium migrates onto the cementum, while the base of the sulcus remains located on the enamel, at the cementoenamel junction or on the root surface. In other words, the base of the epithelial attachment of the gingiva is at the cementoenamel junction in health and gingivitis. This situation changes in periodontitis, where the junctional epithelium migrates apically along the root surface. This concept of attachment level is important when performing periodontal probing and monitoring periodontal disease progression.

ATTACHMENT APPARATUS

The periodontal ligament, cementum, and alveolar and supporting bone constitute the attachment apparatus (Fig. 1–12 ■). The function of these tissues is to support and anchor the teeth within the alveolar process (Hassell 1993).

PERIODONTAL LIGAMENT

The connective tissue that extends from the cementum covering the root surface to the alveolar bone is termed the *periodontal ligament*. The periodontal ligament is primarily composed of collagen fibers and islands of loose connective tissue called *interstitial spaces* where blood vessels, nerves, lymphatics, and cells are embedded in a ground substance (Beertsen, McCulloch, and Sodek 1997). The primary cell of the periodontal ligament is the fibroblast, which synthesizes collagen, collagenase, and ground substance. On one side of the periodontal ligament is the alveolar bone, where osteoblasts reside and are involved in bone formation. The other side of the periodontal ligament is the cementum, where cementoblasts reside and are involved in the formation of cementum.

FIGURE 1–13

Schematic diagram showing the location of the periodontal ligament between the alveolar bone proper and the root cementum. The tooth is joined to the bone by bundles of collagen fibers which can be divided into the following main groups: alveolar crest fibers, horizontal fibers, oblique fibers, interradicular fibers, apical fibers. (From P. F. Fedi, Jr., and A. R. Vernino, *The periodontic syllabus.* Copyright © 2000 by Williams & Wilkins.)

Principal Fiber Groups

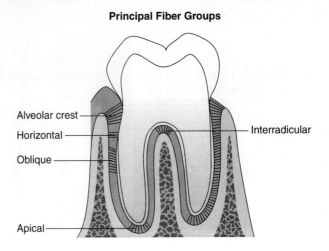

Connective tissue attachment

The primary component of the periodontal ligament is collagen fibers. The fibers are arranged in groups or bundles that blend into one another and are collectively called the *principal fibers* (Fig. 1–13 ■). This constitutes the second type of connective tissue. The principal fibers are a continuation of the gingival fibers or gingival connective tissue attachment (the other type of connective tissue attachment) in the gingiva and are also named according to their direction of insertion and location. Table 1–2 ■ reviews the principal fiber groups (Hassell 1993). The ends of the fibers, which are embedded into alveolar bone and cementum, are termed *Sharpey's fibers.* The first principal fibers formed before the tooth erupts are the alveolar crest fibers. With definitive tooth-to-tooth contact, the oblique fibers mature. Eventually, with the formation of the apical fibers, the periodontal ligament is established. Since the periodontal ligament contains few elastic fibers, it is the wavy configuration of the principal fibers that permits slight movement of the tooth under function (tooth-to-tooth contact). Collagen turnover time is five times faster in the periodontal ligament than in bone or gingiva because of the greater functional demands placed upon it.

Periodontal ligament space

Although the width of the periodontal ligament varies from tooth to tooth and from different areas on the same tooth, the average width is approximately 0.25 mm. Seen radiographically, a tooth that has heavy occlusal loads placed upon it for long periods of time will have a thicker periodontal ligament space. A tooth that is not in function, such as a tooth without an antagonist, will have a narrower periodontal ligament space.

TABLE 1–2			
CLASSIFICATION OF THE PRINCIPAL FIBER GROUPS OF THE PERIODONTAL LIGAMENT			
NAME OF FIBER BUNDLE	**DIRECTION**	**FUNCTION**	**FEATURES**
Alveolar crest	Originates from the cementum and runs apically to insert into the alveolar crest	Resists lateral movement of the tooth and keeps tooth in its socket	The first fibers to be formed before tooth eruption has occurred
Horizontal	Originates from cementum and runs at right angles and inserts into bone	Opposes lateral forces	The second fibers to be formed as soon as the first tooth-to-tooth contact has occurred
Oblique	Found in the middle third of the root apical to the horizontal fibers; originates from cementum and runs coronally and diagonally into bone	Absorbs occlusal forces	The most abundant and thus the principal attachment of the tooth
Apical	Originates from cementum of the apex of the root, spreading out apically and laterally into bone	Resists tipping of the tooth	One of the last fibers to form
Interradicular	From the crest of the interradicular septum extending to the cementum in the furcation area	Resists the forces of luxation (pulling out) and tipping	Lost when bone is destroyed in the furcation area in disease

Functions of the periodontal ligament

The periodontal ligament functions include the following:

1. acts like a suspensory mechanism attaching the tooth to the alveolar bone;
2. acts as a shock absorber transmitting occlusal forces to the bone. Axial placed forces which are parallel to the long axis of the tooth are more easily absorbed than lateral or rotational forces;
3. serves a remodeling function by providing cells that are involved in the formation and resorption of cementum and bone and itself;
4. carries a blood supply to the rest of the periodontium for nutrition;
5. transmits tactile pressure and pain perception via the trigeminal nerve; and
6. allows the feeling of localization to be transmitted through proprioceptive nerve endings (e.g., trigeminal nerve) found in the periodontal ligament. For example, when biting into a hard object, the mouth quickly opens. This quick reflex sensation is a function of the periodontal ligament. The greatest amount of sensory receptors is found in the apical area.

Abnormalities

Histologically, besides collagen fibers, clusters of epithelial cells are found within the periodontal ligament. These clusters are called *epithelial rests of Malassez*. Epithelial rests of Malassez are considered to be remains of epithelium of Hertwig's epithelial root sheath, which plays an important role in the development of the cementum and the shape of the roots. Their presence and function are controversial, but they may play a role in the formation of dental cysts.

Cementicles are calcified bodies of cementum seen in the periodontal ligament of older adults (Fig. 1–12). Either they are attached to the cementum, embedded within the cementum, or not associated with the root. It is unknown if cementicles present any clinical significance.

Cementum

The cementum is a layer of mineralized tissue covering the root of the tooth and is composed of collagen, ground substance, cells, and calcium and phosphate in the form of hydroxyapatite. The primary function of the cementum is to attach the principal fibers to the root surface.

The cementum is a product of the periodontal ligament and forms in layers or increments. As a layer of uncalcified cementoid forms, adjacent cementoblasts found in the periodontal ligament stop producing. When the layer of cementoid becomes 80 to 90% calcified, more cementoid is laid down. Therefore, the cementum is never fully calcified. Cementoid serves a protective function, resisting resorption. Sharpey's fibers are embedded into cementoid allowing for repositioning of the tooth in response to biting forces.

The surface of the cementum is soft and relatively permeable, allowing bacterial byproducts and toxins to easily penetrate the cemental surface. However, it is now recognized that the toxins are actually not as deeply penetrated into the root surface as was once thought (Nakib et al. 1982). The cementum is avascular and does not contain lymph vessels or nerves.

Relationship of cementum and enamel

The relationship of the cementum to the enamel margin varies (Fig. 1–14 ■). In 60 to 65% of the population, the cementum overlaps the enamel. In 30% of the population, the cementum meets exactly with the enamel in an edge-to-edge relationship, and in 5 to 10% of the population, the cementum and enamel do not meet and the dentin is exposed leaving an area of possible sensitivity.

Types of cementum

Two kinds of cementum are identified under the light microscope. Acellular cementum, which is formed before tooth eruption, is found on the coronal two-thirds of the root and is approximately 0.1 mm in thickness, with the cementoenamel junction being the thinnest area. Since acellular cementum does not contain cementocytes, it is not involved in the laying down of new cementum. Cellular cementum, which covers the apical third of the root and furcations, has a thickness of about 0.5 mm and is formed much faster than acellular cementum. Cellular cementum can be laid down on top of acellular cementum or it can comprise the entire thickness of the cementum.

Physiologic features

As teeth wear down (attrition) on either the occlusal surface or incisal edge, there is a compensatory deposition of cellular cementum in the apical area in addition to deposition of bone at the alveolar crest and in the socket. This acts to maintain the vertical dimension of the face and maintain the length of the root. Instead of remod-

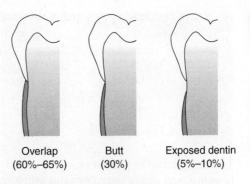

Overlap (60%–65%)   Butt (30%)   Exposed dentin (5%–10%)

FIGURE 1–14

Schematic illustration of the relationships of the cementum to the enamel at the cementoenamel junction. (From P. F. Fedi, Jr, and A. R. Vernino, *The periodontic syllabus.* Copyright © 2000 by Williams & Wilkins.)

eling (resorption and deposition) like bone, cementum is deposited continuously. Cementum thickens with increasing age, but the production of cementum slows.

Cementum does not resorb as readily as bone due to its avascularity and protective layer of cementoid. This property makes orthodontic movement possible without normally resorbing the roots. However, cementum can be resorbed under other circumstances such as inappropriate orthodontic movement, cysts, tumors, trauma, replanted teeth, periapical disease, and periodontal disease or for no known reason. Therefore, instead of resorption followed by deposition, a new layer of cementum is formed on the most superficial or oldest layer.

Abnormalities

Hypercementosis is a condition characterized by an atypical thickening of the cementum. It may be localized to one tooth due to factors such as excessive and rapid orthodontic movement or may result from excessive occlusal force placed on a tooth. It can also involve numerous teeth such as in a systemic hereditary disease like Paget's disease. Usually, the thickening occurs on the apical part or the entire root surface of the cementum.

ALVEOLAR PROCESS

The alveolar process constitutes that part of the maxilla and mandible that forms and supports the sockets or alveoli of the teeth. Periosteum is connective tissue that covers the outer surface of the alveolar process and is well supplied with blood vessels and nerves, some of which enter the bone. Endosteum covers the inner surface of the alveolar process facing the tooth surface.

Parts of the alveolar process

There are two parts to the alveolar process: the alveolar bone proper and the supporting bone. It is important to distinguish between the alveolar process and the alveolar bone proper. The *alveolar bone proper* or cribriform plate is hard compact bone that lines the tooth socket which is contained within the alveolar process (Fig. 1–15 ■). Radiographically, it is referred to as the *lamina dura*. The bone where Sharpey's fibers terminate is called *bundle bone* and is found at the inner surface of the tooth socket. The cribriform plate is perforated by numerous openings that carry blood, nerves, and lymphatics from the bone to the periodontal ligament.

The supporting bone is composed of two parts: compact bone and cancellous bone (also called *spongy* or *trabecular bone*). Compact bone, which covers the alveolar process, consists of buccal (outer) and lingual (inner) cortical plates that are

FIGURE 1-15

A section through the mandible after removal of all teeth. The thin bone lining the tooth socket (cribriform plate or alveolar bone proper) is clearly seen. (Reprinted with permission from A. Schroeder, F. Sutter, D. Buser, and G. Krekeler, *Oral implantology.* Copyright © 1996 by Thieme Medical Publishers, Inc., New York.)

continuous with the cribriform plate (Fig. 1–16a ■). The buccal and lingual cortical plates vary in thickness. Generally, the cortical plate is thicker in the mandible than in the maxilla. In the maxilla, the compact bone is thicker on the palatal than on the buccal surfaces. In the mandible, the bone is thicker in the buccal area of the premolar and molar areas and thinnest in the incisor area.

Cancellous bone fills the area between the buccal and lingual cortical plates and between the alveolar bone proper of adjacent teeth. There may be little or no cancellous bone when there is close root proximity of adjacent teeth. In these cases, the interdental septum is thin and the alveolar bone proper is fused with the cortical plate of bone.

Morphology

The cortical plate of bone covering the roots of the teeth is called *radicular bone.* Interradicular bone is found between roots of the same teeth (e.g., bi- and trifurcation areas of multirooted teeth). The interdental septum or interproximal bone consists of the cribriform plate of two adjacent teeth and some cancellous bone (Fig. 1–16b,c ■). The alveolar bone crest is the most coronal part of the alveolar bone. It is where the outer cortical plate is continuous with and fuses with the cribriform plate. At this area cancellous bone is absent.

Alveolar Bone Crest   The shape of the alveolar bone crest is influenced by the width of the interdental space, stage of eruption, position of the teeth in the arch, and shape of the cementoenamel junction. By following the contour of the cementoenamel junction, the alveolar bone crest is relatively flat in the posterior and more convex and pointed in the anterior. In health, the shape of bone takes on a form where the alveolar bone crest is more coronal than the radicular bone. The slope of the alveolar bone crest follows an imaginary parallel line connecting the cementoenamel junction of adjacent teeth (Ritchey and Orban 1953) and is approximately 2 mm apical to it if the biologic width is taken into consideration (Fig. 1–17 ■), but this relationship may vary.

FIGURE 1–16

(a) Dry skull specimen showing the outer cortical plates of bone covering the roots of the teeth. (b) Dry skull of the maxilla. The cortical plates of bone are removed. a = cancellous bone; b = interdental septum; c = alveolar bone crest. The cortical plates of bone are not present. (c) Dry skull of the mandible: a = cancellous bone; b = interdental bone; c = alveolar bone crest. (Figure 1–16b and c reprinted with permission from A. Schroeder, F. Sutter, D. Buser, and G. Krekeler, *Oral Implantology*. Copyright © 1996 by Thieme Medical Publishers, Inc., New York.)

(a)   (b)

(c)

FIGURE 1–17

The alveolar crest (AC) is parallel to a line connecting the cementoenamel junctions of adjacent teeth, even when a tooth is tilted and the cementoenamel junction on one tooth may be lower than the adjacent tooth.

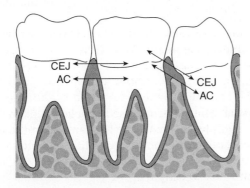

TABLE 1–3		
COMPARISON OF COMPACT AND CANCELLOUS BONE		
	COMPACT BONE	**CANCELLOUS BONE**
Density	Hard and solid	Porous
Structural organization	Osteons (haversian systems)	Trabeculae and bone marrow spaces
Influence from functional forces	None	Increased number of trabeculae with increased function on the tooth

Microscopic anatomy of bone

Bone is a type of connective tissue. The two types of bone, compact and cancellous, are simply different organization of the same histological components (Table 1–3 ■). All bone contains both types of tissues.

The unit of structure of compact bone is the haversian system or osteon. Each haversian system has a central haversian canal that is surrounded by concentrically arranged lamellae or layers of bone. Located between adjacent lamellae are small cavities called lacunae. Each lacunae contains a cell called an osteocyte. Osteocytes communicate with other osteocytes by small canals called canaliculi (Fig. 1–18 ■).

Each haversian canal contains at least one capillary, which supplies oxygen and nutrients and removes carbon dioxide and waste from the osteocyte. Blood vessels reach the canals from larger vessels that are located either on the periosteum or within the marrow spaces. These blood vessels enter the haversian system through Volkmann's canals.

Cancellous bone does not have the same microscopic anatomy as compact bone. Instead of the lamellae being arranged in concentric layers, cancellous bone consists of trabeculae or small supporting plates of bone, which branch and connect with one another to form a meshwork. Between the trabeculae are bone marrow spaces that are filled with bone marrow. The trabeculae have osteocytes embedded as seen in compact bone, but there is no haversian system because blood vessels are close by. The trabeculae serve to give some structure to the cancellous bone and to resist the stresses of occlusal (biting) forces. A tooth without an antagonist is not in function, and therefore it has less bone trabeculae, but larger marrow spaces. In the young, the marrow spaces contain blood-producing cells, whereas in adults, this red marrow is replaced by mostly fatty marrow which does not have blood-forming properties, but still serves as a pathway for blood vessels. In the adult, the maxillary tuberosity and the angle of the mandible are the only areas where red marrow is found.

Ankylosis refers to the fusion of the alveolar bone directly to the root surface without an intervening periodontal ligament.

Composition of bone

The alveolar process is primarily composed of collagen fibers and cells embedded in a ground substance (proteoglycans), which make up the organic component. The inorganic salts of bone are principally calcium and phosphate. The salts allow

FIGURE 1–18	FIGURE 1–19
Diagram showing a section of an haversian system cut in cross section.	Dry skull specimen of a dehiscence (d) showing loss of radicular cortical bone involving the marginal bone and a fenestration (f) with loss of radicular bone but not involving the marginal bone.

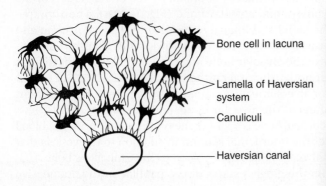

Bone cell in lacuna

Lamella of Haversian system

Canuliculi

Haversian canal

bone to withstand compression. The combination of fibers and salts makes bone exceptionally strong without being brittle. The cells present in the alveolar and supporting bone are

1. osteoblasts, which synthesize and secrete bone;
2. osteocytes, which are osteoblasts that are embedded within lacunae as bone is being laid down; and
3. osteoclasts, which destroy or resorb bone.

Metabolism

Despite its rigid physical characteristic, bone is a vascular tissue and the least stable of all the periodontal tissues. There is a constant remodeling with formation and resorption of bone due to the functional demand placed upon it. This occurs more rapidly in cancellous than compact bone. The normal remodeling of bone occurs by resorption by osteoclasts followed by deposition by osteoblasts. During orthodontic movement, bone is resorbed on the pressure side and laid down on the tension side.

Variations in anatomy

Roots of teeth are usually contained entirely within the alveolar bony plates. Frequently, the bone may not completely encircle prominent roots of teeth that are rotated, in facioversion, in lingoversion, tipped, or crowded. The resulting defects take the form of windows (fenestrations) where the radicular cortical bone is lost except for the most coronal edge or clefts (dehiscences) where the cortical bone, including the marginal bone (most coronal edge of bone), is lost over the root (Fig. 1–19 ■). The etiology of these defects is not definitive. These defects occur more frequently on facial bone than on lingual bone.

Buttressing bone occurs at the margin of bone where it thickens in response to increased functional demands. This is a response to the repair process, with bone resorption and deposition occurring.

PHYSIOLOGY OF THE PERIODONTIUM

Blood that innervates the gingiva is primarily supplied by the blood vessels of the periosteum, periodontal ligament, and alveolar bone (Fig. 1–20 ■). The supraperiosteal vessels run along the facial and lingual surfaces of the alveolar bone and give off many little branches as they make their way toward the gingiva. These finally join with blood vessels of the alveolar bone and periodontal ligament to form a gingival plexus located just under the oral epithelium.

The inferior and superior alveolar arteries supplying the periodontal ligament originate from the apical foramen, the alveolar bone, and the gingiva.

The blood supply to the cortical bone is via branches of the supraperiosteal blood vessels. The vessels that enter the interdental septum in addition to the vessels that supply the remainder of the alveolar bone supply blood to the cancellous bone.

Lymphatic drainage from the gingiva starts in the papillae of the connective tissue and drains into the regional lymph nodes, primarily the submandibular nodes. The lymphatic vessels follow the course of the blood vessels.

The nerves supplying the periodontium branch off from the trigeminal nerve (fifth cranial nerve). The nerves follow the course of the blood vessels that supply blood to the periodontium. Gingival branches of the anterior superior alveolar nerve innervate the gingiva overlying the maxillary incisors and canines. The gingival branches of the middle superior alveolar nerve supply the gingiva around the

FIGURE 1–20

The blood supply to the periodontium comes from three sources:
(1) supraperiosteal blood vessels, (2) blood vessels from the periodontal ligament, and (3) blood vessels of the alveolar process. (Copyright © 1997 by J. Lindhe and T. Karring, Anatomy of the periodontium, in *Clinical periodontology and implant dentistry,* ed. J. Lindhe. Copenhagen: Munksgaard.)

maxillary premolars. The posterior superior alveolar nerve supplies the gingiva around the maxillary molars.

The gingival branches of the inferior alveolar nerve supply the facial gingiva of the mandibular incisors, canines, premolars, and molars. The mental nerve supplies the mandibular facial gingiva of the incisors, canines, and premolars. The gingival branches of the buccal nerve supply the facial gingiva of the mandiublar molars. The lingual nerve supplies the mandibular lingual gingiva.

CHANGES WITH AGING

With increasing age certain changes in the hard- and soft-tissue components of the periodontium occur, as well as a thinning of the gingiva with reduced keratinization. The amount of stippling is either reduced or unchanged. Within the lamina propria, there is a decrease in the number of cells and the gingival fibers become less dense.

Cementum increases in thickness throughout life, with a greater deposition in the apical area in response to the continuing tooth eruption that compensates for tooth attrition.

Cells within the periodontal ligament decrease in number, while the number of elastic fibers increases. The width of the periodontal ligament can be either increased or decreased.

Changes in the alveolar bone occur with aging just as in any other bone in the body. There may be a decrease in vascularity and healing.

A physiologic tendency with increasing age is for the proximal surface contacts of teeth to wear down (attrition), causing the teeth to migrate in a mesial direction (mesial drifting) while retaining tooth-to-tooth contact. Accordingly, bone is laid down on the distal surface, which is the tension side, and bone is resorbed on the mesial surface, which is the pressure side.

SUMMARY

This chapter reviewed the structure and functions of the periodontal soft and hard tissues including the gingiva, periodontal ligament, cementum and supporting and alveolar bone. The periodontium is a dynamic, highly specialized structure that is constantly changing with the demands placed upon it. Knowing the macro and microstructure of the periodontium in health will help to understand the process that leads to pathological destruction.

KEY POINTS

❖ The attachment of the soft and hard tissues to the tooth surface contributes to the stability and health of the periodontium.

❖ The junctional epithelium is a semipermeable membrane involved in the movement of fluids, cells, and substances from the lamina propria into the gingival crevice and vice versa.

❖ The dentogingival unit is involved in the attachment of the gingiva to the tooth.

REFERENCES

Ainamo, J., and A. Talari. 1976. The increase with age of the width of attached gingiva. *J Periodont. Res.* 11:182–188.

Alfano, M. 1974. The origin of gingival fluid. *J. Theor. Biol.* 47:127–136.

Beertsen, W., C. A. G. McCulloch, and J. Sodek. 1997. The periodontal ligament: A unique, multifunctional connective tissue. *Periodontology 2000* 13:20–40.

Gargiulo, A., F. Wentz, and B. Orban. 1961. Dimensions and relations of the dento-gingival junction in humans. *J. Periodontol.* 32:261–267.

Goldman, H. M. 1951. The topography and role of the gingival fibers. *J. Dent. Res.* 30:331–336.

Gordon, J. M., C. B. Walker, J. C. Murphy, J. M. Goodson, and S. S. Socransky. 1981. Tetracycline: Levels achievable in gingival crevice fluid and in vitro effect on subgingival organisms. Part 1. Concentrations in crevicular fluid after repeated doses. *J. Periodontol.* 1993. 52:609–612.

Hassell, T. M. 1993. Tissues and cells of the periodontium. *Periodontology 2000* 3:9–38.

Kornman, K., R. Page, and M. Tonetti. 1997. The host response to the microbial challenge in periodontitis: Assembling the players. *Periodontology 2000* 14:33–53.

Moss-Salentijn, L., and M. Hendricks-Klyvert. 1990. Oral mucosa-epithelium. In *Dental and oral tissues,* ed. L. Moss-Salentijn and M. Hendricks-Klyvert, 27–44. Philadelphia: Lea & Febiger.

Mukherjee, S. 1985. The significance of crevicular fluid. *Compendium Cont. Educ. Dent.* 6:611–616.

Nakib, N., N. M. Bissada, J. W. Simmelink, and S. N. Goldstine. 1982. Endotoxin penetration into root cementum of periodontally healthy and diseased human teeth. *J. Periodontol.* 53:368–378.

Page, R. C., W. F. Ammons, L. R. Schectman, and L. A. Dillingham. 1974. Collagen fibre bundles of the normal marginal gingiva in the marmoset. *Arch. Oral. Biol.* 19:1039–1043.

Ritchey B., and Orban B. 1953. The crests of the interdental alveolar septa. *J. Periodontol.* 24:75–87.

Schroeder, H. E. 1991. Oral mucosa. In *Oral structural biology,* ed. H. E. Schroeder, 350–391. Stuttgart and New York: Georg Thieme Verlag.

Schroeder, H. E., and M. A. Listgarten. 1997. The gingival tissues: The architecture of periodontal protection. *Periodontology 2000* 13:91–120.

Squier, C. A., and M. W. Hill. 1998. Oral mucosa. In *Oral histology,* ed. A. R. Ten Cate. St. Louis: Mosby.

Stern, I. B. 1965. Electron microscopic observations of oral epithelium I. Basal cells and the basement membrane. *Periodontics* 3:224–238.

Tonetti, M. S., M. Imboden, I. L. Gerber, and N. P. Lang. 1995. Compartmentalization of inflammatory cell phenotypes in normal gingiva and peri-implant keratinized mucosa. *J. Clin. Periodontol.* 22:735–742.

SELF-QUIZ

1. Which one of the following structures comprises the attachment apparatus? (pp. 1, 19)

    a. gingiva, cementum, alveolar and supporting bone, periodontal ligament

    b. gingiva, cementum, periodontal ligament

    c. cementum, alveolar and supporting bone, periodontal ligament

    d. cementum, alveolar and supporting bone

2. Which one of the following areas is the width of attached gingiva greatest? (p. 6)

    a. mandibular second premolars

    b. mandibular canines

    c. maxillary lateral incisors

    d. maxillary first premolars

    e. maxillary second molars

3. Which one of the following substances is the primary component of the connective tissue of the periodontium? (p. 14)

    a. gingival crevicular fluid

    b. calcium

    c. collagen

    d. proteoglycans

4. Which one of the following structures directly attaches the junctional epithelium to the enamel? (p. 17)

    a. desmosomes

    b. hemidesmosomes

    c. basal lamina

    d. gingival fibers

5. Which one of the following structures is involved in the attachment of the gingiva to the tooth surface? (p. 17)

    a. alveolar mucosa

    b. dentogingival unit

    c. mucogingival junction

    d. desmosomes

6. Which one of the following structures comprises the biological width? (p. 17)

    a. gingival sulcus, junctional epithelium, gingival connective tissue attachment

    b. gingival sulcus, sulcular epithelium, gingival connective tissue attachment

    c. junctional epithelium, gingival connective tissue attachment

    d. sulcular epithelium, gingival connective tissue attachment

    e. sulcular epithelium, junctional epithelium, principal fibers

7. Which one of the following types of bone lines the tooth socket? (p. 23)

    a. alveolar

    b. interradicular

    c. interdental

    d. trabecular

8. Which one of the following structures is referred to as a *semipermeable membrane?* (p. 12)

    a. junctional epithelium
    b. oral epithelium
    c. sulcular epithelium
    d. lamina propria
    e. cementum

9. All of the following structures are avascular *except* one. Which one is the exception? (p. 22)

    a. enamel
    b. cementum
    c. junctional epithelium
    d. lamina propria

10. Arteries that supply blood and lymphatics to the free gingiva originate from all of the following parts of the periodontium *except* one. Which one is the exception? (p. 28)

    a. supraperiosteal
    b. periodontal ligament
    c. alveolar bone
    d. cementum

PERIODONTAL PATHOLOGY

2

Mea A. Weinberg, D.M.D., M.S.D., R.Ph.
Cheng-Sheng Ho, D.D.S., M.S.

Outline:

Periodontal Disease Activity
Progression of Gingivitis into Periodontitis
The Bacterial-Host Challenge
Oral Defense Mechanisms
The Inflammatory and Immune System
Histopathogenesis of Inflammatory Periodontal Diseases
Pathogenesis of the Periodontal Lesion
Summary
Key Points
References
Self-Quiz

Goal:

To educate the dental hygienist about the tissue and cellular interactions involved in the development of inflammatory periodontal diseases.

Educational Objectives:

Upon completion of this chapter, the reader should be able to:

Discuss three theories of periodontal disease activity;

Discuss the relationship of the inflammatory and immune host responses to inflammatory periodontal diseases;

Describe the course of the progression of gingivitis to periodontitis; and

Distinguish between gingival and periodontal pockets.

KEY WORDS

- periodontitis
- clinical connective tissue attachment loss
- gingivitis
- inflammatory process
- immune response
- periodontal disease activity
- host response
- antigens
- histopathogenesis

*T*he first chapter described the periodontium in the healthy state. This chapter will concentrate on the disease process—the breakdown of the healthy periodontal structures. Periodontal disease pathogenesis is a complex subject, involving a thorough understanding of the clinical and histologic features of the periodontium.

Periodontitis is defined as the loss of clinical connective tissue attachment (also referred to as *clinical attachment loss*). **Clinical connective tissue attachment loss** refers to the pathological detachment of collagen fibers from the cemental surfaces with the concomitant apical migration of the apical part of the junctional epithelium onto the root surface (Armitage 1995). The events leading to clinical connective tissue attachment loss also result in the destruction of alveolar and supporting bone. **Gingivitis** is defined as inflammation confined to the gingiva without clinical connective tissue attachment loss and bone loss. Gingivitis is a direct response to the accumulation of supragingival dental plaque at the gingival margin. The **inflammatory process** involved in the development of gingivitis and periodontitis is influenced by the **immune response** of the individual.

PERIODONTAL DISEASE ACTIVITY

The development of chronic inflammatory periodontal diseases involves a series of host responses or reactions of the body to bacteria present in the dental plaque, which is considered the invader or irritant. Host cells or cells normally found in the body are needed to fight this infection. Examples of host cells include blood cells present in the body, such as macrophages, lymphocytes, and polymorphonuclear leukocytes (PMNs) or, as they are sometimes called, neutrophils. PMNs are a type of white blood cell involved in the host defense system. The host defense is constantly being called upon to ward off attacks of the microorganisms that are colonizing the oral cavity at any given time. This balance of host defense mechanisms against the microbial attack is kept in balance until the microorganisms overtake the defense system, at which time infection and tissue damage develop. It is assumed that host cells mediate the destruction of soft and hard connective tissue because of the reaction to bacteria in the plaque.

Periodontal disease activity (PDA) is defined as the *ongoing* loss of clinical connective tissue attachment and alveolar and supporting bone (Greenstein and Caton 1990) at a certain point in time (e.g., at the clinical examination appointment). Detection of areas in the mouth that are in the active stage of destruction may be important in the implementation of treatment. However, it is extremely difficult to determine at a given time if a site is actively breaking down or will break down in the future.

MODELS OF DISEASE ACTIVITY

Currently, three theories of periodontal disease activity have been described:

- the continuous model theory;
- the random burst theory; and
- the asynchronous multiple burst theory.

The continuous model theory is based on the concept that periodontal destruction is slow and constant until tooth loss and the severity of the disease increase with increasing age (Löe et al. 1986). However, epidemiologic studies have not demonstrated whether destruction is continuous or new diseased sites actually develop (Greenstein and Caton 1990).

The next theory is the random burst theory (Socransky et al. 1984). This theory states that periodontal diseases progress in short bursts of exacerbation (actively losing attachment) followed by a period of remission or quiescence where there is no progressive attachment loss (Socransky et al. 1984; Goodson 1992). Another proposed name for this theory is the episodic burst theory, which reflects the fact that periodontal diseases are site specific and not all sites in the mouth are equally susceptible (Zimmerman 1986).

The third concept, the asynchronous multiple burst hypothesis, states that periodontal disease activity occurs during a limited time period (e.g., acne during childhood may resolve during adulthood) followed by remission (Socransky et al. 1984; Greenstein and Caton 1990).

In reality, all of the above theories may be interacting to explain periodontal disease progression. No one theory alone can explain the disease progression. It cannot be assumed that all sites will continuously get worse. Also, treatment should not wait until a burst of bone destruction has occurred. Periodontal destruction is cumulative over time. Since it is difficult to actually determine if a site is disease active, it is prudent to treat all inflamed sites (Greenstein and Caton 1990).

PROGRESSION OF GINGIVITIS INTO PERIODONTITIS

Gingivitis must precede periodontitis. That is, periodontitis does not develop unless gingivitis existed previously. However, gingivitis may, but does not always, progress to periodontitis.

Why does periodontitis develop in some individuals while in others gingivitis does not progress into periodontitis? Currently, the *exact* cause for the progression of gingivitis into periodontitis is relatively unclear. Approximately 80% of the population is susceptible to periodontal diseases (Brown and Löe 1993). Susceptibility to periodontal diseases involves changes in bacteria-host equilibrium. A failure of this equilibrium results in the initiation of periodontal disease. However, although bacteria are essential to this process, their presence alone is not enough to cause destructive periodontal disease. There must be a decrease in the number of beneficial (good) bacteria such as *Streptococcus* sp., a critical mass of pathogenic (disease-producing) bacteria, a conducive or favorable environment to cause disease, and a susceptible host that reacts to the pathogen. Gingivitis may progress into periodontitis if the host resistance decreases and if bacteria overwhelm the defense system and penetrate soft tissue. Some reasons for a decrease in host resistance include stress, chemotherapy, local tissue trauma, uncontrolled diabetes, leukemia, steroids, and fully developed acquired immunodeficiency syndrome (AIDS).

The **host response** is in nature a defense mechanism. It is a natural response of the body to protect and defend the individual after the person's body has been challenged by an injurious agent such as a bacterium or virus. This same host response

FIGURE 2–1

Pathway of the pathogenesis showing the sequence of events leading to periodontal destruction.

Poor oral hygiene with/without contributing
environmental systemic and acquired factors (a susceptible host)

↓

Accumulation of dental plaque and other antigens
at the gingival margin and in the gingival crevice; bacteria release antigenic
substances through the crevice into the connective tissue

↓

Host's inflammatory and immune systems activated

↙ ↘

Protective
PMN and macrophage phagocytosis;
plasma cell production of antibodies

Destructive
Prostaglandin E_2, cytokines, collagenases
(matrix metalloproteinases (MMPs)) and
lysosomal enzymes cause connective tissue
destruction including bone destruction

that provides protection to host tissues frequently also causes host tissue destruction (Fig. 2–1 ■). When the repair of tissue is greater than its destruction, the tissue starts healing. Fortunately, host tissue destruction usually is not permanent since tissues have a great capacity for healing.

THE BACTERIA-HOST CHALLENGE

MICROBIOLOGY

Bacteria that colonize early on the tooth surface at the gingival margin are predominately supragingival Gram-positive facultative (i.e., can live with or without oxygen) *Streptococci* and *Actinomyces* species. If plaque is not disrupted by toothbrushing and flossing, a more established and varied microbial colony develops. With increasing time and poor plaque control, periodontitis-associated microflora populate the subgingival pocket area, including Gram-negative anaerobes (oxygen intolerant) such as *Fusobacterium nucleatum, Porphyromonas gingivalis, Eikenella corrodens, Actinobacillus actinomycetemcomitans,* and *Prevotella intermedia* (Listgarten 1994). In addition to the subgingival anaerobic bacteria found in the deeper subgingival plaque, the bacteria found in a layer of unattached plaque in direct contact with the junctional epithelium may be or has the potential to become pathogenic and cause disease. Anaerobic bacteria become established as the bacteria multiply and become thicker with less oxygen available to the bacteria. The rate of subgingival plaque recolonization may depend upon supragingival plaque accumulation.

Bacteria, their metabolic wastes or by-products, and toxins they synthesize and release into the subgingival environment are foreign to the body and are termed **antigens.** Long-standing, chronic bacterial accumulation causes an excessive and persistent antigenic stimulus to the host response mechanisms. Thus, while bacteria initiate the disease process, it is enzymes and by-products produced by the host that are actually responsible for most of the breakdown of periodontal tissues. As a side effect, the reactions activated by the host response result in tissue inflammation in which surrounding cells, connective tissue, and bone are destroyed. Thus, host responses are basically protective by destroying antigens, but if the body is overwhelmed then the host responses are destructive, causing soft-and hard-tissue destruction.

Bacterial components

Bacteria release metabolic substances proven to be toxic to cells and tissues. These stimulate the initiation of the inflammatory and immune systems. The following substances are released from bacteria that affect the host:

1. endotoxin, a lipopolysaccharide (also termed lipooligosaccaride), is part of the outer membrane of all Gram-negative bacteria. Endotoxins, which are released when the bacteria die and lysis (break apart), stimulate biologic activities that cause tissue damage and bone destruction;

2. leukotoxin, an exotoxin produced by *Actinobacillus actinomycetemcomitans*, can kill PMNs;

3. bacteria synthesize and release various waste products (by-products) such as ammonia, which is toxic to many host cells, and hydrogen sulfide, which increases the permeability of the epithelium so that antigenic substances can more easily enter the lamina propria; and

4. bacteria synthesize and secrete enzymes, which can break down tissue. Hyaluronidase, an enzyme found in periodontal pockets, may break down or degrade the "cementing substance" between epithelial cells causing widening of the intercellular spaces and increased permeability. Collagenase may break down collagen and proteases degrade the connective tissue ground substance. Host cells such as PMNs and fibroblasts also secrete collagenase. Thus, these enzymes that bacteria and host cells synthesize and release prepare the tissues for absorption of toxic and otherwise harmful bacterial products.

ORAL DEFENSE MECHANISMS

The host interacts with microorganisms at three different areas in the periodontium:

- the supragingival environment;
- the gingival crevice; and
- the gingival connective tissue.

The first attempt at self-protection comes from the supragingival environment. These responses are important in the prevention of the extension of supragingival plaque into the subgingival area (the gingival crevice). Defense mechanisms include:

1. saliva, which contains numerous defensive substances such as antibacterial factors (lysozyme, lactoferrin, lactoperoxidase, myeloperoxidase) and antibodies [secretory immunoglobulin A (sIgA)]. Antibodies called *immunoglobulins* are proteins present in the blood serum and mucosal secretions (e.g., saliva, tears, sweat, nasal fluids) produced following interaction with an antigen;

2. gingival crevicular fluid (GCF) functions as an outward flow cleansing the sulcus. The increased volume of GCF produced during the inflammatory process also serves to deliver more antimicrobial products from the deeper tissue toward the main site of supragingival bacterial

colonization (e.g., tooth surface). These are the first substances to interact with the antigenic challenge (bacteria) to try to neutralize, isolate, or kill it;

3. oral epithelium also serves to prevent bacteria and their by-products from entering the underlying tissues. This is attained by the surface keratin and the close attachment of the epithelial cells; and

4. shedding of epithelial cells from the oral mucosa into the oral cavity.

THE INFLAMMATORY AND IMMUNE SYSTEM

If the body is unsuccessful in eliminating the pathogenic bacteria at the supragingival level, the inflammatory/immune response is further stimulated to eliminate the irritant and prevent the spread of infection. *This system is activated when antigens (e.g., endotoxins, bacterial enzymes, and by-products) present in the plaque mass in the gingival crevice pass through the protective wall of PMNs (leukocyte wall) interposed between the plaque mass and the lining of the gingival crevice and junctional epithelium.* After the antigens cross the junctional epithelial barrier, the deeper tissues are penetrated (Miyasaki 1991; see Fig. 2–2 ■ in this chapter). Only a few bacteria themselves actually enter the connective tissue. Usually, it is the products from the bacteria that enter the tissues while the bacteria remain in the crevice. However, it has been demonstrated that *Actinobacillus actinomycetecomitans, Porphyromonas gingivalis,* and spirochetes invade connective tissue (Renvert et al. 1990; de Graaf, van Winkelhoff, and Goené 1989; Saglie et al. 1982). Activation of the inflammatory/immune system results in the following: (1) elimination or retardation of the invader (bacteria); (2) the limiting of further tissue destruction; and (3) the beginning of healing.

FIGURE 2–2

As the protective wall of neutrophils between the plaque mass and the gingival crevice and junctional epithelium becomes compromised, the inflammatory response becomes magnified by the immune system. Once the antigens in the pocket pass through the wall of white blood cells and touch or penetrate the gingival connective tissue, a burst of immunological response results in gingival tissue, periodontal ligament damage, and alveolar and supporting bone destruction. (Courtesy of Procter & Gamble, Cincinnati, OH.)

THE INFLAMMATORY RESPONSE

The inflammatory response to a bacterial challenge is a nonspecific reaction intended to prevent the spread of invading bacteria and, if possible, destroy the damaging agent. This is accomplished through the process of inflammation.

When bacteria cause irritation to the gingival or periodontal tissues, a series of responses mediated by host defense cells is initiated. First an acute inflammatory response occurs. Table 2–1 ■ lists the cells involved in the inflammatory response. If this is ineffective and the stimulus is not removed and healing does not occur, inflammation becomes chronic and additional defense cells from the immune system become involved. After the events in the periodontal areas subside, the tissues are cleansed, repaired, and rebuilt. Unfortunately, sometimes the damage to some of these tissues is permanent and is present even after the infection is eliminated.

Elements of the inflammatory system

Clinically healthy gingiva that is relatively plaque-free is characterized by a salmon pink color, firm consistency, no bleeding from the gingival crevice, and shallow sulci. In healthy gingiva the junctional epithelium does not have long epithelial ridges and overlies the highly oriented collagen fiber bundles. Although clinically there may appear to be no inflammation, at a microscopic level there may be a mild inflammatory reaction. Thus, in the junctional epithelium of clinically healthy gingiva there are always inflammatory cells, primarily PMNs, which form a protective wall between the epithelium and the bacteria. PMNs constantly migrate from the junctional epithelium into the gingival crevice where the older cells are shed into the oral cavity. With severe inflammation, a greater number of these cells are present.

The inflammatory process

Table 2–2 ■ describes three phases of the inflammatory process. If dental plaque is allowed to accumulate at the gingival margin and is not disrupted, inflammation or gingivitis results. Plaque removal every 48 hours can prevent gingivitis, but if allowed to accumulate for 72 hours, gingivitis will develop (Van Dyke et al. 1999). The gingiva reacts to the bacteria and its products by the first 3 days of plaque accumulation at the gingival margin with signs of acute inflammation. The first inflammatory response to injury is vascular changes in the gingival connective tissue; the epithelium is avascular. Vasodilation of the blood vessels in the connective tissue results in the outflow of blood, fluids, proteins, and cells (PMNs) into the connective tissue (Fig. 2–3 ■). The primary substance responsible for the

TABLE 2–1
KEY ELEMENTS IN THE INFLAMMATORY RESPONSE

- Polymorphonuclear leukocytes (PMNs) or neutrophils
- Macrophages
- Mast cells
- Cytokines
- Serum complement
- Gingival crevicular fluid

TABLE 2–2	
PHASES OF THE INFLAMMATORY PROCESS	
PHASE	**FEATURES**
Acute transient phase	Local vasodilation and increased capillary permeability
Delayed subacute phase	Migration of PMNs and other phagocytic cells into the tissue
Chronic phase	Tissue destruction

Schematic drawing of the relationship of the gingival sulcus to the epithelium and connective tissue in health. Note the dental plaque (P) on the tooth surface at the entrance to the gingival sulcus. Neutrophils are leaving blood vessels in the connective tissue (CT) and moving chemotactically through the semipermeable junctional epithelium (JE) but not through the oral sulcular epithelium (OSE) of the lateral wall of the sulcus. (Copyright © 1997 by Munksgaard, Copenhagen. Reprinted with permission of *Periodontology 2000*.)

vasodilation and increased permeability of the blood vessel wall is histamine, which is released from mast cells found in the connective tissue. Another substance that is involved in the vasodilation is prostaglandins. Prostaglandins are fatty acids found in most cell membranes, are synthesized in large amounts during gingivitis and periodontitis, and may be responsible for the pain and bone loss seen in periodontal diseases (Offenbacher, Heasman, and Collins 1993). Vasodilation clinically shows as gingival edema. Thus, tissue edema or swelling is due to the increase of permeability of blood vessels, which causes the migration and accumulation of cells and fluid from the vessels to surrounding tissue. With the initiation of inflammation, the flow of gingival crevicular fluid increases from the connective tissue out through the junctional epithelium into the gingival crevice. Migration of PMNs through the junctional epithelium into the gingival sulcus and crevicular fluid flow both peak 6 to 12 days after the onset of clinically detectable gingivitis (Kowashi, Jaccard, and Cimasoni 1980; Zappa 1995).

Gingival bleeding at the gingival crevice is an early and important sign of gingival inflammation. When the crevice is probed or stroked, it may bleed immediately because the sulcular epithelium (epithelium lining the sulcus) becomes ulcerated with tears in the epithelial lining. The bleeding on probing comes from the underlying vascular gingival connective tissue (lamina propria), which is engorged with blood because of the disease process (Rizzo 1970).

The Neutrophil: The Phagocytic Cell   The neutrophil has been referred to as a "first line of defense" and the "hallmark of acute inflammation," meaning that it is one of the first defensive cells to be recruited to a site of inflammation. PMNs are the first cells to migrate from inside the blood vessels into the surrounding connective tissue and enter the gingival crevice and junctional epithelium in response to chemotactic substances such as toxins released by the bacteria and complement which are proteins found in the serum (Miyasaki 1991). Chemotaxis is the movement of cells in the direction of a chemical attractant. The PMNs create a wall between swimming, unattached bacteria and the junctional and sulcular epithelium. Once in the tissue, the neutrophil is ready to kill the foreign invader. Once the PMN comes in contact with the bacteria, phagocytosis occurs. The PMN is the major phagocytic cell, whose fast arrival from the blood vessels in the connective tissue into the junctional epithelium and crevice plays an important part in removing bacteria and other foreign substances. Neutrophils live a very short time. They come out of the bone marrow programmed to die in an average of about 5 days. Once at the site of injury, phagocytosis occurs where PMNs recognize the foreign material (bacteria, toxins, and by-products) and "eat and digest" it. Once inside the PMN, the bacteria are degraded by enzymes called *lysosomes*. As the bacteria are engulfed, lysosomal enzymes "leak" out of the cell into the surrounding tissue causing destruction of host tissue. Examples of lysosomal enzymes include collagenase, beta-glucuronidase, and alkaline phosphatase. High levels of these enzymes can be detected in the GCF during periodontitis.

Genetically, impaired PMN function is seen in patients with certain medical conditions. A depressed PMN chemotaxis and depressed phagocytic ability is seen in localized juvenile periodontitis and insulin-dependent diabetes mellitus. A depressed PMN chemotaxis is seen in Chediak-Higashi syndrome, and Papillon-Lefévre syndrome. A decreased number of circulating PMNs are seen in drug-induced agranulocytosis, cyclic neutropenia, and leukemia (Genco and Slots 1984).

The Macrophage: The Other Phagocytic Cell   The other important phagocytic cell is the macrophage. Monocytes (a type of white blood cell) in the blood differentiate or change into macrophages and migrate from the blood vessel into the inflamed connective tissues by chemotaxis and a few continue into the gingival crevice. Similar to PMNs, macrophages kill bacteria by phagocytosis. Although neutrophils and macrophages arrive at the same time at the site of inflammation, neutrophils predominate initially because of their higher concentration in the circulation. The majority of macrophages remain in the inflamed connective tissue for months, where they function to clean up the body's damaged tissue and secrete prostaglandins and cytokines. *Cytokines* are proteins that are involved in regulating the activity of the cells that release them, as well as other cells (Kjeldsen, Holmstrup, and Bendtzen 1993). The major cytokine released by macrophages as a result of phagocytosis is interleukin (IL-1) and tumor necrosis factor (TNF). IL-1 worsens inflammation by stimulating mast cells to release histamine and attracts more PMNs and macrophages into the tissues (Offenbacher 1996). As with PMNs, macrophages can also damage host tissue most likely a result of cytokines. IL-1 can increase the number of osteoclasts, which stimulate bone resorption seen in periodontitis (Tatakis 1993), and stimulates other cells to secrete prostaglandins, which are also involved in bone resorption. TNF is a less potent stimulator of bone resorption (Stashenko et al. 1987).

Phagocytosis: Opsonization   The process of phagocytosis is more effective if opsonins are present. Opsonins are antibodies or complement that bind to the surface of the bacteria, coating the bacteria so they are easier to be identified by PMNs and to be "swallowed."

The Complement System: A Group of Proteins   Besides blood cells (e.g., PMNs) and fluids migrating from the blood vessels into the gingival tissues and crevicular area during inflammation, there is also a series of about twenty to thirty different plasma proteins called the *complement system.* The complement system works together with the rest of the immune system to destroy invaders and to signal to other immune system cells that the attack is occurring. The complement system plays an important role in the inflammatory and immune response by generating chemotactic factors, which attract PMNs, macrophages, and other leukocytes to the inflamed area. Also, it directly kills and lysis (breaks apart) bacteria.

As with everything else in the immune system, the complement system must be activated before it can function. One way it is activated is when antibodies (proteins produced by plasma cells during the immune response) bind to the surface of bacteria (the antigen). This is called the "classical" pathway. The second way is called the "alternative" pathway, whereby endotoxins (lipooligosaccarides) activate the system. A third pathway involves the binding of specific proteins to proteins or carbohydrates on bacteria (Dennison and Van Dyke 1997).

ELEMENTS OF THE IMMUNE SYSTEM

If for any reason inflammation does not subside within several days, it will become a chronic reaction. Usually gingival inflammation progresses quickly into a chronic condition. When the PMNs and macrophages are not strong enough to destroy the invaders, the immune system is further activated, although the inflammatory cells remain in the area.

Activation of the "specific host response" or adaptive immune system is the next line of defense, with the purpose of the host developing immunity or resistance to specific antigens (e.g., bacteria and toxins). There is an interrelationship between the inflammatory and immune reactions. The same reactions and cells seen in the inflammatory level are also seen in the chronic state (e.g., PMNs and macrophages also belong to the immune system), but more cells are involved. There are two parts to the immune reaction: humoral immunity and cellular immunity.

Immune system: Cells

The major cells in the immune system are white blood cells called lymphocytes (Table 2–3 ■). The role of the immune system is to "patrol" the body, identifying foreign pathogens such as bacteria and viruses, cancer cells, or damaged tissue and eliminating them. There are two kinds of lymphocytes that originate in the bone marrow and travel to other areas of the body. In fact, all cells in the inflammatory and immune systems including blood cells are made in the bone marrow from a stem cell. A stem cell is a cell from which all blood cells "stem" or originate. Lymphocytes predominate in the gingival connective tissue (Page and Schroeder 1976). T lymphocytes, also referred to as *T cells*, are the mediators of cellular immunity. B lymphocytes, or *B cells*, are the mediators of humoral immunity.

TABLE 2–3
KEY ELEMENTS IN THE IMMUNE RESPONSE
• B lymphocytes • Antibodies • Macrophages • Cytokines

Humoral immunity

Humoral immune mechanisms are most effective against bacteria such as those found in periodontitis. Although both the humoral and cellular immunity reactions occur almost at the same time, one or the other cells may predominate during a particular stage of periodontal diseases.

B lymphocytes or B cells are so named because much of the early research was done on chickens, in which the bursa (hence "B") of Fabricius is a center of B cell activation; there is no direct equivalent of this bursa in human beings. B cells originate and mature in the bone marrow and then migrate and deposit in the blood and various lymphatic tissues (e.g., lymph nodes).

Humoral Immunity and Periodontal Disease   The following are events depicting the humoral response to plaque accumulated at the gingival margin:

1. in periodontal diseases, bacteria and their products, such as toxins and enzymes, accumulate in the gingival crevice. Then they penetrate through the protective wall of neutrophils and through the junctional epithelium, entering the lamina propria. Once this happens an inflammatory/immune response is set off. As previously stated, if the inflammatory reaction cannot eliminate the antigens effectively, the immune response comes into play;
2. from the tissues, these antigenic substances are carried to the local lymph nodes, probably by macrophages;
3. in the lymph nodes, the macrophages either present the antigens to B cells or the B cells by themselves recognize the antigens. The B cells then transform into plasma cells and memory cells;
4. plasma cells make antibodies in the lymph nodes with the assistance from T_H cells. They also circulate in the blood to seek out and destroy the antigens;
5. the memory B cells remain inactivated, ready to respond should the same antigens appear again;
6. the plasma cells remain in the lymph nodes and secret antibodies into the bloodstream. A local antibody response is also seen in the gingival tissues;
7. the primary antibody produced by the plasma cells is IgG (*Note:* "Ig" stands for immunoglobulin) with lesser amounts of IgM.
   - there are five classes of immunoglobulins found in the serum, secretions, and tissues. IgG and IgM are primarily found in the periodontal tissues and SIgA ("S" stands for secretory) is found in the saliva. IgE is found on mast cells and is responsible for the release of histamine causing vasodilation and allergy. Additionally, there is IgD;
   - antibodies (e.g., IgG) are proteins that directly bind to and neutralize bacterial toxins (foreign antigens) forming an immune complex. This immune complex may activate the complement system or be phagocytosed by PMNs or macrophages for elimination;

8. once the antigens and the surrounding tissue are destroyed, the tissue macrophages phagocytize and digest the debris and stimulate repair; and

9. after the antigens have been eliminated, the short-lived plasma cells disappear into the gingival crevicular fluid and out through the gingival crevice, but the long-lived memory cells remain in circulation and are capable of maturing very rapidly into plasma cells if the antigens are encountered again.

Antibodies to various periodontal pathogens have been found in both serum and gingival crevicular fluids of patients with periodontal diseases (Ebersole and Taubman 1994; Genco and Slots 1984). Immune complex and complement will cause the release of prostaglandins from cell membranes of macrophages and PMNs. Prostaglandins of the E series (PGE_2) are potent stimulators of osteoclast activity responsible for bone resorption. B lymphocytes also release cytokines such as IL-1. Humoral immunity is activated in severe gingivitis and periodontitis. Thus, the proportion of B cells in connective tissue at sites with periodontitis can be as high as 90%.

Cellular immunity

T cells undergo further maturation in the thymus gland located in the chest cavity. From the thymus gland, the T cells migrate into the bloodstream and lymph nodes. From the bloodstream, T cells enter the gingival tissues where they "watch" the tissues. There are three subsets of T cells: The CD 4+ T cells are defined as helper cells (T_H) which upon stimulation secrete cytokines that activate phagocytic cells to destroy target antigens. There is a reduction of CD 4+T_H cells in acquired immunodeficiency syndrome (AIDS) patients. CD 8+ T cells are suppressor cells (T_S) that suppress or inhibit the immune response. Killer T cells (T_k cells) directly kill virus cells by literally making holes in them. Cellular immunity is most effective against fungi, viruses, cancer, and foreign tissue such as transplanted organs and does not play an important role in periodontitis.

Cellular Immunity: Process   When a macrophage presents a foreign antigen to a T cell, it is stimulated to produce more T cells and cytokines. T cells are the target of the human immunodeficiency virus (HIV). AIDS is a manifestation of what happens when T cells are destroyed, showing the importance of T cells for a properly functioning body. This type of response is responsible for organ or tissue rejection in a transplant case. Few lymphocytes within the gingival connective tissue are seen in healthy gingiva, with T lymphocytes mostly seen in gingivitis. The T cells actually kill other cells on contact when the latter are recognized as foreign or have antigens attached. Unfortunately, T cells also have the capacity to contribute to permanent tissue damage by the production of cytokines, which activate macrophages.

HISTOPATHOGENESIS OF INFLAMMATORY PERIODONTAL DISEASES

The **histopathogenesis** of gingivitis and periodontitis is best explained by reviewing the histologic events in the initiation and progression of the gingival lesion as it relates to clinical signs. At the beginning of this chapter, the role of the host immune system in the inflammatory process and periodontal disease progression

	TABLE 2–4		
	PAGE AND SCHROEDER'S STAGES OF PATHOGENESIS OF PERIODONTAL DISEASE		
STAGE	**ONSET TIME AFTER PLAQUE ACCUMULATION**	**HISTOPATHOLOGICAL SIGNS**	**FEATURES**
Initial	2 to 4 Days	Acute inflammation; PMNs, machrophages; vasculitis	Subclinical; no signs of gingivitis; increased flow of GCF
Early	4 to 7 Days	T cell lesion	Clinical signs of gingivitis first seen (redness, bleeding, edema)
Established	2 to 3 Weeks	B cell lesion; plasma cells	Chronic gingivitis
Advanced	Undetermined	Alveolar bone loss, periodontal pocket formation; B cell lesion	Periodontitis

was reviewed. In this section, the microscopic tissue changes seen as a result of periodontal diseases are discussed.

STAGES IN PATHOGENESIS

Page and Schroeder (1976) described the development of periodontal diseases as a progression of inflammation through four different stages: initial lesion, early lesion, established lesion, and advanced lesion (Table 2–4 ■; Fig. 2–4a,b,c,d ■). The initial and early lesions are representative of acute inflammation, while the established lesion is considered to be chronic gingivitis and the advanced lesion is periodontitis (Page and Schroeder 1976). Since there are many factors involved in the initiation and progression of periodontal diseases, it is difficult to exactly pinpoint a clear delineation between the different stages. Also, it is unclear when and if an established lesion develops into an advanced lesion. The inflammatory and immune changes discussed above are involved in the histopathogenesis of periodontal diseases.

Initial lesion (PMN dominated)

The initial lesion develops after 2 to 4 days of plaque accumulation (Page and Schroeder 1976; Löe, Theilade, and Jensen 1965). Dental plaque accumulates on the tooth surface at the free gingival margin level (Fig. 2–4b). The protective wall of PMNs (leukocyte wall) between the plaque mass and the junctional and sulcular epithelium becomes compromised (Miyasaki 1991). Bacterial antigens cross the permeable junctional epithelium and enter the gingival connective tissue. The response of the tissue to the antigens is acute inflammation, developing within minutes of the insult. It is characterized by a dilation of blood vessels within the connective tissue subjacent to the junctional epithelium (Page and Schroeder 1976). There is an increased flow of GCF into the crevice, and migration of PMNs from the connective tissue into the junctional epithelium (Payne et al. 1975) and gingival crevice in response to chemotactic factors released by bacteria and inflammatory cells. There is some loss of collagen in the lamina propria because of the action of collagenase that is replaced with inflammatory cells such as PMNs. This lesion is not clinically seen and is reversible with appropriate oral hygiene (Löe, Theilade, and Jensen 1965).

FIGURE 2–4

Page and Schroeder's histopathologic periodontal lesions. (a) Healthy gingiva. Little supragingival plaque accumulation. A few defense cells, primarily PMNs, migrate through the junctional epithelium into the gingival crevice and out into the oral cavity. (b) Initial lesion: This develops 2 to 4 days after plaque accumulation at the gingival margin. Vasodilation results in an increased emigration of PMNs from the blood vessels into the connective tissue and entering the gingival crevice. This is gingivitis but the lesion is not clinically visible. Early lesion: This lesion appears at the site of the initial lesion within 4 to 7 days following plaque accumulation. The same features seen in the initial lesion appear in the early lesion but they are accentuated with an increased number of PMNs and macrophages. T lymphocytes begin to migrate into the tissue and gingival crevice. A greater area of gingival connective tissue is affected. About 60 to 70% of collagen is destroyed. Acute inflammation features continue in the early lesion. This is still gingivitis. (c) Established lesion: This is characterized by the presence of PMNs, macrophages, and antibody-producing plasma cells (B lymphocytes), which comprise 10 to 30% of the infiltrate. More collagen has been destroyed. The bulk of plaque bacteria and cells in the gingival crevice cause the junctional epithelium to detach from the tooth. The pocket epithelium is mostly derived from junctional epithelium with the formation of epithelial ridges and microulcerations. This is chronic gingivitis and is still reversible if oral hygiene is reinstated. (d) Advanced lesion: This is periodontitis. Plasma cells (> 50%) are the primary cells involved in periodontitis. There is clinical attachment loss with loss of clinical clinical connective tissue attachment to the tooth and apical migration of the junctional (pocket) epithelium, resulting in a periodontal pocket. In addition, alveolar and supporting bone has been destroyed.

Early lesion (T cell dominated)

The early lesion evolves from the initial lesion after approximately 7 days of plaque accumulation and can continue for up to 14 days. Clinically this lesion is observable as gingivitis (Seymour, Powell, and Davies 1979). The presence and accentuation of the features in the initial lesion characterize the early lesion (Fig. 2–4b). PMNs continually migrate from the blood vessels through the junctional epithelium into the gingival crevice, and there is increased gingival crevicular flow. T lymphocytes accumulate immediately subjacent to the junctional epithelium. There is no apparent dividing line between the initial and early lesions. Approximately 60 to 70% of collagen is lost in the connective tissue. Changes start to occur in the junctional epithelium. As a result of the downgrowth of accumulating plaque, the gingival sulcus begins to deepen. This is still an acute gingivitis without clinical connective tissue attachment loss and no bone loss as yet. This lesion is reversible with adequate oral hygiene, healing without adverse consequences.

Established lesion (few B cells/plasma cells)

As adverse clinical conditions progress, the early lesion develops into the chronic or established gingivitis lesion (Page and Schroeder 1976). The gingiva responds to massive accumulations of plaque, which affects a greater area of tissue (Fig. 2–4c). The time period for the initiation of the established lesion has not actually been determined, but it can start within 2 to 3 weeks after plaque accumulation (Page and Schroeder 1976). The manifestations of acute inflammation still persist. Established lesions may persist for months or years without progressing into periodontitis (Page 1986; Zappa 1995). As gingivitis becomes clinically more severe, the proportion of T cells decreases, and B cells and plasma cells increase within the lamina propria (Zappa 1995). More collagen is lost and replaced by an inflammatory cell infiltrate. The gingival fibers are still attached to the root surface; there is no clinical connective tissue attachment loss at this stage. Because of the massive amounts of subgingival plaque that advance in an apical direction, the junctional epithelium detaches laterally from the tooth surface to become pocket epithelium with elongation of epithelial ridges deeper into the connective tissue in an attempt to maintain epithelial integrity (Kinane and Lindhe 1998); this leads to the formation of microulcerations, which may increase its permeability to bacteria and their by-products.

The gingival margin becomes swollen and enlarged, and the gingival margin can be separated easily from the tooth surface, forming a gingival pocket. No alveolar bone loss occurs at this stage. Clinical signs are present and more severe than in the early lesion. Most of the changes that occur in the established lesion are still reversible.

Advanced lesion (plasma cell/antibody dominated)

The advanced lesion is characteristic of periodontitis. The inflammatory infiltrate extends into the alveolar and supporting bone and periodontal ligament (Fig. 2–4d). Periodontal pocket formation occurs with the loss clinical connective tissue attachment to the root surface and the apical migration of the apical aspect of the junctional epithelium along the root surface that was previously occupied by connective tissue; attachment loss occurs. Subsequently there is alveolar and supporting bone loss. The apical and lateral migration of the junctional or pocket epithelium permits extension of subgingival plaque on the root surface. The lymphocytic infiltrate in the subjacent connective tissues is primarily B cells (Seymour and Greenspan 1979). The advanced lesion may become stable or progress continuously (Goodson 1992).

PATHOGENESIS OF THE PERIODONTAL LESION

SEQUENCE OF EVENTS IN POCKET FORMATION

A pocket is defined as a pathologically deepened gingival sulcus (American Academy of Periodontology 1992). The development of a pocket between the root surface and the gingiva includes the transformation of a thin junctional epithelium into a pocket epithelium with the development of microulcerations and epithelial ridges (Müller-Glauser and Schroeder 1982). There are two types of pockets: gingival and periodontal (Fig. 2–5a,b,c,d ■).

The gingival pocket

In early periodontal lesions a gingival pocket, which is also referred to as a *pseudopocket,* is formed. A gingival pocket is formed by gingival enlargement and coronal migration of the gingival margin. There is no loss of clinical connective tissue attachment (the gingival fibers remain attached to the root surface and the junctional epithelium has not migrated apically onto the root surface). Additionally, there is no alveolar and supporting bone loss. Gingival pockets are not true pockets, they are false or "pseudo," which means that the increased height of the gingiva creates an impression that a deep pocket has been formed when probing instruments are used around a tooth. There is no attachment of gingival connective tissue above the cementoenamel junction, and since there is no loss of clinical connective tissue attachment to the root surface, it is not a true pocket. The pocket epithelium extends laterally and detaches from the tooth surface, permitting apical movement of the bacteria in plaque between the tooth and epithelium. A pseudopocket is often seen in drug-induced gingivitis (e.g., gingivitis produced by the use of phenytoin, cyclosporine, and certain calcium channel blockers), severe gingival inflammation, and hormone-induced gingivitis (e.g., during pregnancy or puberty).

The periodontal pocket

As the inflammatory infiltrate progresses from the coronal gingival connective tissue subjacent to the junctional epithelium into the underlying connective tissue, an extensive amount of collagen is destroyed. The detachment of the gingival clinical connective tissue attachment (gingival fibers) to the tooth allows apical migration of the junctional epithelium onto the root surface. Apical migration of the junctional epithelium continues, and as this epithelium separates from the root surface, a periodontal pocket is formed. With increasing periodontal pocket depths, it becomes an ideal environment for plaque accumulation, making it difficult to clean.

There are two types of periodontal pockets: suprabony and infrabony. The difference between the two kinds of pockets lies in the relationship of the base of the pocket or the coronal extent of the junctional epithelium to the alveolar crest and the type of bone destruction (Table 2–5 ■). Bone destruction occurs as the inflammatory infiltrate extends into the alveolar crest and then into the trabecular bone.

FIGURE 2–5

(a) Physiologic periodontium. (b) A gingival pocket or pseudopocket. The gingival margin has migrated coronally, but there is no attachment loss or bone loss. There is a deepened pocket but it is not a true pocket because the depth is due to the coronal position of the gingiva. This type of pocket is seen in gingivitis. (c) A suprabony pocket is a type of periodontal pocket. The deepened pocket is caused by attachment loss. There is also bone loss. The base of the pocket is coronal to the crest of alveolar bone. This type of pocket is seen in periodontitis. (d) An infrabony pocket is another type of periodontal pocket. The base of the pocket is apical to the crest of bone. This type of pocket is seen in periodontitis.

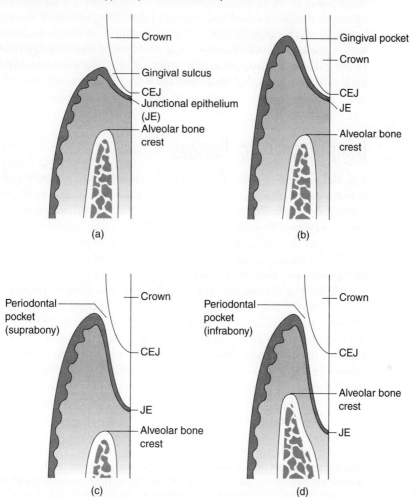

TABLE 2–5

CLASSIFICATION OF POCKETS

TYPE OF POCKET	PATHOGENESIS	RELATIONSHIP OF BASE OF POCKET TO ALVEOLAR CREST	PATTERN OF BONE LOSS
Gingival (pseudopocket) pocket	no clinical connective tissue attachment loss and no bone loss	At the cementoenamel junction	No bone loss
Periodontal pockets: Suprabony pocket	clinical connective tissue attachment loss and bone loss	Coronal to alveolar crest	Horizontal
Infrabony pocket	clinical connective tissue attachment loss and bone loss	Apical to alveolar crest	Vertical or angular

The base of a suprabony pocket (junctional epithelium) is coronal to the crest of bone (Fig. 2–5c), while the base of an infrabony pocket (junctional epithelium) is apical to the crest of bone (Fig. 2–5d). This can be identified on a radiograph when a dense object such as a periodontal probe is placed at the base of the pocket as the radiograph is taken.

Root Surface   The areas of cementum that no longer have gingival or periodontal ligament fibers attached undergo changes. The surface of the cementum is rough because of the detachment of the previous connective tissue. Cementoblasts within the periodontal ligament are no longer present to lay down cementum due to the endotoxin deposition. The surface of cementum becomes rough, easily absorbing endotoxins, bacteria, and their by-products onto and slightly into its surface. This cementum is referred to as *necrotic cementum.*

BONE RESORBING FACTORS

The inflammatory process causes the resorption of alveolar and supporting bone. A consequence of pocket formation and loss of clinical connective tissue attachment is bone resorption. The process of bone loss involves the inflammatory cells previously mentioned in the chapter. As the inflammatory infiltrate destroys more collagen in the connective tissue, the bone is approached.

Three classes of substances are involved in bone resorption: (1) prostaglandins, (2) endotoxins, and (3) cytokines.

Numerous factors can act directly on osteoclasts to stimulate their activity to destroy bone. One of the main mechanisms of bone resorption is through the release of prostaglandins (PGE_2) from macrophages or PMNs (Offenbacher, Heasman, and Collins 1993). Prostaglandins activate resting osteoclasts, increase the number of osteoclasts, increase the number of macrophages, and inhibit bone collagen formation (Offenbacher, Heasman, and Collins 1993). Protaglandins are also produced in bone and have a direct resorptive effect on bone.

Bone resorption can also occur when bacteria release endotoxins, which activate inflammatory cells such as macrophages resulting in the production and release of cytokines such as IL-1 (Schwartz et al. 1997). IL-1 is most important in periodontal destruction (Ishikawa, Nakashima, and Koseki et al. 1997). IL-1 can also stimulate PGE_2 production. Another theory of bone resorption is explained by the role of cytokines and prostaglandins in stimulating collagenase production by PMNs (Reynolds and Meikle 1997). Collagenase is an enzyme that destroys collagen, which is a component of bone.

SITE SPECIFICITY

An important feature of inflammatory periodontal diseases is the site-specific localization of periodontal destruction. Pocket formation and bone loss does not occur in all areas of the dentition at the same time, but it could occur on a few teeth at a time or even on only some aspects of some teeth at any given time, while other teeth are healthy (Carranza 1996). The composition of subgingival plaque samples from different sites in the oral cavity of the same mouth has been shown to be different. These differences have presented a problem for research analysis and treatment response to therapy (Socransky and Haffajee 1997).

RELATIONSHIP OF BONE LOSS AND POCKET FORMATION

Alveolar and supporting bone is destroyed as the pocket develops. Since the level of bone corresponds to previous periodontal destruction and changes in the soft tissue of the pocket wall reflects the present inflammatory condition, the degree of bone loss is not necessarily correlated with the depth of periodontal pockets (Carranza 1996). Radiographically, extensive bone loss can be associated with shallow pocket depths and vice versa. For example, a patient may have had severe periodontitis at one time, but had periodontal treatment that stopped the progression of the disease. Clinically the probing depths are shallow, but radiographically bone loss is evident.

PATTERN OF BONE LOSS

The types of pockets that form and the pattern of bone loss depend on the route the inflammation takes from the gingiva to the underlying supporting structures. The route of extension of the inflammatory infiltrate from the gingiva into the interdental bone is by way of the blood vessels. The interdental bone is resorbed more rapidly than the bundle bone because it is more vascular and less resistant to resorption. Interproximally (between adjacent teeth), inflammation usually spreads along the interdental blood vessels from the gingiva through the crestal bone into the bone marrow spaces extending out to the periodontal ligament fibers (Fig. 2–6a ■). On the facial and lingual surfaces of teeth, the inflammatory infiltrate follows along the supraperiosteal blood vessels located in the periosteum on the outer surface of the bone (Fig. 2–6b ■). Usually, the principal fibers are the most resistant to destruction and are the last to be resorbed.

FIGURE 2–6

(a) The inflammatory infiltrate spreads from the gingiva through the lamina propria into the bone following the most vascular pathway, which is where most of the blood vessels are located. Sometimes the most vascular area (larger blood vessels) is on the side of the alveolar crest, allowing the inflammation to directly enter the periodontal ligament. (b) On the direct facial surface, inflammation extends along the supraperiosteal artery before entering bone. (From Fedi P. R., Jr., and A. R. Vernino, *The periodontic syllabus.* Copyright © 2000 by Williams & Wilkins.)

(a)   (b)

FIGURE 2–7

(a) Horizontal pattern of bone loss between the premolars and second premolar and first molar. Interproximal bone (arrows) is destroyed on both sides of adjacent teeth equally. (b) Left side: Dry skull specimen showing vertical pattern of bone loss and furcation involvement on the mesial aspect of the first molar. Note that the interproximal bone is not flat as with horizontal bone loss. (c) Right side: After the gingiva has been reflected from the tooth and bone, a vertical defect is seen on the mesial aspect of the first molar.

(a)

(b)

(c)

The penetration of the inflammatory infiltrate into the marrow spaces and on the bone surfaces is associated with a loss of the equilibrium (balance) between bone formation and bone resorption, leading to loss of alveolar bone. The pattern of bone loss varies among individual teeth and on different surfaces of the same tooth. Bone destruction can occur on any surface of the tooth. The pattern of bone loss can occur in two different ways:

1. horizontal bone loss when bone resorption occurs from its outer aspect. Bone is lost equally on the surfaces of two adjacent teeth with the interproximal bone level remaining flat (Fig. 2–7a ■) and the deepest portion of the pocket is located coronal to the alveolar crest; or
2. vertical or angular bone loss occurs when the inflammation travels directly from the gingiva into the periodontal ligament and then the bone. The interproximal bone level is not flat and even as in horizontal bone loss. Bone

Vertical bone destruction is classified according to the number of bony walls surrounding the defect. In health there are four bony walls surrounding a tooth: mesial (M), buccal or facial (B), distal (D), and lingual (L). In periodontitis one or more of the bony walls is destroyed. If three bony walls remain, it is called a *three-wall defect.* If the buccal and lingual bony walls remain, it is called a *two-wall defect* or *crater.* If one bony wall remains (e.g., buccal/lingual cortical plate or proximal (mesial, distal) wall of bone), it is called a *one-wall defect.* (Copyright © 1991 by James A. Simonds, D.D.S. Reprinted with permission of *Practical Periodontics.*)

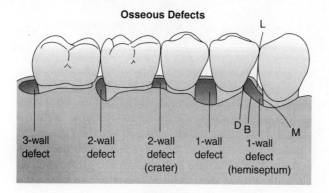

Osseous Defects

loss occurs at different rates around the tooth and is more rapid on one side of the tooth than the other. The base or the deepest portion of the bony defect is apical to the alveolar bone crest creating an infrabony defect (Fig. 2–7b,c ■). The terms *infrabony* and *intrabony* have been used interchangeably to describe all vertical bony defects; however, these terms are frequently misused in the periodontal literature. The term *intra-* translates to mean "within or inside the bone" and *infra-* to mean "below the crest of bone." An infrabony defect is a "generic" term to describe any periodontal vertical bony defect.

Periodontal infrabony defects are classified according to the number of osseous (bony) walls surrounding the pocket (Fig. 2–8 ■). There are four bony interproximal walls surrounding the tooth: the mesial, facial (buccal), distal, and lingual. Most vertical bone loss occurs interproximally, although vertical bone loss does occur on the direct facial and lingual walls. Types of defects include:

1. three-wall bony defect. The three-wall defect has three bony walls remaining interproximally or facially or lingually, with the tooth forming the fourth wall. An *intrabony defect* is a type of three-wall bony defect with specific characteristics (Prichard 1979). As a result of the disease process, the bone lining the infrabony defect, is usually composed of cortical bone. In an intrabony defect, the walls have cancellous bone behind them. The only way to determine if the defect is intrabony is during the surgical procedure when the bone is exposed. Thus, it is incorrect to refer to all infrabony defects as intrabony. A three-wall defect that wraps around the tooth and involves two or more adjacent root surfaces is referred to as a *circumferential defect.*
2. two-wall bony defect. The two-wall defect has two bony walls remaining. An interdental *crater* is the most common angular bony defect. It is a two-wall osseous defect with a buccal and lingual wall remaining.

FIGURE 2–9

The range of bone destruction determines the pattern of bone loss. The area of bone destruction radiates from the plaque mass about 2 mm. (Copyright © 1997 by J. Lindhe and T. Karring, Anatomy of the periodontium, in *Clinical periodontology and implant dentistry*, ed. J. Lindhe. Copenhagen: Munksgaard.)

3. one-wall bony defect. The one-wall defect has one bony wall remaining and usually occurs interdentally. If the remaining wall is the proximal wall, the defect is referred to as a *hemiseptum*.

FACTORS RELATED TO PATTERN OF BONE LOSS

The bone destructive process radiates from the plaque mass, at the base of the periodontal pocket, 1.5 to 2.5 mm circumferentially (Tal 1984) (Fig. 2–9 ■). Within this 2-mm "circle," bone destruction does not occur. Outside this 2-mm "circle," bone destruction occurs. Thus, the width and thickness of the interdental septum primarily determines if the pattern of bone destruction is horizontal or vertical. Bone destruction occurring where there is a wide interdental septum (> 2 mm in width) will most likely not occur across the entire septum and results in a vertical pattern of bone loss. Bone destruction occurring where the interdental septum is narrow (< 2 mm) can be total and results in a horizontal pattern of bone loss.

Teeth such as lower incisors, which have thin facial or lingual cortical plates of bone with little to no cancellous bone between the alveolar bone proper and the outer plate, will usually show a horizontal pattern of bone loss. Molars that have a thick facial cortical plate of bone will usually show a vertical pattern of bone loss.

SUMMARY

The pathway of destruction of inflammatory periodontal diseases is complicated, involving the host inflammatory and immune cells. Ideally, the overall outcome of these reactions is to eliminate harmful pathogens and prevent the spread of infection, while protecting the host tissues.

KEY POINTS

+ Overall, the host defenses are extremely successful in preventing infection around the teeth and in preventing destructive inflammatory periodontal diseases.

+ There are two separate functions that lead to the damage seen in periodontal diseases: (1) direct effects of bacteria (e.g., enzymes, endotoxins) and (2) indirect effects of the body's own immune response.

+ The host immune defense reactions are a double-edged sword; while being protective, they can also cause the host to suffer tissue damage.

+ Bacterial products can enter the connective tissue and cause direct damage, but their effects are limited by the effectiveness of the host response.

+ Weakened host defenses (e.g., because of a systemic disease) will not allow the host to ward off infection; the host will then develop signs and symptoms of destructive periodontal diseases.

+ Neutrophils and macrophages are considered capable and efficient agents of phagocytosis.

+ Clinical signs of gingival inflammation are first evident in the early lesion of gingivitis.

+ B cells/plasma cells predominate in the body's response to periodontitis.

+ Periodontal pocket formation occurs when there is clinical connective tissue attachment loss to the tooth surface with apical migration of the junctional epithelium. The inflammatory events leading to attachment loss also result in alveolar and supporting bone loss.

REFERENCES

American Academy of Periodontology. 1992. *Glossary of periodontal terms* (3rd ed.). Chicago: American Academy of Periodontology.

Armitage, G. C. 1995. Clinical evaluation of periodontal diseases. *Periodontology 2000* 7:39–53.

Brown, L. J., and H. Löe. 1993. Prevalence, extent, severity and progression of periodontal disease. *Periodontology 2000* 2:57–71.

Carranza F. A., Jr. 1996. The periodontal pocket. In *Clinical periodontology* (8th ed.); ed. R. A. Carranza, Jr., and M. G. Newman. 281–313. Philadelphia: W. B. Saunders Co.

de Graaf, J., A. J. van Winkelhoff, and R. J. Goené. 1989. The role of *Actinobacillus actinomycetemcomitans* in periodontal disease. *Infection* 17:269–271.

Dennison, D. K., and T. E. Van Dyke. 1997. The acute inflammatory response and the role of phagocytic cells in periodontal health and disease. *Periodontology 2000* 14:54–78.

Ebersole, J. L., and M. A. Taubman. 1994. The protective nature of host responses in periodontal diseases. *Periodontology 2000* 5:112–141.

Genco, R. J., and J. Slots. 1984. Host response in periodontal diseases. *J. Dental Res.* 63:441–451.

Goodson, J. M. 1992. Diagnosis of periodontitis by physical measurement: Interpretation from episodic disease hypothesis. *J. Periodontol.* 63:373–382.

Greenstein, G., and J. Caton. 1990. Periodontal disease activity: A critical assessment. *J. Periodontol.* 61:543–552.

Ishikawa, I., K. Nakashima, T. Koseki, et al. 1997. Induction of the immune response to periodontopathic bacteria and its role in the pathogenesis of periodontitis. *Periodontology 2000* 14:79–111.

Kinane, D. F., and J. Lindhe. 1998. Pathogenesis of periodontitis. In *Clinical periodontology and implant dentistry*, ed. J. Lindhe, T. Karring, and N. P. Lang. 189–225. Copenhagen: Munksgaard.

Kjeldsen, M., P. Holmstrup, and K. Bendtzen. 1993. Marginal periodontitis and cytokines: A review of the literature. *J. Periodontol.* 64:1013–1022.

Kowashi, Y., F. Jaccard, and G. Cimasoni. 1980. Sulcular polymorphonuclear leukocytes and gingival exudate during experimental gingivitis in man. *J. Periodontol. Res.* 15:151–158.

Listgarten, M. A. 1994. The structure of dental plaque. *Periodontology 2000* 5:52–65.

Löe, H., A. Anerud, H. Boysen, and E. Morrison. 1986. Natural history of periodontal disease in man. Rapid, moderate and no loss of attachment in Sri Lankan laborers 14 to 46 years of age. *J. Clin. Periodontol.* 13:431–440.

Löe, H. J., E. Theilade, and S. B. Jensen. 1965. Experimental gingivitis in man. *J. Periodontol.* 36:177–187.

Miyasaki, K. T. 1991. The neutrophil: Mechanisms of controlling periodontal bacteria. *J. Periodontol.* 62:761–774.

Müller-Glauser, W., and H. H. Schroeder. 1982. The pocket epithelium: A light- and electron-microscopic study. *J. Periodontol.* 53:133–144.

Offenbacher, S., P. A. Heasman, and J. G. Collins. 1993. Modulation of host PGE_2 secretion as a determinant of periodontal disease expression. *J. Periodontol.* 64:432–444.

Offenbacher, S. 1996. Periodontal diseases: Pathogenesis. *Ann. Periodontol.* 1:821–878.

Page, R. C. 1986. Gingivitis. *J. Clin. Periodontol.* 13:345–355.

Page, R. C., and H. E. Schroeder. 1976. Pathogenesis of inflammatory periodontal disease. A summary of current work. *Lab Investigations* 33:235–249.

Payne, W. A., R. C. Page, A. L. Ogilvie, and W. B. Hall. 1975. Histopathologic features of the initial and early stages of experimental gingivitis in man. *J. Periodont. Res.* 10:51–64.

Prichard, J. F. 1979. Management of intrabony defects. In *The diagnosis and treatment of periodontal disease*, ed. J. F. Prichard. 358–361. Philadelphia: W. B. Saunders Co.

Renvert, S., M. Wikström, M. Dahlén, G. Slots, and J. Egelberg. 1990. On the inability of root debridement and periodontal surgery to eliminate *Actinobacillus actinomycemtemcomitans* from periodontal pockets. *J. Clin. Periodontol.* 17:351–355.

Reynolds, J. J., and M. C. Meikle. 1997. Mechanisms of connective tissue matrix destruction in periodontitis. *Periodontology 2000* 14:144–157.

Rizzo, A. 1970. Histologic and immunologic evaluation of antigen penetration into oral tissues after topical application. *J. Periodontol.* 41:210–213.

Saglie, F. R., F. A. Carranza, Jr., M. G. Newman, L. Cheng, and K. J. Lewin. 1982. Identification of tissue-invading bacteria in human periodontal disease. *J. Periodontol. Res.* 17:452–455.

Schwartz, Z., J. Goultschin, D. D. Dean, and B. D. Boyan. 1997. Mechanisms of alveolar bone destruction in periodontitis. *Periodontology 2000* 14:158–172.

Seymour, G. J., R. N. Powell, and W. I. R. Davies. 1979. Conversion of a stable T cell lesion to a progressive B cell lesion in the pathogenesis of chronic inflammatory periodontal disease: An hypothesis. *J. Clin. Periodontol.* 6:267–277.

Seymour, G. J., and J. S. Greenspan. 1979. The phenotypic characterization of lymphocyte subpopulations in established human periodontal disease. *J. Periodont. Res.* 14:39–46.

Socransky, S. S., and A. D. Haffajee. 1997. The nature of periodontal diseases. *Ann. Periodontol.* 2:3–10.

Socransky, S. S., A. D. Haffajee, J. M. Goodson, and J. Lindhe. 1984. New concepts of destructive periodontal diseases. *J. Clin. Periodontol.* 11:21–32.

Stashenko, P., F. E. Dewhirst, W. J. Peros, R. L. Kent, and J. Apo. 1987. Synergistic interactions between interleukin-1, tumor necrosis factor and lymphotoxin in bone resorption. *J. Immunol.* 138:1484–1468.

Tal, H. 1984. Relationship between the interproximal distance of roots and the prevalence of intrabony pockets. *J. Periodontol.* 55:604–607.

Tatakis, D. N. 1993. Interleukin-1 and bone metabolism: A review *J. Periodontol.* 64:416–431.

Van Dyke, T., S. Offenbacher, B. Pihlstrom, M. Putt, and C. Trummel. 1999. What is gingivitis? Current understanding of prevention, treatment, measurement, pathogenesis and relation to periodontitis. *J. International Acad. of Periodontol.* 1:3–10.

Zappa, U. 1995. Histology of the periodontal lesion: implications for diagnosis. *Periodontology 2000* 7:22–38.

Zimmerman, S. O. 1986. Discussion: Attachment level changes in destructive periodontal diseases. *J. Clin. Periodontol.* 13:473–475.

SELF-QUIZ

1. Which one of the following features differentiates periodontitis from gingivitis? (p. 34)

   a. engorged lamina propria
   b. redness of the gingiva
   c. loss of clinical connective tissue attachment
   d. number of bacteria present in the gingival crevice

2. Which one of the following types of cells is primarily recruited in high numbers to the site of acute inflammation? (p. 41)

   a. mast
   b. macrophage
   c. neutrophil
   d. lymphocyte

3. Which one of the following cells is phagocytic? (p. 41)

   a. mast
   b. lymphocyte
   c. macrophage
   d. melanocyte

4. Which one of the following definitions describes a cytokine? (p. 41)

   a. enzymes that destroy collagen
   b. proteins that signal and modify the behavior or actions of cells
   c. fatty acids that increase blood vessel wall permeability
   d. endoxtins involved in phagocytosis of bacteria

5. Which one of the following cells is mainly involved in the body's immune response to invading bacteria? (p. 42)

   a. lymphocytes
   b. mast
   c. macrophages
   d. neutrophils

6. Which periodontal lesion, according to the classification of Page and Schroeder (1976), is characterized by chronic gingival inflammation and the presence of plasma cells? (p. 44)

   a. initial
   b. early
   c. established
   d. advanced

7. Which periodontal lesion, according to the classification of Page and Schroeder (1976), is characterized by attachment loss and bone resorption? (p. 44)

   a. initial
   b. early
   c. established
   d. advanced

8. Which one of the following types of pocket has its base located apical to the alveolar crest as evidenced on a radiograph? (p. 48)

   a. gingival
   b. psuedo
   c. suprabony
   d. infrabony

9. Periodontal diseases are considered a group of infections characterized by destruction of the periodontium. The direct effects of the bacteria and indirect effects by the body's own immune response are primarily responsible for the destruction. (p. 36)

   a. Both statements are TRUE.
   b. Both statements are FALSE.
   c. The first statement is TRUE, the second is FALSE.
   d. The first statement is FALSE, the second is TRUE.

10. The first attempt at self-protection from bacterial invasion comes from which one of the following areas in the oral cavity? (p. 37)

    a. supragingival environment
    b. subgingival environment
    c. gingival connective tissue
    d. tonsillar area

ETIOLOGY OF AND RISK FACTOR ASSESSMENT FOR PERIODONTAL DISEASES

3

Raymond A. Yukna, D.M.D., M.S.
John D. Mason, B.A., D.D.S.

Outline:

Goal:

To introduce the dental hygienist to the concept of risk factors for periodontal diseases and the relationship of periodontal diseases as a risk factor for other medical diseases.

Educational Objectives:

Upon completion of this chapter, the reader should be able to:

Describe dental plaque formation as well as its composition in the supra- and subgingival environment;

Describe the relationship between the mechanisms of bacterial action and host responses in the initiation and progression of periodontal diseases;

List and explain contributing local risk factors;

List and discuss possible systemic risk factors; and

Discuss periodontal diseases as a risk factor for specific disease entities such as diabetes, cardiovascular disease, and preterm low-birth-weight babies.

KEY WORDS

- periodontal diseases
- risk factors
- evidence-based approach
- dental plaque
- microorganisms
- biofilm
- etiology
- genetic
- stress
- diabetes
- smoking
- cardiovascular diseases
- premature
- low birth weight

*J*nflammatory **periodontal diseases** are not a single entity and are not caused by a single causative factor. **Risk factors** are characteristics that have been shown to directly cause periodontal diseases. Causal links are established by longitudinal and cross-sectional studies. Causal relationships are important to identify so that oral disease can be prevented if the risk factor is modifiable. For example, it is accepted that dental plaque causes gingivitis and so is considered a risk factor for gingivitis. A major triad of etiologic and risk factors exists in affecting periodontal health (Table 3–1 ■) (Page et al. 1997): (1) local factors—environmental forces that predispose to inflammatory periodontal diseases; (2) systemic factors—those medical conditions that predispose to inflammatory periodontal diseases; and (3) host factors—the influences of one's own body (e.g., individual susceptibility to disease).

The 1996 World Workshop in Periodontics (Newman 1996; Jeffcoat, McGuire, and Newman 1997) adopted an **evidence-based approach** to assess the effectiveness of a range of diagnostic and treatment options available for periodontal diseases. A consensus was reached that the assessment of risk for developing periodontal diseases is an integral part of recognizing and treating periodontal diseases. Thus, assessment for periodontal diseases fits into the emerging requirement for evidence-based therapy. Evidence-based therapy involves the use of quality research findings in clinical practice and using resources more effectively. The aim of evidence-based dentistry is to encourage the dental practitioner to look for and make sense of the evidence available in order to apply it to everyday clinical problems. *There is now sufficient evidence to support the use of risk assessment techniques to guide clinical decisions in the treatment of periodontal diseases* (Page and Beck 1997).

PRIMARY ETIOLOGY—BACTERIA AND THEIR PRODUCTS

Inflammatory periodontal diseases are initiated and progress as the result of the accumulation of **dental plaque** in the area of the gingival sulcus (Fig. 3–1a,b ■). Dental plaque is defined as a dense, nonmineralized, complex mass of bacterial colonies living in a gel-like intermicrobial matrix. **Microorganisms** besides bacteria can live in this mass, including yeasts and viruses. Other constituents of plaque include cells of various types.

The degree of tissue damage is dependent on the interaction between plaque bacteria and host defense mechanisms. Local contributing factors may encourage the accumulation of dental plaque, and systemic and local modifying factors may alter the host response to the bacterial challenge. However, if dental plaque is reg-

TABLE 3–1
RISK FACTORS FOR PERIODONTAL DISEASES

• Poor oral hygiene	• Male gender
• Tobacco smoking	• Compromised host defense
• Genetics/heredity	• Advancing age
• Stress	• Race, ethnicity
• Past history of periodontitis	• Regularity of dental care
• Systemic diseases	• Interleukin-1 production

(a)   (b)

FIGURE 3–1

Clinical cases of healthy gingiva and inflamed gingiva: (a) healthy gingiva with good color, contour, and texture; (b) inflamed gingiva with bluish red color, puffiness, and altered contour.

ularly removed and not allowed to accumulate, then gingival health can be maintained, in spite of other factors.

BACTERIAL FACTORS

Dental plaque is the major etiologic or risk factor in the initiation and progression of inflammatory periodontal diseases. Löe and coworkers (1965) provided the first direct scientific evidence of the causal relationship between plaque and gingival inflammation. In this classic "experimental gingivitis model" study, when subjects with excellent gingival health and little plaque did not perform oral hygiene procedures for 21 days, plaque accumulation increased and gingivitis developed. Resuming good oral hygiene eliminated dental plaque, resolved gingival inflammation, and restored gingival health. Many other studies have since demonstrated a similar strong positive association between plaque accumulation and the presence of gingivitis.

PLAQUE BIOFILMS

Dental plaque has all of the characteristics of a **biofilm.** Plaque biofilms are defined as matrix-enclosed bacterial populations adherent to each other and/or to surfaces or interfaces (Costerton et al. 1994). Bacteria in the film communicate with one another, build intricate intertwined structures, and even have a primitive circulatory system. Biofilms contain multiple microenvironments that vary greatly in pH, oxygen tension, and availability of specific nutrients. Subgingival plaque biofilm has some loosely attached and unattached bacteria on its surface that contact the adjacent epithelium of the pockets.

MORPHOLOGY/TYPES

Over 500 kinds of bacteria normally inhabit a given patient's mouth, and only about twenty species (< 10%) are considered to be pathogenic for periodontal diseases (Moore and Moore 1994; Fine 1995; see Table 3–2a,b ■). The rest constitute normal oral flora. The mere presence of one or more pathogenic species is not necessarily associated with progressing disease. Both protective host factors and interactions among the components of the dental plaque limit their pathogenicity. For individual

TABLE 3–2A	
NOMENCLATURE OF COMMON PERIODONTAL MICROORGANISMS	
GRAM-POSITIVE BACTERIA	**GRAM-NEGATIVE BACTERIA**
Gram-positive facultative cocci	Gram-negative facultative rods
Streptococcus sanguis, mitis, and *salivarius*	*Eikenella corrodens*
Gram-positive anaerobic cocci	*Capnocytophaga ochracea*
Peptostreptococcus micros	*Actinobacillus actinomycetemcomitans*
Gram-positive facultative rods	Gram-negative obligate anaerobic rods
Actinomyces viscosus, israelii, and *naeslundii*	*Porphyromonas gingivalis*
Corynebacterium matruchotii	*Prevotella intermedia*
Gram-positive obligate anaerobic rod	*Bacteroides forsythus*
Eubacterium lentum	*Fusobacterium nucleatum*
	Gram-negative obligate anaerobic cocci
	Veillonella alcalescens
	Gram-negative anaerobic spirochetes
	Treponema denticola

YEASTS

Candida albicans

TABLE 3–2B	
SPECIFIC BACTERIA ASSOCIATED WITH PERIODONTAL DISEASES	
STRONG EVIDENCE FOR ETIOLOGY	**PRIMARY ASSOCIATION**
Actinobacillus actinomycetemcomitans	Aggressive (early onset) periodontitis
Porphyromonas gingivalis	Chronic (adult) periodontitis
Bacteroides forsythus	Chronic (adult) periodontitis
MODERATE EVIDENCE FOR ETIOLOGY	
Campylobacter rectus	
Eubacterium nodatum	
Fusobacterium nucleatum	
Prevotella intermedia	Pregnancy gingivitis, necrotizing ulcerative periodontal diseases (NUG)
Peptostreptococcus micros	
Streptococcus intermedius-complex	
Treponema denticola	Chronic (adult) periodontitis, necrotizing ulcerative periodontal diseases (NUG)
Capnocytophaga species	Aggressive periodontitis (juvenile periodontitis)

species or groups of bacteria to be considered important in the **etiology** of periodontal diseases, the following criteria are considered important:

1. they are found in high numbers in advancing lesions or sites, and in relatively low numbers at healthy or nonprogressing sites;
2. clinical healing occurs with elimination of the pathogen;
3. they are present prior to clinical changes becoming evident;
4. they create a tissue reaction; and
5. they can be shown to produce disease in experimental animal or human studies.

Bacteria present in the oral cavity come in a wide variety of shapes from round coccoid forms to simple short rods to complicated corkscrew shapes. Both Gram-positive (cell wall intact) and Gram-negative (permeable cell wall) forms are present. Some are oxygen using (aerobic) and some cannot tolerate any oxygen (anaerobic), with many forms being somewhat in between (facultative aerobic,

TABLE 3–3	
HEALTH AND DISEASE ASSOCIATED BACTERIAL CHARACTERISTICS	
HEALTH	**DISEASE**
Gram-positive	Gram-negative
Aerobic	Anaerobic
Nonmotile	Motile
Saccharolytic	Assaccharolytic

microaerophilic, or facultative anaerobic). Within each category are both motile and nonmotile forms. Some bacteria utilize carbohydrates as food (saccharolytic), while others prefer proteins obtained in part from the tissue destruction they cause as a substrate (asaccharolytic). Some bacteria, such as spirochetes, do not readily fit any of these categories. In general terms, health-associated bacteria are Gram-positive, aerobic, saccharolytic, and nonmotile, while disease-associated bacteria tend to be Gram-negative, anaerobic, asaccharolytic, and motile (Table 3–3 ■).

The right combination of bacteria must be present in sufficient numbers to produce periodontal diseases. The presence of beneficial or good bacteria may modify the effects of known pathogens, thereby reducing the likelihood of disease progression. The presence of a single pathogen does not indicate active disease.

In health, the primary bacteria that live in the oral cavity are *Streptococcus sanguis, Streptococcus mitis, Veillonella* sp. *Actinomyces naeslundii,* and *Actinomyces viscosus.* In gingivitis there are increased numbers of all of the bacteria seen in health, especially *Prevotella intermedia* and spirochetes. Table 3–2b lists specific bacteria associated with various forms of periodontal diseases.

MICROORGANISMS OF PLAQUE

The types of microorganisms found in plaque vary among individuals and sites within the mouth. Based upon the surface of the tooth in relationship to the gingival margin, dental plaque can be identified as supragingival or subgingival.

Supragingival plaque

The sequence of events involved in the formation of deposits on teeth starts with the deposition of a pellicle, also called *salivary* or *acquired pellicle.* When the tooth erupts, it has the organic coating of the enamel cuticle. This is lost early due to abrasion or digestion from bacteria. Within seconds after the saliva contacts the natural tooth, a coating of salivary glycoproteins forms on the tooth as an amorphous, tenacious membrane. The pellicle is thought to be acellular in that bacteria are not needed for its formation. The pellicle allows and encourages the colonization of bacteria on the tooth surface, and therefore it participates in plaque formation. Adsorption of bacteria to the pellicle is important since the pellicle is formed from glycoproteins that bind selectively to the tooth, and not all of the bacteria available in the saliva can attach to the pellicle.

The pellicle can form on the surface of the tooth as surface pellicle, or it can adhere in fingerlike projections to the millions of imperfections of the enamel or areas of demineralization. This pellicle is called *subsurface pellicle.* Subsurface pellicle is significant because it connects the protein of the pellicle with the protein of the component of the enamel. The pellicle can be removed during prophylaxis but begins to reform within minutes. The formation is complete in 2 hours.

FIGURE 3–2

Clinical picture of supragingival plaque on teeth made more evident with disclosant.

Bacteria adhere to the tooth surface via molecules called *adhesins* located on the bacterial cell surface. Adhesins that are proteins and that recognize carbohydrate structures are called *lectins.* These adhesins, or lectins, recognize and then link to specific carbohydrate structures in the glycoproteins of the pellicle.

Supragingival Plaque Formation   Plaque formation begins as the bacteria adhere to the pellicle and begin to colonize. The pellicle serves as a nutrient source for the bacteria. As the salivary proteins are metabolized, they release peptides and amino acids.

The general pattern of bacterial succession in supragingival plaque is coccoid forms followed by short rods followed by larger rods and then motile forms including spirochetes. The majority of these bacteria are Gram-positive and aerobic (living entirely in an oxygen environment); however, most aerobic bacteria do not survive on total oxygen but rather are considered facultative, living with or without oxygen. Then a shift toward increased numbers of Gram-negative microorganisms and more motile forms occurs. Supragingival plaque is usually detected by visual inspection of the teeth, with or without disclosing solution (Fig. 3–2 ■).

The initial plaque formation is characterized by the numbers and kinds of bacteria which colonize the pellicle. Phase I, or initiation, begins in 1 to 2 days of plaque accumulation with no removal techniques. The microorganisms form as individual clones that extend both laterally and perpendicularly from the tooth surface to form parallel, palisading layers of bacteria (Fine 1995; Fig. 3–3 ■). The first colonies of bacteria are Gram-positive cocci and short rods, including *Streptococcus mutans* and *Streptococcus sanguis.*

Phase II begins in 2 to 4 days after abstaining from daily toothbrushing or leaving individual areas undisturbed. The early plaque masses provide the base for the next phase of colonies to infiltrate. The next bacteria to form are Gram-positive rods and Gram-negative cocci. The space between the layers of the first plaque provides an anaerobic environment for the arrival of anaerobic and facultative anaerobic (living with or without oxygen) bacteria. The cocci still dominate the plaque; however, filamentous forms and slender rods compete for the space (Fine 1995; Fig. 3–3).

The matrix begins to form around the bacterial colonies derived mainly from salivary material, exudates (e.g., gingival crevicular fluid), and intermicrobials substances. Bacteria can form extracellular polysaccharides (carbohydrates) from sucrose. These glucan, levans, and fructans are significant to the adhesion process

Plaque Formation: Phase I

Clinical — Thin continuous band at gingival margin with a clear zone

Histological — Palisading layers of Gram + bacteria; clonal expansion lateral, perpendicular to tooth

Plaque Formation: Phase II

Clinical — Zone obliterated; marginal band thicker

Histological — Gram + rods and Gram − species; anaerobes begin to occupy interstices

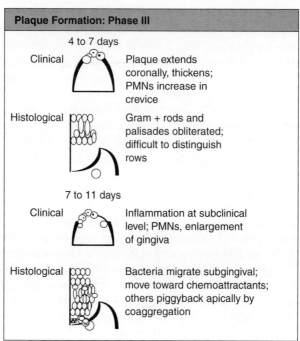

Plaque Formation: Phase III

4 to 7 days

Clinical — Plaque extends coronally, thickens; PMNs increase in crevice

Histological — Gram + rods and palisades obliterated; difficult to distinguish rows

7 to 11 days

Clinical — Inflammation at subclinical level; PMNs, enlargement of gingiva

Histological — Bacteria migrate subgingival; move toward chemoattractants; others piggyback apically by coaggregation

FIGURE 3–3

Illustration of different phases of plaque formation. [From D. Fine, *Periodontology 2000,* 8:89 (1995). Copyright © 1995 by Munksgaard International Publishers Ltd., Copenhagen. Reprinted by permission.]

and their insolubility increases the plaque resistance to removal. The levans and soluble glucans are an energy source for bacteria.

Days 4 to 7 mark Phase III of plaque formation with an increase in the filamentous bacteria. The rods, filaments, and fusobacteria comingle and interact with each other as nonmotile bacteria move with motile bacteria around the gingival margins. As the plaque matures, vibrios and spirochetes can colonize. New plaque

FIGURE 3–4

Electron micrograph of 3-week-old supragingival plaque. The central filament is attached to the enamel surface. (E) The filaments are usually composed of *Actinomyces* sp. or *Fusobacterium nucleatum.* Corncob formati ons extend from the enamel surface and are usually cocci such as *Streptococcus sanguis.* [From M. Listgarten, *J. Periodontol.* 51:1–18 (1976). Copyright 1976 by the American Academy of Periodontology. Reprinted by permission.]

may lie on the surface of mature plaque or spread coronally at the margin. This new plaque is characterized by cocci as before. The filaments at the edge of the plaque serve as binding sites for these cocci and a corncob formation appear (Listgarten, Mayo, and Tremblay 1975; Fig. 3–4 ■). Gram-positive facultative filaments such as *Actinomyces* species bind with cocci such as *Streptococcus sanguis.*

Phase III continues as the plaque continues to mature over days 7 to 11. Due to a change in the environment at the tooth surface, spirochetes continue to multiply and new species such as vibrios appear (Fig. 3–3). The host response to the plaque masses begins with early signs of inflammation observable in the gingiva. This inflammatory response is easily reversed by plaque removal.

Subgingival plaque

Bacteria living without oxygen are considered strict or obligate anaerobes. Anaerobic microbes thrive in the depths of subgingival plaque. As the days progress from 14 to 21, the vibrios and spirochetes remain prevalent in the depths of the mass. The growth, accumulation, and pathogenicity of subgingival plaque are strongly influenced by the presence of supragingival plaque. Inflammation of the gingiva caused by supragingival plaque changes the relationship between the gingival margin and the tooth. In addition, swelling (edema) causes gingival enlargement, which alters the anatomic relationship between the tooth surface and the gingival margin and allows bacteria to invade the subgingival space and to form subgingival dental plaque on the root surface or adjacent to the epithelial tissue in the sulcus (Fig. 3–5 ■). This newly created subgingival space, which is protected from physiologic and mechanical oral cleansing mechanisms, facilitates further bacterial multiplication. The microflora of subgingival plaque is generally more anaerobic, more Gram-negative, more motile, and more asaccharolytic. There are also many motile organisms that are completely unattached to the plaque matrix.

FIGURE 3–5

Histology of shallow pocket with plaque present.

These microbes produce toxins, enzymes, and metabolic products that cause direct injury to the periodontium. More importantly, they act as antigens, and as the host responds to the irritant present, some destruction of the periodontal tissues occurs. Thus, elimination of subgingival plaque is critical to the prevention of periodontal diseases.

Types of Subgingival Plaque Subgingival plaque can be separated into three types based on location: (1) tooth associated (attached), (2) tissue associated, and (3) unattached subgingival plaques have been identified with varying characteristics (Table 3–4 ■; Fig. 3–6 ■). *Unattached Gram-negative anaerobic microorganisms are in close proximity to the epithelium and appear to play an important role in the initiation and progression of periodontitis.* Filaments surrounded by rods can occur, creating a test-tube or bristle brush effect on the surface plaque (Fig. 3–7 ■).

NUTRIENTS

Nutrients from the crevicular fluid in the pocket are readily available, so bacteria that use proteins as energy sources are favored over those that require carbohydrates. For example, hemin-containing compounds found in crevicular fluid enhance the growth of *Porphyromonas* and *Prevotella* species; *Prevotella intermedia* uses menadione, a byproduct of estrogen metabolism. Thus, the final proportions of various bacteria found in the subgingival area are the sum of a large variety of intertwining processes.

TISSUE INVASION

Several studies have shown that plaque bacteria such as *Actinobacillus actinomycetemcomitans, Porphyromonas gingivalis,* and spirochetes can be found

TABLE 3–4
TYPES OF SUBGINGIVAL PLAQUE

TOOTH ASSOCIATED

Densely packed strongly adherent to tooth surface (biofilm)
Gram-positive rods, cocci, and filamentous bacteria
Facultative aerobic or facultative anaerobes
Removed by scaling and root planing
Less virulent (limited ability to cause disease)

TISSUE ASSOCIATED

Loosely packed, loosely adherent to soft tissue wall
Gram-negative, motile, anaerobic
Spirochetes, "bottle brush" types
More virulent (able to cause disease)
Cannot be removed by scaling and root planing; needs to be surgically removed

UNATTACHED

Free swimming in pocket (not a biofilm)
Gram-negative, motile, anaerobic
Spirochetes and others
More virulent (able to cause disease)
Removed by flushing

FIGURE 3–6

Schematic of the three types of subgingival plaque plus the depiction of "invading" microorganisms.

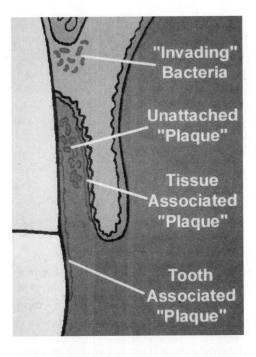

within the tissues, including the epithelium, gingival connective tissues, and the alveolar bone (Saglie et al. 1982; Renvert et al. 1990). Although the bacteria seem to be present in these tissues, they have shown no evidence of local activity or multiplication, so they may be inactive in those locations. In addition, the severity of the periodontal disease and associated tooth mobility, as well as the trauma associated with tooth extraction, suggest that the bacteria may actually be pushed into the tissues, rather than invading. However, invasion of the deeper

FIGURE 3–7

Electron micrograph of subgingival plaque. Subgingival bacteria gather to form a test-tube or bristle brushes configuration composed of Gram-negative rods (bristles) attaching to filamentous bacteria such as *Actinomyces* sp. [From M. Listgarten, *J. Periodotol.* 51:1–18 (1976). Copyright by the Academy of Periodontology. Reprinted with permission.]

periodontal tissues by bacteria may be important to the pathogenesis of certain periodontal diseases (see Chapter 2).

MICROORGANISMS OF DENTAL IMPLANTS

Clinical studies have demonstrated that the microflora of healthy, stable dental implants are similar to that of healthy teeth, while implants that are unstable and failing have bacteria similar to natural teeth with periodontitis (Rams and Link 1983). Dental plaque must be removed around implants just as for natural teeth.

OTHER COMPONENTS OF PLAQUE

Cells

Although bacteria are the primary constituents of plaque, several types of cells are also present. Epithelial cells are found almost universally in samples of plaque in a variety of anatomic forms ranging from cells recently shed from the surface with discrete nuclei and clearly defined cell walls to what may be described as empty "ghosts" of cells filled with bacteria. White blood cells, particularly polymorphonuclear neutrophils (PMNs), are often also found in plaque. Red blood cells are commonly seen in samples taken from tooth surfaces adjacent to pockets with bleeding on probing, indicating a break in the pocket epithelial lining.

OTHER TOOTH-ACCUMULATED MATERIALS

Several other tooth-accumulated materials (TAMs) besides dental plaque and pellicle are found in the region of the gingival sulcus. Food debris is the most commonly found TAM. Materia alba is also a bacterial aggregation with food debris, but it differs from plaque in that it is not strongly adherent to the tooth. There is no definite architecture as with dental plaque, and it is minimally implicated in periodontal diseases. While these tooth-accumulated materials may stain with disclosant and be visible on the tooth surface, they are readily dislodged by rinsing or a water spray, unlike pellicle or dental plaque.

MECHANISMS OF BACTERIAL ACTION

Different combinations of indigenous (living-in-the-mouth) bacteria, rather than just a single species, produce the pathogenic potential necessary to cause progression from gingivitis to destructive periodontitis.

Once pathogenic flora are established, the microorganisms appear to incite destruction of the supporting structures by both direct toxic effects on adjacent tissues and by the indirect activation of host cells.

Direct effect

Cytotoxic Agents   The subgingival unattached plaque has endotoxins, which are lipopolysaccharides (LPS) [now called *lipooligosaccharide* (LOS)]. Lipooligosaccharides, which are found in the cell wall of Gram-negative bacteria, can initiate inflammation, cause soft-tissue destruction, and stimulate bone resorption. Endotoxins are released from the cell wall upon death of Gram-negative bacteria. LOS is found in the cementum of untreated periodontally involved root surfaces.

Enzymes   Many of the bacteria present in the various plaque environments of the sulcus/pocket produce a variety of enzymes, which can adversely affect the gingival and periodontal tissues. These enzymes accumulate in the sulcus and can penetrate through intact epithelium into the deeper tissues. Enyzmes function to destroy the connective tissue by breaking down collagen and ground substance. Some of the enzymes that have been identified as important products of plaque bacteria are shown in Table 3–5 ■.

New information regarding host-mediated degradation (breakdown) of connective tissues has focused on the matrix metalloproteinases (MMPs) (Birkedal-Hansen 1993). This group of structurally similar enzymes is produced by stimulated host cells and includes the collagenases, gelatinases, and stromelysins.

TABLE 3–5
COMMON ENZYMES THAT BREAK DOWN PERIODONTAL TISSUES

Collagenase—this degrades collagen fibers, the major formed elements in the gingiva and periodontal ligament. Produced by both bacteria and the host cells in the body (e.g., PMNs and fibroblasts). Included in the family of enzymes called matrix metalloproteinases (MMPs)

Hyaluronidase—this breaks down hyaluronic acid, an important polysaccharide (carbohydrate) that helps hold tissue and cells together. Can act as a "spreading" factor to increase tissue permeability. This enzyme is also produced both by bacteria and by the host.

Chondroitin sulfatase—this breaks apart chondroitin sulfate, another cell- and tissue-cementing polysaccharide (carbohydrate).

Proteases—a large group of enzymes that contribute to the breakdown of noncollagenous proteins (proteins in the connective tissue other than collagen) and increase capillary permeability.

Elastases—this affects the elastin (elastic) fibers of the mucosa and blood vessels, thereby reducing tissue integrity.

These enzymes are responsible for cleaving the collagen molecule (the major component of connective tissue), degrading proteoglycans (part of the ground substance) and other proteins making up the connective tissues, and causing osteoclastic bone resorption.

Indirect effect

Immunopathologic Mechanisms   Several bacterial antigens induce inflammation in the periodontal tissues by stimulating the immune response. Both the humoral (antibody-based) and the cell-mediated (lymphocyte-based) types of immune responses have been observed in patients with periodontitis. The role of the immunologic response in periodontal disease is not completely understood; however, the potential to cause tissue destruction, as well as to be protective, is apparent. Rather than always being protective, the host immune response may contribute to the tissue destruction. For further discussion see Chapter 2.

Combined mechanisms

While not truly contagious, transmission of pathogenic bacteria has been shown to occur between individuals. *Actinobacillus actinomycetemcomitans* can be transmitted from parent to child and from dogs to humans (Asikainen et al. 1997). There is some evidence that *Porphyromonas gingivalis* is transmitted among individuals in a household including spouses (Asikainen et al. 1997). The most common route of transmission is via saliva.

It is probable that more than one mechanism is involved in the initiation and progression of gingivitis and periodontitis. It is possible that bacterial enzymes and/or cytotoxic substances exert a direct effect on the sulcular and subsulcular tissue, and at the same time initiate an indirect immune response. Therefore, there are multiple mechanisms of action of dental plaque.

LOCAL CONTRIBUTORY RISK FACTORS FOR PERIODONTAL DISEASES

Many local factors can increase plaque deposition and retention, inhibit plaque control, and contribute to the development of gingivitis and periodontitis. These factors are termed *contributory* because they do not by themselves initiate gingival inflammation, but foster increased or long-standing plaque accumulation and make plaque removal more difficult. Awareness of these local risk factors can help the dental hygienist to design more specific plaque-control activities, encourage patients to seek further corrective dental treatment, and contribute to the comprehensive care of periodontal patients.

Perhaps the most significant dentally related local factor strongly associated with an increased probability of developing periodontal disease, but not directly involved in causing the disease, is the presence of established periodontal disease. Sites already or previously affected by periodontitis are at the greatest risk for future episodes (Douglass 1998). More frequent professional care has been shown to reduce the risk.

Histology of calculus with a plaque coating in a deep periodontal pocket.

CALCULUS

Calculus is considered the most important local contributing factor. Calculus is essentially calcified dental plaque, but may form even in the absence of bacteria. Mineralization within plaque initially occurs supragingivally, but the rate of formation varies between individuals. Subgingival calculus forms more slowly in a thinner layer and, being firmly attached to the root, is usually more difficult to remove. Calculus is always covered by plaque and retains toxic bacterial products (Fig. 3–8 ■).

Subgingival calculus is commonly deposited in rings or ledges on root surfaces, but may also appear in a veneer form, and is associated with progressive periodontal disease (Fig. 3–9a,b ■). It is porous and can provide a reservoir of bacteria and endotoxin. Long-term studies of periodontal patients support calculus removal to promote healing and prevent further loss of attachment (Philstrom et al. 1983).

"Tartar" is the common name for dental calculus, and is often used by patients when referring to calculus. The term *tartar* will probably continue to be used for a long time because it is often used in advertising. Products referred to as "tartar control" toothpaste and rinses are popular and reinforce the use of the common name.

Radiographic evaluation of calculus is not an effective diagnostic method. Only about 45% of surfaces with clinically visible calculus are detected radiographically, but tooth surfaces visibly free of calculus show no calculus radiographically (Fig. 3–10a,b ■).

ANATOMIC FACTORS

Dental anatomic factors of importance to the accumulation of dental plaque include root morphology (size and shape) and position of teeth in the arch.

FIGURE 3–9

Clinical photographs of nodular calculus vs. veneer type calculus. (a) Nodular calculus is evident more coronally while (b) veneer-type calculus is often found more apically.

(a)

(b)

FIGURE 3–10

Radiographs of teeth in the same patient (a) with and (b) without calculus evident. Absence of calculus on radiographs does not mean that it is not present clinically (radiographs produce many false negatives).

(a)

(b)

FIGURE 3–11

Clinical photographs of (a) a palatogingival groove with a deep pocket associated with it, and (b) an extracted lateral incisor exhibiting a deep palatal groove.

(a)

(b)

Root morphology

Several deviations in the shape or form of the tooth root can occur, and often contribute to increased plaque accumulation and more severe periodontal disease. Palatal grooves (also called *palatogingival grooves* or *lingual grooves*) are present on about 5 to 8% of maxillary incisors, tend to accumulate plaque, and can become the focus of a narrow deep pocket (Hou & Tsai 1993; see also Fig. 3–11a,b ■). Likewise, plaque may accumulate undisturbed in the deep mesial groove of the upper first premolars.

Enamel in the furcation area of the root surface may manifest as cervical enamel projections (CEPs) or enamel pearls (Fig. 3–12 ■). These ridges of enamel may allow increased plaque accumulation.

Furcation involvements create a complication because they form a cul-de-sac that creates a plaque trap. Difficult access in this protected area fosters increased bacterial deposits and often leads to more severe periodontal disease. Proximal furcations on maxillary molars present particular problems because of even more limited access (Fig. 3–13a,b ■).

Tooth position

Tooth position may influence plaque accumulation and access for oral hygiene and therapy. Most studies that have evaluated the influence of crowding, tilting, rotations, etc., have found that such tooth position anomalies lead to increased plaque accumulation (and more tissue inflammation), especially in patients who

FIGURE 3–12

Clinical photograph of a cervical enamel projection (CEP) at the furcation entrance.

FIGURE 3–13

Clinical photographs of calculus within furcations: (a) dark calculus evident on all internal surfaces of maxillary molar furcations; (b) more veneerlike calculus in internal groove of mesial root of the mandibular molar.

(a)

(b)

FIGURE 3–14

Crowded teeth with in-flammation of the gingiva.

do not have excellent oral hygiene practices (Fig. 3–14 ■). Open contacts allow for food impaction, which may contribute to plaque-induced inflammation.

IATROGENIC FACTORS

There are a number of procedures, techniques, and materials used in dentistry that indirectly, and on occasion directly, contribute to the initiation and/or progress of periodontal disease.

Restorative dentistry

Rough-surfaced and overcontoured amalgams, composites, crowns, bridges, and other types of restorations have been associated with increased gingival inflam-mation and periodontal disease. Plaque accumulation is enhanced by subgingival placement of restorations because of problems with greater surface roughness of the materials, fit of the margin to the remaining tooth structure, and contour of the restoration. Subgingival restorations, especially those with defective or over-hanging margins, may have a profound effect on periodontal health by retaining plaque within a gingival pocket (Fig. 3–15a,b ■).

Injuries to the gingiva can occur during restorative dentistry procedures. For example, a large portion of the interdental papilla can be destroyed by the careless use of a wedge during matrix stabilization. Also, retraction cord, im-pression material, and temporary restorations may result in irreversible damage to the periodontium.

Fixed partial dentures must be designed such that the patient can clean all surfaces of the restoration, including the pontic area. If removable partial den-tures are designed so that they impinge on the soft tissue or they exert torque on the teeth, traumatic injury to the periodontium can occur. In the presence of den-tal plaque, these insults can result in more rapid, more severe destruction of pe-riodontal structures.

Exodontics

Extractions can adversely affect adjacent teeth if their attachment apparatus is damaged. The soft tissue and bone supporting an adjacent tooth can be irre-

Overhanging restorations contributing to more advanced periodontitis: (a) clinical photograph of deficient crown margins exposed at surgery; (b) radiograph of large overhang on mandibular molar resulting in more advanced bone loss on that tooth surface.

(a)

(b)

Clinical photograph of orthodontic bands and brackets with increased plaque and inflammation.

versibly destroyed. Failure to remove calculus from adjacent tooth surfaces during the extraction may negate the chance for proper healing on the adjacent teeth. An environment may be set up that actually fosters plaque accumulation. Frequently, patients stop eating on the side where teeth have been extracted. In addition to the decrease in masticatory (chewing) stimulation to the periodontium, plaque begins to form on those teeth, and patients avoid brushing the area.

Orthodontics

Orthodontic appliances have long been associated with increased plaque accumulation, gingivitis, and caries. Fixed appliances (bands, brackets, and wires) present excellent retentive areas for bacterial growth and can contribute significantly to inflammation. Special attention needs to be paid to these orthodontic plaque-retentive areas. More frequent recalls may be indicated for patients undergoing orthodontic therapy, especially adults (Fig. 3–16 ■).

FIGURE 3–17

Examples of trauma to tissues from home-care procedures due to overzealous use of devices: (a) dental floss lesions between maxillary molars; (b) toothbrush abrasion in cervical area of teeth.

(a)   (b)

TRAUMATIC FACTORS

Trauma to the periodontium from several sources can result in the loss of the attachment apparatus, changes in the local anatomy, and increased plaque accumulation and can contribute to the initiation and progression of periodontal diseases.

Toothbrush trauma

Toothbrush trauma can completely destroy a narrow band of attached gingiva and result in extensive recession. In fact, toothbrush abrasion is one of the two most common factors associated with recession, the other being permanent tooth position. Such abrasion also results in extensive grooving of the root surfaces, creating plaque traps and causing cleaning problems for the patient (Fig. 3–17a,b■).

Factitious disease

Occasionally, patients may persistently gouge or "scratch" their gingiva with their fingernails or other devices (factitious disease). This action usually results in extensive exposure of the root surface and localized inflammation. Although relatively rare, whenever isolated areas of recession are noted and a thorough evaluation fails to identify the etiology of the condition, factitious disease should be considered. The change in the local gingival anatomy often leads to greater plaque accumulation and inflammation (Fig. 3–18■).

Food impaction

Food impaction is one of the more common local factors that may contribute to the initiation and progression of inflammatory periodontal disease. Open contacts, uneven marginal ridges, irregular positions of teeth, and nonphysiologic contours of teeth and restorations can result in the impaction of food on the gingiva and into the gingival sulcus (Fig. 3–19■). The cause of the initial breakdown

FIGURE 3–18

Clinical photograph of a factitious habit; recession area on the mandibular right canine.

FIGURE 3–19

Example of uneven marginal ridges that can cause food impaction. Lower panel shows condition after reshaping of marginal ridges.

in an area of food impaction or food retention is not clear. Forceful wedging of food beneath the gingival tissues may produce inflammation from physical trauma, and/or food retention leads to food degradation and chemical irritation that affords an excellent breeding ground for bacteria that can initiate and perpetuate the disease process.

Chemical injury

Indiscriminate use of topically applied aspirin tablets, strong mouthwashes, and various other topical drugs (including cocaine) may result in ulceration of the gingival tissue. Injuries of this nature are usually transient, but may temporarily interfere with plaque control and contribute to periodontal inflammation (Fig. 3–20 ■).

FIGURE 3–20

Clinical photograph of local cocaine application mimicking an aspirin burn.

Occlusion

In the past, occlusal trauma was considered to be a major factor in the initiation of periodontal diseases. It has been conclusively proven that occlusal trauma does not initiate gingival or periodontal inflammation or pocket formation. Heavy occlusal forces can, however, cause clinical tooth mobility and the radiographic appearance of bone loss. However, these changes involve the periodontal ligament and bone, and not the marginal gingival surface tissues.

Occlusal trauma may increase the rate of progression of periodontitis if plaque-induced inflammation is also present. In this regard, trauma from occlusion acts as a contributing local risk factor in the presence of inflammation, but is not a primary etiologic factor by itself.

PERIODONTAL DISEASES: FUTURE

When teeth are not brushed or flossed properly or frequently enough, plaque microbes accumulate and irritate the gingiva, causing them to swell; if the plaque remains, the swelling may begin to force the gingiva away from the teeth, or to recede. As the bacteria continue to accumulate, the plaque is transformed into calculus. Unless this cycle is broken, more bacteria accumulate within the pockets, creating more inflammation, deeper pockets, and greater bone loss until teeth start to loosen. Without treatment the supporting structures may recede to such an extent that the teeth may be lost. In this manner, current periodontal disease is a local contributing factor for further and future periodontal disease.

SYSTEMIC RISK FACTORS FOR PERIODONTAL DISEASES

While it must be assumed that general health affects a patient's resistance to the development of periodontal diseases, no specific systemic disease has been shown to produce periodontal diseases in the absence of local irritating factors. In fact, the presence of certain systemic conditions may actually enhance or intensify the response to the plaque beyond what would occur if the systemic condition were not present.

While it is not possible to include every systemic disorder that has an impact on periodontal disease progression, numerous conditions potentially modify plaque accumulation and disease progression.

Periodontal diseases are no longer regarded as infections to which everyone is equally susceptible. Research is trying to determine why some patients are more "at risk" than others for destructive periodontal diseases. Although bacteria are essential for the development of periodontitis, they are insufficient by themselves. A susceptible host is also necessary, so host factors play a substantial role. A rather large number of genetic and environmental or acquired factors place individuals at risk for periodontitis (Table 3–1).

GENETICS

It is now known that host susceptibility factors play an important role in high-risk periodontal patients. Evidence for **genetic** control of risk factors for some forms of periodontal disease includes:

1. a consistent association of periodontitis with certain genetically transmitted traits;
2. studies of separated twins with adult onset forms of periodontitis; and
3. genetic studies of early onset forms of periodontitis.

Periodontal diseases can no longer be thought of as a prevalent condition for which all people are at equal risk if they fail to practice good oral hygiene. It appears that microbial and host factors are both important to disease susceptibility, but neither, independently, accounts for all degrees of periodontal disease. Because periodontal diseases are more than likely diverse in etiology, any thought of a universal host risk factor is probably also inappropriate. An association has been found between the susceptibility and severity to periodontitis and the presence of a substance called *interleukin-1* (IL-1). IL-1 is a cytokine released from inflammatory cells in the body. An IL-1 gene-positive patient is about 7 times more likely to develop or have advanced periodontal disease than a gene-negative patient, and this genotype occurs in approximately 30% of the population (Newman 1998).

As with many other diseases, susceptibility to periodontal diseases may, to some extent, be genetically determined. Several congenital diseases with periodontal manifestations have been identified, such as hereditary gingival fibromatosis, cyclic neutropenia, Down syndrome, Papillon-Lefévre syndrome, Chediak-Higashi disease, hypophosphatasia, among others.

It is now clear that genetic factors that act on and modify host responses to the microbial challenge are major determinants of susceptibility to periodontitis, as well as determinants of the rates and extent of disease progression and disease severity. Roughly 50% of the enhanced risk for severe periodontitis can be accounted for by heredity alone. Studies of families with aggressive (early onset) periodontitis and groups of individuals with chronic (adult) periodontitis have shown that certain chromosomes and, in some cases, specific gene loci are linked to enhanced susceptibility for periodontitis (Newman 1998).

Periodontal findings in twins who were reared together or apart have shown a significant genetic component for probing depth, attachment loss, and plaque that could not be explained by differences in family environment such as oral hygiene practices and frequency of dental visits (Michalowicz et al. 1991).

AGE, GENDER, AND RACE

Epidemiologic studies have shown that the incidence (rate of occurrence) of periodontal diseases increases with age (Abdellatif and Burt 1987). This is likely the result of the cumulative effects of bacterial irritation of the tissues over many years, rather than a reduction in host resistance as a function of the aging process. Evidence strongly suggests that periodontal health can be maintained throughout life if local etiologic factors are controlled.

Females are considered to be more susceptible to periodontal diseases than males. However, the National Institute of Dental and Craniofacial Research Survey of Oral Health of Adults in the United States shows that males have a greater incidence and severity of periodontal diseases. This is probably because females see dentists more often and have better oral hygiene practices.

No firm evidence documents that race is a significant risk factor in destructive forms of periodontitis other than as it may be related genetically within particular families.

STRESS

Being under long-term physical and psychological **stress** seems to increase susceptibility to periodontal infection (Table 3–6). Stress (along with depression, financial problems, social isolation, and other psychosocial factors) is another systemic risk factor for periodontitis because it may depress the immune response to periodontal pathogens, thereby increasing the severity of periodontal disease (Genco et al. 1998b). Stressful life events such as divorce, joblessness, and lifestyle factors have been correlated with increased severity of periodontal disease. Stress works in two ways. People under stress change their behavior and may pay less attention to oral hygiene. Also, their bodies increase the production of glucocorticosteroids (hormones made in the body that have antiinflammatory actions and protect against stress) and cortisone, a type of glucocorticosteroid, which results in immunosuppression and a reduced resistance to infection. Stress variables also seem to have an effect on healing.

ENDOCRINE

Diabetes

Diabetes is associated with a reduced ability to cope with infections and with impaired wound healing. The balance of evidence suggests that both insulin-dependent type 1 diabetes and non-insulin-dependent type 2 diabetes carry an increased risk of severe gingivitis and periodontitis (Page and Beck 1997). The relationship between diabetes and periodontal diseases is more likely to be observed in poorly controlled individuals (Nishimura et al. 1998; Taylor et al. 1996). Patients with chronic, poorly controlled diabetes appear to have more attachment loss and bone loss than diabetics with good metabolic control (Safkan-Seppälä and Ainamo 1992).

Elevated blood sugar levels (hyperglycemia) may suppress the host's immune response and lead to poor wound healing and recurrent infections such as multiple or recurrent periodontal abscesses. Impaired polymorphonuclear leukocyte chemotaxis (McMullen et al. 1981; Manouchehr-Pour et al. 1981) and phagocyto-

FIGURE 3–21

Example of pregnancy gingivitis exhibiting proximal puffiness and easy bleeding on probing, reflecting an exaggerated response to local irritants due to hormonal factors.

sis (Cutler et al. 1991) have been implicated as a factor in the predisposition of patients to severe periodontal destruction. Recent evidence indicates that meticulous control of the diabetic state is associated with periodontal health (Grossi and Genco 1998).

Hormones

Gingivitis and periodontitis have been noticed clinically to be more severe in some patients during periods of hormonal change or imbalance (Amar & Chung 1994). In pregnant, pubertal, and postmenopausal patients an exaggerated inflammatory response to local irritation may be evident. Hormonal status in general does have an influence on the inflammatory response.

Pregnancy   While evidence suggests that pregnancy itself may not be associated with an increased risk of periodontitis, pregnant patients often exhibit exaggerated gingival inflammatory changes in the second and third trimesters, sometimes called *pregnancy gingivitis* (Fig. 3–21 ■). Teeth often become more mobile during pregnancy, but return to normal afterwards.

   Similar gingival changes are also seen in patients on oral contraceptives.

Puberty   Hormonal imbalance is also felt to contribute to the increased severity of gingivitis seen at puberty, when there is an exaggerated response to plaque. The mechanisms are probably similar to those present in pregnancy.

Menopause/osteoporosis

Osteoporosis as a result of estrogen depletion causes bone to become more porous, with less trabeculation and decreased thickness of the cortical plate (Jeffcoat 1998). Under sufficient dental plaque stimulus, this can lead to more severe periodontal disease, including tooth loss. A correlation has been found between osteoporosis and both periodontal disease and tooth loss in postmenopausal women (Bando et al. 1998; Jeffcoat 1998), but it is not considered a definitive risk factor.

   Certain risk factors associated with osteoporosis include age, calcium intake (e.g., through the consumption of milk, yogurt, cheese, fish, and calcium supplements), physical activity (e.g., walking, tennis), body build, and smoking status.

FIGURE 3–22

Periodontal lesions associated with HIV infection: (a) inflammation of the gingiva with characteristic lesions; (b) more advanced lesions that resemble necrotizing ulcerative periodontitis (NUP) and that is nonresponsive to typical therapy.

(a)   (b)

In a recent study, Bando et al. (1998) found that normal masticatory function in periodontally healthy postmenopausal women might inhibit or delay the progress of osteoporotic changes in skeletal bone.

HEMATOLOGIC

Several blood dyscrasias have been associated with uncommon, unusual, extreme forms of periodontal diseases. Agranulocytosis and neutropenia (including cyclic neutropenia) are associated with an increased severity of gingivitis and periodontitis as well as necrotic ulcerations. Acute leukemia is characterized by purple-colored gingival enlargement, ulceration, inflammation, and spontaneous severe bleeding. These changes are attributable to infiltration of malignant cells, neutropenia, impaired phagocytosis, platelet deficiency, and decreased effectiveness of associated immune mechanisms. Patients with these medical problems require special attention.

HIV/AIDS

Human immunodeficiency virus (HIV) seropositive individuals appear to be vulnerable to aggressive necrotizing periodontal diseases including linear gingival erythema (LGE), acute necrotizing ulcerative gingivitis (ANUG), and an aggressive necrotizing ulcerative periodontitis (NUP) (Murray 1994). See Chapter 4 and appendix A5 for the newest classification of these diseases. It appears that the degree of immunodeficiency influences the prevalence and severity of these periodontal diseases in the HIV-infected population, and may also influence treatment expectations and prognosis (Fig. 3–22a,b ■).

NUTRITIONAL

Nutritional status

Nutritional deficiencies have not been shown to cause periodontal diseases. Nutrition studies are commonly done by inducing a deprivation state of a single nutrient or a group of related nutrients in laboratory animals that result in decreased formation of the periodontal ligament, bone, and cementum. Very few patients have a diet that is totally lacking in a single nutrient or group of related nutrients; therefore, the information gained from these experimental laboratory studies in animals may not apply to the human clinical situation.

Vitamin deficiencies are probably given more significance in the etiology of periodontal diseases from a clinical standpoint than other nutritional substances. The vitamin most often studied is ascorbic acid (vitamin C), which plays an important role in the normal functions of fibroblasts, osteoblasts, and odontoblasts. When vitamin C levels are greatly reduced, wound healing is impaired.

Some other considerations concerning the diet may be important in the overall dental problems of some patients. Tough or coarse foods do not provide functional stimulation to the gingiva, nor do they help to remove plaque below the contact points or cervical bulge on the teeth.

Patients who regularly eat between meals present a problem in that they constantly provide a food source for the bacteria and may have difficulty in maintaining good oral hygiene.

DRUG INDUCED

Tobacco products

Cigarette **smoking** is a major (and may be the most significant) risk factor for severe periodontal diseases (Table 3–6 ■). Smokers are about 2.5 times more likely to have periodontal destruction than nonsmokers, yet exhibit less gingival bleeding on probing (Tonetti 1998; Krall et al. 1997). A study by Krall et al. (1997) found that current male cigarette smokers had significantly fewer teeth than those men who reported never smoking. The number of missing teeth was positively related to pack/years of cigarette use, age, and coffee consumption and inversely related to level of education. It is more accurate to use the term "pack/years" rather than "pack/day" because it describes the exposure to toxins in a cumulative way. The study also found that current smokers had higher levels of tooth mobility, calculus deposition, and probing depth than men who had never smoked. Former cigarette smokers and men who smoked pipes or cigars were similar to men who never smoked in regard to tooth loss.

Generally, the periodontal status of former smokers has been found to be intermediate between that of never smokers and current smokers (Haber and Kent 1992; Haber et al. 1993). It has been suggested that the past effects of smoking on the periodontium cannot be reversed, but that smoking cessation is beneficial to periodontal health (American Academy of Periodontology, 1999).

Although smoking does not dramatically affect the oral microflora, studies have shown that smoking and tobacco products directly modulate the subgingival microflora by favoring colonization with periodontal pathogens (Grossi et al.

TABLE 3–6
SOCIAL FACTORS
• Tobacco
• Stress
• Alcohol
• Drugs

FIGURE 3–23

Clinical example of smokeless tobacco lesions damaging the periodontium.

1996). Thus, smoking increases the risk for periodontal diseases and interferes with the ability of the gingiva and bone to respond to treatment (Gunsolley et al. 1998; Tonetti 1998). This mechanism is probably through an altered host response. Effects of smoking seem to be related not only to the local effects in the oral cavity (heat, dryness, and increased plaque and calculus deposits), but also to a suppression of the immune system altering the host response to periodontal pathogens. To adequately deal with bacterial infections, functioning neutrophils are necessary. It has been well documented that cigarette smoke can have harmful effects on various neutrophil functions (Kenny et al. 1977). For example, tobacco smoke can impair the chemotaxis and phagocytosis of neutrophils (Lannan et al. 1992). Thus, the PMNs do not function properly in eliminating invasive, pathogenic bacteria. Individuals with alterations in their host defense system would then be more susceptible to periodontal infections by preexisting pathogenic bacteria.

Another problem associated with smoking is that products of cigarette smoke remain on the root surfaces and in the gingival crevicular fluid, thereby providing a reservoir of irritants for the soft tissue and preventing tissue attachment.

Smokeless tobacco for some may be an alternative to cigarette smoking. However, research has shown that smokeless tobacco may also contribute to periodontal diseases and may eventually lead to cancerous changes in the soft tissues (Fig. 3–23 ■). A common finding is gingival recession adjacent to the site of tobacco placement. More research is needed to determine whether smokeless tobacco use is associated with an increased level of plaque-associated gingivitis. New studies have found that cigar and pipe smoking may be as harmful to periodontal tissues as cigarette smoking (Krall, Garvey, and Garcia 1999).

Alcohol

Alcohol abuse may also contribute to periodontal diseases (Table 3–6). Chronic alcohol intake presents an increased risk for periodontitis because of increased bleeding tendencies, poor oral hygiene due to overall neglect, and a tendency to malnutrition. Alcohol consumption is related to increased incidence (Drake, Hunt, and Koch 1995) and prevalence of tooth loss, especially in men (Kranzler et al. 1990; Krall et al. 1997).

FIGURE 3–24

Example of drug-induced gingival overgrowth related to the use of cyclosporine.

Xerostomia due to drugs

Several medications, such as diuretics (antihypertensive drugs) and antidepressant drugs, can cause xerostomia or dry mouth, which can be uncomfortable for the patient, interfere with plaque control, and thereby increase periodontal inflammation (Table 3–6). The reduced salivary flow has also been associated with increased caries.

Gingival overgrowth due to drugs

Gingival enlargement or overgrowth in response to plaque accumulation can be exaggerated by medications such as phenytoin (used for seizures), nifedipine (for cardiovascular problems and hypertension), cyclosporine (in transplant patients), and several others. The alveolar bone and attachment apparatus are not affected by these drugs (Ciancio, 1996; Fig. 3–24 ■).

The areas of enlargement generally begin interproximally, and slowly grow to form triangular tissue masses that eventually unite in a continuous curtain of firm gingival tissue across facial and lingual surfaces. The enlarged tissue interferes with oral hygiene and is often inflamed. Gingival overgrowth has been reported to occur in about 50% of patients receiving phenytoin (Ciancio, Yaffe, and Catz 1972), 15% of patients receiving nifedipine (Barak, Engelberg, and Hiss 1987), and 25% of patients receiving cyclosporine (Daley, Wysocki, and May 1986).

PERIODONTAL DISEASES AS RISK FACTORS
FOR SYSTEMIC CONDITIONS

Although inflammatory periodontal diseases are local infections of the gingiva, it has been shown that the presence of periodontitis may itself be a risk factor for other infections in the body, systemic diseases, and pregnancy-related problems (American Academy of Periodontology, 1998).

DIABETES

Periodontal diseases are responsible for higher levels of blood glucose in diabetics (Grossi and Genco 1998). When these infections are controlled or eliminated in diabetic patients, their insulin requirements can often be reduced. Effective treatment of periodontal diseases can result in a reduced need to gear up tissue metabolism to fight the infection and lower blood sugar levels, thereby reducing insulin requirements and helping in diabetic control. Therefore, control of infections, including periodontal diseases, may be essential to the establishment of good metabolic control in diabetics (American Academy of Periodontology, 1998).

CARDIOVASCULAR DISEASE

Periodontal diseases have been linked with an increased risk for atherosclerosis and thromboembolisms, independent of other risk factors for these **cardiovascular diseases** (Genco et al. 1998a). Men with periodontitis, especially those under age 50, are 25% more likely to develop coronary heart disease (CHD) (American Academy of Periodontology, 1998; Beck 1996). CHD is also inversely related to the number of teeth present. Two different surveys have shown that heart disease is the most common condition shared by periodontitis patients (Umino and Nagao 1993).

The connection between heart attacks and periodontal disease is felt to be so convincing that proper plaque control might actually be an exercise that saves a patient's life. Although it may seem unlikely that an infection in the mouth may result in heart disease, there are several possible links that might explain this association. For example, it is well known that if a person has gum disease, oral bacteria will enter the blood stream even after chewing or tooth brushing. When bacteria from the inflamed gum tissue enter the blood stream they trigger platelets to gather around them in a clump, and possibly infect and obstruct the blood vessels in the heart and the brain. Forty percent of those bacteria, especially *Streptococcus sanguis* and *Porphyromonas gingivalis,* have been traced to the mouth (Genco et al. 1998). Patients have a 50% increased risk for heart disease (DeStefano et al. 1993) and 30% increased risk for stroke if they also have periodontitis.

LOW-BIRTH-WEIGHT BABIES

Women with periodontal disease may be 7 to 8 times more predisposed to deliver **premature** (< 37 weeks) infants with **low birth weight** (< 5.5 lb) (Davenport et al. 1998). Periodontal disease in the mother may be responsible for many of the low-birth-weight, premature births. Current data suggest a relationship between elevated prostaglandin E_2 levels in the gingival crevicular fluid (GCF) as a marker of current periodontal disease activity and decreasing birth weight (Offenbacher et al. 1998). However, there are no studies showing whether treating mothers with periodontal disease will reduce the risk of preterm delivery (Offenbacher and Beck 1998).

RESPIRATORY DISEASES

Patients with periodontal disease may be at risk for respiratory diseases (Hayes et al. 1998). Periodontal disease is added to the list of other risk factors for this problem, including the elderly, people who smoke, and individuals confined to nursing homes or hospitals. Examples of respiratory diseases include pneumonia, bronchitis, and emphysema. Bacteria found in the oral cavity can be taken up into the lung to cause respiratory diseases. In hospital and nursing home environments, there may be less attention paid to oral hygiene. Pneumonia may be the result of infection by anaerobic bacteria, which is a component of dental plaque (American Academy of Periodontology, 1998; Scannapieco and Mylotte 1996)

SUMMARY

Periodontal diseases have multiple risk factors. Therefore, it should not be expected that one risk factor will consistently be associated with the development of this kind of disease, and it should not be expected that control of one risk factor will completely eliminate the risk of developing the disease.

Dental plaque is the primary etiologic factor in periodontal diseases. However, other local and systemic factors play an important role. By taking a thorough health and social history, and correlating known local and systemic risk factors with periodontal clinical findings, clinicians can make patients who are at increased risk aware of the impact of these factors and the influence the factors have on their periodontal condition. Especially when treatment is unsuccessful, reevaluation of primary and secondary risk factors might improve future treatment results.

The Parameters of Care published by the American Academy of Periodontology (2000) suggest that the initial therapy for patients with periodontal inflammation should include the elimination, alteration, or control of risk factors that may contribute to chronic periodontitis. This represents significant progress since it is clear that periodontal diseases are infections initiated by bacteria and may have several associated risk factors. Management of these risk factors is likely to be the most successful approach to preventing periodontitis in the future.

Also, since the presence of periodontitis is recognized as a risk factor for future and more severe periodontal disease, proper diagnosis and therapy of an existing condition is very important in helping prevent future occurrences.

KEY POINTS

✢ Currently, evidence-based dentistry supports the use of risk assessment techniques to guide clinical decisions in the treatment of periodontal diseases.

✢ Important risk factors for periodontal diseases include certain periodontal bacteria, diabetes mellitus, and smoking.

✢ Other risk factors not strongly related but still associated with increased probability of periodontal diseases include aging, gender, genetic predisposition, stress, nutrition, and systemic diseases including immunosuppression.

✢ Inflammatory periodontal diseases are infections caused by bacteria.

✢ Certain secondary local and systemic corisk factors influence the initiation and progression of the disease.

❖ Not only do certain medical conditions predispose individuals to periodontal diseases, but also periodontal diseases predispose people to certain medical conditions.

❖ Attempts to manage risk factors are important in the prevention and treatment of periodontal diseases.

ACKNOWLEDGMENTS

The authors are indebted to Connie Holland Gandy and Marianne Gabb for assistance with the preparation of this chapter.

REFERENCES

Abdellatif, H. M., and B. A. Burt. 1987. An epidemiological investigation into the relative importance of age and oral hygiene status as determinants of periodontitis. *J. Periodontol.* 66:16–33.

Amar, S., and K. M. Chung. 1994. Influence of hormonal variation on the periodontium in women. *Periodontology 2000* 6:79–87.

American Academy of Periodontology. 1998. Periodontal disease as a potential risk factor for systemic disease (position paper). *J. Periodontol.* 69:841–850.

American Academy of Periodontology. 1999. Tobacco use and the periodontal patient (position paper). *J. Periodontol.* 70:1419–1427.

American Academy of Periodontology. Parameters of Care. J. Periodontal 2000; 71(5): 847–883.

Asikainen, S., C. Chen, S. Alaluusua, and J. Slots. 1997. Can one acquire periodontal bacteria and periodontitis from a family member? *J. American Dent. Assoc.* 128:1263–1271.

Bando, K., H. Nitta, M. Matsubara, and I. Ishikawa. 1998. Bone mineral density in periodontally healthy and edentulous postmenopausal women. *Ann. Periodontol.* 3:322–326.

Barak, S., I. S. Engelberg, and J. Hiss. 1987. Gingival hyperplasia caused by nifedipine—histopathologic findings. *J. Periodontol.* 58:639–642.

Beck, J. D. 1996. Periodontal implications: Older adults. *Ann. Periodontol.* 1:322–457.

Birkedal-Hansen, H. 1993. Role of matrix metalloproteinases in human periodontal diseases. *J. Periodontol.* 64:474–484.

Ciancio, S. G. 1996. Medications as risk factors for periodontal disease. *J. Periodontol.* 67:1055–1059.

Ciancio, S. G., S. J. Yaffe, and C. C. Catz. 1972. Gingival hyperplasia and diphenylhydantoin. *J. Periodontol.* 43:411–414.

Costerton, J. W., Z. Lewandowski, D. DeBeer, D. Caldwell, D. Korber, and G. James. 1994. Biofilms, the customized microniche. *J. Bacteriol.* 176:2137–2142.

Cutler, C. W., P. Eke, R. R. Arnold, and T. E. Van Dyke. 1991. Defective neutrophil function in an insulin-dependent diabetic patient. A case report. *J. Periodontol.* 62:394–401.

Daley, T. D., G. P. Wysocki, and C. May. 1986. Clinical and pharmacological correlations in cyclosporin-induced gingival hyerplasia. *Oral Surg. Oral Med. Oral Patho.* 62:417–421.

Davenport, E. S., C. E. C. S. Williams, J. A. C. Sterne, V. Sivapathasundram, J. M. Fearne, and M. A. Curtis. 1998. The East London study of maternal chronic periodontal disease and preterm low birth weight infants: Study design and prevalence data. *Ann. Periodontol.* 3:213–221.

DeStefano, F., R. F. Andda, and H. S. Kahn et al. 1993. Dental disease and risk of coronary heart disease and mortality. *Br. Med. J.* 306:688–691.

Douglass, C. 1998. Risk assessment for periodontal disease in adults. *Oral Care Report* 8:1–11.

Drake, C. W., R. J. Hunt, and G. G. Koch. 1995. Three-year tooth loss among black and white older adults in North Carolina. *J. Dent. Res.* 74:675–680.

Fine, D. 1995. Chemical agents to prevent and regulate plaque development. *Periodontology 2000* 8:87–107.

Genco, R. J., I. Glurich, V. Haraszthy, J. Zambon, and E. DeNardin. 1998a. Overview of risk factors for periodontal disease and implications for diabetes and cardiovascular disease. *Compendium* (special issue) 19:40–45.

Genco, R. J., A. W. Ho, J. Kopman, S. G. Grossi, R. G. Dunford, and L. A. Tedesco. 1998b. Models to evaluate the role of stress in periodontal diseases. *Ann. Periodontol.* 3:288–302.

Grossi, S. G., and R. J. Genco. 1998. Periodontal disease and diabetes mellitus: A two-way relationship. *Ann. Periodontol.* 3:51–61.

Grossi, S. G., F. B. Skrepcinski, T. DeCaro, J. J. Zambon, D. Cummins, and R. J. Genco. 1996. Responses to periodontal therapy in diabetics and smokers. *J. Periodontol.* 67(suppl.):1094–1102.

Gunsolley, J. C., S. M. Quinn, J. Tew, C. M. Gooss, C. N. Brooks, and H. A. Schenkein. 1998. The effect of smoking on individuals with minimal periodontal destruction. *J. Periodontol.* 69:165–170.

Haber, J., and R. L. Kent. 1992. Cigarette smoking in periodontal practice. *J. Periodontol.* 63:100–106.

Haber, J., J. Wattles, M. Crowley, R. Mandell, K. Joshipura, and R. L. Kent. 1993. Evidence for cigarette smoking as a major risk factor for periodontitis. *J. Periodontol.* 64:16–23.

Hayes, C., D. Sparrow, M. Cohen, P. S. Vokonas, and R. I. Garcia. 1998. The association between alveolar bone loss and pulmonary function: The VA dental longitudinal study. *Ann. Periodontol.* 3:257–261.

Hou, G. L., and C. C. Tsai. 1993. Relationship between palato-radicular grooves and localized periodontitis. *J. Clin. Periodontol.* 20:678–682.

Jeffcoat, M. K. 1998. Osteoporosis: A possible modifying factor in oral bone loss. *Ann. Periodontol.* 3:312–321.

Jeffcoat, M. K., M. McGuire, and M. G. Newman. 1997. Evidence-based periodontal treatment: Highlights from the 1996 World Workshop in Periodontics. *J. American Dent. Assoc.* 128:713–724.

Kenny, E. G., J. H. Kraal, S. R. Saxe, and J. Jones. 1977. The effect of cigarette smoke on human oral polymorphonuclear leukocytes. *J. Periodont. Res.* 12:227–234.

Krall, E., A. Garvey, and R. Garcia. 1999. Alveolar bone loss and tooth loss in male cigar and pipe smokers. *J. American Dent. Assoc.* 130:57–64.

Krall, E., C. Hayes, A. J. Garvey, and R. I. Garcia. 1997. Study finds a correlation between smoking and tooth loss. *J. Mass. Dent. Soc.* 46:20–23.

Kranzler, H. R., T. F. Babor, L. Goldstein, and J. Gold. 1990. Dental pathology and alcohol-related indicators in an outpatient clinic sample. *Community Dent. Oral Epidemiol.* 18:204–207.

Lannan, S., A. McLean, and E. Drost et al. 1992. Changes in neutrophil morphology and morphometry following exposure to cigarette smoke. *Int. J. Exp. Pathol.* 73:183–191.

Listgarten, M. A., H. E. Mayo, and R. Tremblay. 1975. Development of dental plaque on epoxy resin crowns in man. A light and electron microscopic study. *J. Periodontol.* 46:10–26.

Löe, H., E. Theilade, and S. Jensen. 1965. Experimental gingivitis in man. *J. Periodontol.* 49:117–187.

Manouchehr-Pour, M., P. J. Spagnuolo, H. M. Rodman, and N. F. Bissada. 1981. Comparison of neutrophil chemotactic response in diabetic patients with mild and severe periodontal disease. *J. Periodontol.* 52:410–414.

McMullen, J. A., T. E. Van Dyke, H. U. Horoszewicz, and R. J. Genco. 1981. Neutrophil chemotaxis in individuals with advanced periodontal disease and a genetic predisposition to diabetes mellitus. *J. Periodontol.* 52:167–173.

Michalowicz, B. S., D. Aeppli, J. G. Virag et al. 1991. A twin study of genetic variation in proportional radiographic alveolar bone height. *J. Dent. Res.* 70:1431–1435.

Moore, W. E. C., and L. V. H. Moore. 1994. The bacteria of periodontal diseases. *Periodontology 2000* 5:66–77.

Murray, P. 1994. Periodontal diseases in patients infected by human immunodeficiency virus. *Periodontology 2000* 6:50–67.

Newman, M. G. 1996. Improved clinical decision making using the evidence-based approach. *Ann. Periodontol.* 1:i–ix.

Newman, M. 1998. Genetic, environmental, and behavioral influences on periodontal infections. *Compendium* (special issue) 19:25–31.

Nishimura, F., K. Takahashi, M. Kurihara, S. Takashiba, and Y. Murayama. 1998. Periodontal disease as a complication of diabetes mellitus. *Ann. Periodontol.* 3:20–29.

Offenbacher, S., and J. D. Beck. 1998. Periodontitis: A potential risk factor for spontaneous preterm birth. *Compendium* (special issue) 19:32–39.

Offenbacher, S., H. L. Jared, P. G. O'Reilly et al. 1998. Potential pathogenic mechanisms of periodontitis-associated pregnancy complication. *Ann. Periodontol;* 3(1): 233–250.

Page, R. C., and J. D. Beck. 1997. Risk assessment for periodontal diseases. *Int. Dent. J.* 47:61–87.

Page, R. C., W. Offenbacher, H. E. Schroeder, G. J. Seymour, and K. S. Kornman. 1997. Advances in the pathogenesis of periodontitis: Summary of developments, clinical implications and future directions. *Periodontology 2000* 14:216–248.

Philstrom, B. L., B. McHugh, and T. H. Oliphant et al. 1983. Comparison of surgical and nonsurgical treatment of periodontal disease. A review of current studies and additional results after 6 1/2 years. *J. Clin. Periodontol.* 10:524–541.

Rams, T. E., and C. C. Link, Jr. 1983. Microbiology of failing dental implants in humans: Electron microscopic observations. *J. Oral Implantol.* 11:93–100.

Renvert, S., M. Wikström, G. Dahlen, J. Slots, and J. Egelberg. 1990. On the inability of root debridement and periodontal surgery to eliminate *Actinobacillus actinomycetemcomitans* from periodontal pockets. *J. Clin. Periodontol.* 17:351–355.

Safkan-Seppälä, B., and J. Ainamo. 1992. Periodontal conditions in insulin-dependent diabetes mellitus. *J. Clin. Periodontol.* 19:24–29.

Saglie, R. F., F. A. Carranza, Jr., M. G. Newman, L. Cheng, and K. J. Lewin. 1982. Identification of tissue-invading bacteria in human periodontal disease. *J. Periodontol. Res.* 17:452–455.

Scannapieco, R. A., and J. M. Mylotte. 1996. Relationships between periodontal disease and bacterial pneumonia. *J. Periodontol.* 67:1114–1122.

Taylor, G. W., B. A. Burt, M. P. Becker, R. J. Genco, M. Shlossman, W. C. Knowler, and D. J. Pettitt. 1996. Severe periodontitis and risk for poor glycemic control in patients with noninsulin-dependent diabetes mellitus. *J. Periodontol.* 67:1085–1093.

Tonetti, M. S. 1998. Cigarette smoking and periodontal diseases: Etiology and management of the disease. *Ann. Periodontol.* 3:88–101.

Umino, M., and M. Nagao. 1993. Systemic disease in elderly dental patients. *Int. Dent. J.* 43:213–218.

SELF-QUIZ

1. All of the following are harmful products produced by bacteria that affect the periodontal tissues *except* one. Which one is the exception? (p. 70)

   a. enzymes
   b. lipooligosaccharides
   c. waste products
   d. crevicular fluid

2. Which one of the following types of bacteria found in subgingival plaque is considered pathogenic for periodontitis? (p. 62)

   a. *Porphyromonas gingivalis*
   b. *Actinomyces viscosis*
   c. *Streptococcus sanguis*
   d. *Corynebacterium matruchotii*

3. Which one of the following is the primary risk factor for periodontal diseases? (p. 60)

   a. dental calculus
   b. dental plaque
   c. diabetes mellitus
   d. HIV/AIDS infection
   e. systemic drugs

4. Which one of the following reasons makes calculus an important local risk factor for periodontal diseases? (p. 72)

   a. it is porous and can provide a reservoir for bacteria
   b. it directly irritates the epithelial lining of the pocket
   c. minerals cause a breakdown in the epithelial attachment
   d. the presence of lipooligosaccharides causes the tissues to erode

5. All of the following anatomic factors may predispose a site to periodontal disease *except* one. Which one is the exception? (p. 72)

   a. tooth position
   b. furcation area
   c. crown surface
   d. root surface

6. Which one of the following evidence exists to support the concept of a genetic predisposition to periodontal diseases? (p. 81)

   a. presence of a specific type of bacteria
   b. increased levels of bacterial enzymes in the blood
   c. association of periodontitis with certain transmitted traits
   d. transmission of bacteria through saliva from mother to child

7. Which one of the following mechanisms explains how increased stress adversely affects the periodontium? (p. 82)

   a. increases in subgingival pathogenic bacteria
   b. increases in estrogen levels results in gingivitis
   c. less compliance with home care of teeth and gums
   d. shifts in the concentration of available endotoxins

8. The hormonal changes associated with pregnancy cause an increased incidence of gingival disease *because* these changes are associated with an increase in sex hormone levels. (p. 83)

   a. Both the statement and the reason are correct and related.
   b. Both the statement and the reason are correct but *not* related.
   c. The statement is correct, but the reason is *not.*
   d. The statement is *not* correct, but the reason is correct.
   e. *Neither* the statement *nor* the reason is correct.

9. Smoking affects the periodontium by which one of the following mechanisms? (p. 85)

   a. decreasing the number of melanocytes
   b. suppressing of the immune system
   c. altering the metabolism of fibroblasts
   d. increasing the amount of fibrotic tissue
   e. decreasing the number of periodontal pathogens

10. Periodontal diseases are thought to be an important risk factor for all of the following medical conditions *except* one. Which one is the exception? (pp. 87–89)

    a. stroke
    b. hypertension
    c. diabetes mellitus
    d. low-birth-weight babies
    e. kidney failure

CLASSIFICATION OF PERIODONTAL DISEASES

Surendra Singh, D.D.S., M.S.

Outline:

Classification System
Gingival Diseases
Periodontitis
Periodontitis Modified by Systemic Factors
Necrotizing Periodontal Diseases/Necrotizing Ulcerative Periodontitis
Peri-Implant Diseases
Summary
Key Points
References
Self-Quiz

Goal:

To provide the dental hygienist with an understanding of the classifications of inflammatory periodontal diseases.

Educational Objectives:

Upon completion of this chapter, the reader should be able to:

Describe the 1999 classification of periodontal diseases;

Discuss the relationship of hormones and medications with periodontal diseases;

Discuss periodontal disease associated with HIV-positive patients; and

Explain the association of periodontal diseases relationship with dental implants.

KEY WORDS

- inflammatory periodontal diseases
- classification systems
- gingivitis
- periodontitis
- peri-implant disease

Inflammatory periodontal diseases are a major cause of tooth loss. Periodontal diseases are not a single disease entity, but a group of lesions affecting the tissues that form the attachment apparatus of a tooth or teeth. These diseases are microbial infections wherein the microorganisms act in concert with a host's reduced capacity to resist disease. To successfully treat periodontal diseases, it is essential that one is able to recognize different types of the diseases. When classifying inflammatory periodontal diseases, it is important to include not only diseases that have primary manifestation and etiology in the periodontium but also periodontal manifestations of systemic diseases. In this chapter a comprehensive classification of chronic inflammatory periodontal diseases or conditions affecting periodontal tissues is presented.

Noninflammatory periodontal diseases are caused by nonplaque-induced factors that effect the periodontium. Included in this group of diseases is occlusal trauma.

CLASSIFICATION SYSTEM

Over the years a number of **classification systems** have been developed to organize and name various disease entities or conditions affecting the periodontium. Currently, two diagnostic classifications exist for periodontal diseases (Tables 4–1■ and 4–2■). In 1989, the American Academy of Periodontology recommended a classification based on the data from periodontal research that is used by the dental community to describe different forms of periodontal diseases (Table 4–1). This was modified in 1992 (American Academy of Periodontology) in a position paper published by the academy to include gingival diseases. The other classification is intended for insurance purposes (Table 4–2) (American Academy of Periodontology 1989). *In 1999 at the International Workshop for a Classification*

TABLE 4–1
1989 CLASSIFICATION OF INFLAMMATORY PERIODONTAL DISEASES

GINGIVAL DISEASES

Gingivitis
- Plaque-associated Gingivitis
- Chronic or long-standing Gingivitis
- Acute Necrotizing Gingivitis
- Steroid Hormone-influenced Gingivitis
- Medication-influenced Gingival Overgrowth
- Desquamative Gingivitis

Periodontitis
- Adult Periodontitis
- Early-Onset Periodontitis
    Prepubertal Periodontitis:
        Generalized
        Localized
    Juvenile Periodontitis:
        Generalized
        Localized
    Rapidly Progressive Periodontitis
- Periodontitis Associated with Systemic Disease
    Necrotizing Ulcerative Periodontitis
- Refractory Periodontitis

Source: American Academy of Periodontology 1989, 1992.

TABLE 4–2		
INSURANCE CLASSIFICATION OF PERIODONTAL DISEASES (ACCORDING TO THE SEVERITY OF DISEASE)		
Case Type I	Gingivitis	Inflammation of the gingiva. There is bleeding on probing. Changes in gingival color, contour, consistency, and surface texture. Shallow probing depths. No bone loss.
Case Type II	Early periodontitis	Inflammation spreads into underlying periodontal structures, with slight bone loss.
Case Type III	Moderate periodontitis	More bone and soft tissue destruction than in Type II. There may be loss of bone in the furcation area of multirooted teeth. Tooth mobility may be a feature.
Case Type IV	Advanced periodontitis	A more advanced stage of Type III. Further bone loss with tooth mobility. Furcation involvement of many multirooted teeth is likely.
Case Type V	Refractory periodontitis	Patients continue to show periodontal breakdown despite appropriate periodontal treatment and optimal home care. These sites most likely appear to be reinfected with periodontal pathogens.

Source: American Academy of Periodontology 1995.

of *Periodental Diseases and Conditions the American Academy of Periodontol-ogy proposed a new classification system* (Armitage, 1999). *This new classification system is not based on the age of the patient at the time of presentation but rather describes distinct forms of periodontal diseases based on clinical, radiographic, and historical data.* The insurance classification of periodontal diseases has been eliminated in the new classification. The American Academy of Periodontology would like this new system to be integrated into dental education as soon as possible. Table 4–3 ■ and appendix 5 reviews this system and compares the old terminology with the new terms (Armitage 1999). The reader should refer to these references when reading this textbook. It should be noted that all the periodontal diseases discussed in this chapter refer to inflammatory periodontal diseases because the conditions are inflammatory in nature where the host's inflammatory and immune responses are triggered by a bacterial insult. Occlusal problems or diseases (e.g., grinding and clenching) related to the periodontium are not inflammatory in nature and will be discussed in Chapter 13.

Gingivitis is an inflammatory lesion, mediated by host/microorganism interactions, which remains limited to the gingival tissues and does not involve the underlying periodontal ligament, cementum, or alveolar and supporting bone (American Academy of Periodontology 1992a). In this broad condition (gingival diseases are summarized in Table 4–1), the apical extent of the junctional epithelium and the coronal gingival connective tissue attachment remain at the cementoenamel junction; hence there is no attachment loss. Gingivitis can affect children, adolescents, and adults.

Gingivitis has been further defined based on clinical manifestations, duration of the disease, and association with either dental plaque or systemic factors such as medical conditions or medications (Page 1986). Some professionals question whether gingivitis should be considered a periodontal disease, since it does not cause loss of significant amounts of periodontal support or tooth mortality (loss). However, most researchers have concluded otherwise (Ranney 1993, 1986; Page 1986).

Periodontitis is an inflammatory lesion mediated by host/microorganism interactions, and results in clinical attachment loss and alveolar and supporting bone loss. Periodontitis primarily affects adults, but children and adolescents can be afflicted (Table 4–1).

TABLE 4–3		
TERMINOLOGY FOR THE NEW CLASSIFICATION OF PERIODONTAL DISEASES		

NEW NAME		OLD NAME
I	Gingival diseases	
	• Gingivitis associated with dental plaque only	• Remains as plaque-associated gingivitis
	• Gingival diseases modified by systemic factors associated with the endocrine system (puberty, pregnancy, menstrual cycle-associated gingivitis, diabetes mellitus)	• Remains as puberty, pregnancy, menstrual-associated gingivitis; diabetes mellitus was not classified before
	• Gingival diseases modified by medications	• Remains as drug-influenced gingivitis
	• Gingival diseases modified by malnutrition	• No prior classification
	• Non-plaque induced gingival diseases (bacterial, viral, and fungal infections; genetic origin, mucocutaneous disorders; allergic reactions; traumatic lesions)	• Previous classification included only desquamative gingivitis
II	Chronic periodontitis; Localized/generalized	Adult periodontitis, prepubertal periodontitis, rapidly progressive periodontitis
III	Aggressive periodontitis: Localized 　　　　　　　　　　　　　　Generalized	Localized juvenile periodontitis (LJP) Generalized juvenile periodontitis (GJP); rapidly progressive periodontitis
IV	Periodontitis as a manifestation of systemic diseases 　- associated with hematological disorders 　- associated with genetic disorders 　- not otherwise specified (NOS)	Remains as before; diseases associated with hematological and genetic disorders
V	Necrotizing periodontal diseases • Necrotizing ulcerative gingivitis (NUG) • Necrotizing ulcerative periodontitis (NUP)	No separate prior classification; NUG and NUP were classified separately
VI	Abscess of the periodontium Gingival abscess, periodontal abscess, periocoronal abscess	No prior classification
VII	Periodontitis associated with endodontic lesions	No prior classification
VIII	Developmental or acquired deformities and conditions • Tooth-related issues, tooth anatomy, dental restoration, endodontic lesions, mucogingival deformities, occlusal trauma, etc.	No prior classification

GINGIVAL DISEASES

Plaque-associated gingivitis

Gingivitis caused by dental plaque is the most common periodontal disease (Page 1985; see also Table 4–4 ■). Dental plaque as the etiology or cause of gingivitis has been confirmed in Löe's classic "Experimental Gingivitis in Man" study (Löe, Theilade and Jensen 1965). Plaque-associated gingivitis begins at the gingival margin and can spread throughout the remaining gingival unit. A plaque-associated gingivitis will not develop unless there are bacteria present (American Academy of Periodontology 1992b); however, the composition of the required oral microflora is not specific (Moore, Moore and Cato 1987). Gingivitis is reversible following the

TABLE 4-4

COMMON FEATURES OF THE PERIODONTAL DISEASES (USING 1989 CLASSIFICATION SYSTEM)

Fig. 4-1 plaque-induced

Fig. 4-2 phenytoin

Fig. 4-3 nifedipine

Fig. 4-4 cyclosporine

DISEASE	PATIENT POPULATION	CLINICAL FEATURES	CAUSES OF THE DISEASE	MICROBIOLOGIC FEATURES
Dental plaque induced gingivitis (Figure 4-1)	Adolescents, adults	Gingival redness, bleeding, and enlargement Absence of clinical attachment loss and bone loss	Inadequate oral hygiene	No specific bacteria are demonstrated although high levels of *Streptococcus sanguis, S. mitis, Fusobacterium nucleatum, Actinomyces viscosus,* and *Veillonella parvula* have been detected
Drug influenced gingivitis (Figures 4-2 to 4-4)	Patients taking phenytoin, calcium channel blockers, cyclosporine	Gingival enlargement or overgrowth Absence of clinical attachment loss and bone loss	Medications and dental plaque	No specific bacteria demonstrated

Continued

TABLE 4–4, CONTINUED

COMMON FEATURES OF THE PERIODONTAL DISEASES

DISEASE	PATIENT POPULATION	CLINICAL FEATURES	CAUSES OF THE DISEASE	MICROBIOLOGIC FEATURES	
Gingival diseases associated with the endocrine system (Figure 4–5)	Pregnant patients, adolescents	Intense gingival inflammation Absence of clinical attachment loss and bone loss	Changes in sex hormone level; exaggerated response to plaque	*Prevotella intermedia*	Fig. 4–5 puberty
Gingival manifestations of systemic conditions, mucocutaneous disorders (Figure 4–6)	These include skin disease including pemphigus, lichen planus, benign mucous membrane pemphigoid (BMMP), and others	Gingiva may appear blotchy red, have blisters or vesicles, or slough (peel) off from the underlying connective tissue	Abnormality in the immune system	None	Fig. 4–6 lichen planus
Chronic periodontitis (Figure 4–7)	Most prevalent in adults but can occur in children and adolescents	Pocket information; bone loss; inflammation	Primary etiologic factor is dental plaque (poor oral hygiene); many other risk factors (e.g., smoking, systemic diseases)	High numbers of *Porphyromonas gingivalis*, *Bacteroides forsythus*, *Prevotella intermedia*, and *Eikenella corrodens*	Fig. 4–7 chronic periodontitis
Generalized aggressive periodontitis	Usually affects persons under 30 years of age	Generalized: Severe gingival inflammation rapid bone destruction affecting at least three permanent teeth other than first molars and incisors	Defect in polymorphonuclear (PMN) and/or macrophage function	Some predominant bacteria include *Prevotella intermedia*, *Actinobacillus actinomycetemcomitans*	Fig. 4–8 aggressive periodontitis in an adolescent (Courtesy of Procter & Gamble, Cincinnati, OH)

Condition		Clinical features	Contributing factors	Microbiology	Figure
Localized aggressive periodontitis (Figure 4–9)	Except for the presence of periodontitis patients are otherwise clinically healthy; circumpubital onset	Sparse amount of plaque and calculus; little inflammation Localized: Incisor and first molar sites	Defect in PMN chemotaxis	*Actinobacillus actinomycetemcomitans Capnocytophaga* species	Fig. 4–9 localized aggressive periodontitis (Courtesy of Procter & Gamble, Cincinnati, OH)
Necrotizing periodontal diseases (NUG) (Figure 4–10)	Young adults	Punched out interdental papillae, pain, and free bleeding	Inadequate oral hygiene; stress; cigarette smoking	Specific bacteria: spirochetes, *Prevotella intermedia, Fusobacterium nucleatum*	Fig. 4–10 NUG (Courtesy of Procter & Gamble, Cincinnati, OH)
Necrotizing periodontal diseases (NUG) (Figure 4–11)	HIV-infected individuals	Distinct red band around marginal gingiva	Immunodeficiency (decrease in CD4+ lymphocytes)	Similar to chronic periodontitis; bacteria: *Porphyromonas gingivalis, Prevotella intermedia, F. nucleatum, Candida albicans* (fungus)	Fig. 4–11 NUG (Courtesy of Procter & Gamble, Cincinnati, OH)
Necrotizing periodontal diseases (NUP) (Figure 4–12)	Patients with HIV infection	Periodontal involvement of deeper structures; rapid loss of bone and spontaneous gingival bleeding	Immunodeficiency	Similar to adult periodontitis; bacteria: *Porphyromonas gingivalis, P. intermedia, F. nucleatum, Candida albicans* (fungus)	Fig. 4–12 NUP (Courtesy of Procter & Gamble, Cincinnati, OH)
Refractory periodontitis	Can occur in any case of periodontal disease	Continued periodontal destruction despite appropriate treatment	Dental plaque	Numerous bacteria; especially high levels of *Bacteroides forsythus, Porphyromonas gingivalis*	

101

removal of dental plaque and maintenance of good oral hygiene self-care. However, if oral hygiene procedures are discontinued and the level of oral hygiene is not adequate, allowing the accumulation of plaque, clinical signs of acute gingivitis develop within 1 to 3 weeks. This classic model of gingivitis induction is used in clinical trials to test antigingivitis oral rinses.

Since the bacteria associated with chronic, long-standing, plaque-induced gingivitis is not very specific, recognition of gingivitis is primarily made clinically. However, the *earliest* changes may not be seen clinically and only histologically under the microscope. With the development of gingivitis, the healthy gingiva changes in color, contour, consistency, and surface texture. Plaque-associated gingivitis starts within the interdental papilla and is clinically characterized by gingival redness, gingival bleeding, swelling, and gingival sensitivity and tenderness (Löe, Theilade, and Jensen 1965; Suzuki 1988).

The features of plaque-induced gingivitis can be summarized as follows:

1. it is related to nonspecific bacteria (although certain types of bacteria are associated with gingivitis, the condition is currently still considered of nonspecific bacterial origin);
2. clinical signs of inflammation are limited to the gingiva;
3. it is reversible to health following the removal of the dental plaque causing it; and
4. even though bacteria are the primary risk factors, secondary factors apparently modify the clinical characteristics of the disease. This has resulted in many subclassifications.

Treatment of gingivitis includes maintenance of adequate oral hygiene self-care and regular professional mechanical debridement.

GINGIVITIS ASSOCIATED WITH MEDICATIONS

Drug-influenced gingivitis

Commonly used drugs can lead to the appearance of gingivitis. There are three types of medications (Table 4–3) that can cause gingival overgrowth or enlargement:

- phenytoin (incidence 50%) used to control convulsive or seizure disorders (Angelopoulos and Goaz 1972; Steinberg and Steinberg 1982; Dongari, McDonnell, and Langlais 1993);
- cyclosporine (incidence about 30%) used for immunosuppressive or anti-rejection therapy when an individual receives an organ transplant (Seymour and Jacobs 1992; Thomason et al. 1995); and
- calcium channel blockers used for the treatment of cardiovascular conditions such as hypertension, angina, and arrhythmias. Although nifedipine was the first calcium channel blocker (Barclay et al. 1992) and is the one most frequently associated with gingival enlargement (incidence about 15%), the condition can occur with any drug in this class (Nishikawa et al. 1991)

There are no specific bacteria associated with this type of gingivitis and no specific risk factors other than poor oral hygiene and use of the medication.

Based on current histological and ultrastructural findings, drug-influenced gingival changes are more accurately referred to as "gingival overgrowth" or "enlargement," rather than "gingival hypertrophy," which is defined as an increase in connective tissue volume, or gingival hyperplasia, which is defined as an abnormal increase in the number of fibroblasts (Hallmon and Rossmann 1999).

The etiology of drug-induced gingival overgrowth is not exactly known. Either there is an excessive production of collagen by gingival fibroblasts, making the gingiva appear thickened or enlarged (Brown, Beaver, and Bottomley 1991), or the action of collagenase, which breaks down collagen, is reduced (Hallmon and Rossmann 1999). The highly active fibroblasts become sensitive to these medications in the presence of inflammation (Brown, Beaver and Bottomley 1991).

Enlargement often occurs within 1 to 3 months after the start of the medication (Nishikawa et al. 1991). Although the amount of the drug used daily and duration of use may be related to the severity of the overgrowth (Addy et al. 1982), several studies have failed to see any relationship between these factors (Hassell and Hefti 1991).

While some clinical studies have shown the level of plaque accumulation affects the severity of the overgrowth, others have shown that, although plaque control and the removal of local irritants is of some benefits for gingival health, these measures alone do not prevent gingival overgrowth (Hefti et al. 1994; Seymour and Smith 1991). It is often difficult to determine whether the increased plaque accumulation preceded the gingival overgrowth or occurred because of ineffective oral hygiene in the presence of enlarged gingiva (Rees 1998). Since hypertension is an adverse side effect of cyclosporine, patients may also be taking a calcium channel blocker such as nifedipine, which may also induce gingival overgrowth. Thus, it is difficult to assess the actual frequency of gingival overgrowth related to the use of cyclosporine (Lundergan 1989).

Gingival diseases modified by systemic factors associated with the endocrine system

Altered hormonal balances elicit an apparent exaggerated response to dental plaque. Hormonal-influenced gingivitis manifests as pregnancy gingivitis, oral contraceptive use gingivitis, and puberty gingivitis (see also Table 4–3 in this chapter). Additionally, the inflammatory response of the gingiva to plaque may be aggravated by poorly controlled plasma glucose levels resulting in a diabetes-associated gingivitis.

Pregnancy gingivitis

Pregnancy gingivitis is inflammation of the gingiva associated with pregnancy. The incidence of gingivitis during pregnancy ranges between 30 and 100%. The effects of pregnancy on *preexisting gingivitis* are seen by the second month of gestation and are most severe in the eighth month at the time of peak hormone levels (Silness and Löe 1963; American Academy of Periodontology 1992b). Pregnant patients with healthy gingiva usually do not develop gingivitis but, if gingivitis or periodontitis is present, the course of the disease is aggravated by pregnancy.

The degree of gingival inflammation is related to the state of oral hygiene of the patient. Accumulation of dental plaque parallels the gingival changes. The severity of the gingivitis is greater in pregnant than in nonpregnant women (Löe 1965) but is not associated with more destructive periodontitis (Cohen et al. 1971). The condition regresses postpartum (Silness and Löe 1963). However, gingivitis during pregnancy can be prevented or be resolved by adequate plaque control starting early in the pregnancy.

Dental plaque present at the gingival margin results in an exaggerated inflammatory response of the gingiva. Tissue inflammation and enlargement seen in pregnancy is not caused by the pregnancy itself but rather by the shifts in the hormonal levels, which aggravate the inflammation. Hormonal changes during pregnancy are due to elevated progesterone and estrogen levels, which in the final gestational month are 10 to 30 times greater than that seen during the normal menstrual cycle (Amar and Chung 1994). Elevations in these steroids, especially progesterone, cause an increased permeability of the blood vessels (microvasculature) (Lindhe and Bränemark 1968) within the lamina propria, resulting in gingival redness, edema, and increased flow of gingival crevicular fluid (Lindhe et al. 1968; Amar and Chung 1994). Subgingival growth of *Prevotella intermedia* is enhanced because this bacterium can substitute progesterone, as well as testosterone and estradiol, as growth factors. Elevated levels of *Prevotella intermedia* are also seen in puberty gingivitis (Kornman and Loesche 1980). Clinically, it presents as a painless protuberant, mushroomlike exophytic mass that is attached to a base at the gingival margin. It will regress or completely disappear postpartum.

Pregnancy gingivitis is not synonymous with a pregnancy tumor. A pregnancy tumor is a nonneoplasm, pyogenic granuloma occurring in a pregnant patient. It arises from an analogue of a dormant (inactive) tumor and is stimulated during pregnancy.

Oral contraceptive use associated gingivitis

The etiology of oral contraceptive-induced gingival inflammation is similar to that seen in pregnancy (Pearlman 1974), since the drugs used contain combinations of estrogen and progesterone that simulate pregnancy. Therefore, the same gingival changes observed during pregnancy are seen with oral contraceptive use (Mealey 1996).

Puberty gingivitis

During puberty, the dramatic elevation in steroid hormones often can cause a gingival response that is similar to what has been described for pregnancy gingivitis. In addition to a rise in hormones, the incidence and severity of gingivitis in adolescents are influenced by a number of factors, including plaque levels, dental caries, mouth breathing, tooth crowding, and tooth eruption (Stamm 1986). The distinguishing feature between plaque-induced gingivitis and puberty gingivitis is the development of gingival inflammation in the presence of a small amount of dental plaque.

Meticulous oral hygiene is the treatment of choice.

Non-plaque-induced gingival diseases
Gingival manifestations of systemic conditions (mucocutaneous disorders)

Mucocutaneous diseases are lesions involving the mucous membranes including the mouth and/or the skin. Oral manifestations of mucocutaneous diseases are seen in erosive lichen planus (Table 4–3), benign mucous membrane pemphigoid, bullous pemphigoid, and pemphigus vulgaris. More adult women than men have been documented with the disease. Oral lesions may involve all or part of the gingiva and other mucous membranes of the oral cavity (Nisengard and Neiders 1981). Gingival involvement may manifest as desquamative gingivitis characterized by desquamation or sloughing (peeling) of the epithelium, leaving a red, painful underlying connective tissue surface (Mariotti 1991). No specific bacteria have been identified. The cause of these mucocutaneous diseases is multifactoral, with some of the diseases being autoimmune in nature whereby the body attacks and destroys its own tissue (Weinberg, Insler, and Campen 1997).

PERIODONTITIS

In 1989 and 1992 the American Academy of Periodontology recommended a classification system containing specific forms of periodontitis. A classification of periodontitis is warranted since each form has a somewhat different history and associated factors. Treatment of periodontitis includes initial therapy (mechanical debridement), oral hygiene instruction, and, when indicated, periodontal surgery.

CHRONIC PERIODONTITIS

The new classification system (Armitage 1999) refers to adult periodontitis as *chronic periodontitis* and does not rely on the age of the patient to make a diagnosis. Chronic periodontitis is the most common form of periodontal disease affecting both adults and adolescents and has a slow rate of progression (Löe et al. 1986). It is directly related to the presence of plaque. There is no sex predilection. Recently, researchers have documented that genetics may play an important noncontrollable risk factor linked to periodontitis (Newman 1998). Chronic periodontitis may be modified by and/or associated with systemic diseases (e.g., diabetes mellitus, HIV infection). Also, other nonsystemic factors such as smoking and stress may modify the progression of periodontitis.

In order for a person to develop periodontitis, gingivitis must have been present. Even though specific bacteria have been identified as related to the disease, it is still considered a nonspecific bacterial infection. Detection of *Porphyromonas gingivalis* indicates a high probability that periodontitis is present (Christersson et al. 1989). Other local risk factors include calculus, overhanging restorations, and other retentive conditions that favor microbial growth, smoking, systemic conditions, hormonal factors, and stress (American Academy of Periodontology 1992b).

Features of chronic periodontitis include pocket formation and alveolar and supporting bone destruction. Tooth mobility may not necessarily be evident.

AGGRESSIVE PERIODONTITIS
(FORMERLY "EARLY ONSET PERIODONTITIS")

According to the American Academy of Periodontology's 1989 classification, early onset periodontitis was further subclassifed into prepubertal periodontitis, juvenile periodontitis, and rapidly progressive periodontitis. Prepubertal and juvenile periodontitis are further divided into localized and generalized forms. At the 1999 International Workshop for a Classification of Periodontal Diseases and Conditions, The American Academy of Periodontology suggested to eliminate the old term "early onset periodontitis" because it was too restrictive in terms of age. Early onset periodontitis included prepubertal periodontitis, juvenile periodontitis and rapidly progressive periodontitis. This form of periodontitis can occur at any age and the disease is not necessarily confined to individuals under age 35. The term "aggressive periodontitis" was chosen since it is less dependent on the age of the individual than "early onset periodontitis" (Tonetti and Mombelli 1999).

Aggressive periodontitis is divided into localized and generalized. Localized aggressive periodontitis replaces the older term "localized juvenile periodontitis (LJP) and generalized aggressive periodontitis replaces the older term "generalized juvenile periodontitis (GLP)". Individuals with aggressive periodontitis have specific clinical and laboratory findings which make it distinctively different from chronic periodontitis. The common features of localized and generalized aggressive periodontitis are (Tonetti and Mombelli 1999):

1. except for the presence of periodontitis, patients are otherwise clinically healthy;
2. rapid attachment loss and bone destruction and;
3. familial disposition.

Secondary features that may be present include:

1. amounts of microbial deposits are inconsistent with the severity of the periodontal tissue destruction;
2. elevated levels of *Actinobacillus actinomycetemcomitans* and, in some populations, *Porphyromonas gingivalis;*
3. progression of attachment loss and bone loss may be self-arresting; and
4. Phagocyte abnormalities.

Features of localized aggressive periodontitis include:

1. Circumpubertal onset; and
2. Localized first molar/incisor presentation with interproximal attachment loss on at least two permanent teeth, one of which is a first molar, and involving no more than two teeth other than first molars and incisors.

Features of generalized aggressive periodontitis include:

1. Usually affecting individuals under 30 years of age, but can be older;
2. Pronounced episodic nature of the destruction of attachment and bone; and
3. Generalized interproximal attachment loss and bone destruction affective at least three permanent teeth other than first molars and incisors.

To these primary classifications, secondary descriptors may be added. For example, risk factors that modify the disease progressive include cigarette smoking, emotional stress, drugs, sex hormones, etc. . . .).

Prepubertal periodontitis

Prepubertal periodontitis (older term) is a rare condition that begins between the time of eruption of the primary teeth and age 4 or 5. The disease occured in both localized and generalized forms. The new terms are localized/generalized aggressive periodontitis. The generalized form affected primary and secondary teeth and was characterized by severe gingival inflammation, rapid bone loss, tooth mobility, and tooth loss. A distinguishing feature that is not seen in chronic periodontitis is the presence of polymorphonuclear (PMN) and macrophage defects (Page et al. 1983b). These white blood cells do not function properly in eliminating the bacteria. Thus, there is a strong genetic or heredity component to this disease. Children with generalized prepubertal periodontitis are more prone to ear, skin, and upper respiratory tract infections (Suzuki 1988).

The localized form affects some of the primary teeth. Plaque accumulation is minimal, there is slight gingival inflammation, and bone loss is not as rapid as in the generalized form. There is usually no accompanying infection. Patients may have either defective PMNs or macrophages, but not both. Predominant bacteria include *Prevotella intermedia* and *Capnocytophaga* species (American Academy of Periodontology 1989).

Juvenile periodontitis

In the newest 1999 classification prepubutal periodontitis associated with a systemic condition is now placed under the heading of "Periodontitis as a Manifestation of Systemic Diseases." Prepubescent children who have periodental destruction without any modifying systemic conditions fits under the heading of "Chronic Periodontitis" or "Aggressive Periodontitis".

Juvenile periodontitis (older term) has its onset around puberty between the ages of 11 and 13 years and persists up to age 20. Although females have been reported to be more likely than males to have juvenile periodontitis, striking differences in gender-specific prevalence rates have not been confirmed in studies with well-defined diagnostic criteria for the patients (Saxby 1984). However, familial tendencies are known to occur for identical twins, parents, and siblings. A wide variation exists in the reported geographic and race distributions. The localized form (localized juvenile periodontitis, LJP) is more common than the generalized form. Under the new system, LJP is called *localized aggressive periodontitis* and the generalized form is called generalized aggressive periodontitis.

Bone loss in localized aggressive periodontitis is limited to permanent first molars and incisors, mainly central incisors (American Academy of Periodontology 1989; see also Table 4–3 in this chapter), and the right and left molars have mirror-image symmetrical bone loss (Kaslick and Chasens 1968), whereas bone loss in the generalized form occurs throughout the entire dentition. The most likely explanation that localizes the attachment loss to the permanent first molars and incisors is because these are the teeth at greatest risk when the disease started, as other permanent teeth are not yet erupted (Ranney 1993).

A unique feature is that the amount of periodontal destruction manifested is not related to the amount of local irritants present. The gingival tissues appear healthy and gingival inflammation is generally less severe due to the apparant lack of dental plaque (Baer 1971; American Academy of Periodontology 1996). High numbers of *Actinobacillus actinomycetemcomitans* in the subgingival pocket are associated with the localized form and they may invade the soft tissue rather than just staying in the pocket. Other microorganisms found in the pocket include the *Capnocytophaga* species, *Porphyromonas gingivalis,* and *Eikenella corrodens.*

There is a defect in PMN chemotaxis and impaired phagocytosis in 70 to 80% of patients (Suzuki et al. 1984). The PMNs are not working properly and arrive late to the diseased site (depressed chemotaxis), so they cannot properly devour the foreign material including bacteria (impaired phagocytosis).

Rapidly progressive periodontitis

Rapidly progressive periodontitis (RPP) (older term) generally affects all teeth; its age of onset is under 30 years (Page et al. 1983a). The newer term is *generalized aggressive periodontitis.* It is found more frequently in females than in males and is characterized by severe gingival inflammation, bleeding, and rapid bone loss (Table 4–3). The majority of patients have a depressed PMN chemotaxis response (Van Dyke, Levine, and Genco 1982). RPP is associated with systemic diseases including insulin-dependent diabetes mellitus, Down syndrome, and acquired immune deficiency syndrome (AIDS). The bacteria found in these sites are similar to chronic periodontitis.

REFRACTORY PERIODONTITIS

Refractory periodontitis is a type of periodontitis wherein adult periodontitis patients previously treated conventionally (periodontal debridement, periodontal surgery, oral hygiene instructions) do not respond favorably to therapy and are considered resistant to treatment. Persistent periodontitis in patients with poor compliance with home care or heavy tobacco use precludes the use of the term *refractory.* These patients more likely have recurrent periodontitis. High numbers of *Prevotella intermedia, Bacteroides forsythus, Fusobacterium nucleatum,* and *Porphyromonas gingivalis* are found in subgingival refractory sites.

Under the new classification system (Armitage 1999), periodontitis associated with refractory conditions has been eliminated as a separate disease category. It was concluded that only a small percentage of periodontitis cases are actually nonresponsive to treatment. Instead, the *refractory* designation could be applied to all forms of periodontitis (e.g., refractory chronic periodontitis, refractory aggressive periodontitis).

PERIODONTITIS MODIFIED BY SYSTEMIC FACTORS

Dental plaque initiates periodontal diseases but the form of disease and its progression is dependent on the host defenses to this challenge. Systemic conditions and environmental exposures may *modify* the normal defenses and influence the outcome of periodontal disease (Kinane 1999). A reduction in the number of function of polymorphonuclear leukocytes (PMNs) usually results in increased rate and severity of periodontal tissue destruction. Additionally, numerous drugs such as phenytoin, nifedipine, and cyclosporine predispose to gingival overgrowth in response to plaque and thus may effect in modifying preexisting periodontitis (Kinane 1999). Several systemic diseases such as Diabetes mellitus, Down syndrome, Papillon-Lefévre syndrome, hyphophosphatasia, Chediak-Higashi syndrome and HIV infection also appear to predispose individuals to periodontitis. These patients also have compromised host responses. Certain environmental conditions or exposures including cigarette smoking and emotional stress may modify periodontitis.

NECROTIZING PERIODONTAL DISEASES/NECROTIZING ULCERATIVE PERIODONTITIS

Necrotizing ulcerative gingivitis

Necrotizing ulcerative gingivitis (NUG) is a rapidly destructive, recurring, noncommunicable gingival infection. Under the new classification (Armitage, 1999), NUG is considered a type of Necrotizing Periodontal Disease limited to the gingival tissues. Additionally, the term "acute" in ANUG is a clinical descriptive term and should not be used as a diagnostic classification (Rowland 1999). NUG is relatively uncommon (incidence 0.1 to 10%) and mostly affects young adults 18 to 30 years old. It is also known as "trench mouth" (during World War I, NUG reached very high levels of incidence and was called "trench mouth" referring to the trenches soldiers inhabited during the war) or "Vincent's infection." In addition to bacteria, other predisposing factors are emotional stress, cigarette smoking, or systemic conditions.

NUG is clinically characterized by small, grey, ulcerative lesions that begin at the tips of the interdental papillae and spread to the gingival margin to form punched-out or cratered lesions. A grayish-white pseudomembrane covering the affected areas may be present. The marginal gingiva is extremely bright red and inflamed. NUG is extremely painful. Patients complain of difficulty eating and a burning sensation in the mouth. There is spontaneous gingival bleeding (i.e., the gingiva bleeds when touched or during eating). There are usually heavy deposits of plaque. These signs and symptoms are sudden in onset, localized, and recurrent. If left untreated, the infection may spread to the underlying periodontal structures. Lymphadenopathy (lymph nodes that are abnormal in size, consistency, or number), fever, and fetid oral odor (foul mouth odor) are variable findings and not always present.

This condition is usually recognized on the basis of clinical signs and symptoms. It has a bacterial origin. Microbiological samples of the affected areas show specific bacteria. High numbers of *Prevotella intermedia*, spirochetes, and *Fusobacterium* sp. have been isolated (Loesche et al. 1982). Spirochetes have been shown to penetrate deep into the connective tissue (Listgarten and Lewis 1967). Normally bacteria stay in the pocket and do not invade the underlying tissues. Thus, NUG is a manifestation of a mixed bacterial infection modified by particular systemic determinants. Necrotizing ulcerative gingivitis may also be the first clinical sign of underlying systemic disease, such as in human immunodeficiency virus (HIV) infection (Murayama et al. 1994).

A complete laboratory work-up is indicated in the management of patients with NUG, especially if a systemic disease is suspected or if the patient does not respond to conventional therapy (Murayama et al. 1994).

Primary herpetic gingivostomatitis must be differentiated from NUG. The primary distinctions are that in primary herpes the patient is usually much younger, elevated temperature is more common, and the patient appears more ill and shows a general malaise. The oral lesions in primary herpes are vesicles that coalesce into ulcers, which occur on the attached gingival and oral mucosa, and the papillae are not "punched out" as in NUG.

HIV-infected patients may present with severe forms of periodontal diseases. These patients are immunodeficient with a specific decrease in CD4+ lymphocytes. Conflicting reports concerning the classification system of HIV-associated periodontal lesions exist. New terminology was proposed in the early 1990s that is recognized by the United States and the rest of the world (EEC-Clearinghouse 1993). *Linear gingival erythema (LGE)* replaces the older term HIV-gingivitis, and *necrotizing ulcerative periodontitis (NUP)* replaces HIV-periodontitis (the latter is discussed later in this chapter). A third subdivision of HIV-associated periodontal diseases was also added, necrotizing ulcerative gingivitis (NUG). In the newest classification system (Armitage 1999) all periodontal conditions related to HIV-infections are grouped together with Necrotizing Periodontal Diseases.

The prevalence of LGE in HIV-infected populations is relatively unknown since the stage of HIV disease varies among the population (Mealey 1996) and more structured studies need to be conducted. Linear gingival erythema is characterized by a distinct band of intense redness along the marginal gingiva extending apically into the attached gingival and alveolar mucosa (Table 4–3). These oral findings do not seem to correspond to supragingival plaque accumulation (Mealey 1996) since removal of dental plaque does not improve the gingival condition as typically seen in chronic, plaque-associated gingivitis. The lesion is confined to the gingiva and does not involve bone loss. Pain is not a prominent feature with this lesion, as it is in ANUG (Winkler and Robertson 1992).

Necrotizing ulcerative gingivitis is characterized by the destruction of one or more interdental papillae that became ulcerated, cratered, and necrotic (Murray 1994), but there is no bone loss. NUG may represent an early form of NUP (Mealey 1996).

It is important for dental practitioners to recognize soft lesions early, since they may be the first signs of HIV infection (Mealey 1996; Winkler and Robertson 1992; Winkler, Grassi, and Murray 1988). Subtle lesions may go unnoticed by the examiner because pain is not a common symptom.

The microorganisms present in the gingival lesions of HIV-positive patients are not similar to the microorganisms found in the gingival lesions of HIV-negative individuals but may be similar to those found in HIV-negative individuals who have adult periodontitis (Mealey 1996; Murray et al. 1991). Implicating pathogens include *Porphyromonas gingivalis (Pg)*, *Prevotella intermedia (Pi)*, *Actinobacillus actinomycetemcomitans (Aa)*, *Fusobacterium nucleatum*, spirochetes, and *Candida albicans* (fungus) (American Academy of Periodontology 1994).

Necrotizing ulcerative periodontitis (NUP) previously replaced the term "HIV-periodontitis." Under the new system (Armitage, 1999) NUP is included with necrotizing periodontal diseases. This form of periodontal disease in the HIV-positive patient may coexist with other forms of periodontitis such as aggressive or chronic periodontitis. NUP is characterized by the extensive necrosis of the gingiva with exposure and rapid destruction of the underlying bone extending past the mucogingival junction. If not successfully treated, NUP can spread into the adjacent maxilla and mandible (Mealey 1996). Compared with NUG, severe pain is a prominent feature (Murray 1994). Essentially all NUP sites bleed on probing, and about 50% of sites show spontaneous bleeding (American Academy of Periodontology 1992b). Extensive clinical attachment loss is common, but deep periodontal pocket formation is not evident (American Academy of Periodontology 1992b).

The microbial population of subgingival sites with NUP is similar to that of adult periodontitis, which is also similar to NUG. This may prove that NUG may be a precursor to the tissue and bone destruction seen in NUP (Murray 1994).

Peri-Implant Diseases

Inflammatory conditions surrounding dental implants are becoming more common today, as more implants are being used. Periodontal disease around implants is not listed in the original or new classification from the American Academy of Periodontology; however, inflammation and periodontal destruction around implants is clinically recognized.

Loss of an implant after successful placement is often due to a bacterial infection. Gram-negative anaerobes, primarily the *Fusobacterium* species and *Prevotella intermedia* are found in the subgingival pockets. **Peri-implant disease** is a collective term for soft-tissue inflammation surrounding an implant. *Peri-implant mucositis* is the term used to describe reversible inflammation in the gingiva around a functioning implant (Albrektsson and Isidor 1994). *Peri-implantitis* is the term used for inflammatory changes in the soft tissues leading to loss of supporting bone around a functioning implant (Albrektsson and Isidor 1994). The primary risk factors for peri-implant diseases is the presence of certain bacteria (Mombelli and Lang 1998).

Treatment of peri-implant diseases is based upon proper clinical and radiographic assessment. It may include periodontal debridement, oral hygiene instruction, mouthrinses, systemic antibiotics, periodontal surgery, or removal of the implant.

Summary

In 1999, a new classification system for periodontal diseases and conditions replaced the 1989 system. This classification, rather than using the age of the patient, describes different forms of periodontal diseases based on clinical presentation. Periodontal diseases are microbial infections that are the outcome of host-bacterial interactions. Periodontal diseases are modified by systemic factors wherein the host has a reduced capacity to resist infection.

Key Points

❖ Inflammatory periodontal diseases are broadly classified into gingivitis and periodontitis.

❖ Gingivitis is a precursor to periodontitis.

✤ Gingivitis is defined as inflammation confined to the gingiva.

✤ Gingivitis is reversible.

✤ Periodontitis is inflammation that extends from the gingiva into the supporting periodontal structures.

✤ Periodontitis is most common in adults, although it does occur in a smaller number of children and adolescents.

✤ Dental plaque is the major risk factor for periodontal diseases; there are other contributory risk factors such as medications, hormones, and systemic diseases.

✤ Inflammatory periodontal diseases are also seen around dental implants.

REFERENCES

Addy, V., J. McElnay, D. Eyre, N. Campbell, and P. D'Arcy. 1982. Risk factors in phenytoin-induced gingival overgrowth. *J. Periodontol.* 54:373–377.

Albrektsson, T., and F. Isidor. 1994. Consensus report of session IV. In *Proceedings of the First European Workshop on Periodontology,* ed. N. P. Lang and T. Karring, 365–369. London: Quintessence.

Amar, S., and K. M. Chung. 1994. Influence of hormonal variation on the periodontium in women. *Periodontology 2000* 6:79–87.

American Academy of Periodontology. 1989. *Proceedings of the World Workshop in Clinical Periodontics,* I-2–I-4. Chicago: The American Academy of Periodontology.

American Academy of Periodontology. 1992a. *Glossary of Periodontal Terms* (3rd ed.). Chicago: The American Academy of Periodontology.

American Academy of Periodontology. 1992b. *The Etiology and Pathogenesis of Periodontal Diseases* (position paper), 1–9. Chicago: The American Academy of Periodontology.

American Academy of Periodontology. 1994. *Periodontal Considerations in the HIV-Positive Patient.* (position paper). Chicago: The American Academy of Periodontology.

American Academy of Periodontology. 1995. *Current Procedural Terminology for Periodontics and Insurance Reporting Manual* (7th ed.). Chicago: The American Academy of Periodontology.

American Academy of Periodontology. 1996. Periodontal diseases of children and adolescents (position paper). *J. Periodontol.* 67:57–62.

Angelopoulos, A. P., and P. W. Goaz. 1972. Incidence of diphenylhydantoin gingival hyperplasia. *Oral Surg. Oral Med. Oral Path.* 34:898–906.

Armitage, G. C. 1999. Development of a classification system for periodontal diseases and conditions. *Ann. Periodontol.* 4:1–6.

Baer, P. N. 1971. The case for periodontosis as a clinical entity. *J. Periodontol.* 42:516–519.

Barclay, S., J. M. Thomason, J. R. Idle, and R. A. Seymour. 1992. The incidence and severity of nifedipine-induced gingival overgrowth. *J. Clin. Periodontol.* 19:311–314.

Brown, R. S., W. T. Beaver, and W. K. Bottomley. 1991. On the mechanisms of drug-induced gingival hyperplasia. *J. Oral Pathol. Med.* 20:201–209.

Christersson, L. A., J. J. Zambon, R. G. Dunford, S. G. Grossi, and R. J. Genco. 1989. Specific subgingival bacteria and diagnosis of gingivitis and periodontitis. *J. Dent. Res.* 68:1633–1639.

Cohen, D. W., J. Shapiro, L. Friedman, G. C. Kyle, and S. Franklin. 1971. A longitudinal investigation of the periodontal changes during pregnancy and fifteen months postpartum. Part III. *J. Periodontol.* 42:653–657.

Dongari, A., H. T. McDonnell, and R. P. Langlais. 1993. Drug-induced gingival overgrowth. *Oral Surg. Oral Med. Oral Pathol.* 76:543–548.

EEC-Clearinghouse on Oral Problems Related to HIV Infections and WHO Collaborating Centre on Oral Manifestations for the Human Immunodeficiency Virus. 1993. Classification and diagnostic criteria for oral lesions in HIV infection. *J. Oral Pathol. Med.* 22:289–291.

Hallmon, W. W., and J. A. Rossmann. 1999. The role of drugs in the pathogenesis of gingival overgrowth. *Periodontology 2000* 21:176–196.

Hassell, T., and A. F. Hefti. 1991. Drug-induced gingival overgrowth: Old problem, new problem. *Crit. Rev. Oral Pathol. Med.* 2:103–137.

Hefti, A. F., A. E. Eshenaur, T. M. Hassell, and C. Stone. 1994. Gingival overgrowth in cyclosporine A treated multiple sclerosis patients. *J. Periodontol.* 65:744–749.

Kaslick, R. S., and A. I. Chasens. 1968. Periodontosis with periodontitis: A clinical study involving young adult males. *Oral Surgery* 25:327–350.

Kinane, D. F. Periodontitis modified by systemic factors. *Ann Periodontal.* 1999; 4:54–63.

Kornman, K. S., and W. J. Loesche. 1980. The subgingival microflora during pregnancy. *J. Periodontol. Res.* 5:111–122.

Lindhe, J., and P. I. Bränemark. 1968. Experimental studies on the etiology of pregnancy gingivitis. *Perio. Abst.* 16:50–51.

Lindhe, J., J. Lindhe, R. Attström, and A. Björn. 1968. Influence of sex hormones on gingival exudation in dogs with chronic gingivitis. *J. Periodont. Res.* 3:279–283.

Listgarten, M. A., and D. W. Lewis. 1967. The distribution of spirochetes in the lesion of acute necrotizing ulcerative gingivitis: An electron microscopic and statistical survey. *J. Periodontol.* 38:379–386.

Löe, H. 1965. Periodontol changes in pregnancy. *J. Periodontol.* 36:209–217.

Löe, H., A. Anerud, H. Boysen, and E. Morrison. 1986. Natural history of periodontal disease in man. Rapid, moderate and no loss of attachment in Sri Lankan Laborers 14 to 46 years of age. *J. Clin. Periodontol.* 13:431–440.

Löe, H., E. Theilade, and S. B. Jensen. 1965. Experimental gingivitis in man. *J. Periodontol.* 36:177–187.

Loeche, W. J., S. A. Syed, and B. E. Laughon et al. 1982. The bacteriology of acute necrotizing ulcerative gingivitis. *J. Periodontol.* 53:223–230.

Lundergan, W. P. 1989. Drug-induced gingival enlargements. Dilantin hyperplasia and beyond. *J. Calif. Dent. Assoc.* 17:48–52.

Mariotti, A. 1991. Desquamative gingivitis: Revisited. *Today's FDA* 3:1C–2C.

Mealey, B. L. 1996. Periodontal implications: Medically compromised patients. *Ann. Periodontol.* 1:256–321.

Mombelli, A., and N. P. Lang. 1998. The diagnosis and treatment of periimplantitis. *Periodontology 2000* 17:63–76.

Moore, L. V. H., W. E. C. Moore, E. P. Cato et al. 1987. Bacteriology of gingivitis. *J. Dent. Res.* 66:989–995.

Murayama, Y., H. Kurihara, A. Nagai, D. Dompkowski, and T. Van Dyke. 1994. Acute necrotizing ulcerative gingivitis: Risk factors involving host defense mechanisms. *Periodontology 2000* 6:116–124.

Murray, P. A. 1994. Periodontal diseases in patients infected by human immunodeficiency virus. *Periodontology 2000* 6:50–67.

Murray, P. A., J. R. Winkler, W. J. Peros, C. K. French, and J. A. Lippke. 1991. DNA probe detection of periodontal pathogens in HIV-associated periodontal lesions. *Oral Microbiol. Immunol.* 6:34–40.

Newman, M. 1998. Genetic, environmental, and behavioral influences on periodontal infections. *Compendium* (special issue) 19:25–31.

Nisengard, R. J., and M. Neiders. 1981. Desquamative lesions of the gingiva. *J. Periodontol.* 52:500–510.

Nishikawa, S., H. Tada, A. Hamasaki et al. 1991. Nifedipine-induced gingival hyperplasia: A clinical and in vitro study. *J. Periodontol.* 62:30–35.

Page, R. C. 1985. Oral health status in the United States. Prevalence of inflammatory periodontal diseases. *J. Dent. Educ.* 49:354–364.

Page, R. C. 1986. Gingivitis. *J. Clin. Periodontol.* 13:245–255.

Page, R. C., L. Altman, J. Ebersole et al. 1983a. Rapidly progressive periodontitis. A distinct clinical condition. *J. Periodontol.* 54:197–209.

Page, R. C., T. Bowen, L. Altman et al. 1983b. Prepubertal periodontitis I. Definition of a clinical disease entity. *J. Periodontol.* 54:257–271.

Pearlman, B. A. 1974. An oral contraceptive drug and gingival enlargement: The relationship between local and systemic factors. *J. Clin. Periodontol.* 1:47–57.

Ranney, R. R. 1986. Discussion: pathogenesis of gingivitis. *J. Clin. Periodontol.* 13:356–359.

Ranney, R. R. 1993. Classification of periodontal diseases. *Periodontology 2000* 2:13–25.

Rees, T. D. 1998. Drugs and oral disorders. *Periodontology 2000* 18:21–36.

Rowland, R. W. Necrotizing ulcerative gingivitis. *Ann Periodontol.* 1999; 4:65–73.

Saxby, M. 1984. Prevalence of juvenile periodontitis in a British school population. *Community Dent. Oral Epidemiol.* 12:185–187.

Seymour, R. A., and D. J. Jacobs. 1992. Cyclosporin and the gingival tissues. *J. Clin. Periodontol.* 19:1–11.

Seymour, R. A., and D. G. Smith. 1991. The effect of a plaque control programme on the incidence and severity of cyclosporin-induced gingival changes. *J. Clin. Periodontol.* 18:107–110.

Silness, J., and H. Löe. 1963. Periodontal disease in pregnancy. *Acta Odontol. Scand.* 21:533–551.

Stamm, J. W. 1986. Epidemiology of gingivitis. *J. Clin. Periodontol.* 13:360–370.

Steinberg, S. C., and A. D. Steinberg. 1982. Phenytoin-induced gingival overgrowth in severely retarded children. *J. Periodontol.* 53:429–433.

Suzuki, J. B. 1988. Diagnosis and classification of periodontal diseases. *Dent. Clin. North America* 32:195–216.

Suzuki, J. B., B. C. Collison, W. A. Falkler, and R. R. Nauman. 1984. Immunologic profile of juvenile periodontitis. II. Neutrophil chemotaxis, phagocytosis and spore germination. *J. Periodontol.* 55:461–467.

Thomason, J. M., R. A. Seymour, J. S. Ellis, P. J. Kelly, G. Parry, J. Dark, and J. R. Idle. 1995. Iatrogenic gingival overgrowth in cardiac transplantation. *J. Periodontol.* 66:742–746.

Tonetti, M. S., Mombelli, A. Early-onset Periodontitis. *Ann. Periodontol.* 1999. 4:39–52.

Van Dyke, T. E., M. J. Levine, and R. J. Genco. 1982. Periodontal diseases and neutrophil abnormalities. In *Host-Parasite Interactions in Periodontal Diseases,* ed. R. J. Genco and S. E. Mergenhagen, 235–245. Washington, DC: American Society for Microbiology.

Weinberg, M. A., M. S. Insler, and R. B. Campen. 1997. Mucocutaneous features of autoimmune blistering diseases. *Oral Surg. Oral Med. Oral Pathol. Oral Radiol. Endod.* 84:517–534.

Winkler, J. R., M. Grassi, and P. A. Murray. 1988. Clinical description and etiology of HIV-associated periodontal diseases. In *Perspectives on Oral Manifestations of AIDS,* ed. P. B. Robertson and J. S. Greenspan, 49–70. Littleton, MA: PSG Publishing.

Winkler, J. R., and P. B. Robertson. 1992. Periodontal disease associated with HIV infection. *Oral Surg. Oral Med. Oral Pathol.* 73:145–150.

SELF-QUIZ

1. Which one of the following features describes chronic periodontitis? (p. 105)

    a. occurs primarily in children

    b. no attachment loss or bone loss occurs

    c. bone loss does not occur

    d. risk factors include pathogenic bacteria and smoking

2. The latest classification of periodontal diseases is based on all of the following factors except one. Which one is the exception? (pp. 97–98)

    a. age of patient

    b. clinical presentation

    c. radiographic survey

    d. historical data

3. All of the following medications are contributing risk factors in causing gingival enlargement *except* one. Which one is the exception? (p. 102)

    a. phenytoin

    b. cyclosporine

    c. ibuprofen

    d. nifedipine

4. Which one of the following periodontal diseases is described by having inflammation of the gingiva without loss of clinical connective tissue attachment? (p. 97)

   a. dental plaque-induced gingivitis

   b. chronic periodontitis

   c. aggressive periodontitis

   d. refractory periodontitis

   e. necrotizing ulcerative periodontitis

5. Which one of the following forms of periodontitis is associated with a chemotactic defective in the polymorphonuclear leukocytes? (pp. 106–107)

   a. dental plaque-induced gingivitis

   b. chronic periodontitis

   c. puberty gingivitis

   d. localized aggressive periodontitis

   e. drug-influenced gingivitis

6. Which one of the following bacteria is found in high numbers in localized juvenile periodontitis (localized aggressive periodontitis)? (pp. 106–107)

   a. *Porphyromonas gingivalis*

   b. *Prevotella intermedia*

   c. *Actinomyces viscosus*

   d. *Actinobacillus actinomycetemcomitans*

   e. *Streptococcus sanguis*

7. In the latest 1999 classification of periodontal diseases, which one of the following terms replaces adult periodontitis? (p. 98)

   a. aggressive periodontitis

   b. necrotizing ulcerative periodontitis

   c. chronic periodontitis

   d. refractory periodontitis

   e. recurrent periodontitis

8. Which one of the following is a term used to describe reversible inflammation in the gingiva around a functioning implant? (p. 110)

   a. peri-implantitis

   b. peri-implant mucositis

   c. localized aggressive periodontitis

   d. generalized aggressive periodontitis

9. Which one of the following statements describes an HIV-positive patient with necrotizing periodontal disease? (p. 109)

   a. higher prevalence in females than males

   b. higher incidence of skin lesions

   c. microbial profile is similar in noninfected periodontally involved patients*

   d. geographic distribution shows a higher prevalence in the Eastern U.S.

10. Which one of the following bacteria is found in high numbers in pregnancy gingivitis? (p. 103)

   a. *Streptococcus sanguis*

   b. *Prevotella intermedia*

   c. *Veillonella parvula*

   d. *Porphyromonas gingivalis*

EPIDEMIOLOGY OF PERIODONTAL DISEASES

5

Mary Elizabeth Aichelmann-Reidy, D.D.S.

Outline:

Introduction and Definitions
Indices
Accuracy of Methodology
Prevalence of Periodontal Diseases
Incidence and Disease Progression
Epidemiologic Variables
Treatment Needs
Future Trends
Key Points
References
Self-Quiz

Goal:

To provide the dental hygienist with an understanding of the prevalence, extent, and severity of periodontal diseases in the population.

Educational Objectives:

Upon completion of this chapter, the reader should be able to:

Describe epidemiology and its descriptive terms: prevalence, incidence, extent, and severity;

Explain the significance of epidemiologic data to future treatment;

Describe the role of indices in private practice and population surveys;

Describe the prevalence and incidence of periodontal diseases;

Identify risk factors and risk indicators for periodontal diseases; and

Discuss future periodontal treatment needs and future trends that may have an impact on the dental hygiene practice.

KEY WORDS

- epidemiology
- risk factors
- periodontal diseases
- population surveys
- prevalence
- incidence
- severity
- extent
- indices
- risk indicators
- risk factors

INTRODUCTION AND DEFINITIONS

*E*pidemiology is the study of health and disease in the human population. It requires knowing the distribution and occurrence of the study disease. The rationale for the study of epidemiology is to identify events and **risk factors** in populations that lead to disease so that future health problems can be anticipated, prevented, and controlled. A risk factor is an event or characteristic associated with a given disease. It is important to identify risk factors so that health care measures can target people at risk for a particular disease, perhaps altering the future course of the disease.

Epidemiologic studies focus on populations rather than individuals. Much of what we know about **periodontal diseases** comes from national or **population surveys.** Population surveys evaluate representative samples of individuals within a study population to assess the true risk for disease and quantify how many individuals are or will be affected by disease. This quantification of disease is referred to as *disease prevalence* and *incidence.* **Prevalence** is the proportion or number of individuals in a population having the disease (old and new cases) at a given time. **Incidence** is defined as the rate of new cases occurring within a certain period of time. Disease prevalence and incidence can only be understood by looking at a large number of individuals within a population. Population surveys also provide insight into the **severity** and **extent** of a particular disease, say, periodontal disease, in populations. *Severity* is defined as the degree or amount of periodontal disease involvement and quantifies the amount of attachment loss, bone loss, or probing depth (Oliver, Brown, and Löe 1998). The *extent* of periodontal disease refers to the number or percentage of diseased teeth or sites per individual.

Epidemiologic research is used to detect the underlying patterns of a disease and its associated factors to help find the cause of the disease. Trends are detectable when data collected from large numbers of individuals from within a study population are combined. Because numerous subjects must be examined, multiple examiners are needed to collect the data. Each examiner must use the same methodology as other examiners, examine subjects in a similar way, and report the results with clearly defined measures. For a survey to be useful, the clinical assessments must be standardized so that population means (averages) can be determined.

Epidemiologic data are collected through the use of a specific methodology that differs from patient evaluations in private practice. For example, complete, full-mouth periodontal examinations, which are necessary to establish an individual's diagnosis and to determine treatment needs, are too time consuming for use on a large scale in an epidemiologic survey. The survey methods used to evaluate periodontal diseases in a population usually involve screening tools designed to quantify and simplify the disease assessment. These tools are referred to as **indices** (singular: *index*). An *index* is a numerical expression of values, with upper and lower limits, that is used to describe a specific condition. Indices are used in both clinical practice and research as the system of measurement for collecting data. They provide the private practitioner with information for patient treatment planning and the researcher with information about the prevalence and incidence of disease.

SIGNIFICANCE OF INDICES

Epidemiology is used to identify disease patterns, and indices are the measurement systems used for collecting the necessary data. For the study of periodontal diseases, assessments of plaque, calculus, gingival inflammation, periodontal attachment level, bleeding, and mobility are necessary to determine individual disease status. An index is a tool for standardized data collection and can measure the presence, absence, or severity of a disease condition on a specific tooth, area, or whole mouth and then can be extrapolated to the population. Unlike subjective clinician assessments of parameters of disease, an index is a numerical expression given to conditions that can then be quantified, tabulated, and used in comparisons to predict disease patterns, progression, and trends in study populations.

For example, if a dental hygienist examines a patient and subjectively describes the condition oral cleanliness in the mouth as "a fair amount of plaque and calculus on the teeth," this description could be interpreted differently by another clinician and might be interpreted as light or moderate plaque levels. Terms such as *fair, light, moderate,* and *heavy* have different meaning for different practitioners and therefore need to be standardized. The use of indices can help to standardize and reproduce findings for comparison of patient progression in private practice and are essential for collection of data in large population surveys so that comparisons and tabulations can be made with consistent and clearly defined measures.

Dentists and dental hygienists formulate treatment plans based on full-mouth data collection. Becoming aware of the periodontal problem, assessing its severity, and presenting the findings to the patient require the practitioner to record and chart data in formats that can be compared over time. Periodontal charting forms and indices tabulate the measurements to be interpreted for treatment plans. However, it is not possible to complete individual assessments in large epidemiologic studies; instead indices of a representation sample from the population are used.

Indices measure disease outcomes and so measure past disease. When a dental hygienist supplements a patient's clinical examination with index scores to monitor patient conditions over time, these data, along with information gleaned from population surveys, can help the clinician predict future disease progression and establish a prognosis for the individual patient. Dental hygienists and dentists also must learn to use indices compared over time to project the progress of disease in each individual, since disease progression cannot be irrefutably established and must be estimated as a continuous process.

CRITERIA FOR INDICES

There are many types of indices a practitioner can select from depending on the specific method of data collection and the meaning to be given to the data collected. When selecting an index or set of indices, the following properties should be considered:

1. Simplicity or ease of use is critical to provide a fast and reproducible
   method to collect the data. Reproducibility creates a reliable instrument

that can be used by different examiners or the same examiner over time to produce the same results.

2. The index should be quick to perform and practical. Whether in the field for research purposes or in a dental practice, the method of data collection must not be time-consuming, costly, or involve many instruments.

3. Sensitivity requires the index to detect small changes. Sensitivity determines if the disease is really present and can be seen. A true-positive result would indicate that the disease or condition exists.

4. Validity provides the correlation of the disease with the measure employed. If bleeding on probing is to be measured, then the index can be confounded by other variables such as probing pressure, spontaneous bleeding, or instrumentation differences. A valid index must measure what it intended to measure.

There is no perfect index or one that assesses all categories of inquiry. There are numerous indices, and the practitioner must select the best ones to represent the disease under examination or the health of the patient. There are over 40 types of indices in periodontics. They fall into four general categories: oral hygiene indices (plaque and calculus), gingival indices, periodontal (destruction) indices, and treatment needs indices. An overview of historically important and commonly used indices is presented in Table 5–1 ■ and will be reviewed briefly below.

PLAQUE AND DEBRIS INDICES

Oral cleanliness is quantified by indices that measure plaque and debris and indices that measure calculus. Since plaque is considered the primary cause or risk factor of periodontal diseases, methods of measuring plaque (debris) are important epidemiologically and are useful to practitioners treating the disease. Many plaque indices are used today. Some are meant simply as screening tools in clinical practice to assess home-care practices, whereas others are designed to quantify and locate plaque as needed for the evaluation of plaque-control devices or products before and after use.

One of the simplest methods of monitoring patient plaque levels is the use of the O'Leary Plaque Index (O'Leary, Drake, and Naylor 1972), also called the *plaque control record*. A visual record of plaque control is made using a disclosing agent. A diagram is made of plaque-covered surfaces that can be shared with patients to visually help them identify problem areas and focus their efforts at home. O'Leary, Drake, and Naylor (1972) recommended reduction of plaque levels to 10% of the available tooth surfaces as the patient's goal for home-care mastery.

Other common plaque indices are the Plaque Index (PlI) (Silness and Löe 1964), the Debris Index (DI-S) of the Simplified Oral Hygiene Index (Greene 1967), and the modified Quigley-Hein Plaque Index (Turesky, Gilmore, and Glickman 1970). These plaque indices provide subjective numerical values that quantify the amount of plaque present, unlike the O'Leary Index, which merely indicates the presence or absence of plaque and is most suited for patient education and motivation in private practice rather than epidemiologic surveys.

The Plaque Index (PlI) (Silness and Löe 1964) scores the plaque thickness along the gingival margin of the tooth, whereas the Debris Index (DS-I) measures plaque surface area. The Debris Index is a component of the Simplified Oral Hygiene Index (OHI-S) developed by Greene and Vermillion (1964). The other component of the OHI-S is a Calculus Index (CI-S). The OHI-S is used primarily for epidemiologic and longitudinal dental studies.

Another plaque index used more specifically for clinical trials is the Turesky Modification of the Quigley-Hein Index (Turesky, Gilmore, and Glickman 1970). Plaque is assessed on all facial and lingual tooth surfaces (excluding third molars) after disclosing agent is applied. The additional scoring categories of this index allow researchers to quantify improvement or change in plaque levels after the use of a plaque-control device or topical antimicrobial. Both the modified Quigley-Hein Index and the Plaque Index (PII) are suitable for the evaluation of topical antimicrobials and plaque-removal devices (Fischman 1986).

In summary, a number of plaque indices are used today. Four plaque indices were presented, and each serves different purposes. The plaque control record (O'Leary, Drake, and Naylor 1972) is used most commonly in periodontal practice, whereas the others are used more frequently in clinical trials and population surveys. Plaque indices are employed in epidemiologic surveys to elucidate the oral cleanliness of the population and how it relates to the presentation of periodontal disease in that population. Another measure of oral cleanliness is the quantification of calculus using a calculus index.

CALCULUS INDICES

In clinical practice, calculus is not monitored by a numeric index, but in epidemiologic surveys, calculus indices find common use. Numerous methods have been devised to quantify this deposit, and three commonly used calculus indices will be presented here (see Table 5–1).

The simplified Calculus Index (CS-1), which is part of the OHI-S mentioned previously (Greene 1967), is valuable for epidemiologic surveys and longitudinal studies and quantifies calculus by location and surface area. Another common calculus evaluation is the Volpe Manhold Calculus Assessment (Volpe, Manhold, and Hazen 1965; Volpe, Kupczak, and King 1967), which measures the height and dimension of the calculus present. It was designed originally for use on the lingual surfaces of the mandibular incisors but can be used throughout the mouth.

National epidemiologic studies, conducted through the National Institute of Dental Research (NIDR), have developed and used their own calculus index (Miller et al. 1987). The NIDR Index merely indicates the presence or absence of calculus supragingivally or subgingivally. This index was used for the third National Health and Nutrition Examination Survey (NHANES III), conducted by the National Center for the Health Statistics in collaboration with the National Institute for Dental Research from 1988 to 1991.

GINGIVAL INDICES

The epidemiologic tool used to quickly assess gingival inflammation is the gingival index. A gingival index is designed to measure the degree of visible inflammation of the gingival tissues. Visible signs of gingival inflammation, including bleeding, redness, and swelling, are accepted clinical signs of inflammation and also have been incorporated into indices for evaluation of the periodontal status of individuals and populations.

The Gingival Index (GI) of Löe and Silness (Löe, 1967) is based on the subjective assessment of the visual indicators of gingival inflammation. The degree of inflammation is subdivided into three categories, with moderate inflammation determined by the presence of bleeding and severe inflammation determined by

TABLE 5–1

INDICES USED FOR PERIODONTAL DISEASE ASSESSMENTS

INDEX	TYPE OF MEASURE	TEETH MEASURED	METHOD OF MEASUREMENT	SCALE OF MEASUREMENT	PURPOSE	ADVANTAGES	DISADVANTAGES	USES
O'Leary (O'Leary, Drake, and Naylor, 1972)	Plaque	All teeth are scored at the cervical third of the tooth. Four surfaces of each tooth (M, B, D, L,) are measured.	A plaque record is made by marking a tooth diagram with the surface location of plaque. Mark each tooth surface with plaque as positive (disclosing agent used).	Calculation: Surfaces with plaque divided by the total number of surfaces. Multiply by 100 to get the percent of surfaces with plaque. Patient goal of 10% or less of plaque is ideal.	Visual record of plaque distribution; shows patients where they are insufficient in plaque removal; patient motivation.	Complete assessment of all tooth surfaces to determine areas of cleaning deficiency.	Will not pick up changes in plaque quantity at each tooth surface; time-consuming.	Private practice.
Plaque Index (PlI) (Silness and Löe, 1964)	Plaque	All teeth (distal, facial, mesial, lingual) or selected teeth.	Sweep a probe along the tooth surface at the gingival margin. (No disclosing agent is used.) The score (0, 1, 2, or 3) per tooth is obtained by summing the four different surface scores and dividing by four. Adding each tooth score and dividing by the number of teeth evaluated generates a patient score. Excellent: 0 Poor: 2.0–3.0	0 No plaque 1 A thinly adherent layer of plaque visible only when a probe is run across the tooth 2 A visible layer of plaque which is thin to moderately thick 3 Heavy plaque accumulation in the crevice and the gingival margin	Measures the thickness or amount of plaque along the gingival margin.	Good for research purposes because qualitative changes can be measured; not as time-consuming if selected teeth are used.	Somewhat subjective; limited to the cervical portion of the tooth, not for patient motivation.	Clinical studies, epidemiologic surveys.
Simplified Debris Index (DI-S) of the Simplified Oral Hygiene Index (OHI-S) (Greene and Vermillion 1964)	Soft debris	Six tooth surfaces per mouth are scored: facial surfaces of teeth nos. 3,8,14,24, and lingual surfaces of teeth nos. 19,30. If the first molars are missing, choose the first fully erupted tooth distal to the second premolar.	Each tooth is divided into gingival, middle, and incisal thirds. Scoring is done by moving a no. 23 explorer from the incisal third toward the gingival third of the tooth. No disclosing agent is used. Score as 0, 1, 2, 3. Calculation:	0 No stain or debris 1 Soft deposit covering ≤ 1/3 of the surface or the presence of extrinsic stain 2 Soft deposit covering more than 1/3 but less than 2/3 of the tooth surface 3 Soft deposit covering > 2/3 of the tooth surface.	Measures plaque surface area.	Measures the quantity of debris rather than the presence or absence; not as time-consuming.	Somewhat subjective.	Epidemiologic and research projects.

Index	Type	Teeth Scored	Scoring/Calculation	Measures	Advantages	Uses
Turesky Modification of the Quigley-Hein Index (Turesky, Gilmore, and Glickman 1970)	Plaque	Facial and lingual surfaces of all teeth excluding the third molars.	total of surface scores divided by the number of surfaces scored Good score: 0.0–0.6 Poor score: 1.9–3.0 Score as 0, 1, 2, 3, 4, 5. Disclosing agent is used. Calculation: Total of all scores divided by the number of surfaces examined	0 No plaque 1 Flecks of plaque at the cervical margin 2 Thin, continuous band of plaque (≤ 1 mm) at the cervical margin 3 Band of plaque wider than a 1 mm but covering less than 1/3 of crown. 4 Plaque covering at least 1/3 but less than 2/3 of the crown 5 Plaque covering more than 2/3 of the crown	Measures surface area of plaque.	The additional scoring categories allow the researcher to quantify improvement or change in plaque levels after the use of a plaque-control device or topical antimicrobial.	Somewhat subjective; time-consuming.	Index of choice in clinical trials.
Simplified Calculus Index (CI-S); part of the OHI-S (Greene 1967)	Calculus	Six tooth surfaces per mouth are scored: facial surfaces of teeth nos. 3, 8, 14, 24, and lingual surfaces of teeth nos. 19, 30. If the first molars are missing, choose the first fully erupted tooth distal to the second premolar.	Score as 0, 1, 2, 3. Calculation: total calculus scores divided by the number of surfaces scored. To tabulate the total OHI-S, add the DI-S + CI-S. Combined OHI-S: Good: 0.0–0–1.2 Poor: 3.1–6.0	0 No calculus present 1 Supragingival calculus covering $\leq$ 1/3 of the exposed tooth 2 Supragingival calculus covering more than 1/3 but 2/3 or less of exposed tooth or separate flecks of subgingival calculus in the cervical region 3 Supragingival calculus covering more than 2/3 of exposed tooth or a continuous heavy band of subgingival calculus	Quantifies calculus.	Well-defined criteria, allows for interexaminer reproducibility.	Combines location and quantity.	Epidemiologic and longitudinal studies.

Continued

TABLE 5–1, *CONTINUED*

INDICES USED FOR PERIODONTAL DISEASE ASSESSMENTS

INDEX	TYPE OF MEASURE	TEETH MEASURED	METHOD OF MEASUREMENT	SCALE OF MEASUREMENT	PURPOSE	ADVANTAGES	DISADVANTAGES	USES
Volpe Manhold Calculus Assessment (Volpe, Manhold, and Hazen 1965)	Calculus	Mandibular incisors and cuspids (lingual surfaces).	With a probe, the coronal extension of supragingival calculus is measured in millimeters. Three readings are made bisecting the dimension of calculus at the direct lingual and mesial and distal line angles. These readings are averaged to generate a tooth score, and the individual tooth scores are averaged to provide the total patient score.	Readings are scored in millimeter markings from the probe.	Measures the height or dimension of calculus.	Ability to measure the rate of calculus formation.	Difficult to master.	Clinical studies and epidemiologic studies.
Calculus Index of the National Institute of Dental Research (Miller et al. 1987)	Calculus	Mesiobuccal and midbuccal surfaces of all fully erupted permanent teeth present in two randomly selected quadrants (one mandibular and the other maxillary).	Detected by explorer or probe.	0 No calculus 1 Supragingival calculus only (calculus on the crown and root not extending more than 1 mm below the gingival margin) 2 Subgingival calculus is detected with or without supragingival calculus	Presence or absence and location supra- or subgingival.	Simple.	Unable to quantify amount of calculus.	Used in the National Health and Nutrition and Examination Survey (NHANES III).
Gingival Index (GI) (Löe 1967)	Gingival inflammation	Four gingival areas (buccal, mesial, distal, and lingual) for all teeth or select teeth.	Probe is inserted into the gingival crevice and moved with a sweeping along the pocket wall. Probe is also pressed lightly against the gingiva to determine its firmness. Calculation: Each of the four gingival areas per	0 Normal gingiva 1 Mild inflammation with slight changes in color and edema (swelling); no bleeding on probing 2 Moderate inflammation with redness, edema, and glazing; bleeding on probing	Measures severity of gingivitis.	Can detect change in degree of inflammation.	Somewhat subjective, time-consuming.	Epidemiologic and clinical studies.

Index	What is measured	Sites examined	Scoring and calculation	Purpose	Advantages	Disadvantages	Uses
(continued)			3 Severe inflammation with marked redness and edema; tendency to spontaneously bleed. tooth is given a GI score of 0 to 3. Total the scores for each area and divide by the number of teeth scored. Good: 0.0–1.0 Fair: 1.1–2.0 Poor: 2.1–3.0				
Sulcus Bleeding Index (Mühlemann and Son 1971)	Gingival inflammation	Three gingival areas (facial and lingual marginal gingival and mesial and distal interdental papillae) for all teeth.	Insert probe in the sulcus and withdraw it. Wait 30 seconds to score the area. Calculation: Total the scores for each tooth, and divide by the number of teeth. 0 Healthy appearance with no bleeding on probing 1 Healthy but with bleeding on probing 2 Bleeding on probing and color change but no swelling 3 Bleeding on probing, color change, and slight edema 4 Bleeding on probing and obvious swelling with or without color change 5 Bleeding on probing and spontaneous bleeding and color change, marked swelling with or without ulceration	Presence or absence and severity of gingival inflammation.	Less subjective, more gradations of severe inflammation.	Criticized for scores beyond clinical gingivitis.	Clinical and epidemiologic studies.
Periodontal Index (PI) (Russell 1967)	Inflammation, pocket depth, tooth mobility (visual assessment, without periodontal probing)	All teeth.	Each tooth is given a score from 0 (no disease) to 8 (severe disease) Calculation: Add up the scores for all teeth, and divide by the number of teeth scored. 0.0–0.2: normal periodontal condition 0.3–0.9: simple gingivitis 0–1.9: early destructive periodontitis 1.6–5.0: established periodontitis 3.8–8.0: terminal disease 0 Tooth with healthy periodontium 1 Mild gingivitis, localized and does not involve the entire tooth 2 Gingivitis encircling the entire tooth 6 Gingivitis with pocket formation with no loss of function or mobility 8 Advanced destruction with tooth mobility	Measures the severity of the periodontal condition.	Objective measures.	Visual assessment that often underestimates disease; evaluates both gingivitis and periodontitis in the same index.	National epidemiologic surveys including the National Health and Nutrition Examination Survey (1971–1974).

Continued

TABLE 5–1, CONTINUED

INDICES USED FOR PERIODONTAL DISEASE ASSESSMENTS

INDEX	TYPE OF MEASURE	TEETH MEASURED	METHOD OF MEASUREMENT	SCALE OF MEASUREMENT	PURPOSE	ADVANTAGES	DISADVANTAGES	USES
Community Periodontal Index of Treatment Needs (Ainamo et al. 1982)	Periodontal pockets, calculus, gingival bleeding	Ten teeth: 2, 3, 8, 14, 15, 18, 19, 24, 30, 31	A 0.5-mm ball-tip probe with demarcations for shallow (3.5-mm) and deep (5.5-mm) pockets (CIPTN probe) is used to detect and record the presence of bleeding, calculus, and periodontal pockets. The individual is scored by sextant assigning the worst tooth score per sextant as the overall sextant score. Treatment needs are assigned based on the highest code received by each sextant. 0 No further therapy needed. 1 Patient only requires oral home-care instruction 2 Patient requires oral hygiene improvement and professional scaling 3 Patient requires oral hygiene improvement and professional scaling 4 Patient requires complex treatment (scaling and root planing with dental anesthesia and may require periodontal surgery)	Code 0: No pocketing or inflammation Code 1: Bleeding on probing Code 2: Calculus present Code 3: Pocketing extending in to the black area of the probe (4–5 mm) Code 4: Pocketing extending beyond the black area of the probe (≥6 mm)	Measures severity of the periodontal condition and treatment needs.	Simple.	Only selective teeth are measured, which may underestimate the disease.	Epidemiologic surveys (specifically designed by the WHO to compare population surveys internationally).

Periodontal Screening and Recording (PSR) (AAP 1992)	Periodontal pockets, calculus, bleeding, and defective restorations	Mouth is divided into sextants. All teeth are measured.	Each tooth in the sextant is probed, and the tooth with the worst score determines the sextant score. The highest-scoring sextant determines the individual's overall management. If two or more sextants have a score of 3 or any one sextant has a score of 4, then a complete periodontal charting is advised. Scores of 0 or 1 require preventive measures inclusive of home-care instructions. Scores of 2 or greater require the patient to have additional professional cleaning and correction of defective restorations.	Code 0–No calculus, defective margins, or bleeding, and the black band of the probe is completely visible (probing depth less than 3.5 mm) Code 1–No calculus or defective margins, but there is bleeding, and the black band of the probe is completely visible Code 2–Supragingival or subgingival calculus or defective markings are present, but the black band is still visible Code 3–Calculus, defective restorations, and bleeding may or may not be present, and the black band is partly visible (probing depth more than 3.5 mm but less than 5.5 mm) Code 4–The black band of the probe is not visible (probing depth more than 5.5 mm) An asterisk (*) is added if any additional pathology is present, such as furcations.	Screening of periodontal disease in private practice.	Simplifies the charting of an individual's periodontal condition when extensive treatment is not required.	Cannot be substituted for a complete periodontal charting necessary for the treatment of periodontitis patients.	Private practice.

spontaneous bleeding. The GI historically has been used for epidemiologic studies. Lobene et al. (1986) modified this index for use in clinical trials evaluating plaque-control products. The Modified Gingival Index (Lobene et al. 1986) assesses gingival health by looking only at qualitative changes in the gingiva. Unlike the GI, which uses bleeding as an indicator of increasing severity of gingival inflammation, this index does not use bleeding on probing and has more gradations. The Modified Gingival Index is scored to pick up subtle changes earlier with four different scores for gingival inflammation.

Other gingival indices based primarily on bleeding include the Sulcus Bleeding Index (Mühlemann and Son 1971) and the Interdental Bleeding Index (Caton and Polson 1985). One of the first indices to be based on bleeding is the Sulcus Bleeding Index. Gingival bleeding as a measure of gingival inflammation is considered a more objective measure, whereas gingival color and consistency are more subjective. For this index, gingival bleeding is determined by gently inserting a probe in the sulcus and withdrawing it. Mühlemann and Son based the Sulcus Bleeding Index on bleeding being the earliest symptom of gingivitis, but it has been criticized because distinctions are made beyond the clinical point of gingivitis.

A novel approach to determining bleeding is the use of a wooden interdental cleaner rather than a periodontal probe. The Interdental Bleeding Index (Caton and Polson 1985) uses interdental cleaners to evaluate bleeding in the midproximal gingival tissues where periodontal changes are most likely to be found. The interdental cleaner is inserted between teeth and removed, depressing the interdental papilla 1 to 2 mm. Fifteen seconds after insertion and removal, bleeding is recorded.

In an attempt to achieve a more objective measure, gingival bleeding is being used increasingly for the determination of gingival changes in epidemiologic studies. The presence or absence of bleeding has been used in current demographic studies, in the NIDR Adult Survey (1985–1986) (Brown, Oliver, and Löe 1989), and in NHANES III (1988–1991) (Brown, Brunelle, and Kingman 1996). Gingival bleeding also has been used to monitor patient home oral hygiene practices. The percentage of bleeding sites is considered a more accurate representation of the patient's true level of daily home care. Bleeding and gingival indices also have been monitored along with individual attachment levels and pocket bacteria to find markers or predictors of disease activity.

Indices of Periodontal Destruction

Another essential measure employed in epidemiologic studies is evaluation of periodontal destruction. Indices of periodontal destruction are designed to measure disease severity and extent by observing the outcomes of periodontal destruction. This is done by measuring clinical attachment loss and probing depth and recording bone loss and loss of function. Current national studies use direct measures of these disease outcomes. These measures are taken at the midbuccal and mesiobuccal levels of all fully erupted teeth (Brown, Brunelle, and Kingman 1996). Even though current national surveys do not employ periodontal indices or directly measure the outcome of destruction, much of the historical data pertinent to periodontal diseases in the United States have been compiled using periodontal indices.

The Periodontal Index (PI) (Russell 1967) has been a standard measure for the large national surveys that are responsible for early views of periodontal disease prevalence and incidence in the United States. The PI is a visual index and does not use a periodontal probe. The presence of inflammation, pocket formation, and loss of function is assessed visually as criteria for numeric scoring of teeth.

Two additional indices of epidemiologic importance evaluate periodontal destruction and designate treatment needs. The Community Periodontal Index of Treatment Needs (CPITN) (Ainamo et al. 1982) was developed by an initiative of the World Health Organization (WHO) expressly for population studies. Its primary focus is to assess treatment needs.

The CPITN was modified to the Periodontal Screening and Recording (PSR) system for general-practice use. The PSR system was developed to evaluate individual treatment needs and to be used as a quick screening tool to document new patient periodontal findings in lieu of a complete periodontal charting. It has been endorsed by the American Academy of Periodontology and the American Dental Association as a quick and easy method to record the periodontal status of a patient in the private-practice setting. This screening tool reduces the number of patients that need a complete periodontal charting simply by identifying those with periodontal treatment needs and therefore the need for a complete periodontal charting.

The CPITN probe is used in the PSR system, and the same parameters employed by the CPITN are evaluated—bleeding, calculus, and probing depth. The CPITN probe has a ball tip to aid in calculus detection and a black band that demarcates probing depth from 3.5 to 5.5 mm. It was developed to increase the recognition and treatment of periodontal disease in the general dental practice. Generation of the PSR score is the responsibility of the dental hygienist, especially for recall visits.

ACCURACY OF METHODOLOGY

Thus far the tools used for assessing the periodontal condition in epidemiologic studies have been described. These tools define or identify individuals within a population with periodontal disease. The sampling methodology for population studies differs from that used in clinical periodontics and can influence the accuracy of the data obtained. Epidemiologic data-collection tools do not measure all the periodontal findings a clinician might use to establish a diagnosis and prognosis, such as furcation involvement or tooth mobility. Population studies, because of their large sample sizes, use indices as assessment tools, unlike diagnostic evaluations in clinical practice, and thus only score a portion of the mouth. To streamline the examination process, partial mouth scores are incorporated into indices. Partial mouth observations improve study efficiency but reduce the accuracy of overall reporting of periodontal disease prevalence and incidence.

For example, the CPITN measures only ten teeth in the mouth. Baelum et al. (1993) found that the prevalence of teeth with moderate to deep pockets was underreported in the partial mouth scores of the CPITN. This was especially true for severe periodontal conditions. In another report, Baelum et al. (1995) concluded that the CPITN scores tend to underestimate prevalence and severity in younger age groups and overestimate the same in the elderly. The methodology employed by the NIDR for the most recent survey, NHANES III, also involves a partial mouth evaluation. As described earlier, periodontal probing is performed in half the mouth. When half-mouth and full-mouth scores were compared (Hunt and Fann 1991), the results were similar. Half-mouth examination was considered accurate in estimating the prevalence of periodontal disease but still underestimated the percentage of the population with more advanced disease (periodontal attachment loss). A review by Papapanou (1996) concluded that the current NIDR methodology is inadequate because it is a combination of partial scores (e.g., only two sites per tooth are measured in only one-half of the mouth). Papapanou contended that the location of the pocket and the number of probing measures could have a profound influence on the outcome of the study. Partly because previous studies comparing half-mouth scores with full-mouth scores had used partial scores for their comparison, not all probing sites encircling a tooth were measured. When combining partial mouth scores with measures at only the midbuccal and mesiobuccal sites, current methodology actually could produce a mean percentage underestimation of deep pockets of 40% and an underestimation of the prevalence of these deep pockets of 58%.

The validity of an index in describing a population also can be affected by tooth loss. Missing teeth may have been the ones most severely affected by periodontitis. Since they are no longer present to be measured, there is a built-in selection bias for the healthier teeth still present, potentially underestimating both severity and prevalence of the disease (periodontitis). Thus the overall reliability of an index is affected by the method of data collection. It is difficult to have one tool that will be representative, accurate, and efficient at the same time for all periodontal measures. Historical and modern data are based on methodologies that have been criticized, but some researchers contend that they still render an adequate estimation of disease.

PREVALENCE OF PERIODONTAL DISEASES

National surveys have helped build our knowledge of the prevalence, severity, and extent of periodontal diseases in the United States. Based on the results of these surveys, the commonly accepted model for periodontal diseases has changed and evolved. Historically, periodontal disease was considered inevitable, and all individuals were susceptible to advanced periodontal disease, gingivitis being its precursor. In essence, periodontal disease was considered universal, and the susceptibility to periodontitis increased with age (Waerhaug 1966).

Information gathered from more recent national surveys, however, suggests otherwise. More severe disease (advanced periodontitis) was found in only 5 to 20% of adults (U.S. Public Health Service 1987), and moderate disease (periodontitis) was found in the majority of adults (U.S. Public Health Service 1987). Thus only a few individuals will be susceptible to advanced disease. Today, periodontitis is not considered part of the aging process but occurs because of the interaction of bacteria and the immune response of the individual.

PREVALENCE OF GINGIVITIS

Gingivitis is a common form of periodontal disease found in individuals of all ages; it can even occur in early childhood (Ayers, Abrama, and Lausten 1979). In the U.S. Health and Resources and Service Administration (HRSA) study of 1981 (Brown, Oliver, and Löe 1989), 54% of adults over age 18 were affected with gingivitis involving at least six or more teeth. Another national study of employed adults between the ages of 18 and 64, the NIDR Adult Survey (1985–1986), reported less gingivitis, finding that 44% of the sample had gingivitis (defined by gingival bleeding) (Miller et al. 1987). The average involvement was 2.7 sites per person, and the extent of gingivitis increased with age. In the more recent NHANES III study (Brown, Brunelle, and Kingman 1996), gingival bleeding was present in

63% of those examined, and 12% of all sites examined bled on probing. Gingivitis was slightly more prevalent in teenagers (13–17 years). The extent was similar among all age groups, ranging from 10 to 15% of the sites examined. Plaque and calculus deposits correlated with the prevalence of gingivitis, and subgingival calculus were found in 67% of the population and at 22% of the sites evaluated.

When compared with earlier national surveys, *gingivitis has declined in the United States most likely due to the current focus on oral hygiene as part of a daily personal hygiene routine* (Burt 1996). In the early 1960s, visual assessments revealed that 85% of men and 79% of women had gingivitis. Current surveys report that 63% of the population has gingival bleeding and that gingivitis is found in 44 to 54% of the population. This differs considerably from reports from Third World countries, where gingivitis in the presence of extensive plaque and calculus is considered normal among adults (Löe et al. 1978).

PREVALENCE OF PERIODONTITIS

Chronic periodontitis, a more severe form of periodontal disease, commonly is not found among young individuals and is more prevalent with age. The NHANES III study (Brown, Brunelle, and Kingman 1996) ($n=7447$ surveyed) found that over 90% of individuals over age 13 had some attachment loss, with only 15% of the population having advanced disease (defined as 5 mm or more of attachment loss). If the definition of attachment loss were limited to 3 mm or more, the prevalence was 40%. One-quarter of the individuals surveyed showed moderate attachment loss (3–4 mm). With increasing age, the prevalence of moderate and severe attachment loss increased, but the prevalence of pockets 4 mm or greater and 6 mm or greater in size remained the same. Since the extent and prevalence of attachment loss were found to increase with age and the prevalence of 4-mm or greater pocket depths did not, increased gingival recession was deemed responsible for the increased attachment loss experienced with age (Oliver, Brown, and Löe 1998).

In the HRSA survey (Brown, Oliver, and Löe 1989), periodontitis (at least one tooth with a pocket 4 mm or deeper) was found in 36% of the 7078 individuals examined. The prevalence of the disease increased with age. Twenty-nine percent of individuals in the 19- to 44-year age group were affected, whereas almost 50% of individuals 45 years of age or older were affected. The percentage of elderly individuals (65 and older) with pockets was similar to that of the 45- to 64-year age group, although the number of teeth present decreased. Periodontitis, when present, usually involved only a few teeth, and advanced periodontitis was relatively rare.

In the NIDR study of employed adults between the ages of 18 and 64 years (Brown Oliver, and Löe et al. 1990), almost all had some attachment loss, with 44% experiencing attachment loss of 3 mm or more. Moderate pocket depths (4–6 mm) were present in only 13.4% of those examined, generally affecting only one to two sites. More advanced disease again was considered rare and was found in only 0.6% of the study population. Males experienced more disease than females, and blacks were more affected than whites.

In the NHANES III study (Brown, Brunelle, and Kingman 1996), racial and gender differences were reported as well. Females overall were in better periodontal health than their male counterparts, and non-Hispanic whites had less periodontal disease than non-Hispanic blacks or Mexican-Americans. Overall, the United States has a relatively low prevalence and severity of periodontal disease compared with the rest of the world, and the severity and extent of disease have declined in the past thirty years (Oliver, Brown, and Löe 1998).

PREVALENCE OF AGGRESSIVE PERIODONTITIS

The prevalence of aggressive periodontitis (replaces the older term "early-onset periodontitis"), has been estimated to be less than 1% of the general population (Papapanou 1996). It is considered a rare form of periodontal disease. A review of national population studies indicates that approximately 3.6% of individuals between the ages of 18 to 34 years (NIDR Adult Survey, 1985–1986; Oliver, Brown, and Löe 1998) have moderate periodontal disease. Among 14- to 17-year-olds (Löe and Brown 1991), the prevalence of all forms of aggressive periodontitis was 2.27%, 0.53% were affected by localized aggressive periodontitis, (older term is localized juvenile periodontitis) and 0.13% were estimated to be affected by generalized aggressive periodontitis (replaces the older term "generalized juvenile periodontitis").

Racial differences also have been reported. Blacks were affected more often than whites by all forms of aggressive periodontitis. Ironically, racial and gender prevalences reported by recent national surveys do not match diagnostic criteria used to define and distinguish forms of aggressive periodontitis from chronic periodontitis. In a national (NIDR) study of over 11,000 adolescents between the ages of 14 to 17, gender differences existed and were influenced by race. For example, black males were 2.9 times more likely to have localized aggressive periodontitis than black females, and white females were more frequently affected by localized aggressive periodontitis than white males by the same amount. Males, in general, were 4.3 times more likely to have generalized juvenile (aggressive) periodontitis than females. When these results were extrapolated to the racial mix of the U.S. population in general, about 87,000 cases of localized and generalized aggressive periodontitis were estimated among 13 million 14- to 17-year-olds (Oliver, Brown, and Löe 1998).

Traditionally, black females have been reported to be 2 to 3 times more likely to have aggressive periodontitis than white females. *It has been suggested that clinical trials and case reports used to establish this racial and gender predilection may have been skewed by ascertainment bias because more females will seek dental treatment and participate in clinical trials than males* (Oliver, Brown, and Löe 1998). Thus a national survey that does not start out with this selection bias may more accurately reflect the national population prevalence.

In summary, the national status of periodontal disease has been gleaned by three recent national surveys: the NIDR, NHANES III, and HRSA surveys. About 50% of all American adults have gingivitis involving three to four teeth. Periodontitis is experienced in over 90% of the population over 13 years of age, but only 15% have severe disease. There is a specific small subset of the population that has more advanced disease. Aggressive periodontitis is considered a rare disease in the United States and affects only 0.53 to 3.6% of individuals under age 35. Overall, the national prevalence of gingivitis has declined over the past thirty years, but the prevalence of periodontitis has remained the same, and only the severity of disease has decreased (Capilouto and Douglass 1988).

INCIDENCE AND DISEASE PROGRESSION

National surveys used to estimate disease prevalence are *cross-sectional,* which means that the study population is evaluated at only one point in time. To determine the natural progression of periodontal diseases, *longitudinal* studies are necessary, where individuals are examined at multiple intervals. Few longitudinal studies are available because of the difficulty of conducting them. In a 15-year longitudinal study by Löe et al. (1986), 480 Sri Lankan tea workers with untreated disease were evaluated. About 8% had rapid progression of their periodontitis, and most had a moderate rate of disease progression. A small portion of this population (11%) showed no progression beyond gingivitis despite the presence of heavy plaque and calculus.

A parallel study run in Norway (Löe et al. 1978) showed a different rate of disease progression. No cases of aggressive (juvenile) periodontitis were found, unlike the Sri Lankan study. The mean annual rate of attachment loss was 0.08 mm for interproximal and 0.1 mm for buccal surfaces as individuals approached 40 years of age. In patients with moderate periodontitis, progression occurred slowly at any given site. The rate of periodontal destruction did not increase with age, and therefore, the progression of periodontitis (extent and severity) appeared to be slow and continuous in this population.

In a report by Beck, Koch, and Offenbacher (1994) detailing a longitudinal study of adults identified with extensive attachment loss between the ages of 65 and 80 years in North Carolina, additional evidence of slow disease progression also can be found. Only 12% of this population experienced 3 mm or more of attachment loss on one or more teeth during the 3-year study period. Again, it appears that subjects with a past history of periodontitis can be quite resistant to future disease (breakdown). Future attachment loss was associated with greater baseline probing depths, but the vast majority of sites that lost attachment had probing depths of 3 mm or less at baseline. Individuals who experienced attachment loss in the first 18 months of the study were more likely to experience attachment loss in the subsequent 18-month period.

Racial differences also were detected. Blacks tended to experience more attachment loss during both 18-month periods of the study. Only 45% of blacks had no attachment loss during the 3-year period, whereas 63% of whites were free of attachment loss. Despite having advanced attachment loss at the outset of the study, both blacks and whites had a high frequency of no further disease progression. Similarly, adult subjects with gingivitis monitored over a 3-year period had no detectable increase in probing depth (Listgarten, Schifter, and Laster 1985). In a review by Stamm (1986), the incidence of gingivitis was greatest at puberty, declined through age 17, and then remained steady.

These studies imply that only select individuals or a small portion of the population will have new disease or disease progression. In another U.S. study by Löe and Brown (1991), only a small portion of the study population had the highest rate of disease progression, as noted by attachment loss; this subset of the population was identified with aggressive periodontitis. In the Beck, Koch, and Offenbacher (1994) study of elderly adults, disease progression was more likely when extensive bone loss and tooth loss were experienced at a young age, again alluding to a specific subset of the population with a higher incidence of disease. In sum, only a small portion of the population will experience incidence and progression of severe attachment loss. This attachment loss will not progress at the same rate but may be episodic. The progression of periodontal disease appears to be influenced by education level, socioeconomic factors, gender, and race. These variables will be discussed in the next section of this chapter.

EPIDEMIOLOGIC VARIABLES

RISK INDICATORS

Risk indicators are demographic, behavioral, and socioeconomic characteristics that are associated with disease but not considered causal for the disease. Aging is considered a risk indicator for periodontal disease, but does not cause periodontal disease. With increasing age, the prevalence of periodontal disease increases, but the aging process is not responsible for the disease. It is believed that there is more disease with age because there is more exposure to plaque-induced inflammation over time. Other characteristics associated with an increased frequency of disease are the level of education, gender, and race. Females have less periodontal disease than males (Sheiham and Striffler 1970). Caucasians (Anglo-Saxon) were found to have less periodontal disease than Hispanics, Mexicans, Indians, and African-Americans. It is hypothesized that these differences are due to the availability and use of dental services, oral home care, and preventive practices. For example, the higher levels of periodontal disease reported in males versus females are attributed to higher levels of plaque and less use of dental services. More education, higher income, and dental insurance reduce the risk of oral disease. Where extensive plaque, calculus, and gingival inflammation are considered normal among adults in Third World countries, an association is found with less education and low income, and generally, there is more attachment loss than in industrial nations of the Western world.

RISK FACTORS

Risk factors are characteristics that have been shown to directly cause periodontal disease. Causal links are established by longitudinal and cross-sectional studies. It is important to identify causal relationships so that oral disease can be prevented if a risk factor is modifiable. For example, it is accepted that dental plaque causes gingivitis, and thus plaque is considered a risk factor for gingivitis. Poor oral hygiene has been correlated strongly with periodontal disease. The NHANES I data showed an inverse relationship between tooth loss and good oral hygiene. The periodontal index (PI) and oral hygiene (OHI-S) index scores were significantly better in individuals with the least tooth loss (Burt, Ismail, and Eklund 1985). However, the causal relationship is not clear-cut with periodontitis. Supragingival plaque and supragingival calculus are not as strongly correlated with periodontitis as with gingivitis (Bakdash 1994, Löe et al. 1978). In a recent appraisal by Oliver, Brown, and Löe (1998), the presence of subgingival calculus appeared to be a better predictor of periodontitis but was not considered causal because there was an inconsistent relationship among the epidemiologic data regarding oral hygiene, plaque and calculus, and periodontitis. Sites with dental calculus frequently do not bleed or display attachment loss. In the NHANES III survey (Brown, Brunelle, and Kingman 1996), no bleeding was found 88% of the time when subgingival calculus was present. Additionally, gingivitis does not always progress to periodontitis, which means that periodontitis will not always occur in the presence of plaque and calculus. One could infer from this inconsistency that poor oral hygiene is an important risk factor in individuals who are more susceptible based on their immune response to bacterial plaque.

Other risk factors for periodontitis are diabetes and tobacco use. The prevalence and extent of periodontal pockets are greater in diabetics than in nondiabetics. This is especially true for poorly controlled diabetics, who experience more attachment and bone loss than well-controlled diabetics with similar plaque levels (Seppälä, Seppälä, and Ainamo 1993). Oliver and Tervonen (1994) outlined diabetes as a risk factor for extensive, severe periodontitis when the individual's diabetes is poorly controlled and the individual has extensive subgingival calculus from poor home care and lack of professional cleanings. In a recent report (Taylor et al. 1998), subjects with non-insulin-dependent diabetes mellitus (NIDDM) had more severe alveolar bone loss progression over a 2-year period than those without NIDDM.

Smoking has been well documented as a risk factor for periodontitis. An early National Health and Nutrition Survey (NHANES I) in 1971–1974 first demonstrated the relationship between smoking and periodontitis (Ismail, Burt, and Eklund 1983) in the United States. More recent longitudinal studies confirm this relationship. One longitudinal study showed that smokers lost proximal bone twice as fast as nonsmokers (Bolin et al. 1993). Even when plaque accumulation is minimal, smokers have more teeth with deeper pockets and alveolar bone loss than nonsmokers (Bergström and Eliasson 1987, Bergström and Floderus-Myrhed 1983). In a 3-year study conducted by Beck, Koch, and Offenbacher (1995), disease was more likely to progress if the subject was a cigarette smoker, had the presence of gram-negative anaerobes in his or her subgingival microflora (especially *Porphyromonas gingivalis*), or had financial stress. All led to an increased risk for disease progression. Thus it is apparent that microflora and stress could be considered risk factors for periodontitis. Currently, these factors are being explored.

Another longitudinal study running from 1959 to 1985 in Tecumseh, Michigan (Ismail et al. 1990), reported age, smoking, and the presence of tooth mobility as risk markers for future attachment loss (2 mm or more). It has been hypothesized (Papapanou 1996) that periodontitis actually may have different factors associated with its initiation than those involved in its progression. Multiple factors may play a role in the induction and progression of periodontal disease. The commonly accepted risk factors are lack of oral cleanliness, smoking, and systemic disease (diabetes). Specific subgingival bacteria and socioeconomic stress also have been linked causally to periodontal disease through epidemiologic studies, but further evaluation is ongoing. Gender, race, and age may play a role in disease expression but are not causally linked to periodontal disease.

TREATMENT NEEDS

Information provided by epidemiologic surveys regarding gingival bleeding (gingival inflammation), subgingival calculus, and probing depths of 4 mm or greater is of great importance to the dental hygienist. These data represent clinical parameters used to decide when treatment of periodontal disease is necessary. Most individuals will need periodontal preventive care (Oliver, Brown, and Löe 1998), which is provided by the hygienist. Over 90% of people surveyed (NHANES III) have attachment loss, and only 15% of the population has advanced disease, suggesting that much of the treatment needs of the United States can be fulfilled by hygienists. More extensive, severe disease is found among minorities and those with less income and education. However, these are the same individuals who are less likely to seek or perceive the need for dental services. Tooth loss due to periodontal disease remains high in the United States (Brown, Oliver, and Löe 1989). *This suggests that public awareness and education about the preventive services of dental hygienists are paramount if those individuals who are most affected are to be treated before tooth loss due to periodontitis occurs.*

FUTURE TRENDS

The hygienist in the general dentist's office plays an important role in the treatment of periodontal patients. The general dentist office handles the management of early and some moderate cases of periodontitis, with delegation of preventive care to the hygienist. Prevention and education are important responsibilities of the dental hygienist. As epidemiologic studies elaborate and refine the interrelationship between periodontal infections and the systemic health of the patient, hygienists will need to include this information in patient education sessions. The impact of periodontal disease on the overall health of a patient has been the subject of recent news media attention. Periodontal infections as risk factors for other diseases such as coronary heart disease and preterm low-birth-weight babies and its interrelationship with diabetes will most likely trigger increased demand for dental hygiene services. As patient awareness of periodontal disease and its systemic implications increases, more individuals will specifically seek the preventive and periodontal scaling services of the dental hygienist.

Further, there should be an increased prevalence of periodontal disease because edentulism has declined in the last twenty years. More people will retain more teeth, and thus more teeth will be exposed to plaque-related inflammation for more time, increasing the probability of periodontitis and gingivitis. In light of this, despite the decreased severity of disease from past generations, the disease level should still persist and the demand for dental hygiene services remain high.

KEY POINTS

- Epidemiologic measurements used to assess periodontal diseases include plaque, calculus, gingival, and periodontal indices.
- Indices measure past disease activity rather than current disease activity or future periodontal breakdown.
- Gingivitis is the most common form of periodontal disease.
- Aggressive periodontitis is not common in the general population.
- Chronic periodontitis is prevalent in the general population.
- Numerous contributory risk factors influence the development and prevalence of periodontal diseases.

REFERENCES

Ainamo, J., D. Barmes, G. Beargie, T. Cutress, and J. Martin. 1982. Development of the World Health Organization (WHO) Community Periodontal Index of Treatment Needs (CPITN). *Int. Dent. J.* 32:281–291.

Ayers, C., A. Abrama, and L. Lausten. 1979. Oral health assessment of inner city preschoolers. *Dent. Hygiene* 53:465–468.

Baelum, V., F. Manji, G. Fejerskov, and D. Wansola. 1993. Validity of CPITN's assumptions of hierarchical occurrence of periodontal conditions in a Kenyan population aged 15–65 years. *Commun. Dent. Oral Epidemiol.* 21:347–353.

Baelum, V., F. Manji, P. Wanzala, and O. Fejerskov. 1995. Relationship between CPITN and periodontal attachment loss findings in an adult population. *J. Clin. Periodontol.* 22:146–152.

Bakdash, B. 1994. Oral hygiene and compliance as risk factors in periodontitis. *J. Periodontol.* 65:539–544.

Beck, J., G. Koch, and S. Offenbacher. 1994. Attachment loss trend over 3 years in community-dwelling older adults. *J. Periodontol.* 65:737–743.

Beck, J., G. Koch, and S. Offenbacher. 1995. Incidence of attachment loss over 3 years in older adults: New and progressing lesions. *Commun. Dent. Oral Epidemiol.* 23:291–296.

Bergström, J., and S. Eliasson. 1987. Cigarette smoking and alveolar bone height in subjects with high standard oral hygiene. *J. Clin. Periodontol.* 14:466–469.

Bergström, J., and B. Floderus-Myrhed. 1983. Co-twin study of the relationship between smoking and some periodontal disease factors. *Commun. Dent. Oral Epidemiol.* 11:113–116.

Bolin, A., G. Eklund, L. Frithiof, and S. Lavstedt. 1993. The effect of changed smoking habits on marginal alveolar bone loss: A longitudinal study. *Swed. Dent. J.* 17:211–216.

Brown, L., J. Brunelle, and A. Kingman. 1996. Periodontal status in the United States, 1988–91: Prevalence, extent, and demographic variation. *J. Dent. Res.* 75 (spec issue): 672–683.

Brown, L., R. Oliver, and H. Löe. 1990. Evaluating periodontal status of U.S. employed adults. *J. Am. Dent. Assoc.* 121:226–232.

Brown, L., R. Oliver, and H. Löe. 1989. Periodontal diseases in the U.S. in 1981: Prevalence, severity, extent and role in tooth mortality. *J. Periodontol.* 60:363–371.

Burt, B. 1996. Epidemiology of periodontal diseases. *J. Periodontol.* 67:935–945.

Burt, B., A. Ismail, and S. Eklund. 1985. Periodontal disease, tooth loss and oral hygiene among older Americans. *Commun. Dent. Oral Epidemiol.* 13(2):93–96.

Capilouto, M., and C. Douglass. 1988. Trends in the prevalence and severity of periodontal disease in the US: A public health problem? *J. Public Health Dent.* 48:245–251.

Caton, J., and A. Polson. 1985. The Interdental Bleeding Index: A simplified procedure for monitoring gingival health. *Comp. Cont. Educ. Dent.* 6:88–92.

Fischman, S. 1986. Current status of indices of plaque. *J. Clin. Periodontol.* 13:371–374.

Greene, J. 1967. The Oral Hygiene Index. Development and uses. *J. Periodontol.* 38:625–637.

Greene, J., and J. Vermillion. 1964. The Simplified Oral Hygiene Index. *J. Am. Dent. Assoc.* 68:7–13.

Hunt, R., and S. Fann. 1991. Effect of examining half the teeth in a partial periodontal recording of older adults. *J. Dent. Res.* 70:1380–1385.

Ismail, A., E. Morrison, B. Burt, R. Cafesse, and M. Kavanaugh. 1990. Natural history of periodontal disease in adults: Findings from the Tecumseh Periodontal Disease Study, 1959–1987. *J. Dent. Res.* 69(2):430–435.

Ismail, A., B. Burt, and S. Eklund. 1983. Epidmiologic patterns of smoking and periodontal disease in the United States. *J. Am. Dent. Assoc.* 106:617–621.

Listgarten, M., C. Schifter, and L. Laster. 1985. Three-year longitudinal study of the periodontal status of an adult population with gingivitis. *J. Clin. Periodontol.* 12:225–238.

Lobene, R., T. Weatherford, N. Ross, R. Lam, and L. Menaker. 1986. A modified gingival index for use in clinical trials. *Clin. Prev. Dent.* 8(1):3–6.

Löe, H., and L. Brown. 1991. Early-onset periodontitis in the United States of America. *J. Periodontol.* 62:608–616.

Löe, H., A. Anerud, H. Boysen, and E. Morrison. 1986. Natural history of periodontal disease in man: Rapid, moderate and no loss of attachment in Sri Lankan laborers 14–46 years of age. *J. Clin. Periodontol.* 13:431–446.

Löe, H., A. Anerud, H. Boysen, and M. Smith. 1978. The natural history of periodontal disease in man: The rate of periodontal destruction before 40 years of age. *J. Periodontol.* 49(12):607–620.

Löe, H. the gingival index, the plaque index, and the retention index. Systems (Part II). *J. Periodontol* 1967: 38:610–616.

Miller, A., J. Brunelle, J. Carlos, Brown, L. J., and Löe, H. 1987. Oral Health of the United States Adults. National findings 1985–1986. Bethesda, MD: U.S. Public Health Service, U.S. Dept. of Health and Human Services.

Mühlemann, H. R., and S. Son. 1971. Gingival sulcus bleeding: A leading symptom in initial gingivitis. *Helv. Odont. Acta* 15:107–113.

O'Leary, T. J., R. Drake, and J. Naylor. 1972. The Plaque Control Record. *J. Periodontol.* 43(1):38.

Oliver, R., L. Brown, and H. Löe. 1998. Periodontal disease in the United States population. *J. Periodontol.* 69:269–278.

Oliver, R., and T. Tervonen. 1994. Diabetes: A risk factor for periodontitis in adults. *J. Periodontol.* 65:530–538.

Papapanou, P. 1996. Annals of Periodontology, Section 1A: Periodontal diseases: Epidemiology. 1996 World Workshop in Periodontics, Lansdowne, VA.

Russell, A. L. 1967. The Periodontal Index. *J. Periodontol.* 38:585–591.

Seppälä, B., M. Seppälä, and J. Ainamo. 1993. A longitudinal study on insulin-dependent diabetes mellitus and periodontal disease. *J. Clin. Periodontol.* 20:161–165.

Sheiham, A., and D. Striffler. 1970. A comparison of four epidemiological methods of assessing periodontal disease: I. Population findings. *J. Periodont. Res.* 5:148–154.

Silness, J., and H. Löe. 1964. Periodontal disease in pregnancy: II. Correlation between oral hygiene and periodontal condition. *Acta Odontol. Scand.* 22:121–135.

Stamm, J. 1986. Epidemiology of gingivitis. *J. Clin. Periodontol.* 13:360–366.

Taylor, G. W., B. A. Burt, M. P. Becker, R. J. Genco, M. Schlossman, W. C. Knowler, and D. J. Pettitt. 1998. Non-insulin-dependent diabetes and the progression of bone loss over a two-year period. *J. Periodontol.* 68:76–83.

Turesky, S., N. Gilmore, and I. Glickman. 1970. Reduced plaque formation by the chloromethyl analogue of victamine C. *J. Periodontol.* 41:41–43.

U.S. Public Health Service NIDR. 1987. *Oral Health in United States Adults: National Findings* (NIH Publication No. 87-2868), pp. 1–168. Bethesda, MD: National Institute of Health, NIDR.

Volpe, A., L. Kupczak, and W. King. 1967. In vivo calculus assessment: III. Scoring techniques, rate of calculus formation, partial mouth exams versus full mouth exams, and intra-examiner reproducibility. *Periodontics* 5:184–193.

Volpe, A., J. H. Manhold, and S. P. Hazen. 1965. In vivo calculus assessment: I. A method and its examiner reproducibility. *J. Periodontol.* 36:292–298.

Waerhaug, J. 1966. Epidemiology of periodontal disease: A review of literature. In *World Workshop in Periodontics,* pp. 179–212. Ann Arbor, MI: University of Michigan.

Self-Quiz

1. Which one of the following modalities would best determine disease prevalence? (p. 116)

   a. comprehensive periodontal charting

   b. epidemiologic population surveys

   c. patient questionnaires

   d. national dental hygiene expenditures

2. Which one of the following terms describes the rate of new cases of peri- odontal disease occurring in a given time period? (p. 116)

   a. prevalence

   b. incidence

   c. severity

   d. extent

   e. index

3. An individual has been identified with advanced attachment loss at one point in time. It is highly unlikely (infrequent) that this individual will again experience rapid attachment loss (≥ 3 mm) within the next three years? (p. 129)

   a. The first statement is true, and the second statement is false.

   b. The first statement is false, and the second statement is true.

   c. Both statements are true.

   d. Both statements are false.

4. Which one of the following indices is best used to monitor a patient's plaque control in private dental practice? (pp. 118–119, Table 5–1)

   a. Quigley-Hein Plaque Index

   b. Plaque Record (O'Leary)

   c. Periodontal Screening and Recording (PSR) System

   d. Sulcus Bleeding Index

5. Which one of the following best measures the *severity* of periodontal dis- ease in a population? (pp. 116–118)

   a. radiographs

   b. intraoral cameras

   c. indices

   d. surgical costs

6. All of the following are risk factors for periodontal disease *except* one. Which one is the exception? (p. 132)

   a. age

   b. smoking

   c. diabetes

   d. oral cleanliness

7. A risk indicator differs from a risk factor in that there is no causal rela- tionship of the associated characteristic with the disease. Low income and less education are risk indicators for periodontal disease. (pp. 132–133)

   a. The first statement is true, and the second statement is false.

   b. The first statement is false, and the second statement is true.

   c. Both statements are true.

   d. Both statements are false.

8. According to recent surveys, which of the following percentages of the U.S. adult population has severe periodontal disease (advanced periodontitis)? (p. 129)

    a. 5–20
    b. 40–50
    c. 70–80
    d. 90–100

9. Which one of the following describes how has the prevalence of gingivitis changed over the past thirty years? (pp. 128–129)

    a. increased
    b. decreased
    c. remained the same
    d. increased in the first ten years and then decreased

10. Which one of the following describes the prevalence of aggressive periodontitis in the general population? (p. 130)

    a. rare
    b. frequent
    c. universal
    d. nonexistent

MEDICAL HISTORY:

The patient is a 65-year-old male who states he is in perfect health and goes to his physician once a year for a check-up. His blood pressure is 135/84 and he has a pulse of 72. He is 5 feet 9 inches tall and weighs 195 lb (88.6 kg). He denies taking any medications, including over-the-counter products. Occasionally he takes one aspirin when he has a headache.

CHIEF COMPLAINT:

"My gums look red and they bleed when I brush hard."

DENTAL HISTORY:

The patient has not seen a dentist in the last 3 years because he states he is too busy with work and he thinks the condition of his gingiva is due to brushing too hard. He brushes twice a day but does not floss.

SOCIAL HISTORY:

The patient is married with two grown-up children. He is the head of an investment company and travels frequently. The patient has smoked 1 pack of cigarettes a day for 30 years (30 pack/years) and drinks one or two cocktails every night at dinner as well as beer on the weekends.

ORAL HYGIENE STATUS:

The patient has poor oral hygiene. An examination revealed generalized supra/subgingival plaque and calculus.

DENTAL EXAM:

The patient is missing all third molars.

GINGIVAL EXAM:

The gingiva is red and edematous. There is generalized gingival recession.

PERIODONTAL EXAM:

Periodontal probing depths range from 3 to 8 mm, with the deepest depths being on the maxillary molars. Radiographic survey reveals generalized bone loss with vertical bony defects on the mesial surface of the mandibular left first and second molar.

CASE STUDY

INTERPRETATION

PATIENT PROBLEM	BASIS FOR DISCUSSION	QUESTIONS (Q)/ANSWERS (A)	CHAPTER LOCATION
Gingiva is red and bleeds	Inflammation is present	Q) What causes the erythema and bleeding?	2
		A) Erythema is caused by vascular proliferation. Sites that bleed have a greater area of inflamed gingival connective tissue	
Smokes	Patient needs to stop smoking. Talk to patient about a smoking cessation program.	Q) Does smoking affect the periodontium?	3
		A) Smoking is an important risk factor for inflammatory periodontal diseases. Smokers have greater probing depths, clinical attachment loss, and bone loss. Smoking can also impair the chemotaxis and phagocytosis of neutrophils.	
Drinks	Patient needs to stop or reduce alcohol consumption.	Q) Does alcohol affect the periodontium?	3
		A) Chronic alcohol intake presents an increased risk for periodontitis because of increased bleeding tendencies, poor oral hygiene due to overall neglect, and a tendency to malnutrition.	
Patient has poor oral hygiene	Generalized plaque accumulation	Q) What type of assessment procedure will best help the patient understand and improve his oral hygiene status?	5
		A) A plaque index. The O'Leary, Drake and Naylor Plaque Control Record shows the distribution rather than the amount of plaque. This will help to motivate the patient by showing him where most of plaque accumulates.	
Generalized periodontal pockets and bone loss	Patient has generalized mild gingivitis and generalized moderate with localized areas of severe chronic periodontitis.	Q) What is the etiology of the periodontal pockets and the bone loss?	2

PATIENT PROBLEM	BASIS FOR DISCUSSION	QUESTIONS (Q)/ANSWERS (A)	CHAPTER LOCATION
		A) The primary risk factor for periodontal diseases is dental plaque or biofilms. Bacteria and host cells synthesize toxins, by-products, and enzymes that cause bone destruction and pocket formation. Periodontal pockets form when the apical part of the junctional epithelium migrates apically along the root surface. This happens when the gingival fibers (gingival connective tissue attachment) is destroyed. This is referred to as attachment loss.	

1. All of the following are contributing factors for this patient's periodontal condition *except* one. Which one is the exception? (p. 60)

    a. pathogenic bacteria
    b. dental calculus
    c. smoking
    d. alcohol
    e. aspirin

2. Which one of the following types of pockets is found on the mesial surface of the mandibular left first molar? (p. 49)

    a. gingival
    b. pseudo
    c. suprabony *base of pocket is coronal to crest of bone*
    d. infrabony *base of sulcus pocket is apical to crestal bone.*

3. Which one of the following cells *predominate* in the area immediately below the junctional epithelium in this patient? (p. 45)

    a. mast
    b. melanocytes
    c. T lymphocytes
    d. B lymphocytes

4. Which one of the following parts of the periodontium is responsible for keeping the patient's mandibular left second molar in the tooth socket? (p. 19)

    a. gingival fibers
    b. periodontal ligament fibers
    c. alveolar bone proper
    d. junctional epithelium

CASE STUDY

✱TBQ

5. Which one of the following findings is most consistent with gingival inflammation in this patient? (p. 41)

   a. bleeding on probing
   b. redness of the gingiva
   c. deep probing depths
   d. vertical bone loss

6. Which one of the following classification of periodontal diseases (American Academy of Periodontology) is characteristic of this patient? (pp. 99–101)

   a. plaque-induced gingivitis
   b. localized aggressive periodontitis
   c. generalized aggressive periodontitis
   d. chronic periodontitis
   e. necrotizing ulcerative periodontitis

7. High numbers of which of the following bacteria are most likely evident in this patient? (p. 62)

   a. *Candida albicans*
   b. *Streptococcus sanguis*
   c. *Fusobacterium nucleatum*
   d. *Porphyromonas gingivalis*

8. All of the following features characterize this patient's periodontal condition *except* one. Which one is the exception? (pp. 45–47)

   a. apical migration of the junctional epithelium
   b. increased width of the attached gingiva
   c. supporting and alveolar bone loss
   d. loss of gingival connective tissue attachment

9. Which one of the following features in this patient is possibly responsible for a decrease in function of neutrophils? (p. 85)

   a. increased age
   b. cigarette smoking
   c. alcohol drinking
   d. high blood pressure
   e. aspirin tablets

10. Which one of the following substances is *most* likely the *direct* cause of the bone loss that has occurred in this patient? (pp. 50, 70)

   a. lipooligosaccharides and enzymes
   b. bacterial waste products and enzymes
   c. cigarette smoke and dental calculus
   d. dental calculus and alcohol

PERIODONTAL DISEASES: THE ASSESSMENT PHASE

Section II

PATIENT ASSESSMENT

Outline:

I. DENTAL HYGIENE PROCESS OF CARE FOR THE PERIODONTAL PATIENT

Cheryl Westphal, R.D.H., M.S.

Goal:

To provide the dental hygienist with information on the procedures of patient care.

Educational Objectives:

Upon completion of this chapter section, the reader should be able to:

List and discuss five phases of the dental hygiene process for periodontal patient care;

Explain the importance of stating the goals for periodontal patient care; and

Discuss the difference between a dental diagnosis and a dental hygiene diagnosis.

DENTAL HYGIENE: PROCEDURES FOR PATIENT CARE

The purpose of the dental hygiene process of care is to provide a framework within which the individualized needs of the patient can be met. The dental hygiene process of care is an assessment process involving five phases (Mueller-Joseph and Petersen 1995) of a search for clues leading up to the identification and classification of the nature of the disease and the steps in patient care needed to alleviate the problem (DeGowin 1994; Bates, Bickley, and Hoekelman 1995):

1. assessment;
2. dental hygiene diagnosis;
3. planning;
4. implementation; and
5. evaluation.

KEY WORDS

- assessment
- subjective data
- objective data
- dental hygiene diagnosis
- treatment plan
- implementation
- evaluation
- documentation

ASSESSMENT

Assessment is the gathering of all relevant information concerning the patient including medical/dental history, vital signs, extraoral and intraoral examination, periodontal and dental examination, radiographs, indices, and risk assessments

146

(e.g., patient use of tobacco, presence of systemic caries). In the patient history assessment, clues are symptoms, which are abnormalities experienced by the patient. Information obtained by observations of and statements made by the patient are termed **subjective data.** In the clinical examination, on the other hand, clues are signs, which are abnormalities perceived by the practitioner. Information obtained from observations of the patient and statements made by the practitioner are termed **objective data.**

Data collection starts with taking down the medical/dental history, followed by the intra/extraoral examination, restorative charting, gingival assessment, periodontal assessment, oral hygiene evaluation, radiographs, and additional diagnostic laboratory tests if required.

DENTAL HYGIENE DIAGNOSIS

After the data are collected, the dental hygienist reviews and analyzes the information. A **dental hygiene diagnosis** differs from a dental diagnosis, since a dental diagnosis gives a name to the disease and the dental hygiene diagnosis identifies the patient's actual or potential response to the disease process (Mueller-Joseph and Peterson 1995). *The purpose of a dental hygiene diagnosis is to keep the planning of patient care centered on problems or conditions that are responsive to dental hygiene intervention* (Mueller-Joseph and Peterson 1995). For example, a patient has inflamed gingiva, but no bone loss is shown on the radiographs. The dentist will make a dental diagnosis of gingivitis, whereas *the dental hygiene diagnosis focuses on educating the patient on the need and benefit* (Mueller-Joseph and Peterson 1995) of proper plaque control to reduce supragingival plaque accumulation. The dental hygienist should also understand the need to disrupt the pathogenic bacteria so that a more beneficial microflora will populate the tooth/soft tissue area.

After the disease is diagnosed, the practitioner should determine the cause so that a treatment plan can be established that will eliminate or control the condition. The dental hygienist should know why the patient developed the condition in order for appropriate treatment to be rendered. For example, a patient complains of tooth pain. The dental hygienist assesses the situation and asks questions of the patient to determine whether the pain occurs with cold or hot foods or liquids. The dental hygienist can then determine the etiologic factor for this condition and develop a plan to eliminate the pain.

PLANNING

Planning is the establishment of realistic goals and treatment strategies to facilitate optimal oral health. A **treatment plan** involves the development of a written treatment plan for the patient's individual needs based on data collection and assessment. Alternative options should be included in the plan that may be implemented instead of the ideal plan if the patient is in poor health, if the patient is not compliant or motivated to follow the ideal plan, or if the patient cannot afford the ideal treatment. The treatment plan must be presented to the patient and agreed upon before any treatment is started. An appropriate sequence of treatments must be stated. Developing a plan involves knowledge from a variety of disciplines besides dental hygiene, including behavioral sciences, pharmacology, anatomy and physiology, chemistry, and microbiology. Critical thinking and decision-making skills are necessary to provide effective and efficient dental hygiene services.

When developing a dental care plan, the *goal* or *end result* of treatment must be stated (Mueller-Joseph and Petersen 1995). The goal is a statement that addresses and identifies the purpose for implementing dental care. The individualized plan also identifies the *interventions* necessary to meet the health care goals of the patient. Interventions are procedures carried out by the dental hygienist to help the patient reach the desired goal. For example, let us say that a dental diagnosis is pregnancy gingivitis. The dental hygiene diagnosis is gingival inflammation related to the elevated hormonal levels and inadequate home care of the teeth and gums by the patient. The aims of dental hygiene treatment are to reduce plaque levels by oral hygiene instruction and educate the patient on the influence of plaque and hormones on overall dental health. Dental hygiene intervention deals with the disruption of plaque by mechanical debridement.

IMPLEMENTATION

Once the care plan is presented to the patient and an informed consent form is signed by the patient and dentist, treatment commences. This **implementation** phase includes (1) preparing the operatory for the patient; (2) using proper infection control procedures; (3) carrying out periodontal debridement procedures; (4) implementing pain management procedures; (5) applying chemotherapeutic agents; (6) carrying out fluoride therapy; (7) undertaking coronal polishing; (8) teaching the patient proper care of oral prostheses; (9) teaching the patient proper care and maintenance of restorations; (10) providing the patient with health education and preventive counseling; (11) providing the patient with nutritional counseling; and (12) documenting the process properly.

EVALUATION

The **evaluation** phase of therapy deals with feedback on the effectiveness of the treatment and procedures. This phase occurs after treatment has been completed, when the patient returns for a follow-up visit a few weeks after the nonsurgical periodontal therapy (initial therapy or Phase I therapy) or surgical therapy has been completed, or for periodontal maintenance (recall) procedures.

SOCIAL, ECONOMIC, AND CULTURAL CONSIDERATIONS

From the moment the patient enters the care cycle within the practice, the whole person is assessed to understand aspects such as her or his health background, health beliefs, cultural background, social and economic background, educational background, and work-related issues. These factors play an important role when determining a home-care regime for the person that will yield compliance.

A review of the patient's dental and medical history from the viewpoint of social and economic concerns provides insight as to the patient's ability to afford subsequent dental follow-up home-care regimes. Often factors such as people's beliefs about the role they should play in their own health care and the part their bad habits play in causing periodontal disease will impact upon their desire to maintain their oral health after surgery or other extensive dental care. A complete discussion with the patient is crucial to elicit the information instead of a nonverbal form of the medical history questionnaire often done without any review of these factors.

TECHNOLOGY AND DOCUMENTATION

Since data collection is an ongoing process, an appropriate method of written and visual **documentation** is required. The intraoral camera is a recent technological advance that can be used to document various findings before and after the treatment procedure. The practitioner is able to view and record such conditions as plaque retention sites, gingival conditions, faulty margins or caries, and stain or other deposits. The recordings can then be utilized to explain the condition and create a historical file that can be placed in the patient's file and used to show the patient any progress or degeneration of the periodontal condition being treated at subsequent appointments. Many different manufacturers exist that offer systems of computers and cameras available for chairside use. The intraoral camera can be employed during the charting, oral soft tissue exam, or oral hygiene evaluation to involve the patient in the process and discuss the findings. Currently the great majority of practitioners who use intraoral video cameras do not have those cameras integrated with their computer systems, although the number who do is growing. This involves converting the images to a digital format using specialized software. Although some practitioners do not feel the need to permanently save images after case presentation, doing so is a valuable tool in terms of educating patients and increasing the likelihood that the recommended treatment procedures will be performed.

Computer technology is becoming essential for the treatment record, appointment planning, recare visit booking, and patient documentation parts of running a dental practice. Oral hygiene evaluations as part of the computer record of the patient offer an array of visual presentations, which can enhance treatment planning and patient compliance with the recommended procedures. Patients can be shown a pictorial display of their probing depths, caries, gum and tooth recession, other gingival involvement, or potential treatment outcomes of surgery or prosthetic replacements.

KEY POINTS

- Five components of the dental hygiene process enable the dental hygienist to identify the patient's periodontal problem, to determine the cause of the problem, and then to treat the problem.
- An intraoral camera can be useful to point out areas of recession, plaque-retentive sites, bleeding points, and restorations.
- Documentation is an integral part of the dental hygiene process; good documentation in the patient's chart is of utmost importance.

REFERENCES

Bates, B., L. S. Bickley, and R. A. Hoekelman. 1995. *A pocket guide to physical examination and history taking.* 2d ed., Philadelphia: J. B. Lippincott Company.

DeGowin, R. L. 1994. *DeGowin & DeGowin's diagnostic examination,* 3–4. New York: McGraw-Hill.

Chapter: The Dental Hygiene Process of Care pp. 1–19. Editors are Mueller-Joseph, L., and M. Petersen. 1995. The dental hygiene process of care. In *Dental hygiene process: Diagnosis and care planning.* Albany, NY: Delmar Publishers.

SELF-QUIZ

1. All of the following are components of the dental hygiene process *except* one. Which one is the exception? (p. 146)

   a. assessment
   b. dental diagnosis
   c. treatment planning
   d. implementation
   e. evaluation

2. Which one of the following reasons is important for determining the individual goals for periodontal patient care? (pp. 147–148)

   a. establishes a rapport with the patient
   b. emphasizes the need for prevention in the care of the patient
   c. identifies the purpose for treating the patient
   d. evaluates for treatment needs after the first appointment

3. Which one of the following statements explains the purpose of a dental hygiene diagnosis? (p. 147)

   a. keeps the planning of patient care centered on problems or conditions that are responsive to dental hygiene intervention
   b. helps the dental hygienist determine the need for additional radiographs
   c. identifies the type of periodontal disease
   d. anticipates the effectiveness in achieving the desired outcome of therapy

4. Before undergoing any periodontal treatment, every patient should have his/her mouth and dentition photographed with an intraoral camera *because* the intraoral camera is an important part of documentation. (p. 149)

   a. Both the statement and the reason are correct and related.
   b. Both the statement and the reason are correct but *not* related.
   c. The statement is correct, but the reason is *not.*
   d. The statement is *not* correct, but the reason is correct.
   e. *Neither* the statement *nor* the reason is correct.

5. Which of the following reasons best explains the purpose of evaluation of periodontal therapy? (p. 148)

   a. determines the need for additional periodontal intervention
   b. deals with the feedback on the effectiveness of treatment
   c. identifies the type of disease present
   d. allows the dental hygienist to introduce oral hygiene care products for home use

II. PATIENT HISTORY

Ann M. Goodwin, R.D.H., M.S.
Rosemary DeRosa Hays, R.D.H., M.S.

Goal:

To provide the dental hygienist with information on the patient history-taking process.

Educational Objectives:

Upon completion of this chapter section, the reader should be able to:

Explain the importance of data collection;

Evaluate the importance of total health assessment in providing periodontal services;

Discuss the importance of interviewing and questioning the patient; and

Discuss the implications of the chief complaint and medical history in planning periodontal treatment.

The patient's first visit is the time to collect subjective data. A complete **dental/medical history** is an essential aspect of this initial evaluation. It is here that the dental hygienist becomes an advantageous partner in the health-care evaluation process. Interview the patient for his or her history, which is divided into the personal profile, social history, chief complaint, history of the present illness, medical history, family history, and dental history. The collective diagnostic information developed through this interview provides a basis for future comparisons to evaluate the progress of disease, the efficacy of treatment, and the appearance of new findings. Therefore, taking the patient history is a mandatory first step in the treatment process.

THE INTERVIEW

The **interview process,** so critical to the successful completion of the dental and medical history, demands a high level of communication between the patient and the dental hygienist. If done properly, an interview helps establish a rapport between the dental hygienist and the patient. History taking can be accomplished through a questionnaire, a patient interview, or a combination of both. The most practical and successful method for assessing the health status of a patient is a combination questionnaire and interview.

KEY WORDS
- dental/medical history
- interview process
- chief complaint

During the interview, open-ended questions such as "What changes in your health or medications have occurred since your last dental visit?" or "What in your mouth bothers you?" open doors to gaining more pertinent information. If good rapport develops, the patient will feel more comfortable, and as the interview progresses, he or she will volunteer more information. Open-ended questions put patients more at ease. Nevertheless, closed-ended questions also are necessary, such as "When was your last dental visit?" These types of questions do not require much responding from the patient; rather, they can be answered usually in one sentence.

PERSONAL PROFILE

The obvious place to begin the interview is by asking questions concerning the patient's identity. This *personal profile* consists of the patient's name, age, address, occupation, and telephone number. Some of this information is needed for identification purposes, while the patient's age and sex may be useful in the classification of the periodontal disease. Document the name, address, and telephone number of the patient's physician, which will be useful if consultation is necessary.

SOCIAL HISTORY

The *social history* includes the patient's occupation, lifestyle, marital status, diet, and use of alcohol and tobacco, both smoking and chewing tobacco. Habits such as cigarette smoking or use of smokeless tobacco should be noted because they are potential risk factors for periodontal diseases.

Cigarette smoking is reported in pack/years, which is determined by multiplying the number of packs of cigarettes smoked per day by the number of years the patient has smoked. Documenting the amount of smoking in pack/years gives a better understanding of the total exposure of nicotine during the lifetime of an individual. For example, if a person smoked one pack every day for 10 years, this is 10 pack/years.

The patient's lifestyle, including family and social structure, attitudes, and behaviors, is part of the social history. A patient's social perceptions, priorities, amount of stress, and ideas on aesthetics provide clues to compliance with dental care. A dental hygienist can work toward changing a patient's attitudes and behaviors by understanding the patient's cultural differences, motivation, patience, education, and expectations.

CHIEF COMPLAINT

The next step is to ask the patient to identify his or her **chief complaint (CC)**. The patient should state in his or her own words why he or she is seeking treatment. Determination of the CC assists in the identification of any ongoing disease process. Symptoms of periodontal problems include pressure in the gingiva or jaw or itchy gingiva. Signs of periodontal disease include bleeding, halitosis (bad breath), and/or tooth mobility. Given the insidious nature of periodontal diseases, many patients have no idea there is a problem. If the patient's CC involves something other than periodontal disease, that must be treated first before any other dental treatment is rendered.

HISTORY OF PRESENT ILLNESS

The history of the CC expands on the patient's awareness of the problem and is also referred to as the *history of present illness.* The dental hygienist should inquire how long the patient's problem has existed, any previous treatment(s), and if this problem has occurred before. For instance, if the patient's CC is "bleeding from the gums," the dental hygienist should ask about the onset, cause, location, and duration of the bleeding.

MEDICAL HISTORY

The current and past status of the patient's general health, or *medical history,* should be the next area of investigation. A questionnaire, an interview, or a combination of questionnaire and interview can be used to accomplish this. Sometimes, however, a simple telephone call to the patient prior to the first appointment may screen for potential medical problems. A written questionnaire provides a baseline for treatment, whereas an interview provides both personal contact with the patient and supplementary information that may contribute to a more comprehensive evaluation. It is important to listen closely to the patient and have a genuine interest in what is said in order to provide insight, accuracy, and clarity in the history (McDaniel et al. 1995). Allowing the patient to describe symptoms or complaints at length encourages trust and fosters a sympathetic professional relationship, but it is only necessary to record the relevant facts and details.

The interview should close with an open-ended question inviting discussion of details of the history. Before the interview ends, the hygienist should review the written questionnaire to ensure that all the information recorded on the form is complete and accurate and that nothing has been omitted inadvertently. Many patients do not understand the terminology used on the form because of either language difficulties or different cultural and educational backgrounds (Jolly 1994).

There are many standard medical history forms. They vary in length, content, and format depending on the setting for which they are designed. The American Dental Association (ADA) Medical History Form* and Medical History interview* universally known and recognized as comprehensive (Figs. 6–1 ■, 6–2 ■). It should be completed during the first appointment and reviewed at each subsequent visit. All questions on the form must be answered, and any positive responses can be highlighted or marked in red so that later they can be easily seen and reviewed. (Table 6–1 ■).

The medical history includes the date of the patient's last physical examination, a review of organ systems (ROS) to determine any medical conditions the patient may have, and a list of any medications the patient is taking. The ROS assists in the identification of diseases that are associated with the physical systems of the body. Questions can then be addressed to specific diseases, including the dates and duration of illness. A high percentage of dental patients have medical conditions that can have an affect on a clinician's therapeutic decisions (Peacock and Carson 1995).

Questions concerning current medication use and drug allergies are crucial because the answers may have a direct effect on any treatment the dentist eventually

---

*American Dental Association: Medical History Form (S-500) and Medical History Interview (S-502), ADA Department of Salable Materials, 211 East Chicago Avenue, Chicago, IL 60611-2678.

Table 6-1
Medical History Interpretation

QUESTION	REASON FOR QUESTION	TREATMENT PLAN MODIFICATION
Date Name Address Telephone (home and business): Social Security Number:	To establish when the initial visit occurred; for office management, records, and insurance purposes	None
Occupation	To determine any etiologic factors associated with the general health of patient To determine educational status of patient	None
Date of birth	To determine age of patient for legal considerations, appointment times, and age-related oral conditions and/or healing factors	May warrant parental or guardian approval and signature Appointment scheduling considerations
Height and weight	Necessary for medication dosages A change in weight may indicate an underlying disease process	Nutritional counseling
Name of spouse and closest relation and telephone numbers	Office records Emergency situations	None
"Are you in good health?" "Has there been any change in your health within the last year?"	To obtain subjective summary of patient's concerns and medical conditions	If any significant changes in medical status, consultation with the patient's physician may be necessary If no changes in medical status, proceed with treatment
Last physical examination Physician's name and address Are you under the care of a physician? Hospitalizations in past 5 years?	To determine how often patient seeks health care To disclose a medical problem To consult and refer for any medical problem To contact physician in an emergency	Premedication requirements Medical consultation
Use of prescription or non-prescription medicines	Identification of medications that may affect the oral cavity Identification of drug-drug or drug-food interactions	Confirm with physician if any modifications are necessary prior to dental treatment
Rheumatic heart disease or heart murmur Damaged heart valves or artificial heart valves	Infective endocarditis	Necessary premedication prior to dental treatment recommended by the American Heart Association (see appendix 1A)
Cardiovascular disease (heart trouble, heart attack, angina, coronary insufficiency, coronary occlusion, high blood pressure, arteriosclerosis, stroke)	To indicate patients who are presently taking anticoagulants and aspirin Gingiva overgrowth caused by calcium channel blockers Drugs causing xerostomia Periodontal disease	Minimal stress and shorter appointments Possible medical consultation prior to dental treatment Caution with use of vasoconstrictors in local anesthetics Salivary substitutes and fluoride rinses for xerostomia Minimize tissue trauma Chair positioning Bleeding tendency due to anticoagulants
Cardiac pacemaker	Date of pacemaker insertion	Medical consultation

Condition	History/Findings	Dental Management Considerations
Allergy to medications	Identification of agent (e.g., antibiotics) With medications, be certain it is a true allergy and not a side effect of the drug (e.g., nausea with codeine is a side effect not an allergy)	Avoidance of allergic agents Emergency preparation
Sinus trouble	Headaches or discomfort in the maxilla, including teeth	Radiographic findings to determine sinus positioning for periodontal surgery
Asthma or hay fever	Breathing difficulties/airway obstruction Allergic background When was last attack?	Sulfite-containing local anesthetics are contraindicated for asthmatics Aspirin, barbituates, and narcotics are contraindicated in asthmatics Have inhalant on bracket table
Fainting spells	History of high blood pressure Fear and anxiety	Consultation with physician Minimal stress Chair positioning
Persistent diarrhea or weight loss	Determine underlying conditions causing signs and symptoms	Medical consultation for chronic condition.
Diabetes mellitus	Increases susceptibility to periodontal disease Time of day of appointment Importance of the timing of food intake and medication compliance Lower resistance to infection and possible oral ulcers Decreased healing response	Need frequent maintenance appointments Optimal oral hygiene Minimize tissue trauma Medical consultation for undiagnosed but symptomatic conditions Have sugar available in some form in case of insulin reaction Prophylactic antibiotic medication may be warranted for an uncontrolled diabetic
Hepatitis, jaundice, or liver disease	Determine type of hepatitis Bleeding problems Faulty drug metabolism Laboratory findings Vaccination of health care professionals with hepatitis B (HBV) vaccine	Postpone treatment for patients with active disease Nutritional and oral hygiene emphasis
AIDS (acquired immunodeficiency syndrome) or HIV (human immunodeficiency virus) infection	Identify undiagnosed cases through medical history findings and/or chronic signs and symptoms Laboratory results necessary for all diagnosed patients prior to any dental treatment HBV	Prophylactic antibiotic therapy is contraindicated for surgical and/or any invasive procedures in the severely immune-suppressed patient Complete oral examination identifying any new lesions and/or signs and symptoms that will indicate disease progression Use of Prophy jet, sonic, or ultrasonic instruments is contraindicated
Thyroid problems	Determine type of thyroid disease and medications Monitor blood pressure	Avoidance of epinephrine when treating uncontrolled hyperthyroidism
Respiratory problems (emphysema, bronchitis)	Patient should have medication inhaler at each dental appointment Chair positioning Smoking	Use of the ultrasonic and air abrasives is contraindicated

Continued

TABLE 6-1, CONTINUED

MEDICAL HISTORY INTERPRETATION

QUESTION	REASON FOR QUESTION	TREATMENT PLAN MODIFICATION
Arthritis or painful, swollen joints	Temporomandibular joint (TMJ) involvement Possible increased bleeding time for those patients taking aspirin and nonsteroidal anti-inflammatory medications	Short appointments Chair positioning Appointment time Possible antibiotic premedication for prosthetic joint
Stomach ulcer or hyperacidity	Any medications Stress management	Aspirin and ibuprofen are contraindicated
Kidney trouble	Determine type of kidney disease and current medications Dialysis treatment Kidney transplant Hepatitis carrier Anemia Hypertension Prone to infection and lack of healing Lack of stress tolerance	Antibiotic premedications Monitor blood pressure Bleeding tendency if anemic
Tuberculosis	Establish active or passive disease status Duration of disease Highly contagious Laboratory findings Identify undiagnosed cases through medical history findings and/or chronic signs and symptoms Lowered resistance to infection	Postpone treatment for patients with active disease Use of air abrasives and sonic and ultrasonic devices and nitrous oxide–oxygen analgesia is contraindicated Possible use of high-efficiency mask
Persistent cough or cough that produces blood	Tuberculosis Carcinoma Smoking Emphysema Gastrointestinal conditions	Medical consultation Compromised respiration Chair positioning
Persistent swollen glands in the neck	Immunosuppressive diseases Upper respiratory and infectious diseases	Consultation with physician
Low blood pressure	Monitor blood pressure Dietary and eating habits Exercise regime Dizziness or lightheadedness	Chair positioning Limited stress tolerance
Sexually transmitted diseases	Identification of oral lesions Reinfection	Medical consultation When cases are active, give dental care only in emergencies Use of air abrasives and ultrasonic devices is contraindicated

Condition	Considerations	Dental Management
Epilepsy or other neurologic disease	Drug-induced gingival enlargement Seizure episodes Syncope Emergency care for seizures	Optimum oral hygiene Minimal dental stress Sedation Medications can make patient drowsy, less alert Medical consultation Anticonvulsant drug therapy/side effects, e.g., gingival bleeding, xerostomia, gingival overgrowth
Problems with mental health	Possible medications may cause side effects, e.g., drowsiness, xerostomia Increased periodontal disease and caries	Medical consultation Treatment plans must be coordinated with psychiatric disorder Minimize stress Nitrous oxide–oxygen analgesia is contraindicated
Cancer	History of type, therapy/medication, metastasis, and remission status Side effects of head and neck radiation on oral cavity, e.g., xerostomia and dental caries Compromised healing Treatment and care of any dental disease prior to cancer therapy Hypersensitivity of teeth and oral tissues Oral lesions and infections	Optimal oral hygiene Salivary substitutes for xerostomia Medical consultation Laboratory tests (blood counts) prior to dental treatment Fluoride therapy for increased caries incidence and hypersensitivity Possible antibiotic premedication for anticancer chemotherapy Caution against further dental radiation Palliative treatment for any oral lesions Chlorhexidine rinses for control of plaque and candidiasis
Abnormal bleeding	Association with prior dental treatment Use of any anticoagulants Reveal an underlying history of hepatitis, HIV infection, kidney problems, transplants, blood diseases	Possible laboratory tests Avoid aspirin, aspirin-containing compounds, and nonsteroidal anti-inflammatory drugs (NSAIDs) Medical consultation
Anemia	Identify type of anemia and medications being used Identify oral lesions and symptoms associated with the disease	Avoid general anesthesia for severe anemia Palliative treatment for any oral lesions Delayed healing Laboratory tests Optimal oral hygiene maintenance and frequent recall visits
Treatment for a tumor or growth	Benign or malignant? What kind of treatment was given? Location, description, and duration of tumor or growth	Susceptibility to infection and/or bleeding Medical consultation Conservative treatment if malignancy exists
Women: Pregnancy Nursing Birth control pills	What trimester of pregnancy? Any complications associated with pregnancy Gingivitis influenced by hormones Elevated blood pressure Some antibiotic medication may interfere with the efficacy of birth control pills	Gingival bleeding problems Chair positioning Conservative treatment during the first trimester Avoid x-rays

Source: Adapted from Darby and Walsh (1995).

157

FIGURE 6–1

Medical history form. (Copyright 1988 American Dental Association; reprinted with permission of ADA Publishing Co., Inc., Chicago, IL)

Medical History Form

Date _____

Name _____ Home Phone (_____) _____
     Last   First   Middle

Address _____ Business Phone (_____) _____
       Number, Street

City _____ State _____ Zip Code _____

Occupation _____ Social Security No. _____

Date of Birth ___/___/___ Sex M F Height _____ Weight _____ Single _____ Married _____
      mo. day yr.

Name of Spouse _____ Closest Relative _____ Phone (_____) _____

If you are completing this form for another person, what is your relationship to that person? _____

Referred by _____

For the following questions, *circle yes or no*, whichever applies. Your answers are for our records only and will be considered confidential. Please note that during your initial visit you will be asked some questions about your responses to this questionnaire and there may be additional questions concerning your health.

1. Are you in good health?	Yes	No
2. Has there been any change in your general health within the past year?	Yes	No
3. My last physical examination was on _____		
4. Are you now under the care of a physician?	Yes	No
If so, what is the condition being treated? _____		
5. The name and address of my physician(s) is _____		
6. Have you had any serious illness, operation, or been hospitalized in the past 5 years?	Yes	No
If so, what was the illness or problem? _____		
7. Are you taking any medicine(s) including non-prescription medicine?.	Yes	No
If so, what medicine(s) are you taking? _____		
8. Do you have or have you had any of the following diseases or problems?		
a. Damaged heart valves or artificial heart valves, including heart murmur or rheumatic heart disease	Yes	No
b. Cardiovascular disease (heart trouble, heart attack, angina, coronary insufficiency, coronary occlusion, high blood pressure, arteriosclerosis, stroke)	Yes	No
1. Do you have chest pain upon exertion?	Yes	No
2. Are you ever short of breath after mild exercise or when lying down?.	Yes	No
3. Do your ankles swell?	Yes	No
4. Do you have inborn heart defects?	Yes	No
5. Do you have a cardiac pacemaker?	Yes	No
c. Allergy	Yes	No
d. Sinus trouble	Yes	No
e. Asthma or hay fever	Yes	No
f. Fainting spells or seizures	Yes	No
g. Persistent diarrhea or recent weight loss	Yes	No
h. Diabetes	Yes	No
i. Hepatitis, jaundice or liver disease	Yes	No
j. AIDS or HIV infection	Yes	No
k. Thyroid problems	Yes	No
l. Respiratory problems, emphysema, bronchitis, etc.	Yes	No
m. Arthritis or painful swollen joints	Yes	No
n. Stomach ulcer or hyperacidity	Yes	No
o. Kidney trouble	Yes	No
p. Tuberculosis	Yes	No
q. Persistent cough or cough that produces blood	Yes	No
r. Persistent swollen glands in neck	Yes	No
s. Low blood pressure	Yes	No
t. Sexually transmitted disease	Yes	No
u. Epilepsy or other neurological disease	Yes	No
v. Problems with mental health	Yes	No
w. Cancer	Yes	No
x. Problems of the immune system	Yes	No

SAMPLE

(over)

FIGURE 6–1, CONTINUED

Medical history form. (Copyright 1988 American Dental Association; reprinted with permission of ADA Publishing Co., Inc., Chicago, IL)

9.	Have you had abnormal bleeding?.	Yes	No
	a. Have you ever required a blood transfusion?.	Yes	No
10.	Do you have any blood disorder such as anemia?	Yes	No
11.	Have you ever had any treatment for a tumor or growth?	Yes	No
12.	Are you allergic or have you had a reaction to:		
	a. Local anesthetics	Yes	No
	b. Penicillin or other antibiotics	Yes	No
	c. Sulfa drugs .	Yes	No
	d. Barbiturates, sedatives, or sleeping pills	Yes	No
	e. Aspirin	Yes	No
	f. Iodine	Yes	No
	g. Codeine or other narcotics	Yes	No
	h. Other _____		
13.	Have you had any serious trouble associated with any previous dental treatment?	Yes	No
	If so, explain _____		
14.	Do you have any disease, condition, or problem not listed above that you think I should know about?	Yes	No
	If so, explain _____		
15.	Are you wearing contact lenses?	Yes	No
16.	Are you wearing removable dental appliances?	Yes	No

Women

17.	Are you pregnant?	Yes	No
18.	Do you have any problems associated with your menstrual period?	Yes	No
19.	Are you nursing?	Yes	No
20.	Are you taking birth control pills?	Yes	No

Chief Dental Complaint _____

I certify that I have read and understand the above. I acknowledge that my questions, if any, about the inquiries set forth above have been answered to my satisfaction. I will not hold my dentist, or any other member of his/her staff, responsible for any errors or omissions that I may have made in the completion of this form.

_____
Signature of Patient

For completion by the dentist.
Comments on patient interview concerning medical history: _____

Significant findings from questionnaire or oral interview: _____

Dental management considerations: _____

_____   _____
(Date)   Signature of Dentist

Medical history update:

Date	Comments	Signature
_____	_____	_____
_____	_____	_____
_____	_____	_____
_____	_____	_____

FIGURE 6–2

Medical history interview. (Copyright 1992 American Dental Association; reprinted with permission of ADA Publishing Co., Inc., Chicago, IL)

MEDICAL HISTORY INTERVIEW

Date_____

Part I *(to be completed by patient or guardian)*

Name_____ Home Phone (_____) _____

Address_____ Business Phone (_____) _____

City_____ State_____ Zip Code_____

Occupation_____ Social Security No._____

Date of Birth_____ Sex   M   F   Height_____ Weight_____ Single____ Married____

Name of Spouse_____ Closest Relative_____ Phone (_____) _____

If the person completing this form is other than the patient, what is his/her relationship to the patient?_____

Referred by_____

Part II *(to be completed by dentist)*

A. CHIEF COMPLAINT

_____

B. DENTAL HISTORY

Frequency of visits to dentist_____

Type of care received_____

Difficulties with past treatment_____

Adverse reactions to local anesthetics, latex gloves, rubber dam_____

Date of most recent dental radiographic exam_____

C. MEDICAL HISTORY

Are you now or have you been under the care of a physician during the past 12 months?_____

Last time at physician_____ For what purpose?_____

Physician_____ Physician's Phone No._____

Do you have any known allergies or sensitivities?_____

Do you take any medications at the present time?_____

Females only: Do you take oral contraceptives?_____ Are you pregnant?_____

Have you noted a change in your menstrual pattern?_____

D. FAMILY HISTORY

(Have any members of your family ever been treated for the conditions listed or any other medical problems?)

Diabetes_____ High blood pressure_____ Heart problem_____ Seizures_____

Other_____

E. SOCIAL HISTORY

Smoking_____ Alcohol_____ Other_____

S-502

160

FIGURE 6–2, CONTINUED

Medical history interview. (Copyright 1992 American Dental Association; reprinted with permission of ADA Publishing Co., Inc., Chicago, IL)

F. REVIEW OF SYSTEMS (Have you ever had or do you now have any of the conditions listed?)

I. Skin
Itching_____
Rash_____
Ulcers_____
Pigmentations_____
Lack or loss of body hair_____

II. Extremities
Varicose veins_____
Swollen, painful joints_____
Muscle weakness, pain_____
Bone deformity, fracture_____
Prosthetic joints_____

III. Eyes
Blurring of vision_____
Double vision_____
Drooping of eyelid_____
Glaucoma_____

IV. Ear, Nose, Throat
Earache_____
Hearing loss_____
Frequent nosebleeds_____
Sinusitis)_____
Frequent sore throat_____
Hoarseness_____

V. Respiratory
Cough, blood in sputum_____
Emphysema, bronchitis_____
Wheezing, asthma_____
Tuberculosis, exposure to_____

VI. Cardiac
Shortness of breath_____
Pain, pressure in chest_____
Swelling of ankles_____
High, low blood pressure_____
Rheumatic, scarlet fever_____
Heart murmur, attack_____
Prosthetic valves/pacemakers_____

VII. Gastrointestinal
Difficulty swallowing_____
Abdominal pain, ulcers_____
Hepatitis, jaundice_____
Liver disease_____

VIII. Genitourinary
Difficulty, pain on urination_____
Blood in urine_____
Excessive urination_____
Kidney infections_____
Sexually transmitted diseases_____

IX. Endocrine
Thyroid trouble_____
Weight change_____
Diabetes_____
Excessive thirst_____

X. Hematopoietic
Easy bruising, excessive bleeding_____
Persistent lymphadenopathy_____
G6PD deficiency_____
Anemia_____
HIV infection, AIDS_____
Leukemia, problems with immune system_____
Spleen problems_____

XI. Neurologic
Frequent headaches_____
Dizziness, fainting_____
Epilepsy, fits_____
Neuritis, neuralgia_____
Parasthesias, numbness_____
Paralysis_____

XII. Psychiatric
Nervousness_____
Irritability_____
Depression, excessive worry_____
Nervous breakdown_____

XIII. Growth or Tumor
Radiotherapy/chemotherapy_____

I certify that any and all questions I had about the inquiries above have been answered to my satisfaction. I was asked all of the questions on this form and I have answered these questions truthfully and completely. I will not hold my dentist, or any other member of his/her staff, responsible for any errors or omissions that I may have made.

_____   _____
date   signature of patient

_____   _____
date   signature of guardian (where applicable)

Comments on patient interview concerning medical history:_____

_____

Significant findings from questionnaire or oral interview:_____

_____

Dental management considerations:_____

_____

_____   _____
(date)   (signature of dentist)

Medical History Update:

Date   Comments   Signature

_____   _____   _____

_____   _____   _____

_____   _____   _____

prescribes. Both prescription and over-the-counter medications the patient is taking should be recorded. The name, dosage, and indications also should be written on the form. The hygienist should look especially for any potential drug-drug or drug-food interactions. Adverse side effects (undesirable effects of the drug on the body) of certain medications may be the source of dental problems. For example, antidepressant and antihypertensive medications may cause xerostomia, or dry mouth. Some medications for hypertension or epileptic seizures may cause enlargement of the gingiva, which can result in plaque-control problems. Absorption from the intestines of certain antibiotics such as tetracycline is delayed with food and calcium-containing products including milk and other dairy products. Consultation with the patient's physician may be necessary. If the patient does not know the names of the medications, ask him or her to bring the containers to the next office visit. If a patient is regularly taking medication for diabetes or hypertension, it is extremely important to ask if he or she took the medication as prescribed on that day; if so, the dosage and frequency of usage should be noted on the form. Sometimes a patient may forget to take high blood pressure (antihypertensive) medication and present with uncontrolled blood pressure. If this is the case, the hygienist should contact the patient's physician.

The medical history may uncover other conditions that can have an affect on periodontal health or treatment, such as diabetes mellitus, leukemia, or acquired immunodeficiency syndrome (AIDS) (Neff 1997). If the patient is suspected of being medically compromised, consultation with the patient's physician is indicated (Little and Falace 1997), and a written release should be obtained from the patient before treatment begins.

Infective endocarditis is of particular concern in dental care. Infective endocarditis is an infection of the tissue lining of the heart that can result in damage to the heart valves. Any dental procedure that causes bleeding could allow bacteria to enter the bloodstream, resulting in bacteremia. Before initiating any dental treatment that may cause bleeding in patients who are susceptible to developing infective endocarditis, proper antibiotic protection should be administered. The American Heart Association (AHA) recommends a prophylactic antibiotic regimen for such patients (see appendix A1). Because specific recommendations vary depending on the individual patient's condition, the dental hygienist should collaborate with the dentist and/or patient's physician to determine the appropriate premedication therapy. It is the responsibility of the dental hygienist, however, to screen for susceptible patients by taking a complete health history.

The medical history form is a legal document that provides a past and present profile of the patient's health. After the medical history is complete, the document must be dated and signed by the patient and the dentist, and at each future visit, the form should be updated. The patient should review this information and sign the form again. A new form should be filled out yearly. Indelible ink, preferably black (because it will copy better than blue), should be used. If the patient is a minor, a parent or legal guardian should date and sign the form.

FAMILY HISTORY

The *family history* consists of the present and past medical illnesses of family members. Such a record may help to identify disease trends in the family that are risk factors for dental/periodontal diseases such as diabetes and ischemic heart disease.

DENTAL HISTORY

The *dental history* includes past and present dental treatments, past dental problems, oral habits, nutritional profile, past response to treatment, and oral hygiene status. This information is collected by way of a written form and an interview with the patient. There are numerous dental history forms, each tailored to fit the setting of a particular office or clinic. Table 6–2 ■ is one type of dental history form available.

TABLE 6–2
SAMPLE DENTAL HISTORY FORM

1. Date of last dental examination.
2. Reason for this visit.
3. Date of last x-rays taken.
4. Do you have any pain in your mouth?
5. Do you have difficulty chewing food?
6. Does food catch between your teeth?
7. Have you ever had any serious trouble associated with any dental treatment (e.g., pain, bad experience)?
8. Do your gums bleed when you brush?
9. How often do you brush your teeth?
10. What other aids do you use (floss, bridge cleaners, rubber tips)?
11. Do you live in an area with fluoridated water?
12. Do you use any of the following products at home:

    <u>Yes</u>   <u>No</u>

    a. Fluoride toothpaste
    b. Fluoride rinse/gel
    c. Other antimicrobials   Describe _____
13. Have you ever had any of the following (if unsure, ask the hygienist to describe these treatments):

    <u>Yes</u>   <u>No</u>

    a. Periodontal treatment or surgery
    b. Orthodontic treatment
    c. Extractions
    d. Endodontic treatment
    e. Dental implants   If yes, when _____
                              If yes, explain _____
14. Have you ever had any type of reaction to:

    <u>Yes</u>   <u>No</u>

    a. Local anesthesia
    b. Rubber dam
    c. Latex gloves
                              If yes, when _____
15. How do you feel about your teeth?
16. Do you have a habit of:

    <u>Yes</u>   <u>No</u>

    a. Clenching or grinding your teeth
    b. Chewing cheek or lip
    c. Breathing through mouth
    d. Thumbsucking
    e. Nail biting or biting objects
    f. Smoking
17. Do you use any of the following:

	Amount per Day	Used for How Many Years	What Year Did You Quit
a. Cigarette	_____	_____	_____
b. Cigar	_____	_____	_____
c. Pipe	_____	_____	_____
d. Chew	_____	_____	_____
e. Snuff	_____	_____	_____

18. What smoking-cessation efforts have you tried? When?

The past dental history often provides insight into previous dental experiences, pleasant or unpleasant, in all areas of dentistry, including oral surgery, periodontics, restorative dentistry, endodontics, and orthodontics. Experiences with local anesthetics and nitrous oxide should be recorded. Questions especially pertinent to the dental hygiene visit include those regarding the patient's last dental visit, what was done, and how long since the last prophylaxis.

A nutritional or diet profile of the patient is helpful in assisting the dental hygienist in recognizing a caries-prone diet. During the interview, the dental hygienist can suggest ways in which the patient can alter his or her diet to promote better dental health.

Past dental history also provides information on the patient's dental health values. The periodontal history may be significant. For example, a patient should be asked if previous periodontal surgery was performed (make sure he or she understands what periodontal surgery is). The patient may respond that he or she has had periodontal surgery twice in the past year. On further questioning, it may become apparent that the patient returned to the dental office only once for a periodontal maintenance appointment. This information suggests that the patient is noncompliant with oral hygiene self-care and dental visits.

Other areas to explore include the patient's attitude toward dental care and the present surroundings and the level desire for treatment. Question the patient on what specific oral hygiene regimen he or she follows, including the types of products used. Question the patient on what kind of toothbrush (e.g., soft, medium, or hard bristled), dental floss, and mouthrinse he or she uses. The frequency of product use should be documented, as well as compliance with recommended periodontal maintenance appointments.

SUMMARY

The initial step performed on a periodontal patient is to obtain a complete dental/medical history. Dermination and recording of medications the patient is taking is important since certain drugs affect the periodontium and severe drug interactions can occur. Other risk factors such as the amount of cigarettes smoked should also be recorded.

KEY POINTS

❖ The interviewing process establishes rapport with the patient.

❖ Medical diseases and medications can affect conditions in the mouth.

❖ Update a patient's dental/medical history at every appointment.

REFERENCES

Darby, M. L., and M. M. Walsh. 1995. *Dental hygiene theory and practice,* 249–280. Philadelphia: W. B. Saunders.

Jolly, D. E. 1994. Evaluation of the medical history. *Dent. Clin. North Am.* 38(3):361–380.

Little, J. W., and D. A. Falace. 1997. *Dental management of the medically compromised patient,* 4th ed., 79–102. St. Louis: Mosby–Year Book.

McDaniel, T. F., D. Miller, R. Jones, and M. Davis. 1995. Assessing patient willingness to reveal health history information. *J. Am. Dent. Assoc.* 126:375–379.

Neff, L. 1997. Oral health and systemic disease. *Access* 11(3):29–34.

Peacock, M. E., and R. E. Carson. 1995. Frequency of self-reported medical conditions in periodontal patients. *J. Periodontol.* 66:1004–1007.

Wilkens, E. M. 1994. *Clinical practice of the dental hygienist,* 7th ed., 93–101. Philadelphia: Lea and Febiger.

SELF-QUIZ

1. Which one of the following information collected from the patient is subjective? (pp. 147, 151)

   a. medical history
   b. dental examination
   c. periodontal examination
   d. radiographic survey
   e. oral hygiene evaluation

2. Which one of the following statements explains the importance of patient information collected during the interview? (p. 151)

   a. anticipates patient's attitude about periodontal care
   b. determines the number of visits for the patient
   c. allows the patient to voice their opinions about treatment.
   d. provides a basis for future comparison

3. Which one of the following actions should a dental hygienist take before periodontal treatment is started if the patient cannot remember the names of the mediations he or she is taking? (p. 162)

   a. Call the patient's pharmacist to confirm the medications.
   b. Call the patient's physician to confirm the medications.
   c. Tell the patient to bring the containers to the next appointment.
   d. Tell the patient to call home.

4. On which one of the following parts of the interview does the history of present illness expand? (p. 152)

   a. chief complaint
   b. dietary profile
   c. medical history
   d. social history
   e. dental history

5. All the following types of communications are *most* appropriate to determine the medical history of a patient *except* one. Which one is the exception? (pp. 151–152)

   a. telephone
   b. questionnaire
   c. interview
   d. computer

III. CLINICAL EXAMINATION
A. EXTRAORAL/INTRAORAL EXAMINATION/DENTAL EVALUATION

Ann M. Goodwin, R.D.H., M.S.
Rosemary DeRosa Hays, R.D.H., M.S.

Goal:

To educate the dental hygienist on the clinical components of a dental examination and how it relates to the periodontal condition.

Educational Objectives:

Upon completion of this chapter subsection, the reader should be able to:

Discuss the role of the dental hygienist in evaluating the dental and oral hygiene status of a patient;

Describe the importance of performing an intraoral and extraoral examination;

Describe the components of the dental examination; and

Explain how the findings of the dental evaluation relate to the recognition of periodontal diseases.

KEY WORDS

- oral cancer
- dental charting
- caries
- dental implants
- occlusion
- tooth wear
- parafunctional habits
- dental anomalies
- dentinal hypersensitivity

After completing the patient history, the next aspect of patient assessment involves the collection of objective data by means of a physical examination of the patient. The dental hygienist's tools for this task include the intraoral/extraoral examination, the dental evaluation, the oral hygiene evaluation, the gingival assessment, and the periodontal examination. This section focuses on the intraoral/extraoral examination and the dental evaluation. The section concludes with a brief discussion of dental hypersensitivity.

Extraoral/Intraoral Examination

There are five steps to an extraoral and intraoral examination: inspection, palpation, percussion, auscultation, and olfaction. *Inspection* involves using the eyes to observe the patient. *Palpation* is the action of feeling by the sense of touch. *Auscultation* is the act of listening to sounds from different parts of the body [e.g., using the stethoscope to hear temporomandibular joint (TMJ) sounds on opening]. *Percussion* is the process of striking a part of the body (e.g., detection of the source of a painful tooth) to give off a sound. *Olfaction* involves using the nose to smell odors on the breath such as alcohol or the fruity breath of diabetes mellitus.

In the overall appraisal, the dental hygienist should examine the patient's gait, eyes, lips, skin, and head and neck area. Check for lymphadenopathy or lymph nodes that are abnormal in size, consistency, or number. The TMJ also should be examined.

The overall assessment also includes determination of the patient's vital signs. Vital signs include blood pressure, pulse rate, and respiration rate and provide immediate evidence of the patient's basic physiologic functions. Vital signs should be taken at every dental appointment.

The intraoral examination involves screening for **oral cancer** by examining the tongue, gingiva, lining mucosa, and hard palate for color, bleeding, enlargements, and the presence of pain. It is not within the scope of this textbook to thoroughly discuss the components of the extraoral/intraoral examination.

Dental Evaluation

Dental evaluation begins with a general assessment of the dentition. **Dental charting** is done and analyzed not only for existing restorations, periodontal factors, and needed care but also for the impact of each finding on gingival health. The dental hygienist must examine overhangs, food impaction sites, crown contours, bridge abutments (a tooth or implant used for support and retention of a crown or removable partial denture), and pontics (a missing tooth that is replaced with a restoration and for which there are no roots) as possible plaque-retention sites and evaluate the success of the patient in cleansing these areas. Table 6–3 ■ lists the components of the dental evaluation. Identification of these areas and any resulting

TABLE 6–3
COMPONENTS OF THE DENTAL EVALUATION

- Number of teeth present or absent
- Evaluation of the teeth for dental and root caries
- Restorative status: presence and condition of existing restorations
- Dental implants
- Malpositioning and proximal contact relationships
- Occlusion
- Intraoral appliances
- Conditions of tooth wear
- Parafunctional habits
- Dental anomalies
- Dentinal hypersensitivity

dental needs will allow for sequential planning, proper instrumentation, and continual recording and updating of the patient's clinical services.

EVALUATE THE NUMBER OF TEETH

The dental hygienist should begin by determining which teeth are present or missing in the dentition and charting the findings. Information provided by the past dental history, patient interview, and radiographic findings will enable the dental hygienist to determine whether missing teeth were missing at birth, are impacted, or have been extracted due to periodontal, endodontic, or restorative problems. The history of extractions should be discussed to determine the patient's attitude toward dental health and the incidence of dental disease.

CARIES

Clinical evidence of dental **caries** may be detected first visually, through a change in tooth color, and then by tactile instrumentation and radiographs, fiberoptics, or other transilluminating devices. The standard method for classifying dental caries is G. V. Black's classification system. Types of dental caries are described by location. Pit and fissure caries frequently is found in the grooves and crevices of occlusal, lingual, and buccal surfaces. Smooth-surface caries is found on the facial, lingual, and interproximal surfaces of teeth.

Root-surface caries is found on the roots of teeth. This is of particular concern in periodontal therapy because of an increased accumulation of plaque due to loss of anatomic tooth structure and difficulty in removing tooth-accumulated materials (e.g., bacterial plaque, calculus, and stains) from that location. Several risk factors predispose to root caries: (1) gingival recession, which exposes the cementum to the oral environment (causes of gingival recession include periodontal disease and postperiodontal surgery; the number of teeth with gingival recession increases with age only because the teeth have been in the mouth longer), (2) xerostomia, particularly in the elderly due to systemic medication, which may decrease salivary flow, (3) head and neck radiation, resulting in xerostomia, (4) advanced age, because of age-related reduction in salivary gland function, (5) lack of fluoride, and (6) smoking and poor general health status or multiple medication use (smokers and patients on multiple medications had a significantly higher prevalence of root caries than nonsmokers and patients in good health; Ravald and Birkhed 1992, Page 1998).

Root caries is detected clinically by visual inspection and/or use of an explorer or periodontal probe. There are two classifications of root caries. Root caries either can be apparent on an exposed root surface (Fig. 6–3 ■), where the gingival margin has receded onto the root surface below the caries, or has developed in a pocket, with the gingival tissue covering the root area in a way that makes detection of the caries more difficult. Root caries is preventable with rigorous oral self-care and professional care.

RESTORATIVE STATUS

Existing dental restorations should be evaluated for defective or overcontoured surfaces, overhanging margins, and proximal contacts. Ill-fitting removable prosthetic appliances, including clasps, also should be noted. Patients complaints of

FIGURE 6–3

Gingival recession allows for visibility of root caries on the palatal surface of the maxillary first molar.

floss breaking or shredding may indicate a defective restorative margin. Noting any inadequacies is of particular concern in the periodontal assessment. Any dental restoration should follow the contour of the original tooth, and there should be a tight, firm contact point between the restoration and the adjacent tooth. Overhangs and open margins are conducive to plaque retention, impede oral hygiene, hinder proper scaling and root planing, affect probing accuracy, and can contribute to gingival inflammation and periodontal breakdown. At each appointment, the dental hygienist should update and record any changes that will influence ongoing treatment and continuity of care.

DENTAL IMPLANTS

Dental implants and their prosthetic suprastructures present a vast array of dental configurations conducive to plaque retention. Patient complaints about an implant should be addressed as soon as possible (Wilson 1996). Methods of examination of dental implants and peri-implant tissues (Fig. 6–4 ■) are reviewed in Chapter 16.

MALPOSITIONING AND PROXIMAL CONTACT RELATIONSHIPS

Evaluation of malposed teeth should include teeth that are in facial or lingual version when compared with the normal alignment of existing dentition. Malpositioning can have an effect on oral hygiene and the integrity of a sound periodontium. Tooth crowding can occur anywhere in the dentition. Crowding of teeth may encourage food impaction and plaque accumulation by compromising oral hygiene and consequently exacerbating gingival inflammation (Fig. 6–5 ■). Crowding of teeth per se does not cause or accelerate periodontal tissue destruction, but crowding does make oral hygiene difficult, resulting in the accumulation of bacterial plaque and calculus, and this can then start the process of tissue destruction.

Often a missing tooth may cause the adjacent tooth to tip mesially. When the crown tips or tilts into the edentulous space, causing the gingival on the mesial surface to bunch up, a plaque trap is created. When proximal contact is lost, for

FIGURE 6–4

Dental implants replacing the maxillary left central and lateral incisor, canine, and first premolar. Check the tissues around implants and implant stability.

FIGURE 6–5

Crowding of the mandibular incisors decreases the efficiency of oral hygiene practices.

example, after an extraction, teeth can drift or shift physiologically (both crown and root movement) into the edentulous space. Tipped (just the crown moves, whereas the root is stationary) and drifted teeth (the entire tooth has moved) can lead to uneven marginal ridges. If a tooth is missing, the opposing tooth may extrude into the edentulous space (Fig. 6–6 ■). In such a situation, the tooth will be coronal to the line of occlusion. When a tooth is apical to the occlusal plane, it is said to be *intruded.* Frequently, a tilted or extruded tooth is associated with a plunger cusp, which is a pronounced cusp with steep inclined planes that causes a wedging effect on the interproximal area of the opposite arch. This may lead to food impaction and inflamed tissues.

Contacts between teeth should be checked using dental floss. The patient may complain of food impaction where there is an open contact or disastema between two adjacent teeth. Open contacts develop because of (1) congenital tooth abnormalities, (2) teeth that are extruded beyond the occlusal plane, (3) loss of support from an adjacent tooth, and (4) loss of bone support around a tooth (causing the tooth to move and lose adjacent tooth contact; Fig. 6–7 ■).

FIGURE 6–6

The maxillary first molar is ankylosed and never fully erupted. This tooth is intruded. The mandibular first molar is extruded above the occlusal plane. Uneven marginal ridges result from this occlusal problem.

FIGURE 6–7

Numerous diastemas in the maxillary arch were caused by loss of bony support.

Adjacent marginal ridges should be at the same level. Uneven marginal ridges due to extrusion or intrusion of a tooth produce a poor tooth contact relationship, which results in loss of protection of the interdental papillae from food impaction or trauma.

OCCLUSION

Occlusion describes the contact relationship of teeth in function and dysfunction and is defined as any contact between the incisal or occlusal surfaces of the maxillary and mandibular teeth. It consists of all tooth contacts during swallowing and chewing. *Centric occlusion* (CO) is defined as maximal intercuspation or contact of the maxillary and mandibular teeth. The *centric relation* (CR) is the most retruded (posterior) position of the mandible in relation to the maxilla from which lateral movements of the jaw can be made.

An "ideal" or normal occlusion occurs where the arrangement of teeth is considered to be most correct. This is to say, on closing the mouth, all upper and lower teeth come together at the same time and there are no crowded, malposited, or tipped teeth. Few patients have an ideal or normal occlusion. Usually, there are deviations from normal. Any deviation from the ideal or normal occlusion, for example, crowding, malposited, or tipped teeth, is referred to as *malocclusion*. However, malocclusion does not necessarily indicate occlusal disease. Classification of the various forms of malocclusion is done with Edward H. Angle's principles of defining occlusion. This classification is based on the interdigitation of the maxillary and mandibular teeth. Malpositioning is described in terms of crowding of individual teeth or groups of teeth. Figure 6–8■ describes the three classes of mal-

FIGURE 6–8

Classification of malocclusion: Angle's classification.

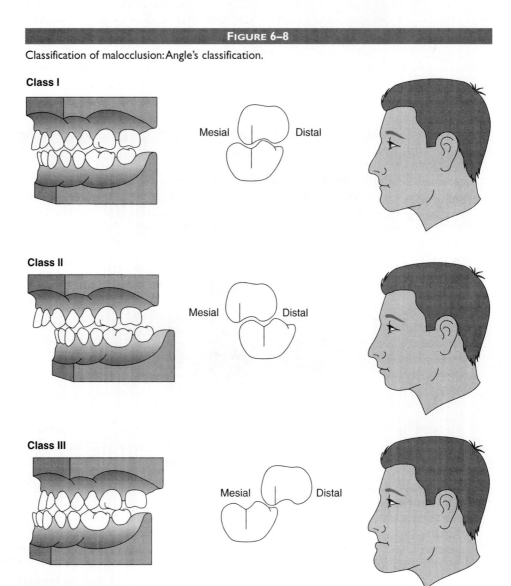

Class I

Mesial   Distal

Class II

Mesial   Distal

Class III

Mesial   Distal

occlusion. If the maxillary first molar is missing, the maxillary canine is used. The use of study casts to provide a better indication of occlusion is sometimes required. The main purpose for using this classification is for diagnostic consistency and treatment planning because malocclusion is a contributing risk factor for inflammatory periodontal diseases.

Functional occlusion consists of teeth that are in function when the mandible moves in lateral and protrusive excursions or movements. Lateral movements are defined by the direction in which the mandible is moving (Fig. 6–9 ■). If the mandible moves to the left, the movement is called a *left working movement,* and the left side of the arch is known as the *working side.* In a left working movement, the right side is known as the *nonworking (balancing) side.* If the mandible moves to the right, the movement is called a *right working movement,* and the right side of the arch is then referred to as the working side. The left side is referred to as the nonworking (balancing) side. For some patients, a lateral movement results in contacts between the posterior teeth on the working side. This is called *group function* (Fig. 6–10 ■). For other patients, a lateral movement results in contact only between the maxillary and mandibular canines on the working side. This is called *canine protection* or *canine guidance* (see Fig. 6–11 ■). It is generally believed that during lateral movements there should be no tooth contact on the nonworking side. However, balancing side contacts are probably prevalent in most patients. Denture wearers need tooth-to-tooth contacts on both the working and nonworking sides for the dentures to function effectively.

Protrusive occlusion is movement of the mandible in a direction anterior to centric occlusion (Fig. 6–11). Guidance for this movement should be on the anterior teeth, and edge-to-edge contact of the incisors should be possible. Any posterior contact during protrusive occlusion is considered undesirable.

Prematurity, or *premature contact* (also called an *occlusal interference*), occurs when there are interferences to closure of opposing teeth. In other words, individual teeth touch the opposing teeth before full closure in centric occlusion and prevent the other teeth in the arch from achieving contact. Premature contact

---

FIGURE 6–9

Illustration of centric occlusion (*center*). Teeth close together with even pressure on both sides of the mouth. In right working movement (*left*), the mandible moves to the right. In left working movement (*right*), the mandible moves to the left.

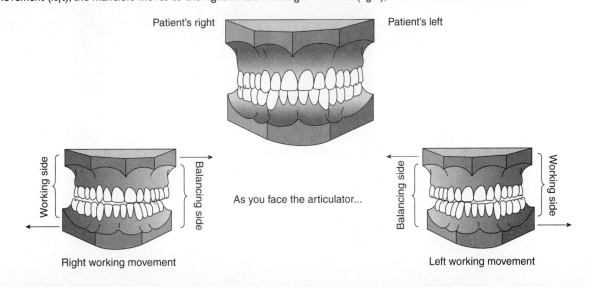

Patient's right   Patient's left

Working side   Balancing side

As you face the articulator...

Balancing side   Working side

Right working movement   Left working movement

FIGURE 6–10

Group function: Lateral movement results in contact of all posterior teeth (*top*). Canine guidance: Lateral movement results in contact between the maxillary and mandibular canines (*bottom*).

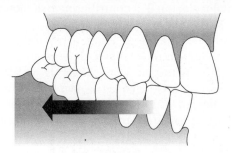

Right working movement
All posterior teeth are in contact: group function

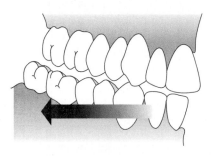

Right working movement
Only the canines are in contact: canine protection

FIGURE 6–11

Protrusive occlusion (movement): Mandible moves forward from centric occlusion so that there is contact of the incisors.

also can occur during lateral movements, either on the working side or on the non-working side. Posterior interference is seen frequently with an extruded or tipped tooth. A classic example of a prematurity occurs when an amalgam filling is too high (placed above the line of occlusion), and on biting down, the patient feels as though that particular area is touching first. Therefore, in this situation, one or

FIGURE 6–12

A deep overbite causes the mandibular incisors to touch the palatal gingiva of the maxillary anterior area.

more teeth are touching the occlusal surface rather than all the teeth touching simultaneously.

Cases where patients have occlusions that are not ideal but are symptom-free and their dentition "survives" or "adapts" to this deviated occlusion are referred to as *physiologic occlusion. Pathologic occlusion* occurs when patients show evidence or signs and have symptoms of occlusal disease (Goldman and Cohen 1980). This is reviewed in Chapter 13.

Overbite (amount of vertical overlap of anterior teeth) and *overjet* (horizontal protrusion of upper teeth beyond the lower) are measured with a periodontal probe. Normally, the incisal edges of the lower incisors and the cingulum of the upper incisors establish the stops necessary to maintain tooth position. A deep overbite can occur as a result of skeletal relationship, extrusion or migration of teeth, or if posterior teeth are missing causing the anterior teeth to handle the occlusal load. Overclosure of anterior teeth can cause trauma to the gingiva of the maxillary and/or mandibular anterior teeth (Fig. 6–12■). This is referred to as *traumatic overbite.* An *open bite* occurs when anterior and/or posterior maxillary and mandibular teeth do not occlude.

INTRAORAL APPLIANCES

Orthodontics, retainers, and splinting wires often present difficulty in cleansing the areas through normal toothbrushing and flossing techniques. Once plaque builds around such appliances and the gingival tissue response occurs with edema and gingival overgrowth, the condition becomes even more difficult to manage. Determining the need for altered home care through a complete oral hygiene analysis can prevent future inflammatory responses.

CONDITIONS OF TOOTH WEAR

Conditions and situations that may account for loss of tooth structure include dental attrition, abrasion, and erosion. Usually, the intraoral examination coupled with a patient interview will reveal the type of **tooth wear** and its causes.

Figure 6–13

(a) Attrition of the maxillary teeth due to buxism. (b) Note that the brownish dentin is exposed as a result of enamel loss.

(a)   (b)

Attrition is the loss of tooth structure as a result of tooth-to-tooth contact. Causes include a parafunctional habit such as bruxism (unconscious clenching or grinding of teeth), constant chewing of abrasive foods, the normal wear of tooth structure by physiologic masticatory (chewing) forces, or the mesial drifting of teeth due to the normal aging process. It is important to recognize a bruxing habit in patients who are undergoing restorative care. Contact between a natural tooth and a porcelain crown surface results in rapid wear of the tooth because porcelain is a very hard material. It is best to have tooth-to-artificial-crown contacts on a metallic surface or a highly polished porcelain surface. Attrition is found most often on the incisal/occlusal surfaces of teeth (Fig. 6–13a,b ■) but also is found on proximal tooth surfaces that are flat, as seen with mesial drifting. Attrition also occurs as *wear facets,* which are small, smooth, polished, flat surfaces on the enamel where there is heavy tooth contact. Usually wear facets are seen on the side of a tooth cusp.

Abrasion is the abnormal mechanical wearing away of tooth structure for reasons other than mastication. Frequently, it is evident on exposed cementum as a notch apical to the cementoenamel junction (Fig. 6–14 ■). Examples of abrasion include excessive force from improper toothbrushing techniques, (Dyer, Addy, Newcombe 2000) use of a hard-bristle toothbrush and very abrasive dentifrices. Abrasion also can occur on the incisal/occlusal surfaces when an object such as a pin or pipe is held between the teeth for many years.

Erosion is the chemical wearing away of tooth structure, usually enamel (Fig. 6–15 ■). It is caused by dietary acids (e.g., acidic beverages, lemons) and gastric juices coming from regurgitation or vomiting, as seen in bulimia. Location of the erosion cannot be considered pathognomonic (a direct cause) for certain etiologic factors, although if erosion is present on the palatal surfaces of maxillary incisors, it is most likely due to gastric juices. Traditionally, erosion is proportionally greater in younger patients, but erosion may increase with age as the salivary flow rate decreases.

Parafunctional habits

Parafunctional habits are activities of the masticatory (chewing) system that are beyond the normal range of function. Chewing and swallowing are normal as opposed to grinding and clenching, which are abnormal. *Bruxism* is the unconscious

FIGURE 6–14

V- or U-shaped notching at the exposed cervical root surface just apical to the cementoenamel junction. This pattern of tooth wear (abrasion) may be associated with improper toothbrushing technique.

FIGURE 6–15

Erosion in a 35-year-old woman who was bulimic. Chronic vomiting wore away the enamel on the palatal surfaces of the maxillary anterior teeth, creating a shiny, smooth surface.

grinding and/or clenching of the teeth when the patient is not swallowing or chewing. During sleep, it is called *nocturnal bruxism* and is often associated with stressful situations. While most patients show signs of bruxism, only 5 to 20% are consciously aware of it (Hallmon et al. 1996). The early signs of bruxism may go undetected, but with increased duration, intensity, and direction of the habit, wear facets will be visible on tooth surfaces and tooth mobility may be seen (Attansio 1991). Initially, this increase in functional demand will be accommodated by the periodontium. Other changes include cusp fractures, increased thermal sensitivity, and increased tooth mobility, which can resolve when the parafunctional action is discontinued. Other examples of parafunctional habits include nail biting, tongue thrusting, and chewing of foreign objects between the teeth such as bobby pins, nails, pipes, and pencils.

Tongue thrusting or thumb sucking often creates a class II, division I malocclusion with an anterior and posterior open bite (Fig. 6–16 ■). During swallowing, the tongue is placed between the maxillary and mandibular anterior teeth and on

FIGURE 6–16

An anterior open bite caused by tongue thrusting.

the sides rather than on the hard palate near the rugae. The lips and chin muscles contract, visualized as a massive grimace. Tongue thrusting eventually can lead to a mouth breathing habit, which may cause a localized gingival inflammation of the maxillary and mandibular incisor region that is unrelated to plaque accumulation. In addition, the lips will be dry and parted at rest.

Parafunctional activity can produce symptoms from the musculature or TMJ. Palpation of the muscles of mastication can detect muscle spasms or pain. Parafunctional habits may lead to occlusal trauma. *Occlusal trauma* is defined as injury to the attachment apparatus as a result of excessive occlusal force.

DENTAL ANOMALIES

Knowledge of dental morphology, supplemented by radiographs and the patient's dental history, is needed to identify anomalies. An *anomaly* is defined as a deviation from normal tooth development or function. Examples of **dental anomalies** include cervical enamel projections (CEPs), enamel pearls, and palatogingival grooves.

The palatogingival groove of maxillary incisors, more often lateral than central incisors (Hou and Tsai 1993), has been described as a predisposing factor to localized periodontal disease. The groove originates in the cingulum and extends mesially or distally in an apical direction along the root surface (Fig. 6–17a,b ■) and can involve the entire root. The groove acts as a plaque trap, making the plaque inaccessible to oral hygiene. Because approximately 8% of patients exhibit this defect, dental hygienists should be aware of its existence (Robison and Cooley 1988). Patients who have this condition often will have a deep pocket associated with the area.

A CEP is an extension of enamel from the cementoenamel junction apically to the entrance of the furcation, which may predispose the area to plaque accumulation and periodontal destruction within the furcation (Machtei et al. 1996; Fig. 6–18 ■). It may be difficult to detect a CEP clinically because the area is covered by gingiva. The highest incidence of CEPs is on the buccal aspect of the mandibular second molars.

FIGURE 6–17

(a) Palatogingival groove extending from cingulum on the palatal surface of the maxillary lateral incisior onto the root surface. (b) The probing depth is 6 mm.

(a)

(b)

FIGURE 6–18

A cervical enamel projection (CEP) on a mandibular molar. (Courtesy of Dr. Raymond Yukna.)

An enamel pearl is similar to a CEP except that it consists of a clump of enamel most commonly located in the bifurcation of molar roots just apical to the cementoenamel junction (Fig. 6–19 ■). It also contributes to plaque accumulation and sometimes is mistaken for calculus.

Dental hygienists must be aware of these tooth anomalies and their importance of their presence in the etiology of local periodontal breakdown. The earlier these conditions are recognized, the better is the outcome of treatment.

FIGURE 6–19

Enamel pearl located at the lingual bifurcation on the mandibular first molar resembles a pearl. It is a potential plaque trap.

DENTINAL HYPERSENSITIVITY

Many patients experience **dentinal hypersensitivity** as a painful response to an irritation where roots are exposed. Dentinal hypersensitivity is a transient, sharp pain arising from exposed dentin in response to a stimulus; it does not last very long. Hypersensitivity will vary in intensity from very mild to excruciatingly painful. Some patients can tolerate the pain, whereas others simply cannot endure it.

ETIOLOGY OF DENTINAL HYPERSENSITIVITY

Although not all patients with exposed dentin experience dentinal or root surface hypersensitivity, an estimated 10 to 25% of people in the United States complain of some type of acute or chronic dentinal hypersensitivity resulting from vigorous toothbrushing, thermal stimulus, mechanical periodontal debridement, or periodontal surgery that exposes the root surfaces.

While there are numerous theories explaining the etiology of hypersensitive tooth surfaces, the most prevalent theory is the hydrodynamic explanation (Paine, Slots, and Rich 1998). This theory states that the fluid in the exposed dentinal tubules contracts or expands when an external stimulus is applied. The pain experienced is due to this minute fluid movement within the tubules.

The most common situation in which hypersensitivity occurs is as follows: Initially, gingival recession occurs, in which the gingival margin migrates apically as a result of trauma or forceful toothbrushing, and this exposes the underlying cementum. The thin cementum can be worn away easily by the abrasive agents in dentifrices or from mechanical root debridement, which exposes the underlying dentin and the open dentinal tubules. Usually the pain is instigated by thermal changes such as cold air or cold foods (ice cream or a cold drink), a mechanical stimulus such as toothbrushing or touch with an instrument or other object, or a chemical stimulus such as sweets.

IDENTIFICATION

It is important to rule out any dental pathology. The dental hygienist can be among the first practitioners to recognize dentinal hypersensitivity. A patient usually complains of a tooth that hurts but will not say, "I have a hypersensitive tooth." If a patient cannot identify a specific tooth, then the problem probably is not a hypersensitive tooth but rather a root or crown fracture, leaking restorations, or teeth in hyperfunction. If the patient points to a tooth, the dental hygienist should ask further questions pertaining to various risk factors.

Testing for sensitivity should be a part of the initial examination and should include something that can be used as a baseline measurement of sensitivity. The air-blast test is one method of assessing hypersensitivity. The area should be dried before using the air syringe. Most patients who have gingival recession should have sensitivity tests. It also may be important to do pretreatment sensitivity tests before periodontal therapy (e.g., instrumentation, periodontal surgery) so that it can be determined if any posttherapy sensitivity was present before treatment or has resulted from the treatment.

SUMMARY

The dental examination follows the medical/dental history and is an intricate step in assessing baseline data and dental care of the patient. With a thorough and systematic approach to the dental examination, risk factors can be identified that will aid in the appropriate treatment planning needs of the patient.

KEY POINTS

❖ The dental examination involves identification of contributory local risk factors for periodontal diseases.

❖ Individual teeth and the entire dentition are examined for deviations.

❖ Dentinal hypersensitivity is a common complaint. Identification of the causes will help in its treatment.

REFERENCES

Dyer D, Addy M, Newcombe R. Studies invitro of Abrasion by different manual toothbrush heads and a standard toothpaste. J Clin Periodontal 2000; 27:99–103.

Goldman, H. M., and W. D. Cohen (eds.). 1980. Occulsal adjustment, 1065–1111. In: *Periodontal therapy,* 6th ed. St. Louis: C. V. Mosby.

Hallmon, W. W., F. A. Carranza, C. L. Drisko, J. W. Rapley, and P. Robinson. 1996. Occlusion. In: *Periodontal literature review.* Chicago American Academy of Periodontology.

Hou, G. L., and C. C. Tsai. 1993. Relationship between palato-radicular grooves and localized periodontitis. *J. Clin. Periodontol.* 20:668–682.

Machtei, E. E., S. M. Wasenstein, B. Peretz, and D. Laufer. 1996. The relationship between cervical enamel projection and class II furcation defects in humans. *Quintessence Int.* 28:315–320.

Page, R. 1998. Risk assessment for root caries in adults. *Oral Care Rep.* 8:7.

Paine, M. L., J. Slots, and S. K. Rich. 1998. Fluoride use in periodontal therapy: A review of the literature. *J. Am. Dent. Assoc.* 129:69–66.

Ravald, N., and D. Birkhed. 1992. Prediction of root caries in periodontally treated patients maintained with different fluoride programmes. *Caries Res.* 26:450–458.

Robison, S. F., and R. L. Cooley. 1988. Palatogingival groove lesions: Recognition and treatment. *Gen. Dent.* 36:340–342.

Wilson, T. G. 1996. A typical maintenance visit for patients with dental implants. *Periodontology 2000* 12:29.

Self-Quiz

1. Which one of the following risk factors is characteristic for root caries? (p. 168)

    a. smoking
    b. xerostomia
    c. parafunctional habit
    d. alcohol consumption

2. Which one of the following methods best detects root caries? (p. 168)

    a. explorer #23
    b. radiographs
    c. rinsing with a disclosing agent
    d. brushing with an abrasive dentifrice

3. Which one of the following classifications of tooth wear occurs when a patient continuously bites on a pipe? (p. 176)

    a. attrition
    b. erosion
    c. abrasion
    d. fracture

4. All the following habits are considered parafunctional *except* one. Which one is the exception? (pp. 176–178)

    a. tongue thrusting
    b. night bruxism
    c. clenching
    d. eating

5. Which one of the following terms describes the action of feeling by the sense of touch? (p. 167)

    a. inspection
    b. palpation
    c. percussion
    d. olfaction

B. ORAL HYGIENE EVALUATION

Cheryl Westphal, R.D.H., M.S.

Goal:

To provide the dental hygienist with the knowledge to perform an oral hygiene evaluation for the purpose of assessing the presence of tooth-accumulated materials and their effect on the periodontium and the overall periodontal treatment plan.

Educational Objectives:

Upon completion of this chapter subsection, the reader should be able to:

Describe the significance of dental plaque on gingival health;

Discuss calculus formation and its effects on gingival health;

Describe the types of stains and their significance to oral hygiene;

Determine the use and effectiveness of disclosing solutions for assessing gingival health; and

Plan oral hygiene education and resulting services based on the extent and location of tooth-accumulated materials.

*T*he oral hygiene evaluation involves examination of the dentition for the presence of such tooth-accumulated materials as plaque, calculus, and stain. The dental hygienist is the professional primarily responsible for determining the patient's oral hygiene status, and this assessment will be the basis for the dental hygiene treatment plan, patient education, and treatment.

The oral cavity must be evaluated completely in order to plan the needed dental and dental hygiene services and educational emphasis for the patient or consumer of wellness. Therefore, the oral hygiene evaluation could be defined by its many component parts, each part is related to the next in planning the total process of care. All the areas discussed in this subsection are significant to the assessment process and integral to the reevaluation and continuing care needs of the patient or consumer.

Given the vast number of findings in the oral cavity, it is necessary for the dental hygienist to apply sound judgment and employ accurate recording methods and reproducible charting so as to facilitate comparison of the findings from one data point to another. As will be seen, various tools are available for such evaluations, and a number of recording devices have been developed.

KEY WORDS
• dental plaque
• supragingival plaque
• subgingival plaque
• calculus
• tooth stains
• halitosis
• xerostomia

DENTAL PLAQUE

CLINICAL SIGNIFICANCE

Because **dental plaque** or plaque biofilm is the major risk factor for periodontal disease, it is incumbent on the dental hygienist to understand its formation, distribution, removal, and prevention. Dental plaque can be described in terms of its composition, location, ability to adhere to the tooth surface, and the microbial colonies it contains. A complete understanding of the significance of this film will assist the dental hygienist in planning future patient care.

In determining why plaque is the major risk factor for periodontal disease, studies have proven that the microbial colonies present in plaque are the cause of periodontal infections found in both the soft and hard tissues of the periodontium. Löe and his colleagues proved that there is a direct relationship between dental plaque and periodontal diseases (Löe, Theilade, and Jensen 1965). This study has formed the basis of much research on the affects of microbial colonies on gingival health. Some of these studies have shown that removal of dental plaque restores gingival health, and thus there is ample evidence to suggest the need to remove the causal colonies before the infections begin.

Dental plaque is an accumulation of bacteria and other microorganisms and cells on tooth surfaces or on other oral tissues. It is often described as a "sticky film" because of its ability to adhere to the tooth surface and resist rinsing away. *Plaque* most often is synonymous with *bacterial plaque* because it is a dense mass of microbial colonies in a gel-like matrix. However, since plaque contains other microorganisms, it is more accurately termed *microbial* or *dental plaque* or plaque biofilm. Dental plaque is usually invisible, unless stained with a disclosing agent (Fig. 6–20a,b ■) or until the microbial colonies accumulate enough for them to appear as a cheesy-white irregular mass on the tooth surface.

FIGURE 6–20

(a) Supragingival plaque on teeth is visible because of its thickness. (b) This same dentition after use of a disclosing solution.

(a)   (b)

LOCATION OF DENTAL PLAQUE

Supragingival plaque exists on the clinical crown of natural teeth, as well as on restorations, prosthetic teeth, orthodontics appliances, or removable appliances or dentures. **Subgingival plaque** adheres to the irregular surfaces of the cementoenamel junction or the cementum depending on the location of the gingival margin. *Fissure plaque* is seen in the pits and fissures of crowns. At times, an entire tooth surface can be covered with plaque, and the plaque can extend continuously to the subgingival area.

PLAQUE FORMATION

Dental plaque mostly consists of bacterial colonies, but other microorganisms such as viruses, yeast, protozoa, or mycoplasmas can be found. Bacterial colonization has become the primary focus in understanding plaque because of its etiologic role in periodontal disease. One cubic millimeter of plaque may contain more than 10^8, or 100 million, organisms, with hundreds of different species.

Microorganisms initially colonize the mouth during birth, acquired naturally from the mother. In addition, bacteria come to reside in the mouth from such sources as the atmosphere, food, human contact, family members, and animals such as pets (Asikainen et al. 1997). When a tooth begins to erupt, it is exposed to saliva, which contains all the acquired bacteria. At this point, the formation of dental plaque begins (Newman and Listgarten 1999).

Recording of supragingival plaque

Recording a plaque index is essential before, during, and after periodontal therapy. In a dental office setting, it is advisable to choose a plaque index (see Chapter 3) that will enhance patient self-care education. The plaque control record (O'Leary, Drake, and Naylor 1972) demonstrates the distribution of plaque on the cervical areas of teeth. This index shows where the patient is missing with toothbrushing and hopefully will motivate the patient to improve his or her brushing technique.

DENTAL CALCULUS

CLINICAL SIGNIFICANCE

Plaque has been identified as the primary risk factor for periodontal diseases, yet the importance of **calculus** as a contributor to the disease cannot be denied. *Tartar* is synonymous with *calculus* in the laypersons' terminology. *Tartar* is used to describe the sediment or crust on the side of a wine cask. The term was coined by a Swiss-German physician who identified all stony accretions in humans as tartars because they were similar in composition of the potassium bitartrate deposits on wine casks (Mandel 1990). The term *calculus* is a Latin-rooted word meaning "pebble" or "stone." Needless to say, the population has become more aware of the word *tartar* because of the advertising of "tartar control" toothpaste and rinses.

The population is more aware of plaque and its relationship to gingivitis than it is of subgingival plaque and its relationship to periodontitis. Awareness is still lacking in the need to remove plaque to prevent periodontal disease and how to remove supragingival and subgingival plaque. The situation becomes increasingly confusing when descriptions are added of mineralized plaque becoming calculus or of loosely adherent plaque residing on top of mineralized calculus. Because calculus that forms above the gingival margin is both hard and visible, it has become the focus of consumers for removal based for aesthetic reasons. Rather than being a mechanical irritant, as was once thought (Carranza 1996), calculus contributes to the accumulation of plaque by having a porous surface. It is unknown if calculus covered with bacterial plaque is more damaging to tissues than plaque alone (Mandel 1995).

Dental calculus can be defined as mineralized plaque, although calculus has been shown to result in germ-free animals. As with plaque, described according to its location in relationship to the gingival margin, calculus is also described as supragingival and subgingival. The mineralization process occurs separately for supragingival and subgingival plaque, and because of this, varying amounts of calculus can be found in the supragingival and subgingival areas.

Supragingival calculus can occur on any clinical crown, exposed root surface, prosthesis, or restoration. It is associated most frequently with sites that are adjacent to a salivary source, such as the parotid gland (maxillary molar area) or floor of the mouth and salivary caruncle (lingual surfaces of mandibular anterior teeth; Fig. 6–21a,b ■). Any retention site, such as a maligned tooth, a missed area of plaque removal, or an area where mastication does not remove all debris, is a primary site for supragingival calculus formation. The mineral components of calculus are derived from saliva.

The formation of supragingival calculus occurs in layers beginning closest to the tooth. The minerals are deposited within 24 to 72 hours of plaque formation. Minerals from the saliva are deposited in the plaque matrix and around the filamentous bacteria. The process can take approximately 12 days or less for rapid formers. The actual mineralization process can occur in as few as 24 to 48 hours.

FIGURE 6–21

(a) Supragingival calculus on the maxillary first molar opposite Stensen's duct. (b) Supragingival calculus on the lingual surface of the mandibular anteriors in relation to the opening or orifice of the submandibular and sublingual salivary glands.

(a)

(b)

Formation time varies according to the individual, the contents of the saliva, and the ability to remove plaque on all surfaces or various retention sites.

Subgingival calculus is derived from gingival crevicular fluid and any inflammatory exudates. There are more minerals available as the inflammatory process continues, and the calculus contains more calcium, magnesium, and fluoride than supragingival calculus (Mandel 1990). It most often forms in rings around the roots of the tooth or in ledges.

The mineralization process continues as crystals of hydroxyapatite, brushite, and whitlockite form. These crystals have different proportions of calcium and phosphate in combination with other ions, such as magnesium, zinc, fluoride, and other carbonates (Ellwood, Melling, and Rutter 1979). The crystals form in the matrix and then on the surface of the bacteria; finally, they calcify the bacteria.

Other differences in subgingival calculus and supragingival calculus are the hardness of the calculus and the difficulty in removing it. Supragingival calculus is 30% mineralized, whereas subgingival calculus is 60% mineralized. Subgingival calculus is more difficult to remove because of this hardness. The color of the two calculus types varies from yellow-white for supragingival calculus to the gray or black for subgingival calculus. Unless the subgingival calculus is minutely visible at the gingival margin, this coloration adds little to its removal. The gray or black color derives from the bacterial and blood pigments.

The structure of calculus was described as layers in supragingival calculus. These layers build into incremental lines on the surfaces of a tooth. The surface of the calculus is irregular and rough. Plaque accumulates on the surface of the calculus. It can lodge in the pits and valleys of the calculus surface. In the subgingival calculus the outer surface may be less calcified. Again, subgingival plaque can accumulate. In either case, the plaque on the surface of the calculus contains living bacteria and is detrimental to the tissue. In this sense, calculus is a contributing risk factor for periodontal diseases. The calculus acts as an irritant to the gingival margin or the sulcular tissue. The overlying bacterial plaque continues to be the etiologic factor in periodontal disease.

Because of the complex attachment of calculus to root surfaces, removal is difficult. Four modes of attachment of subgingival calculus to root surfaces have been recognized (Zander 1953):

1. attachment by means of mechanical locking into irregularities in the cementum;
2. attachment into areas of cementum resorption;
3. attachment by means of an organic pellicle; and
4. attachment by penetration into bacteria (not accepted by all researchers).

TOOTH STAINS

DEVELOPMENT AND SIGNIFICANCE

Tooth stains are discolorations on or within tooth surfaces. Depending on its origin, the stain can be classified as *exogenous* or *endogenous*. Depending on its location, the stain can be *intrinsic* if it is internal to the hard tissue or *extrinsic* if it is external to the surface. Exogenous stains are derived from external sources and often are thought to reside on the outer surface of the tooth. They come from chromogenic (producing color or pigment) bacteria, foods, or chemicals. Endogenous stains are incorporated into the structure of the tooth and cannot be removed by surface polishing. Combinations of these classifications can exist, so stains can be exogenous and extrinsic or endogenous and intrinsic (Table 6–4 ■).

TYPES OF INTRINSIC STAINS

Endogenous stains are always intrinsic because they come from within the tooth and therefore are incorporated into the tooth structure. Examples include (Goldstein and Garber 1995)

1. a nonvital tooth where the pulpal contents have discolored the enamel (this could have resulted from deep dental caries);
2. an older patient in whom the teeth appear "yellowish brown" from dentin exposure (with aging, the enamel becomes thinner, exposing the darker color of the underlying dentin);
3. ingestion of excessive fluoride (fluorosis) between the third month of pregnancy and 8 years of age (the teeth appear as whitish opaque to brownish);
4. ingestion of the antibiotic tetracycline during calcification of the developing teeth.

Women should not take tetracycline after the second trimester of pregnancy, and children up to 8 years of age also should not be given tetracycline. Minocycline, a semisynthetic derivative of tetracycline, can cause discoloration in adult teeth. Discoloration depends on concentration (the more tetracycline ingested, the more discoloration). Initially, a yellow fluorescent color is seen that changes to a nonfluorescent grayish brown color.

Extrinsic stains may become intrinsic if they are incorporated into the enamel or dentin, as in amalgam leakage or tobacco stain embedded into the enamel surface.

TYPES OF EXTRINSIC STAINS

Yellow stain can cause the tooth to appear yellowish or dull. It is associated with the color of the underlying plaque and can be removed by plaque removal. Brown-black stain can be seen in coffee or tea drinkers who do not brush enough to remove the tannin. Plaque does not have to be present, since the pellicle may take on the brown staining alone. Increasing brushing frequency or changing the toothpaste to a more abrasive one may be all that is needed to control the staining. Chewing tobacco often penetrates microcracks in the enamel, resulting in a dark brown-black stain.

Smoking tobacco can produce a stain that is light to dark brown and leathery. It will follow the distribution of the plaque or lodge on the tooth surface most exposed to the tar products of combustion. The stain can cover the cervical third of the tooth or expand to cover the central third as well. It is mostly on the lingual surfaces but can be in the pits and fissures as well. Some tobacco staining can be so severe that it will incorporate in the irregular surfaces of the enamel or exposed dentin. The exogenous, extrinsic stain becomes subsurface and intrinsic, and it increases with neglect. After removal of the extrinsic stain by polishing, increased frequency of plaque removal is required for maintenance. Intrinsic stains may require bleaching for removal.

TABLE 6-4

CLASSIFICATION OF COMMON TOOTH STAIN

STAIN	ORIGIN	TREATMENT	FIGURE
Intrinsic stains Brownish red, bluish black	Nonvital pulp	Root canal treatment, tooth leaching	brownish stain
Grayish brown	Tetracycline	Vital tooth bleaching	grayish-brown stain
Whitish brown Localized	Decalcification	Restore with a restoration; use sodium fluoride (0.05%) rinse	
Generalized	Excessive fluoride ingestion during enamel formation (fluorosis)	Restorative care or no treatment necessary	whitish-brown stain
Yellowish brown	Dentin exposure	No treatment necessary	yellowish-brown stain

How old was this person when this happen?

Continued

189

TABLE 6–4, CONTINUED
CLASSIFICATION OF COMMON TOOTH STAIN

STAIN	ORIGIN	TREATMENT	FEATURE
Extrinsic stains			
Brown	Tobacco (nicotine)	Remove with scaling and tooth polishing	brown (tobacco) stain
	Coffee or tea (tannins)	Remove with scaling and tooth polishing	
	Chlorhexidine oral rinse, stannous fluoride dentifrice or rinse	Remove with scaling and tooth polishing Brush dorsal surface of tongue	brown (chlorhexidine) stain
Black line	Gram-positive rods	Remove with scaling and tooth polishing	blackline stain
Green stain	Chromogenic bacteria	No scaling, polish with mild abrasive	

Black-line stain is a black line that follows in continuous fashion, the facial and lingual gingival margin. It has virtually no thickness and is only 1 mm wide. It usually traverses 1 mm above the gingival margin. This stain is associated with the gram-positive rod of *Actinomyces* species (Slots 1974). Even though this bacterium is present, the stain is not associated with poor oral hygiene. The microorganisms embed in an adherent matrix and attach to the pellicle. The stain is common in women and children and occurs naturally. Meticulous home care is required to reduce the quantity or frequency of black stain.

Green stain is light or yellowish green to very dark green. The composition comes from chromogenic bacteria and fungi, decomposed hemoglobin (blood), and some inorganic elements. The stain is common in children, occurring on the gingival half of the facial surfaces of the maxillary anterior teeth and extending to the proximal surfaces. The stain can occur as a small curved line following the gingival margin or become a diffused smear covering the facial surface. The enamel under the stain is often rough and demineralized, which encourages plaque retention. Plaque and stain removal through polishing is necessary, yet prevention of recurrence depends on meticulous home care.

Chlorhexidine, used in oral rinses to control plaque and gingivitis, discolors the teeth with a yellow-brown stain on the proximal surfaces, on restorations, and on the tongue (Löe and Schlott 1970). In approximately 50% of patients, staining occurs within a few days after starting the rinse. The cause of the staining is unclear, but it may be the result of a reaction with foods containing aldehydes or ketones. Although the staining is not permanent, it is a significant side effect that may deter routine compliance. Polishing the enamel or exposed root surfaces removes the stain. Often a patient will have staining only interproximally and not on the direct facial or lingual surfaces. This indicates that the patient practices good oral self-care.

SIGNIFICANCE OF STAINS

The significance of stains relates to the rough surfaces they may create and the resulting plaque retention sites. Stains can adhere directly to a tooth, discolor the pellicle and plaque, or become part of the tooth.

If either of the first two occur, the tooth surface could have an overlay of stain. This is cosmetic at first until it increases in thickness. If plaque adheres to the stain, the same gingival response occurs. The stain needs to be removed in order to promote oral cleanliness and eliminate possible plaque retention sites.

The key to choosing a removal process is identification of the stain by source and location. Analysis of the color is not always the only determinant of source. Some colors, such as brown, may represent poor hygiene, tobacco use, tea or coffee consumption, or dental fluorosis. The analysis also must determine if the stain resides on the surface and can be removed by polishing or is intrinsic and must be removed by tooth bleaching.

HALITOSIS

Halitosis, also called *breath malodor* or simply *bad breath,* is caused by the production of volatile sulfur compounds, primarily methyl mercaptan and hydrogen sulfide, on the breath. A thorough medical history is necessary to rule out a systemic disease as the cause. Oral risk factors include periodontal disease, inadequate oral hygiene, **xerostomia** (dry mouth), gross caries, retained food particles, tongue coatings, oral cancer, gingivitis, periodontitis, and mouth infections. Nonoral risk factors include aging, alcohol and tobacco use, consumption of strong foods (e.g., onion or garlic), and upper respiratory and gastrointestinal problems (Page 1997). However, one study found that only 1% of individuals with halitosis actually had a gastrointestinal condition (Delanghe et al. 1999). Bad breath on awakening in the morning is the result of reduced salivary flow during the night and the lack of tongue and cheek movement to assist in removal of food particles (Young, Oxtoby, and Field 1993).

Treatment of halitosis depends on the cause. In patients in whom oral factors are involved, dental care is indicated. Brushing the tongue may change the oral flora to one that does not produce odor. A review of nutritional factors or use of sugarless products to control odor may be required. Mouth rinses for cosmetic purposes may be used to "freshen" the breath. These cosmetic mouth rinses do not claim to be antibacterial, however. In patients in whom nonoral or medical factors are suspected, referral to a physician is required. A portable monitor that measures sulfide and mercaptans may provide chairside bad breath testing. This information may be used to access the effectiveness of treatment (Rosenberg et al. 1991).

PERIODONTAL HEALTH: MOTIVATION AND BEHAVIOR AND SUMMARY

Since dental and periodontal health is taking on increasing importance for both patients and family members, evaluation of a patient's motivation and behavior in terms of oral self-care is important in the overall treatment plan.

In the process of evaluating a patient's oral hygiene, it is necessary to assess the clinical aspects of oral hygiene as well as relating the patient's attitude toward oral hygiene and his or her commitment to oral hygiene practices.

KEY POINTS

✤ The removal of plaque through daily plaque-control practices and professional cleanings is important in controlling subgingival plaque formation.

✤ Recognition and identification of tooth stains is determined from the medical and dental history, food diary of the patient, and oral hygiene habits.

✤ There are numerous periodontal and medical causes of bad breath that need to be explored to effectively treat halitosis.

REFERENCES

Asikainen, S., C. Chen, S. Alaluusua, and J. Slots. 1997. Can one acquire periodontal bacteria and periodontitis from a family member? *J. Am. Dent. Assoc.* 128:1263–1271.

Carranza, F. A., Jr. 1996. Dental calculus. In: *Clinical periodontology,* F. A. Carranza, Jr., and M. G. Newman (eds.), 8th ed., 150–160. Philadelphia: W. B. Saunders.

Delanghe, G., J. Ghyselen, C. Bollen, D. van Steenberghe, B. Vanderkerckhove, and L. Feenstra. 1999. An inventory of patients response to treatment at a multidisciplinary breath odor clinic. *Quintessence Int.* 30:307–310.

Ellwood, D., J. Melling, and P. Rutter. 1979. The accumulation of organisms on the teeth. In: Society for General Microbiology (ed.): *Adhesion of micro-organisms to surfaces,* 137–164. New York: Academic Press.

Goldstein, R. E., and D. A. Garber. 1995. *Complete dental bleaching,* 2–13. Chicago: Quintessence.

Löe, H., and C. Schlott. 1970. The effect of mouthrinses and topical application of chlorhexidine on the development of dental plaque and gingivitis in man. *J. Periodont. Res.* 5:79–83.

Löe, H., E. Theilade, and S. E. Jensen. 1965. Experimental gingivitis in man. *J. Periodontol.* 36:177–187.

Mandel, I. D. 1990. Dental calculus (calcified dental plaque). In: *Contemporary periodontics,* R. J. Genco, H. M. Goldman, and D. W. Cohen (eds.), 135–146. St. Louis: C. V. Mosby.

Mandel, I. D. 1995. Calculus update: Prevalence, pathogenicity and prevention. *J. Am. Dent. Assoc.* 126:573–580.

Newman, H. N., and M. A. Listgarten. 1999. The development of dental plaque: From preeruptive primary cuticle to acquired pellicle to dental plaque to calculus formation. In: N. O. Harris and F. Garcia-Godoy (eds.): *Primary preventive dentistry,* 5th ed., 21–39. Stamford, CT: Appleton and Lange.

O'Leary, T. J., R. B. Drake, and J. E. Naylor. 1972. The plaque control record. *J. Periodontol.* 43:38.

Page, R. C. 1997. Causes of halitosis. *Oral Care Rep.* 7(4):7–8.

Rosenberg, M., I. Septon, I. Eli, R. Bar-Ness, I. Gelernter, S. Brenner, and J. Gabbay. 1991. Halitosis measurement by an industrial sulfide monitor. *J. Periodontol.* 62:487–489.

Slots, J. 1974. The microflora of black stain on human primary teeth. *Scand. J. Dent. Res.* 82:484.

Young, K., A. Oxtoby, and E. Field. 1993. Halitosis: A review. *Dental Update (UK)* (March):57.

Zander, H. 1953. The attachment of calculus to root surfaces. *J. Periodontol.* 24:16–19.

SELF-QUIZ

1. Löe and co-workers proved that there is a direct relationship between dental plaque and periodontal diseases because the removal of dental plaque improves gingival health. (p. 184)

   a. Both the statement and reason are correct and related.

   b. Both the statement and reason are correct but not related.

   c. The statement is correct, but the reason is not.

   d. The statement is not correct, but the reason is correct.

   e. Neither the statement nor reason is correct.

2. Which one of the following sources accounts for the mineralization of subgingival calculus? (p. 187)

   a. salivary proteins
   b. crevicular fluid
   c. dental plaque
   d. acquired pellicle

3. Which one of the following reasons explains the finding of supragingival calculus on the lingual surfaces of the mandibular incisors? (p. 186)

   a. difficulty in cleaning the area with a toothbrush
   b. inability of efficient salivary flow to that area
   c. presence of the parotid duct
   d. presence of Warton's duct

4. Which one of the following extrinsic stains is related to chromogenic bacteria? (p. 191)

   a. black
   b. brown
   c. green
   d. yellow

5. All visible stains have to be removed from the tooth surfaces because stains are harmful to the teeth? (p. 191)

   a. *Both* the statement and the reason are correct and related.
   b. *Both* the statement and the reason are correct but *not* related.
   c. The statement is correct, but the reason is *not.*
   d. The statement is *not* correct, but the reason is correct.
   e. *Neither* the statement *nor* the reason is correct.

C. Gingival Assessment

Eva M. Lupovici, R.D.H., M.S.

Goal:

To provide the dental hygienist with knowledge of the clinical and histologic features of gingival changes in disease.

Learning Objectives:

Upon completion of this chapter subsection, the reader should be able to:

Describe the rationale for performing a gingival assessment as part of the patient evaluation;

Describe the clinical features of the gingiva in health and disease;

Evaluate the procedures used in performing a gingival assessment;

Explain bleeding at the gingival margin versus bleeding on probing; and

Recognize and discuss factors found in gingival assessment procedures that may be predictors of future disease activity.

Traditional diagnostic procedures are divided into two components: detection of inflammation and assessment of damage to periodontal tissues (Armitage 1996). Detection of inflammation will be discussed in this subsection, and the next subsection addresses the resulting damage to the periodontium.

In considering the status of the periodontium, practitioners frequently state that the tissue is either "normal" or "diseased," with no in-between stage. In medicine as well as in dentistry, however, there is a range of normality. Slight deviations from the healthy norm can fall within the range of normality for an individual.

OBJECTIVES OF A GINGIVAL ASSESSMENT

The purpose of performing a **gingival assessment** is to evaluate the condition of the gingival tissues and to determine inflammatory and noninflammatory changes. Gingival assessment is one of the essential steps in identifying **inflammatory periodontal diseases.** The accurate recording of initial examination findings is essential in formulating an appropriate treatment plan, as a baseline comparison with future clinical findings after the initial phase of therapy is completed, and in subsequent periodontal maintenance visits.

KEY WORDS

- gingival assessment
- inflammatory periodontal diseases
- risk factors

Risk Factors for Gingival Diseases

The inflammatory process occurs in response to the presence of irritation to the tissues caused by dental plaque. Inflammation is the host's response to the irritation, which stimulates tissue repair. However, as noted in Chapter 3, additional **risk factors** predispose a host to gingival or periodontal diseases. Host susceptibility to periodontal diseases should be considered if inflammation is not resolved after treatment. Having knowledge of all the potential risk factors is important in providing the appropriate treatment.

Risk factors for gingival inflammation or gingival enlargement include the following:

1. changes in hormone levels, as seen in pregnancy, menopause, puberty, or use of oral contraceptives;
2. systemic diseases, such as diabetes mellitus, leukemia, or human immunodeficiency virus (HIV) infection;
3. eruption of the permanent dentition; and
4. certain drugs including phenytoin, cyclosporine, and calcium channel blockers.

Clinical Assessment Procedures

When examining the interdental papillae and gingival margin, the dental hygienist should compare them with adjacent areas. These are the first areas that are affected clinically by inflammation. In the presence of inflammation, gingival tissue manifests some or all of the following five cardinal signs: redness (*rubor*), swelling (*tumor*), and heat (*calor*). Pain (*dolor*) and loss of function (*functio laesa*) may not be present until the advanced stages of periodontal disease. If inflammation is not resolved, then the inflammatory infiltrate progresses into the attached gingiva and alveolar mucosa. Since the alveolar mucosa is composed of loose connective tissue, the inflammatory infiltrate travels through it more quickly than through the attached gingiva, which is composed of dense connective tissue.

Color

The entire mouth should be examined visually, not just the anterior portions of the oral cavity. In health, the color of the gingiva is salmon pink. Color is determined by the degree of vascularity, epithelial keratinization, presence of melanin, and thickness of the epithelium. In the presence of inflammation, the color of the tissues can be various shades of red (erythema) or light to whitish pink, depending on the chronicity of the lesion. Initially, there is a bright red color, which can change to deeper red or bluish red (cyanotic) or pale white in severe periodontal disease. *Tissue redness should not be used as the sole indicator of inflammation, nor is it strongly associated with or a predictor for future periodontal disease activity (PDA)* (Halazonetis, Haffajee, and Socransky 1989). However, the *absence of gingival redness is more indicative of the absence of disease* (Lang et al. 1990).

Gingiva color may appear to be healthy superficially at clinical examination and still be diseased because the site of inflammation is deep within the tissues and not seen at the gingival margin until after the disease progresses. Conversely, individuals with thin oral epithelium may have a healthy gingiva that is red in color.

Within the norm range, healthy gingiva varies in color. In certain dark-skinned individuals such as Asians, African descendants, and Mediterranean people, the gingiva will appear to have a light brown to black pigmentation due to the presence of melanin (Table 6–5 ■). Another cause for variation in gingival color may be an amalgam restoration. The metals from an amalgam restoration may absorb into the gingiva causing a bluish gray color. This is termed an *amalgam tattoo*. This condition causes discoloration of the gingiva (Fig. 6–22 ■) but is not inflammatory in nature, and the gingiva is considered to be healthy.

CONTOUR

Examining the contour of the gingiva is the next phase of the gingival assessment (see Table 6–5). Gingival contour is determined by the shapes and positions of the teeth, alignment of the teeth, location and size of the contact area, size of the gingival embrasure, and soft-tissue inflammation. Therefore, the contour of the gingiva will vary from anterior to posterior areas and between individual teeth.

Marginal gingiva and interdental papillae

In health, the marginal gingiva (or free gingival margin) is knife-edged in contour. In disease, the margins become rolled or rounded due to destruction of the circular fibers.

Interdental papillae in healthy gingiva are tightly tucked into the gingival embrasures. Papillae of anterior teeth are pyramidal in shape because they follow the cementoenamel junction (CEJ) and contact areas, which are narrow. Papillae of posterior teeth are flatter because the CEJ is flatter and the contact areas are wider. In disease, the papillae become bulbous or enlarged because of edema. The papillae may be cratered where there is a depression between the facial and lingual papillae or blunted where the tip of the papilla is absent and there is an open gingival embrasure. Blunting of the gingiva also may be due to noninflammatory causes such as overuse or misuse of interdental cleaning aids. It may be caused in response to the use of an interdental brush in areas where the interdental papilla completely fills the gingival embrasure. Changes in the contour of the gingiva can reflect current or past periodontal tissue destruction.

Gingival clefts

In examining gingival contour, the dental hygienist may observe a gingival cleft or a pseudocleft. A gingival cleft is a V-shaped slit that extends apically from the gingival margin. A gingival cleft may be caused by many factors, such as incorrect toothbrushing, improper flossing (flossing cleft), or a break through the gingiva around a tooth as a result of pocket formation. Gingival clefts can resolve spontaneously or may require periodontal surgery.

A pseudocleft is a gingival cleft that occurs when adjacent papillae become enlarged to the point that they join each other at the center of the tooth (see Table 6–5). This is not a true cleft because there is no marginal tissue destruction. Pseudocleft is seen commonly in patients with crowding of teeth or in patients with severely enlarged gingiva who are taking certain medications such as

TABLE 6–5

CLINICAL AND HISTOLOGIC CHANGES SEEN IN HEALTH AND GINGIVITIS

CLINICAL FEATURES	HISTOLOGIC FEATURES	FIGURE
COLOR		
In *health,* the gingiva is salmon pink.	Presence of keratin.	1 salmon pink gingiva
Pigmentation	Indicates the production of melanin by melanocytes; this does not indicate the presence of inflammation or disease.	2 pigmented gingiva
In *acute inflammation,* the tissues exhibit various shades of red (fiery red); in *chronic inflammation,* the gingiva may be a bluish red (cyanotic or magenta), or pale white.	Redness is due to increased vasodilation (engorged blood vessels) resulting in locally increased blood flow. As the condition worsens, the bluish red color is due to stagnation of blood in the vessels. The pale white color is due to the repair process with excessive collagen formation.	3 inflamed gingiva
CONTOUR		
Free gingival margin Knife-edged	Intact gingiva fibers firmly brace the gingiva to the tooth.	4 knife-edged free gingiva margins
Rolled or rounded	Destruction of gingival fibers.	5 rolled free gingiva margins
Gingival cleft	Narrow slit in the gingiva starting at the gingival margin; probably associated with tooth position in the arch or the beginning of pocket formation; not related to occlusal forces, as once thought.	6 gingival cleft

Interdental papillae

Pyramidal or pointed (flatter in posterior)

Papillae completely fill in gingival embrasure; no tissue destruction.

7 pyramidal papillae

Bulbous

Enlarged papillae due to accumulation of fluid in the tissue; the papilla is not tucked in the gingival embrasure but partly covers the enamel.

8 bulbous papillae

Blunted

Destruction of the tip of the papilla.

9 blunted papillae

Absent

Destruction of the entire papilla; occurs where there is a diastema.

10 absent papillae

Cratered

Destruction of the tissue between the papillae; a "concavity"

11 cratered papillae

CONSISTENCY

Firm and resilient

Intact collagen fibers in the lamina propria give the gingiva its firm consistency. Tissues are easily compressed with a blunt instrument.

12 firm gingiva

Continued

TABLE 6–5, CONTINUED
CLINICAL AND HISTOLOGIC CHANGES SEEN IN HEALTH AND GINGIVITIS

CLINICAL FEATURES	HISTOLOGIC FEATURES	FIGURE
CONSISTENCY		
Edematous	Loss of collagen and vascular permeability resulting in fluid accumulation in the surrounding tissue.	 13 edematous gingiva
Fibrotic	Reparative process whereby the fibroblasts in tissue in an attempt to heal produce and secrete excessive collagen. Tissue becomes hard and nonresilient. Tissue is not compressible.	 14 fibrotic gingiva
Retractable	Loss of collagen fibers. Papillae and margins are easily retracted by a blast of air.	 15 retractable gingiva
SURFACE TEXTURE		
Stippling	Stippling results from the intersecting epithelial ridges on the undersurface of the epithelium. An excessive amount of stippling is seen in chronic inflammation.	 16 stippling
Shiny and smooth	Can occur in health or disease. In disease, loss of stippling occurs because of accumulation of fluid in the underlying gingival connective tissue.	 17 loss of stippling

FIGURE 6-22

An amalgam tattoo is seen on the lingual surface near the second premolar. Note the bluish gray color. This is healthy gingiva.

phenytoin, cyclosporine, or nifedipine. Additionally, coronal migration of the gingival margin caused by the gingival overgrowth results in the formation of a pseudopocket or gingival pocket.

CONSISTENCY

The consistency of the gingiva is examined by lightly pressing the side of the periodontal probe against the marginal and interdental gingiva. *Consistency* refers to the firmness of the underlying connective tissue. In health, the gingiva is firm and resilient when pressed. As stated earlier, inflammatory changes occur within the vascular connective tissue of the gingiva, and when edema is present, the tissue will "pit" and not rebound quickly when the periodontal probe is applied lightly. Edema causes gingival enlargement, resulting in the formation of a gingival pocket or pseudopocket. Firm, resilient gingiva may not be an indicator of health, however, as seen with fibrotic gingiva. On examination, fibrotic gingiva will be hard and will not show a"pit" when tested with a periodontal probe.

Recent studies have found that smokers have the same or less gingival inflammation than nonsmokers (American Academy of Periodontology 1996, Stafne 1997). However, the gingival consistency in smokers tends to be fibrotic with rolled gingival margins. Smoking or smokeless tobacco chewing causes the tissue to become hyperkeratinized with an abnormal whitish thickening of the keratin layer of the epithelium. Following smoking cessation, the gingiva returns to its condition prior to smoking (Haber 1994).

During the disease process, the collagen fibers are destroyed, causing the gingiva to be retractable or flaccid (see Table 6–5). Once the inflammation is eliminated and controlled, the collagen fibers may re-form and unite the gingiva to the tooth.

SURFACE TEXTURE

Surface texture is assessed by drying the attached gingiva with gauze and observing the surface for stippling. Clinically, stippling is described as having an appearance similar to the outside peel of an orange. The presence or absence of stippling does not necessarily indicate the health status of the gingiva. Stippling is present in health and in chronic inflammation when the gingiva becomes fibrotic. In chronic inflammation, the presence of stippling represents tissue scarring. Edematous gingival tissue may retain stippling. In the absence of stippling, the gingiva is described as being smooth or shiny.

Size: Gingival Enlargement

The size of the gingiva is influenced by several factors, such as cellular and intercellular elements and vascular supply. In gingival overgrowth or enlargement, the free gingival margin is located coronal to its normal position at or slightly coronal to the CEJ. Gingival enlargement can be the result of a tissue response to inflammation caused by dental plaque, hormonal imbalance in pregnancy and puberty, side effects of certain medications, mouth breathing, and iatrogenic dentistry such as poorly contoured crowns.

Hormonal and Drug-Influenced Gingivitis

Hormonal changes

Clinically, gingivitis in pregnancy is characterized by either generalized or localized inflammation to the gingival papillae, which show a sharp demarcation from the attached gingiva. The inflammation or swelling can spread to involve the marginal gingiva. The gingiva is bright red and edematous, with a shiny, smooth surface. The molars show the most inflammation, followed by the premolars and the incisors (Silness and Löe 1963).

In more severe cases, pregnancy tumors also may occur, but these are not considered a true neoplasm; they are an inflammatory reaction to the dental plaque. Actually, a pyogenic granuloma occurring in a pregnant patient is called a *pregnancy tumor.* This swelling appears mainly in the anterior facial areas of the mouth. It is a mass of tissue that protrudes outward. It is deep red and edematous.

Postpartum, these gingival conditions usually regress to their status during the second month of pregnancy. Most of the gingival changes seen during pregnancy can be prevented by removal of plaque and meticulous home care.

Gingival inflammation during pregnancy is not exclusive to pregnancy. Similar gingival changes, except for pregnancy tumors, are seen in adolescents as *puberty gingivitis.* These patients develop massive gingival enlargement that recurs even in the presence of little plaque. After puberty, the enlargement regresses, but total disappearance only occurs after all local irritants are removed.

Drug-influenced gingival enlargement

Clinically, drug-induced gingivitis is seen as a generalized overgrowth of the gingiva, especially of the interdental papillae on the facial gingiva, of the maxillary and mandibular teeth, particularly the anterior sextent, and does not often occur in edentulous areas (Figs. 6–23 ■, 6–24 ■). Enlargement of the gingiva may result in malpositioning of teeth and interference with normal chewing, speech, and oral hygiene (Pihlstrom 1990). The gingival tissue in cyclosporine-induced overgrowth tends to be more soft, red or bluish red, and fragile, and it bleeds more easily on probing than tissue undergoing phenytoin-induced overgrowth (Hallmon and Rossmann 1999).

FIGURE 6–23

A 38-year-old woman taking phenytoin for seizures for the last 3 years. Note the generalized gingival enlargement, especially the interdental papillae.

FIGURE 6–24

A 56-year-old woman taking nifedipine for hypertension. Note the enlargement of the interdental papillae. The enlarged papillae take on a lobulated or nodular appearance.

In most cases, maintaining strict plaque control can prevent this enlargement, but surgical intervention frequently is required to obtain physiologic gingival contours and aesthetics.

MOUTH BREATHING

The alternative drying and wetting of the gingiva during mouth breathing promotes an inflammatory response causing gingival enlargement from the maxillary canine to the canine. The appearance of the gingiva, especially the palatal surface, is usually shiny and red in color.

MAXILLARY TUBEROSITY

Gingival enlargement of the maxillary tuberosity is not considered to be a disease state. The enlargement is developmental in origin.

HEREDITARY GINGIVAL FIBROMATOSIS

Hereditary gingival fibromatosis is a rare form of severe gingival enlargement seen commonly in children beginning with the eruption of either the primary or permanent dentition. The etiology is unknown, but heredity is most likely involved, and many such patients are mentally retarded. Gingival enlargement is generalized throughout the mouth, involving both the papillae and the marginal gingiva. The teeth may be completely covered by tissue overgrowth, preventing eruption.

GINGIVAL BLEEDING

The next step in the gingival examination is to determine the presence of marginal bleeding. This can be done by several methods, including stroking the lining of the sulcus or inserting a wooden or plastic wedge to assess proximal bleeding (Caton and Polson 1985). If the stroke method is used, the probe is placed within the gingival crevice and is dragged from one interproximal space to the other interproximal space on the same tooth. Any bleeding seen within 30 seconds is labeled as a bleeding site. Bleeding measured at the gingival margin or crevice is often indicative of gingival inflammation. On the other hand, bleeding on probing (bleeding coming from a pocket during periodontal probing) indicates a deeper inflammatory involvement. In private practice or a clinic setting, bleeding on probing usually is recorded as being either absent or present by placing a red dot over the site that bleeds. For research purposes, a bleeding index is used to standardize measurements. It is important to note that bleeding may be masked if the gingiva is fibrotic.

Bleeding occurs when there is disruption of the sulcular and junctional epithelium allowing for passage of blood or exudate from the lamina propria into the sulcus. The epithelium is avascular and receives its blood supply and nutrients from the underlying vascular lamina propria. When the epithelium becomes inflamed, it reacts by forming microulcerations. Thus, sweeping the lining of the crevice or probing allows for blood to pass through from the engorged and newly formed blood vessels in the lamina propria subjacent to the epithelium.

Bleeding traditionally is accepted as an *objective* clinical sign of inflammation; however, some visually inflamed gingival sites do not bleed. Therefore, it can be stated that bleeding is not always an early sign of gingival inflammation, and the actual mechanisms responsible for bleeding probably are not truly understood. In addition, the presence of bleeding from a periodontitis site is a poor predictor of future attachment loss (Armitage 1996). On the other hand, *the absence of bleeding is strongly indicative of low levels of inflammation* (Lang et al. 1990) *and high periodontal stability* (Goodson 1992). Gingival bleeding has been related to increased gingival crevicular fluid flow rate, which is associated with the presence of inflammation (Armitage 1996). Another limitation of the use of bleeding as an inflammatory parameter is the possibility that healthy tissues may bleed on stimulation or probing (Lang et al. 1990) when excessive probing forces are used or improper toothbrushing methods or improper use of interdental cleaning aids has occurred. Thus the dental hygienist must discriminate between bleeding sites that are inflamed and those which bleed for other reasons. In order to eliminate bleeding, the pathologic process must be changed. Traditionally, altering plaque levels by periodontal debridement and improved oral hygiene has been successful, especially in the reduction of gingivitis.

DOCUMENTATION AND SUMMARY

After the gingival assessment is completed, the findings are summarized according to location, distribution, and severity of the gingival changes. The findings can be either localized or generalized (localized to certain areas such as the mandibular lingual teeth or generalized throughout the entire mouth). Distribution is either marginal, papillary, or diffuse. If the marginal gingiva is affected, it is called *marginal inflammation*. If the interdental papillae is affected, it is called *papillary inflammation*. If the free, attached, and/or alveolar mucosa is affected, it is referred to as *diffuse*. Severity is classified as mild, moderate, or severe.

KEY POINTS

✢ The purpose of performing a gingival evaluation is to determine the status of the gingiva and the presence or absence of gingival inflammation and/or gingival enlargement.

✢ Gingival enlargement can be due to an inflammatory response to dental plaque or to certain drugs.

✢ The steps involved in a gingival evaluation include assessing for gingival color, contour, consistency, surface texture, size, and bleeding.

✢ The absence of bleeding indicates periodontal stability.

REFERENCES

American Academy of Periodontology. 1996. Tobacco use and the periodontal patient. *J. Periodontol.* 67:51–56.

Armitage, G. C. 1996. Periodontal diseases: Diagnosis. *Ann. Periodontol.* 1:37–215.

Caton, J., and A. Polson. 1985. The interdental bleeding index: A simplified procedure for monitoring gingival health. *Compend. Contin. Educ. Dent.* 6:88–92.

Goodson, J. M. 1992. Diagnosis of periodontitis by physical measurement: Interpretation from episodic disease hypothesis. *J. Periodontol.* 63:373–382.

Haber, J. 1994. Cigarette smoking: A major risk factor for periodontitis. *Compend. Contin. Educ. Dent.* 15:1002, 1004–1008, 1014.

Hallmon, W. W., and J. A. Rossmann. 1999. The role of drugs in the pathogenesis of gingival overgrowth. *Periodontology 2000* 21:176–196.

Halazonetis, T. D., A. D. Haffajee, and S. S. Socransky. 1989. Relationship of clinical parameters to attachment loss in subsets of subjects with destructive periodontal diseases. *J. Clin. Periodontol.* 16:563–568.

Lang, N. P., R. Adler, A. Joss, and S. Nyman. 1990. Absence of bleeding on probing: An indicator of periodontal stability. *J. Clin. Periodontol.* 17:714–721.

Pihlstrom, B. L. 1990. Prevention and treatment of Dilantin®-associated gingival enlargement. *Compend. Contin. Educ. Dent.* 11(suppl 14):S506–S510.

Silness, J., and H. Löe. 1963. Periodontal disease in pregnancy. *Acta Odontol. Scand.* 21:533–551.

Stafne, E. E. 1997. Cigarette smoking and periodontal disease: The benefits of smoking cessation. *Northwest Dent.* (Sept.–Oct.): 25–29.

SELF-QUIZ

1. Which one of the following features describe the gingival appearance in a patient who is a 30 pack/years smoker? (p. 201)

   a. red gingiva and cratered interdental papillae
   b. red gingiva and bulbous gingival margins
   c. whitish gingiva and absent interdental papillae
   d. whitish gingiva and rolled, receded gingival margins

2. Which one of the following considerations must be addressed by the dental hygienist when performing a gingival assessment? (p. 195)

   a. determine inflammatory gingival changes
   b. evaluate periodontal disease activity
   c. assess destruction of supporting and alveolar bone.
   d. evaluate probing depth changes.

3. Which one of the following statements is related to bleeding on probing or sulcular stimulation? (p. 204)

   a. The absence of bleeding is strongly indicative of low levels of inflammation.
   b. The presence of bleeding from a periodontitis site is a good predictor for future attachment loss.
   c. All visually inflamed gingival sites bleed.
   d. Bleeding occurs when there is disruption of the oral epithelium.

4. All of the following factors are related to gingival enlargement *except* one. Which one is the exception? (p. 202)

   a. gingival inflammation
   b. hormonal changes
   c. cigarette smoking
   d. mouth breathing
   e. nifedipine

5. Tissue redness should be used as the primary indicator of inflammation *because* it is strongly associated with future periodontal disease activity. (p. 196)

   a. *Both* the statement and the reason are correct and related.
   b. *Both* the statement and the reason are correct but *not* related.
   c. The statement is correct, but the reason is *not.*
   d. The statement is *not* correct, but the reason is correct.
   e. *Neither* the statement *nor* the reason is correct.

D. PERIODONTAL ASSESSMENT

Theodore L. West, D.D.S., M.D.S.

Goal:

To provide the dental hygienist with the basic elements for performing a periodontal examination.

Educational Objectives:

Upon completion of this chapter subsection, the reader should be able to:

Explain the purposes for performing a periodontal assessment;

Describe the components of a periodontal assessment;

Explain the clinical significance of each component of a periodontal assessment;

Discuss the significance of measuring clinical attachment loss versus probing depths; and

Compare and contrast several factors that can affect the accuracy of probe readings.

<table>
<tr><th>KEY WORDS</th></tr>
<tr><td>

- screening
- periodontal assessment
- monitoring
- outcome measure
- periodontal disease severity
- periodontal disease activity
- clinical attachment level
- clinical attachment loss

</td></tr>
</table>

$\mathcal{T}$he periodontal examination performed by a dental hygienist has many purposes. First, large population groups in health fairs, schools, hospitals, clinics, and other institutions may need to be examined rapidly for periodontal diseases requiring further evaluation and subsequent treatment—the periodontal **screening**. For visual detection of periodontal diseases, rapid screening can be performed with as little instrumentation as two disposable wooden tongue blades and a flashlight to evaluate tooth loss, migration, and mobility; gingival recession, redness, suppuration, and swelling; and calculus and plaque levels. Essentially, screening is done in a single visit to differentiate between health and disease.

RATIONALE FOR PERIODONTAL ASSESSMENT

A more thorough examination requires a mouth mirror, a periodontal probe, and radiographs. The **periodontal assessment** includes complete medical and dental histories, and the recording of gingival findings, probing depths, clinical attachment levels, tooth mobility, tooth malposition, level of oral hygiene, occlusal relationships, and bone levels.

This periodontal assessment provides the baseline for the long-term **monitoring** of periodontal disease activity. Such monitoring is often performed by the dental hygienist from one to four times a year at the periodontal maintenance visit. Such monitoring for increases in clinical attachment loss, gingival recession, swelling, bleeding, tooth mobility, etc., because of the episodic and recurrent nature of periodontal diseases, is vitally necessary if the patient is to be maintained in a state of periodontal health. It often becomes the dental hygienist's responsibility to find and point out areas of recurrent periodontal disease activity in a patient's mouth.

Finally, the periodontal assessment examination should be used by the practitioner as an **outcome measure** to evaluate the success of periodontal treatment and the need for and frequency of periodontal maintenance visits.

It seems likely that some general dental practices do not adequately assess periodontal diseases (McFall et al. 1988). In a study of almost 2500 patient records from 36 general practices, radiographic bone loss was seen in over half the film sets. However, in only one in five records was there a periodontal diagnostic entry or a notation about pocket formation. This random sample of adult patient records had very infrequent recordings of bleeding, recession, furcation invasions, pocketing, tooth mobility, etc. These findings can be compared with an epidemiologic study in the same state of North Carolina (Bawden and DeFriese 1981) that indicated that 55 to 75% of the adult population was affected by periodontal disease.

If periodontal disease assessment in the general dental practice is inadequate, then it certainly must follow that the monitoring of periodontal disease progression becomes an impossibility. It seems probable that the burden for assessing and monitoring periodontal diseases in a general practice may fall, to a greater or lesser extent, on the shoulders of the dental hygienist.

Although periodontal diseases occur primarily in the adult population, they also can occur in young people, occasionally in a very severe form. Therefore, a periodontal evaluation should be performed for all patients regardless of their age. A national survey of over 2600 individuals 19 years of age and older, using a mouth mirror, explorer, and periodontal probe, showed 28% with periodontitis, 53.9% with gingivitis, and only 17.3% free of periodontal disease in the youngest group (19–44 years). In the 45 to 64 age group, only 8.3% were free of periodontal disease, and 47.6% had pocket depths of 4 mm or more (Brown, Oliver, and Löe 1989). Periodontal diseases have now been associated with increased risk for heart disease, stroke, diabetic complications, and premature, low-birth-weight babies. Since race, socioeconomic factors, nutrition, tobacco use, and various systemic diseases can further increase the prevalence of periodontal diseases at any age, the importance of the periodontal examination is obvious.

Periodontal disease severity represents the total destruction and healing that occur during the lifetime of a tooth (Jeffcoat 1994). It is the status of the periodontium or extent of tissue damage at the time of the examination (Lamster et al. 1993) and is determined by visual inspection, single measurements of probing depths, and evaluating radiographs for bone loss.

Periodontal disease activity, which is different from periodontal disease severity, is defined as the current or ongoing (at the time of the examination) loss of soft-tissue attachment, specifically destruction of the gingival fibers and apical migration of the junctional epithelium with subsequent alveolar bone loss. Periodontal disease activity is usually seen as episodic periods of exacerbation or active periodontal tissue destruction (loss of connective tissue attachment and alveolar bone) with intervening periods of quiescence or disease inactivity (Jeffcoat 1994, Lamster et al. 1993, Greenstein and Caton 1990). Periodontal disease activity is difficult to determine because it is a measurement of the continued breakdown of periodontal pockets between two points in time (separated by several weeks to months). Destruction must have occurred at some time between these two measurements.

While periodontal probing and radiographic assessment are retrospective views of disease activity and cannot identify an active disease site from a inactive one (nor accurately predict future destruction), they are still the foundation on which the classification of the disease and its treatment is made (Haffajee, Socransky, and Goodson 1983). The clinical importance of distinguishing between a progressive or active periodontal lesion and a stable or inactive lesion is apparent. Therefore, more sophisticated techniques and assessments have been introduced recently that are designed to determine current periodontal disease activity and/or if a site will break down in the future (Williams, Beck, and Offenbacher 1996). For a review of these adjunctive assessment tests, see Chapter 8.

PERIODONTAL TERMINOLOGY

PERIODONTAL PROBING DEPTHS

Screening method

Periodontal probing is the most commonly used physical screening method for measuring the depth of the gingival crevice and the clinical attachment level. *Periodontal probing is a clinical approximation of the depth of a gingival sulcus or periodontal pocket* (Armitage 1995). Measurement of probing depths allows the practitioner to make certain presumptions about the state of health of the periodontium. Periodontal pockets are the result of the destruction of the coronal part of the junctional epithelium and the connective tissue attachment to the tooth surface at the apical aspect of the junctional epithelium (Fig. 6–25a,b ■). The clinical significance of having pockets greater than 5 mm in depth is that such pockets may be difficult or impossible for the dental team to maintain in a state of health even with a patient's best oral hygiene self-care efforts and frequent professional cleanings.

Clinically, *probing depth* is defined as the distance from the gingival margin to the most apical extent of the probe or where physical resistance of the probe is met. This approximates the level of soft tissue attachment (junctional epithelium) to the tooth. In healthy gingiva the free gingival margin is approximately 0.5 to 2 mm coronal to the cementoenamel junction (CEJ).

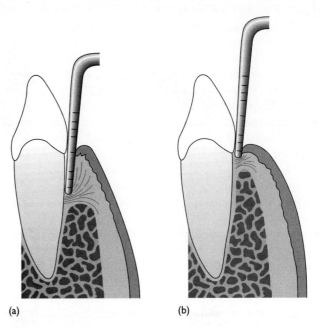

FIGURE 6–25

Probing depth measurement. (a) Deep pocket with apical migration of the junctional epithelium and bone loss. Probing depth is 6 mm. (b) Shallow probing depth (2 mm). There is no attachment loss or bone loss.

(a)   (b)

It should be noted that here we are using the term *probing depth* rather than *pocket depth* because what is being probed could be a pocket or a sulcus. This text will continue to use the term *probing depth* unless otherwise indicated.

Limitations of Probing   In health, the apical extent of the periodontal probe routinely penetrates the coronal to middle portion of the junctional epithelium (Listgarten, Mao, and Robinson 1976; Spray et al. 1978; Robinson and Vitek 1979). When the gingiva is inflamed, the probe can transverse the junctional epithelium to deeper levels within the tissue. It can stop at, enter, or go through the lamina propria to the alveolar bone crest. Thus this measurement may be greater than the actual tissue destruction. Therefore, the clinical probing depth noted may be greater than the histologic probing depth due to probe penetration of inflamed tissue (Armitage, Svanberg, and Löe 1977).

Probing depth measurements have several inherent limitations besides the degree of gingival inflammation (Robinson and Vitek 1979). The apical extent of probe penetration depends on the force used to probe (van der Velden 1979), variations in placement and angulation of the probe, the site being probed, the type of probe used, the size of the probe (Keagle et al. 1989), and tooth anatomy. Other factors that influence the accuracy of probing include the presence of calculus, the visibility of the area, and the level of patient sensitivity. Despite these limitations, periodontal probing remains the most accurate and widely used method of assessing periodontal destruction. When done carefully, a probing difference of 2 mm or more can be clinically meaningful.

Disease Progression   Periodontal probing is important in determining past periodontal disease activity and is used to evaluate the results of periodontal treatment. Single probing measurements do not adequately reflect periodontal disease progression; they only signify past disease activity or the severity of attachment or bone loss at one point in time. Therefore, serial probing measurements must be

Schematic illustrations showing the different positions of the gingival margin. (a) Periodontal health. (b–d) The junctional epithelium has migrated onto the root surface. (Dimensions and relations of the dentogingival junction in humans. Gargiulo A. W.; Wentz, F. M., Orban B. Copyright by the American Academy of Periodontology, Chicago IL; reprinted with permission of the *Journal of Periodontology* 1961; 32: 261–267.)

A. Sulcus depth
B. Attached epithelium
C. Apical point of epithelial attachment below cementoenamel junction
D. Bottom of sulcus from cementoenamel junction
E. Cementoenamel junction to alveolar bone
F. Deepest point of epithelial attachment to alveolar bone

(a)

(b)

(c)

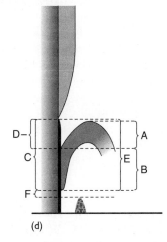
(d)

done (e.g., at periodontal maintenance visits) and compared with previous measurements to determine whether the disease is progressing (Jeffcoat 1994).

Probing depth measurements therefore are good for identifying areas that are potential therapeutic problems on a site-by-site basis (Armitage 1995) and to determine the type of treatment needed. However, in longitudinal monitoring (e.g., at periodontal maintenance visits) for disease progression, probing depths are not reliable in determining the amount of detachment of the soft tissues from the root surface because the gingival margin may change its position over time due to gingival recession or gingival enlargement. This was first described in 1961 by Garguilo, Wentz, and Orban (Fig. 6–26a,b,c,d ■).

Level of attachment

Clinical attachment level (CAL) is the distance from the CEJ to the most apical extent of the periodontal probe or where resistance is met. Clinical attachment level is a clinical approximation of the loss of connective tissue attachment from the root surface (Armitage 1996). *Measuring the level of attachment of the base of the pocket on the tooth surface gives a better indication of the severity of periodontal disease.*

Since the position of the gingival margin changes over time, probing depth measurements are not reliable for determining the extent of detachment of soft tissue from the root surfaces. Measurement of the clinical attachment level is the reference method used to establish disease progression. The CEJ is a stable reference point that does not move over time. If the stationary point used is a part of the tooth other than the CEJ (e.g. cusp tip or restoration), the term used is *relative attachment level.* Although probing depth measurements are considered to be less valid for monitoring disease progression, they still should be considered as a clinical measure (Reddy 1997; Carlos, Brunelle, and Wolfe 1987).

When performing a periodontal charting, it is advisable to measure probing depths and to record the location of the free gingival margin. Future comparisons can then determine disease activity. In addition, the position of the gingival margin relative to the CEJ should be drawn on the chart.

Clinical Connective Tissue Attachment Loss   Attachment level measurements determine the amount of attachment loss if it has occurred on a tooth. **Clinical attachment loss** is defined as the pathologic detachment of the gingival collagen fibers from the root surface with the concomitant apical migration of the junctional epithelium along the root surface. Supporting and alveolar bone resorption also occurs as a result of the inflammatory events, but is a consequence of the attachment loss.

The CAL must take into account the probing depth and location of the gingival margin. A significant increase in CALs is the gold standard for measurement of periodontal disease activity at a given site (Goodson 1986). *Currently, a change in clinical attachment level of between 2 and 3 mm, measured at different examination visits, must occur before a site can be labeled disease-active.*

Individuals who have extensive attachment loss also may have gingival recession, but if they have shallow probing depths and no bleeding, they are considered to have a healthy periodontium and not periodontitis at that point in time. Such patients could have been treated successfully and the disease progression stopped, or they may be in remission with no disease activity present.

OTHER USES OF THE PERIODONTAL PROBE

The periodontal probe can be used not only to determine the level of the soft tissue attachment to a tooth but also to establish the presence of bleeding, the location of the mucogingival junction, the amount of gingival recession, the width of keratinized/attached gingiva, and the consistency of the gingiva.

CONTROLLED-FORCE PROBES

Within the past decade, automated pressure-sensitive or controlled-force probes have been developed that provide a fixed 20- to 25-g probing force in order to reduce examiner error and to make changes of less than 2 mm clinically meaningful. Examples of these probes include the Florida probe (Florida Probe® Corporation, Gainesville, FL) and the Interprobe™ (The Dental Probe Inc., Richmond, VA). Most such probes are connected to a computer for storage of data (see Fig. 6–27 ■). Automated recording of the CEJ also has been developed.

FIGURE 6–27

Example of a periodontal chart generated from a controlled-force probe. (Courtesy of Florida Probe Corporation, Gainesville, FL, *www.floridaprobe.com*.)

Copyright 1996-97 by Florida Probe Corporation, Gainesville, Florida

Continued

FIGURE 6–27, CONTINUED

Example of a periodontal chart generated from a controlled-force probe. (Courtesy of Florida Probe Corporation, Gainesville, FL, *www.floridaprobe.com*.)

FLORIDA PROBE®

Chart #:
Name:
Examiner:
Examination Date:

Tests Performed: ☒Recession ☒Probing,Bleeding,Suppuration
☒Furcation ☒Plaque ☒Mobility

Tooth #	DB		B			MB		ML		L			DL		
1	2.8 B		2.4	R=2	F=1 P	2.4		1.4	F=0	1.6	R=3		2 B		F=0	M=1
2	2.2		1.6	R=1	F=0	1.6	P	3.8	F=0	2.2B	R=3	P	2.6		F=0	M=1
3	2	P	1.4	R=1	F=0	2.4 B	P	2.4 BS	F=0	2	R=2		2.4		F=0	M=0
4	2.8	P	2.6	R=0		1.4		1.8		2.6	R=1		2			M=0
5	2 B	F=0 P	3	R=1		1.6	F=0	2.2		1.8	R=1		2.6			M=0
6	2.4		1.0	R=0		2		2.8		2.4	R=0	P	2.8 B			M=0
7	2.4		1.4	R=0		2.4		1		0.4	R=0.0		0.8			M=0
8	0.8		0.8	R=0		1.4		1.4		1.4	R=0.0		1			M=0
	MB		B			DB		DL		L			ML			
9	1		2.2	R=0		2		0.8		0.8	R=0.0		1			M=0
10	1.4		1	R=0		1		0.6		0.4	R=1		0.6			M=0
11	2.6		2.4 B	R=1	P	2.2	P	1.2		2.8	R=1		2.4			M=0
12	1	F=0 P	2.6	R=1		1.2 BS	F=0 P	2.8		2.2	R=2	P	2.4			M=0
13																
14	1.2		2.6	R=1	F=0	2.4		3.2 B	F=0	2.2 S	R=1	P	1.4 S		F=0	M=0
15	2.6		2	R=2	F=0	2 B	P	2 BS	F=0	1.6 S	R=2	P	1.8		F=0	M=0
16	3		2.6	R=2	F=0	4.8 S	P	2.2 B	F=0	2.6	R=2	P	2.4		F=0	M=1
17	2.6		2.6	R=2̸	F=0 P	4	P	3.4		2.4 B	R=2	F=0 P	2			M=1
18	1.2		0.6		F=0 P	1.6 BS	P	1.6		0.6	R=2	F=0 P	1			M=0
19	1.4		1.2	R=2	F=1	2.0		2.8 S		3.2	R=2	F=0 P	2.2 B			M=0
20	0.6	P	1.6	R=2		1.4 B		1.8		2.4	R=1		2.2			M=0
21	1.0	P	1.2	R=2		1		2		2.4	R=1		2.0			M=0
22	2.2		1.4 B	R=0		0.6		1		1.4	R=0		2			M=0
23	0.8		1.6	R=0		0.8		1		1	R=0.0		0.6			M=0
24	0.4		1.6	R=0		1.8		1		1	R=0.0		1.8			M=0
	DB		B			MB		ML		L			DL			
25	1		0.8	R=0.0		0.8		2		2	R=0		2.6			M=0
26	1.6		1.2	R=0.0		0.6		0.8 B		2.2	R=1		1.4			M=0
27	1	P	1	R=2		0.8		2.2		1.2	R=2		1.8			M=0
28	4.6		2.6	S R=0		2		2.6		2.8	R=2	P	2.8			M=0
29	1.2		1.2	R=1		1.8		2		1.6 BS	R=2		2.6			M=0
30																
31	2.0	P	3	S R=2	F=1 P	2.4 BS		2.6		2.6	R=1	F=0	2.4			M=1
32	1.6 B		2.0	R=2	F=0 P	2.6		1.6		0.4	R=1	F=0	2.2			M=1

Plaque Index Scores

All surfaces:	26%
Molar:	45%
Inter-proximal:	26%
Buccal Lingual:	26%
Buccal:	20%
Lingual:	33%

Probing Summary

30 Teeth   22 Bleeding sites   13 Suppurating
11 sites progressing deeper by at least 1mm.
5 moderate sites with 2 progressing deeper by at least 1mm.
0 severe sites with 0 progressing deeper by at least 1mm.
3 furcations were found.
6 teeth were found to have some degree of mobility.

With automated probing, the loss of tactile sense inherent in manual probing has been shown to increase rather than decrease probing errors. This is especially true in probing the patient with untreated periodontitis in whom subgingival calculus deposits are present. In the treated patient, controlled-force probing has been shown to be more accurate in some studies but not in others (Armitage 1996).

Although the Florida probe has been used in a number of research studies to reduce the interexaminer error and the Interprobe was designed for routine clinical practice, their use has not been widely accepted. The automated probing examination may be more time consuming when compared with manual probing with no clear advantage of increased accuracy. It seems likely, however, that rapid, accurate, and easy-to-use automated probes will be available in the near future.

EXAMINATION TECHNIQUES

PERIODONTAL PROBING DEPTHS

To assess the probing depth, six measurements are recorded for each tooth, three on the facial surface (mesiofacial, facial, distofacial) and three on the lingual surface (mesiolingual, lingual, distolingual). It is best to develop a standardized sequence when probing. For instance, probing should start on the facial tooth surfaces of the maxillary right quadrant, proceeding to the maxillary left quadrant, then to the palatal surfaces of the maxillary right quadrant, then to the maxillary left quadrant, and finally to the mandibular quadrants in the same sequence. The probe is "walked" in approximately 1-mm increments to follow the level of attachment (Fig. 6–28 ■). Spot probing is not adequate for a thorough periodontal examination. When a reading is between two millimeter marks on the probe, the higher reading is used.

FIGURE 6–28

Walking the probe around the tooth allows exploration of the morphology of the gingival crevice. (Reprinted with permission of Procter & Gamble, Cincinnati, OH.)

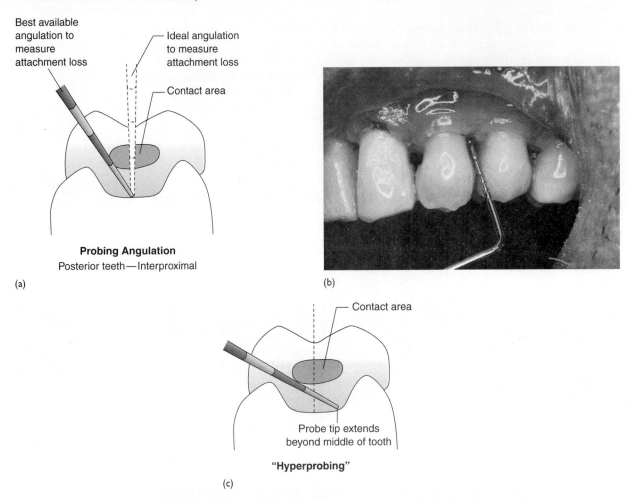

FIGURE 6–29

(a) Correct probe angulation on a posterior tooth. Probe inserts under the contact area into the col. (Courtesy of James A. Simonds, D.M.D., *Practical Periodontics,* Copyright 1991. Continental Education. Santa Rosa, CA.) (b) Clinically, the probe is angled to reach the col. (c) Incorrect probe angulation. (Courtesy of James A. Simonds, D.M.D., *Practical Periodontics,* Copyright 1991. Continental Education. Santa Rosa, CA)

Best available angulation to measure attachment loss

Ideal angulation to measure attachment loss

Contact area

Probing Angulation
Posterior teeth—Interproximal

(a)

(b)

Contact area

Probe tip extends beyond middle of tooth

"Hyperprobing"

(c)

Most errors occur in interproximal readings. When probing interproximal sites on posterior teeth, the probe is angled slightly so that the tip of the probe reaches the col area, just under the contact area of the tooth (Fig. 6–29a,b,c ■). When probing interproximal sites on anterior teeth, the probe needs to be parallel to the long axis of the tooth but at the same time should be as close to the interproximal area and not at the line angle (Fig. 6–30 ■). The probe is parallel to the long axis of all teeth on the facial and lingual surfaces.

Bleeding sites

In clinical practice, the primary value of bleeding on probing as a diagnostic sign is that its presence indicates that the tissues are inflamed and not healthy (Armitage 1995). Bleeding points should be recorded on the chart with a small red

FIGURE 6–30

Correct probe placement on an anterior tooth. Probe is not angled, but it must reach interproximally with the shank against the teeth.

dot over the probing depth measurement. Bleeding on probing indicates inflammation in the deeper tissues, whereas bleeding or stroking the gingival crevice indicates gingivitis. *Sites that bleed with deep pockets and clinical attachment loss are at greater risk for future tissue destruction and should be monitored* (Lang and Löe 1993, Lang, Joss, and Nyman 1990). Sites that do not bleed on probing are likely not breaking down.

CLINICAL ATTACHMENT LEVEL

To assess the CALs, two measurements are needed: probing depth and the distance of the gingival margin from the CEJ at each of the six sites around the tooth. If gingival recession is present (Fig. 6–31a ■), the CAL is determined by adding the gingival recession value and the probing depth. If there is gingival overgrowth or a pseudopocket (see Fig. 6–31b ■), the CAL is determined by subtracting the amount of gingiva (in millimeters) coronal to the CEJ from the probing depth measurement gingival corona to CEJ distance from the probing depth. If the free gingival margin is located at the CEJ (see Fig. 6–31c ■), the CAL is equal to the probing depth. There is more tissue destruction or loss of attachment when gingival recession is present. When the attachment loss is 5 mm or greater with deep periodontal pockets, the patient should be referred to a specialist.

Another method to determine the CAL is to give a negative number to the amount of recession and then subtract it from the probing depth. A positive number is given to the amount of gingival overgrowth and then subtracted from the probing depth.

Repeated measurements, when done in this manner, have been shown in numerous studies to be reproducible to within ±1 mm 90% of the time and within ±2 mm 99% of the time (Armitage 1996). Attachment loss of more than 2 mm has become the gold standard for the assessment of periodontal disease progression (Armitage 1996). This change is necessary to take into consideration the inherent errors, as mentioned earlier, in periodontal probing.

FIGURE 6–31

Probing depth versus clinical attachment level. Probing depth is the distance from the free gingival margin to the attached gingival tissues. Clinical attachment level is the distance from the CEJ to the attached gingival tissues. When the free gingival margin is apical to the CEJ (a), add the amount of recession to the probing depth [3 mm + probing depth (2 mm) = 5 mm clinical attachment level]. When the free gingival margin is coronal to the CEJ (b), the distance to the CEJ is measured and subtracted from the probing depth (5 mm probing depth −2 mm gingival enlargement = 3 mm clinical attachment level). (c) When the free gingival margin is at the CEJ, the probing depth equals the clinical attachment level (2 mm probing depth = 2 mm clinical attachment level).

(a)

(b)

(c)

PERIODONTAL SCREENING AND RECORDING

The Periodontal Screening and Recording (PSR) system provides a rapid, 2- to 3-minute periodontal screening examination to be performed by a dentist or hygienist for the detection of periodontal diseases and monitoring of the periodontal patient. This system was developed by the American Dental Association and the American Academy of Periodontology with financial support from the Procter & Gamble Company. PSR indicates when a more comprehensive full-mouth periodontal examination should be done. Implants are examined in the same way as natural teeth.

The key component of the system is a thin, plastic or metal, ball-end periodontal probe. The ball tip enhances patient comfort and aids in detecting overhanging margins and subgingival calculus. The probe has a colored band extending from 3.5 to 5.5 mm for classifying pocket depth. The mouth is divided into six sextants or sections. Although six sites are probed on each tooth as in a conventional periodontal examination, only the deepest site in each sextant is scored and recorded in the patient's chart. The PSR code score is determined by how much of the colored band is visible when the PSR probe is placed in the gingival crevice (Fig. 6–32a ■).

The following are the codes used:

Code 0: Colored probe area completely visible; no bleeding; no calculus or roughness

Code 1: Colored probe area completely visible; bleeding; no calculus or roughness

Code 2: Colored probe area completely visible; bleeding; calculus and/or roughness

Code 3: Colored probe area partially visible (4–5 mm depth)

Code 4: Colored probe area submerged completely (>5.5 mm depth)

An asterisk is used to denote a furcation defect, tooth mobility, mucogingival involvement, or soft tissue recession.

The treatment of patients is based on their sextant scores (see Fig. 32b,c ■). A code 3 or code 4 indicates that a more comprehensive periodontal examination and charting of the affected sextant is required to determine the treatment. When this system is used in the long-term monitoring of periodontal patients whose deep probing sites are being maintained nonsurgically, recording the tooth number and attachment level alongside the PSR coding box facilitates rapid monitoring of these sites at each periodontal maintenance visit.

SUPPURATION

Suppuration, also referred to as *purulent exudate* or *pus,* is a clinical feature of inflammation. Pus is composed of dead cells, polymorphonuclear leukocytes (PMNs or neutrophils), and tissue fluids. The presence of suppuration indicates an ongoing infection in the periodontal pocket. Pus can be detected visually coming from the pocket by either probing the gingival crevice or using digital pressure from the base of the crevice on the outer surface of the gingiva moving in a coronal direction.

TOOTH MOBILITY

Tooth mobility is classified as either physiologic or pathologic. Physiologic movement of a tooth is limited to the width of the periodontal ligament space. All teeth have some degree of physiologic mobility that occurs with normal function. The range of physiologic mobility varies according to the time of the day and the tooth. It is most evident on teeth with short roots, such as mandibular incisors, and early in the morning. Increased tooth mobility in the hours just after awakening is due to slight extrusion of the tooth as a result of limited occlusal contact during sleep (Carranza 1996).

Pathologic mobility of teeth results from bone loss, gingival inflammation, periapical pathology, hormonal imbalance (e.g., pregnancy gingivitis), or occlusal trauma, where excessive occlusal forces are placed on a tooth. Periodontal disease can be advanced without any evidence of increased tooth mobility. Therefore, the

FIGURE 6–32

PSR system. (Courtesy of the American Dental Association, Chicago, IL.) (a) Code 0, code 1, code 2, code 3, code 4.

(a)

FIGURE 6–32, CONTINUED

PSR system. (Courtesy of the American Dental Association, Chicago, IL) (b) A box chart is used to record the scores for each sextant. (c) Treatment implication for code 2 involves oral hygiene instructions and subgingival plaque removal. (Courtesy of ADA.)

(b)

(c)

TABLE 6–6

CLASSIFICATION OF PATHOLOGIC MOBILITY (MILLER'S CLASSIFICATION)

I. First distinguishable sign of tooth movement in a facial/lingual direction
II. Movement of the crown in a facial/lingual direction up to 1 mm
III. Movement of the crown in a facial/lingual direction more than 1 mm and/or depressed in a vertical direction

severity of tooth mobility is not always due to the amount of bone loss. Since tooth mobility may not result from periodontal problems, identification of the cause is important so that the appropriate treatment can be rendered.

Measurement of tooth mobility

The degree of mobility can be measured either manually or with electronic devices. Although the most common classification for measuring pathologic tooth mobility is the Miller classification, it remains very subjective. Mobility is assessed by using the handles of two hand instruments on the facial and lingual aspects of the crown and applying force. The Miller classification is summarized in Table 6–6 (Miller 1950). Mobility requires treatment when the patient feels discomfort or when the mobility increases over time.

FREMITUS

Fremitus is the vibrational movement of a tooth under occlusal forces. Fremitus is determined by gently placing the index finger on the facial surfaces of the maxillary teeth while instructing the patient to tap the teeth together and grind them side to side. Only the maxillary teeth are checked for fremitus because the arch is fixed where as the mandibular arch is moving.

FIGURE 6–33

Pathologic tooth migration in a 26-year-old woman with rapidly progressive periodontitis. The patient complained of flaring and increasing space between the maxillary central incisors.

The amount of fremitus is subjective, but the following guide can be used:

+ (slight vibrations can be felt);

++ (obvious, palpable vibrations can be felt, but movement of the tooth is barely visible); or

+++ (visible movement is seen).

Fremitus should be eliminated by occlusal adjustment by means of, say, selective grinding.

PATHOLOGIC TOOTH MIGRATION

Pathologic tooth migration is defined as the movement of teeth due to the disruption of forces that normally maintain physiologic tooth position. Tooth movement can occur in any direction. Clinically, this may be seen as increased spacing between teeth, dramatic overjet of anterior teeth (anterior flaring), rotation of teeth, or extrusion where tooth migration occurs in an occlusal or incisal direction (Fig. 6–33 ■). Usually tooth mobility is also present. Any of these symptoms is a common chief complaint of a patient that may prompt a professional evaluation. As part of the clinical examination, it is important to ask the patient if spaces between the teeth have increased over time or if they have always been present. It is important to recognize signs and symptoms of pathologic migration and determine the cause of the problem in order to render appropriate treatment.

Periodontal disease destruction of the attachment apparatus plays a major role in the etiology of pathologic migration (Towfighi et al. 1997). Other contributing factors include parafunctional habits such as tongue thrusting or bruxism, teeth adjacent to edentulous areas, and drug-induced gingival enlargement.

FURCATION INVOLVEMENT

A *furcation* or *furca* is the area of root division on multirooted teeth, including the maxillary first and second molars, maxillary first premolar, and mandibular first and second molars. The third molars usually have fused conical roots. Since the maxillary molars have three roots (mesiobuccal, distofacial, palatal), they are

FIGURE 6–34

Dry-skull specimen of a furcation involvement on the mandibular molars. Root trunk length is the distance from the CEJ to the entrance (roof) of the furca.

ROOT TRUNK

ROOF
OF FURCA

tirfurcated. There are three furcation entrances: mesial, distal, and buccal. The mandibular molars are bifurcated; that is, they have two roots (mesial and distal). There are two furcation entrances: buccal and lingual. The maxillary first premolar is also bifurcated, having a buccal and lingual root. There are two furcation entrances: mesial and distal.

Furcation involvement occurs when interradicular bone (bone between the root branches of the same tooth) destruction occurs. Furcation involvement is affected by factors such as the length of the root trunk and the presence of root concavities, which create a plaque trap. The root trunk is the area on the tooth from the CEJ to the roof or entrance of the furca (Fig. 6–34 ■). As seen radiographically, high furcation with a short root trunk will have a greater chance of interradicular bone destruction early in the disease process than a low furcation with a long root trunk. The average root trunk length on a maxillary molar is about 4 mm at the mesial, 5 mm at the distal, and 4 mm at the buccal furcation. The root trunk length of the mandibular molar is 3 mm on the buccal aspect and 4 mm on the lingual aspect (Gher and Dunlap 1985; Dunlap and Gher 1985). This suggests that a minimum of 5 mm of attachment loss on a molar may result in early furcation involvement.

Classification of furcation involvement

The clinical detection of furcation involvements is important because it is difficult for both the patient and the dental hygienist to effectively clean these areas. Radiographic interpretation does not allow sufficient detection of furcation involvement. The anatomy of the tooth and location of the furca are determined from both the radiograph and clinical examination. The pattern of interradicular bone loss is both horizontal and vertical. Although many classifications of horizontal furcation involvement have been suggested, Glickman's classification is described in Table 6–7 ■. Classification of vertical bone loss (Tarnow and Fletcher 1984) is described in Fig. 6–35 ■.

Technique for locating furcation involvements

A calibrated curved Nabers probe is used to clinically locate the furcation entrances and degree of horizontal pattern of bone destruction (Fig. 6–36a ■). In the

TABLE 6–7

GLICKMAN'S CLASSIFICATION OF FURCATION INVOLVEMENT
(HORIZONTAL PATTERN OF BONE DESTRUCTION)

Grade I Involvement: Pocket formation into the fluting of the furca, but the interradicualr bone is intact. No gross or radiographic evidence of bone loss. This is recorded on the periodontal chart as ∧

Grade II Involvement: Interradicular bone is destroyed on one or more aspects of the furcation, but a portion of alveolar bone and periodontal ligament remains intact. This is recorded on the periodontal chart as △

Grade III Involvement: The furcation is occluded by gingiva but the interradicular bone has been destroyed so that a probe can be passed through from one surface to the other. This is recorded on the periodontal chart as ▲

Grade IV Involvement: The periodontium is destroyed to such a degree that the furcation is open and exposed and clinically visible. ▲

Source: From Carranza, F.A., and H. H. Takei. 1996. Treatment of furcation involvement and combined periodontal-endodontic therapy. In: F.A. Carranza and M. G. Newman (eds.): *Clinical periodontology,* 640. Philadelphia: W. B. Saunders. Illustrations courtesy of James A. Simonds, D.D.S., Copyright 1991 *Practical Periodontics.* Continental Education. Santa Rosa, CA.

FIGURE 6–35

Schematic drawing of a mandibular molar demonstrating the vertical classification of furcation involvement. The amount of vertical bone loss is determined from the roof of the furca apically.
(Reprinted with permission from the American Academy of Periodontology. Copyright 1984 *J. Periodontol.* 1983;55:283–284.) Tarnow D., Fletcher P. Classification of the vertical component of furcation involvement.

Root trunk

Grade A 1–3 mm

Grade B 4–6 mm

Grade C 7 mm +

FIGURE 6–36

(a) Placement of the Nabers probe in determining the presence of a buccal furcation. Note that the handle is parallel to the occlusal plane. (b) Nabers probe placed to determine the presence of a mesial furcation of a maxillary molar. Note that the handle
is parallel to the long axis of the tooth when probing interproximal furcations.

(a)   (b)

maxillary molar, the mesial furcation is not centered. The entrance is usually located about two-thirds of the buccal-lingual width toward the palatal aspect of the
tooth (see Fig. 6–36b ■). Thus the mesial furcation is approached from the palatal
side. The distal furcation is centered equally from the buccal and palatal aspects
of the tooth (in the interproximal area), and thus the Nabers probe can be positioned from either the buccal or palatal side. The instrument handle is placed parallel to the long axis of the tooth. When a furcation defect is found, it is noted in
the chart on the involved root. Furcations thus can be classified according to their
horizontal and vertical component of bone loss, for example, IIA.

Cervical enamel projections

Cervical enamel projections (CEPs) are extensions of enamel toward and often into the furcation area. This area is thought to be a plaque trap, enhancing plaque accumulation. This area may be more prone to attachment loss because instead of a connective tissue attachment, the periodontal attachment on enamel will be via a junctional epithelium, which may not be as strong (Easly and Drennan 1969). However, it has been demonstrated that an epithelial attachment may be just as resistant as a connective tissue attachment to inflammatory disease.

GINGIVAL POSITION

In health, the free gingival margin is located approximately 0.5 to 2 mm coronal to the CEJ. *Gingival recession* (also called *gingival atrophy*) is defined as a shift in the gingival margin apical to the CEJ with exposure of the root surface to the oral environment. Actually, since the soft tissue margin may not always be composed of gingiva, the term *soft tissue recession* rather than *gingival recession* may be more appropriate. However, since this is currently not universally accepted, this text will continue to use *gingival recession* (Wennström 1996). Gingival recession may be localized to one tooth or generalized throughout the mouth. Usually the facial surface is involved, but all other tooth surfaces could be involved as well.

Measurement of gingival recession

Visible recession, which is seen clinically, is measured from the CEJ to the gingival margin and represents the apparent position of the gingiva. Hidden recession, which is covered by the gingiva and therefore not visible, can only be measured by placing a periodontal probe at the level of attachment. This represents the actual position of the gingiva or the level of soft tissue attachment (junctional epithelium) to the tooth surface (Carranza 1996; Fig. 6–37 ■). The visible recession added to the hidden recession equals the clinical attachment level. The clinical importance of measuring recession is often overlooked. There can be loss of attachment or gingival recession without a corresponding increase in probing depth. This often can be misleading, and it could be assumed that there is no tissue destruction occurring when actually there is.

Etiology of gingival recession

The principal predisposing factor that determines whether recession occurs is the anatomy of the area, specifically the thickness of the alveolar bone and overlying gingiva. The etiology of gingival recession is multifactoral. Etiologic factors include:

1. mechanical trauma: soft tissue trauma from overzealous toothbrushing;
2. orthodontic movement;
3. dental procedures;
4. crown margins;
5. clasps from partial dentures;
6. destructive inflammatory periodontal disease, where there is loss of attachment (destruction of gingival fibers and apical migration of the junctional epithelium; Fig. 6–38 ■);
7. tooth malposition (rotated, lingually or facially displaced teeth), where the alveolar bone over a prominent root such as a maxillary canine is thin or absent;

FIGURE 6–37

Diagram showing visible and hidden recession. Clinically, visible recession is determined by measuring with a periodontal probe from the CEJ to the free gingival margin. Hidden recession corresponds to the probing depth. The visible recession measurement added to the hidden recession measurement equals the clinical attachment level (CAL). (Reprinted with permission from James A. Simonds, D.M.D. *Practical Periodontics,* Continental Education. Santa Rosa, CA. Copyright 1991.)

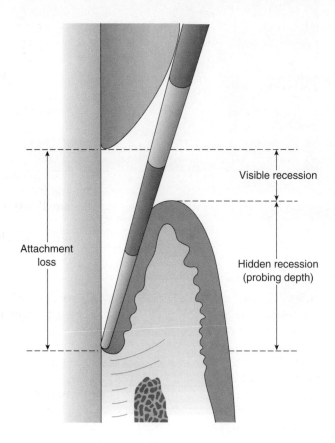

8. periodontal therapy (periodontal debridement or surgery), where tissue shrinkage has occurred;
9. oral habits causing injury to the gingiva such as fingernail biting;
10. anatomic variations that may accelerate gingival recession include a high frenum attachment pulling the free gingival margin (Fig. 6–39 ■);
11. occlusal trauma (this has been suggested to cause gingival recession but has not been demonstrated; Carranza 1996); and
12. cigarette smoking and chewing tobacco (Fig. 6–40 ■), but the exact mechanism is has not been elucidated (Gunsolley et al. 1998).

It is imperative that the cause be determined in individual cases so that the progressive nature of the recession can be controlled and interceptive therapy initiated if necessary. Gingival recession can be seen in healthy gingiva; inflammation may or may not be present. The association with age does not necessarily suggest a physiologic effect of aging on recession. It may just reflect the fact that older people have been subject to the force of brushing for longer periods of time (Joshipura, Kent, and DePaola 1994).

FIGURE 6–38

Gingival recession in a refractory periodontitis patient. Note the presence of inflammation and suppuration. Gingival recession is due to the disease process.

FIGURE 6–39

Recession on the mandibular incisors caused by the high frenum attachment pulling on the free gingival margin. Note the heavy accumulation of plaque and calculus.

Clinical significance of gingival recession

Identification of gingival recession has clinical significance. Root surfaces exposed to the oral environment are more vulnerable to the development of root caries. The thin layer of cementum on the exposed root surface may wear away easily, exposing the underlying dental tubules to the oral environment. Fluid in the exposed dentinal tubules contracts or expands when an external stimulus such as cold or touch is applied. This may stimulate nerves to produce pain. In addition, the col shape changes when gingival recession is present. If the interdental area is open so that no col exists, the facial and palatal gingiva become continuous and keratinized. Thus interproximal recession may create areas of food impaction.

Pathogenesis

The pathogenesis of gingival recession is debatable. As mentioned earlier, it has been considered perhaps to be a normal physiologic process that occurs with in-

FIGURE 6–40

A 45-year-old man who placed chewing tobacco in the facial vestible of the anterior teeth. Note the gingival recession on the anterior teeth.

creasing age, but there is limited documentation to uphold this concept. Others consider it to be a pathologic condition. When the free gingiva is thin, the inflammatory lesion will occupy and degrade the entire connective tissue portion, resulting in collapse of the free gingiva (Wennström 1994). If there is less than 1 mm or more of attached gingiva, the free gingival margin may be movable, which allows microorganisms to enter into the crevice, initiating an inflammatory response.

The amount of attached gingiva needed for gingival health is controversial. Experimental studies (Wennström and Lindhe 1983a, 1983b) have failed to consistently support the concept of a minimal width of gingiva for maintenance of periodontal health.

MUCOGINGIVAL CONSIDERATIONS

A *mucogingival involvement or defect* is defined as a discrepancy in the relationship between the free gingival margin and the mucogingival junction. Pathology or loss of attachment may not be involved. Common mucogingival conditions may be the result of

1. gingival recession resulting in inadequate or diminished attached gingiva;
2. probing depths extending to or beyond the mucogingival junction into the alveolar mucosa (Fig. 6–41 ■); and
3. anatomical variations that may complicate the management of these conditions, including a high frenum attachment pulling the gingival margin away from the tooth surface (see Fig. 6–39) (surgical intervention may be necessary to augment the amount of attached gingiva and correct the mucogingival problem).

Mucogingival examination

A thorough mucogingival examination using appropriate screening techniques and recording the free gingival margin and mucogingival junction on the chart is necessary to detect these conditions. This also enables the practitioner to monitor the progressive nature at future periodontal maintenance visits so that appropriate treatment can be rendered. While radiographs are not used in the identification of

FIGURE 6–41

There is no attached gingiva present on this tooth. This is a mucogingival defect.

FIGURE 6–42

(*Left probe*) Determination of the amount of gingiva (free + attached) by measuring from the free gingival margin to the mucogingival junction. (*Right probe*) Determination of the amount of attached gingiva by subtracting the probing depth (free gingiva) from the total width of gingiva.

[Handwritten margin note: recession + pocket depth — (CEJ to mucoging. junct) = clinical attachment level]

mucogingival problems, appropriate radiographs may be used as part of a preoperative appraisal.

Recording the free gingival margin on the chart will identify the presence or absence of gingival recession or overgrowth. Recession on all six tooth surfaces should be recorded. It is important to measure the amount of recession (in millimeters) because it provides information for determining total attachment loss.

The next step in the mucogingival examination is to determine the total width or height of keratinized gingiva. The width of keratinized gingiva is determined by measuring with a periodontal probe the distance from the gingival margin to the mucogingival junction. The width of attached gingiva is determined by subtracting the probing depth (free gingiva) from the amount of keratinized gingiva (Fig. 6–42 ■). Mucogingival involvement exists when no attached gingiva is present on a tooth. To establish the position of the mucogingival junction, move the side of the periodontal probe gently across the alveolar mucosa in an apical-coronal direction until the tissue stops moving (Fig. 6–43 ■). At this point, elastic fibers are not present, and attached gingiva is coronal to the mucogingival junction. Other methods include the visual method. The problem with this technique is that with inflammation, the gingiva is red, and it will be difficult to differentiate between the red alveolar mucosa and the gingiva. Another method is to pull the lip outward, and the mucogingival junction is seen at the point of tension. This is sometimes misleading, and the actual location of the mucogingival junction is not always distinguished.

FIGURE 6–43

The periodontal probe is gently placed on the alveolar mucosa and moved coronally until the tissue does not move. This is the mucogingival junction.

—no attached gingiva

FIGURE 6–44

A 40-year-old patient exhibiting delayed passive eruption. Note that the gingival margin is on the cervical bulge of the enamel.

too much attached gingiva

teeth look "short"

To determine if any frenal attachments are encroaching on the gingival margin, retract the cheeks and lips laterally by pulling with the thumb and index finger, and watch for movement of the gingival margin in the frenal attachment area.

Delayed passive eruption

Delayed passive eruption occurs in adults when the free gingival margin failed to migrate apically toward the CEJ and still remains on or near the cervical bulge of the enamel, creating a "gummy smile" (Fig. 6–44 ■). This condition is also seen in children up to the time of completed eruption of permanent teeth. This is a normal situation, and the process of passive eruption ultimately will move the free gingival margin apically.

DOCUMENTATION AND SUMMARY

Documentation of clinical findings is done on a periodontal chart. Many types of charts are available. An example of a chart is given in Fig. 6–45 ■. It is important to accurately date and record all clinical findings for legal reasons and to permit the comparison of pretreatment measurements with posttreatment values. Documentation includes the medical and dental histories, chief complaint, oral hygiene evaluation (plaque index), and gingival and periodontal evaluations.

FIGURE 6–45

A periodontal charting form that records initial and final probing depths, clinical attachment levels, tooth mobility, bleeding points, furcation involvement, and gingival recession. (Courtesy of the Department of Oral Biology, School of Dental Medicine, State University of New York at Buffalo, Buffalo, NY)

PERIODONTICS RECORD

FILE NO. ☐ ☐ ☐ ☐ ☐ ☐

NAME	BIRTHDATE	CLINICIAN	EXAM DATE

CHIEF PERIODONTAL COMPLAINT

ORAL HYGIENE METHODS
Current:

Rx:

HISTORY OF PERIODONTAL ILLNESS

PLAQUE INDEX (P.I.)

Date							
P.I.							

PREVIOUS PERIO (prophylaxis, other perio, inc. dates)

HABIT HISTORY

OCCLUSAL OBSERVATIONS

Arch Rel. (angle):　　　　Overbite:　　　Overjet:
Teeth in fremitus:
C.R. ⟶ C.O.:
C.O. ⟶ P.:
P.:
R.L. working:
　　non-working:
L.L. working:
　　non-working:
TMD:

RADIOGRAPHIC FINDINGS

B

SOFT TISSUE EXAM

ETIOLOGY

Local Factors:

GINGIVAL EXAM (color, form, density, bleeding on probing, etc.)

Microbiological Findings:

Occlusal Factors:

Systemic Factors:

DIAGNOSIS

TREATMENT PLAN

PRE-TREATMENT PROGNOSIS

SYSTEMIC FACTORS OF IMPORTANCE IN TREATMENT

FIGURE 6–45, CONTINUED

A periodontal charting form that records initial and final probing depths, clinical attachment levels, tooth mobility, bleeding points, furcation involvement, and gingival recession. (Courtesy of the Department of Oral Biology, School of Dental Medicine, State University of New York at Buffalo, Buffalo, NY)

PERIODONTAL EXAMINATION

PATIENT'S NAME:_____ DATE:_____

Findings from the periodontal examination should be interpreted together with the medical, dental, oral hygiene, gingival, and radiographic assessments. Recording of clinical attachment level is important for long-term monitoring of patients for periodontal destruction.

KEY POINTS

✧ All new and maintaining patients should receive a periodontal examination.

✧ Probing depth is measured from the gingival margin to wherever the tip of the probe stops (in the junctional epithelium).

✧ Clinical attachment level is measured from the CEJ to the apical extent of the probe and is a more accurate long-term measurement for disease progression than probing depths.

REFERENCES

Armitage, G. C. 1995. Clinical evaluation of periodontal diseases. *Periodontology 2000* 7:39–52.

Armitage, G. C. 1996. Periodontal diseases: diagnosis. *Ann. Periodontol.* 1:37–215.

Armitage, G. C., G. K. Svanberg, and H. Löe. 1977. Microscopic evaluation of clinical measurements of connective tissue attachment levels. *J. Clin. Peridontol.* 4:173–190.

Bawden, J. W., and G. H. DeFriese (eds.). 1981. *Planning for dental care on a statewide basis: The North Carolina Dental Manpower Project.* Chapel Hill, NC: The Dental Foundation of North Carolina.

Brown, L. J., R. C. Oliver, and H. Löe. 1989. Periodontal diseases in the U.S. in 1981: Prevalence, severity, extent, and role in tooth mortality. *J. Periodontol.* 60:363–380.

Carlos, J. P., J. A. Brunelle, and M. D. Wolfe. 1987. Attachment loss versus pocket depth as indicators of periodontal disease: A methodologic note. *J. Periodont. Res.* 22:524–525.

Carranza, F. A. 1996. Clinical diagnosis. In: *Clinical periodontology,* F. A. Carranza and M. G. Newman (eds.), 8th ed., 344–362. Philadelphia: W. B. Saunders.

Dunlap, R. M., and M. E. Gher. 1985. Root surface measurements of the mandibular first molar. *J. Periodontol.* 56:234–238.

Easly, J. R., and G. A. Drennan. 1969. Morphological classification of the furca. *J. Can. Dent. Assoc.* 35:105–107.

Garguilo, A. W., F. M. Wentz, and B. Orban. 1961. Dimensions and relations of the dentogingival junction in humans. *J. Periodontol.* 32:261–267.

Gher, M. E., and R. W. Dunlap. 1985. Linear variation of the root surface area of the maxillary first molar. *J. Periodontol.* 56:39–43.

Goodson, J. M. 1986. Clinical measurements of periodontitis. *J. Clin. Periodontol.* 13:446–455.

Greenstein, G., and J. Caton. 1990. Periodontal disease activity: A critical assessment. *J. Periodontol.* 61:543–552.

Gunsolley, J. C., S. M. Quinn, J. Tew, C. M. Gooss, C. M. Brooks, and H. A. Schenkein. 1998. The effect of smoking on individuals with minimal periodontal destruction. *J. Periodontol.* 69:165–170.

Haffajee, A. D., S. S. Socransky, and J. M. Goodson. 1983. Clinical parameters as predictors of destructive periodontal disease activity. *J. Clin. Periodontol.* 10:257–265.

Jeffcoat, M. K. 1994. Current concepts in periodontal disease testing. *J. Am. Dent. Assoc.* 125:1071–1078.

Joshipura, K. J., R. L. Kent, and P. F. DePaola. 1994. Gingival recession: Intra-oral distribution and associated factors. *J. Periodontol.* 65:864–871.

Keagle, J. G., J. J. Garnick, J. R. Searle, G. E. King, and P. K. Morse. 1989. Gingival resistance to probing forces: I. Determination of optimal probe diameter. *J. Periodontol.* 60:167–171.

Lamster, I. B., R. S. Celenti, H. H. Jans, J. B. Fine, and J. T. Grbic 1993. Current status of tests for periodontal disease. *Adv. Dent. Res.* 7:182–190.

Lang, N. P., and H. Löe. 1993. Clinical management of periodontal diseases. *Periodontology 2000* 2:128–139.

Lang, N. P., A. R. Joss, and S. Nyman. 1990. Absence of bleeding on probing: An indicator of periodontal stability. *J. Clin. Periodontol.* 17:714–721.

Listgarten, M. A., R. Mao, and P. J. Robinson. 1976. Periodontal probing and the relationship of the probe tip to periodontal tissues. *J. Periodontol.* 47:511–513.

McFall, W. T., Jr., J. D. Bader, G. R. Rozier, and D. Ramsey. 1988. Presence of periodontal data in patient records of general practitioners. *J. Periodontol.* 59:445–449.

Miller, S. C. 1950. *Textbook of periodontia,* 3d ed., 125. Philadelphia: Blakiston.

Reddy, M. S. 1997. The use of periodontal probes and radiographs in clinical trials of diagnostic tests. *Ann. Periodontol.* 2:113–122.

Robinson, P. J., and R. M. Vitaek. 1979. The relationship between gingival inflammation and resistance to probe penetration. *J. Periodont. Res.* 14:230–243.

Spray, J. R., J. J. Garnick, L. R. Doles, and J. J. Klawitter. 1978. Microscopic demonstration of the position of periodontal probes. *J. Periodontol.* 49:148–152.

Tarnow, D., and P. Fletcher. 1984. Classification of the vertical component of furcation involvement. *J. Periodontol.* 55:283–284.

Towfighi, P. P., M. A. Brunsvold, A. T. Storey, et al. 1997. Pathologic migration of anterior teeth in patients with moderate to severe periodontitis. *J. Periodontol.* 68:967–972.

van der Velden, U. 1979. Probing force and the relationship of the probe tip to the periodontal tissues. *J. Clin. Periodontol.* 6:106–114.

Wennström, J. L. 1994. Mucogingival surgery. In: *Proceedings of the 1st European Workshop on Periodontology,* N. P. Lang and T. Karring (eds.), 193–199. London: Quintessence Books.

Wennström, J. L. 1996. Mucogingival therapy. *Ann. Periodontol.* 1:671–701.

Wennström, J. L., and J. Lindhe. 1983a. Plaque-induced gingival inflammation in the absence of attached gingiva in dogs. *J. Clin. Periodontol.* 10:266–276.

Wennström, J. L., and J. Lindhe. 1983b. The role of attached gingiva for maintenance of periodontal health: Healing following excisional and grafting procedures in dogs. *J. Clin. Periodontol.* 10:206–221.

Williams, R. C., J. D. Beck, and S. N. Offenbacher. 1996. The impact of new technologies on the diagnosis and treatment of periodontal disease: A look to the future. *J. Clin. Periodontol.* 23:299–305.

SELF-QUIZ

1. Which one of the following reasons explains why measuring the clinical attachment levels (CALs) is a more reliable method for determing clinical attachment loss overtime than probing depth measurements? (p. 211)

   a. less penetration into the junctional epithelium occurs

   b. a stable reference point is used (e.g. CEJ)

   c. more mesuring points are used on the tooth

   d. less bleeding occurs at periodontal active sites

2. Which one of the following instruments is best to measure the amount of horizontal bone loss in a furcation? (p. 223)

    a. periodontal probe
    b. Nabers probe
    c. no. 11/12 explorer
    d. CH3 explorer

3. Which one of the following techniques describes how visible recession is recorded? (p. 226)

    a. Use a periodontal probe to measure from the cementoenamel junction to the free gingival margin.
    b. Use a periodontal probe to measure from the free gingival margin to the base of the pocket.
    c. Use an explorer to determine the location of the cementoenamel junction.
    d. Use an explorer to determine the apical extent of the junctional epithelium.

4. Which one of the following conditions is related to gingival recession? (pp. 226–227)

    a. grinding and clenching of teeth
    b. tongue thrusting
    c. tooth malposition
    d. mouth breathing

5. Which one of the following is a cause of a mucogingival involvement or defect? (p. 229)
    a. mouth rinses with a high alcohol content
    b. brushing with a hard bristle toothbrush
    c. inadequate amount or width of attached gingiva
    d. inadequate amount or width of alveolar mucosa

RADIOLOGY AND PERIODONTAL TREATMENT

7

Herbert Frommer, D.D.S.

Outline:

Goal:

To provide the dental hygienist with a radiology background that is used in conjunction with clinical data to recognize and classify periodontal diseases.

Educational Objectives:

Upon completion of this chapter, the reader should be able to:

Recognize and discuss the periodontal structures seen on a radiograph;

Discuss the rationale for radiographs in periodontics;

Explain the features of conventional and computer-based digital imaging;

List and discuss the benefits and limitations of radiographs used in periodontics;

Explain the radiographic improvements aimed at decreasing patient radiation exposure; and

Discuss the types of radiographs used in the treatment planning and evaluation of implants.

KEY WORDS

- full-mouth survey
- conventional radiographs
- exposure time
- paralleling technique
- direct digital radiography
- computed tomographic (CT) scans

237

INTRODUCTION

*T*he proper classification, evaluation, and treatment of the periodontal diseases can be accomplished only with a combination of radiographic and clinical examinations (Fig. 7–1 ■). One must be aware of the diagnostic limitations of radiographs because periodontal diseases have both soft tissue and bony components. Soft-tissue changes such as inflammation, gingival enlargement, and recession cannot be seen on radiographs because such tissues are radiolucent and therefore appear black. Owing to the superimposition of the buccal and lingual alveolar bone plates, bone loss in some areas also may not be seen. Radiographs essentially portray a three-dimensional disease process in two planes. This point must be kept in mind when viewing radiographs because the appearance can be very misleading.

Despite these limitations, a proper periodontal classification cannot be made without a **full-mouth survey.** Radiographs serve to (1) identify predisposing factors, (2) detect early to moderate bone changes where treatment can preserve the dentition, (3) approximate the amount of bone loss and its location, (4) help in evaluating the prognosis of affected teeth and the restorative needs of these teeth, and (5) serve as baseline data and as a means to evaluate posttreatment results.

This chapter will discuss the role of **conventional radiographs** (i.e., radiographs taken on film with an x-ray machine) and computer-based image processing (i.e., the use of a computer to display and enhance images of teeth and bone).

CONVENTIONAL RADIOGRAPHS: INTRAORAL TECHNIQUE

PARAMETERS

The three parameters, or choices, that the dental professional selects at the control panel of an x-ray machine are kilovoltage, milliamperage, and exposure time. Understanding the effect of each of these parameters on the diagnostic x-ray beam

FIGURE 7–1

Radiographs are used to obtain a visual image of the bone and teeth or dental implants. (Courtesy of Procter & Gamble, Cincinnati, OH)

is important and will help in making a correct classification of the disease process (i.e., dental hygiene diagnosis).

Kilovoltage   The amount of penetration of the x-ray beam is controlled by the kilovoltage. The suitable range for dental radiography is 65 to 100 kilovolt peak (kVp). This range is determined by the density of the objects to be radiographed (e.g., teeth, bone). Kilovoltage settings above 100 kVp result in overpenetration, and settings below 45 kVp would result in underpenetration. Kilovoltage settings in the range of 45 to 65 kVp, although producing a diagnostic beam, are never used because of the excess secondary radiation that results.

The question to be answered is: "Within the acceptable kilovoltage range, what kilovoltage is most appropriate for periodontal diagnosis?" The answer is determined by the degree of density and contrast that is most diagnostic for the clinician. *Density* is the degree of blackness on a film, and *contrast* is the difference in the degrees of blackness between adjacent areas.

Radiographs have a high degree of (short scale) contrast when low kilovolt-peak settings are used. The x-ray photons either penetrate the tissue or are absorbed—a sort of yes or no, black or white reaction. When higher kilovolt-peak settings are used, there is less contrast, and the overall tone of the radiograph is gray (Fig. 7–2 ■). This occurs because there is much more partial penetration with the resulting long-scale contrast. Such low contrast is not as satisfying visually as high contrast, but early changes in object density such as early bone loss may be seen in the gradations of gray as a result of more selective penetration, which is not present in high-contrast films. Theoretically, therefore, higher kilovolt-peak settings with their resulting long-scale contrast produce better results in terms of periodontal diagnosis. A number of clinicians, however, feel that the human eye is not capable of seeing these very subtle gray changes and recommend using 75 kVp, where bony changes are distinguished more easily.

Milliamperage   The milliamperage setting controls the number of x-rays generated in a given exposure time. As noted above, the kilovoltage determines the *quality* (penetration) of the x-rays produced, but the milliamperage determines the *quantity* of x-rays produced.

It is more precise, however, to consider the concept of milliampere seconds (mAs) than milliamperage alone because the milliamperage setting and duration

FIGURE 7–2

Selection of settings. (Courtesy of Procter & Gamble, Cincinnati, OH)

of exposure are interdependent values. In order to make a diagnostic exposure, different types of film need different milliamperage-second settings, and this is determined by the sensitivity of the film and the focal distance of the film. If the milliamperage setting is increased, then the **exposure time** can be reduced. For example, an exposure, at a given kilovolt-peak setting, of 1 s using 10 mA is 10 mAs. A 2-s exposure at the same kilovolt-peak setting using 5 mA would produce an identical film because the resulting exposure is again 10 mAs ($10 \times 1 = 10$ and $5 \times 2 = 10$). Both patients would receive the same amount of radiation. The only advantage of the higher milliamperage is the decrease in exposure time, which lessens the chance of patient movement. Common practice today is to use short exposure times at a magnitude of 6 impulses (1/10 s), so patient movement is less of a factor (see below). This reduction in exposure time to 1/10 s alone, however, will not prevent patient movement or gagging; it just facilitates obtaining the radiograph before such movement occurs. Thus it is apparent that it makes no diagnostic and little technical difference if we work at 5, 6, 7, 10, or 15 mA. It should be pointed out that conventional dental x-ray machines do not have milliamperage settings higher than 15 because of heat limitations within the tube.

Dental x-ray machines do not emit a continuous stream of radiation when an exposure is made; rather, they emit a series of radiation impulses. The number of impulses depends on the number of cycles per second in the electric current being used. With 60-cycle alternating current, which is standard, there are 60 x-ray pulses per second. Newer-generation x-ray machines have timer dials calibrated in impulses, not in seconds. On the timer dial, 15 would mean 15 impulses or 15/60-s exposure. These extremely short exposure times can only be controlled by an electric timer. The old mechanical timers are not this precise, and all x-ray machines should have electronic timers that are capable of delivering short, accurate exposure times.

FILM TYPE

Even with the introduction of digital radiographs, film remains by far the most commonly used image receptor in dentistry. In periodontal diagnostic radiology, the most commonly used sizes are number 1 (narrow anterior), number 2 (adult size), and number 3 (long bitewing). Number 2 film with either loops or stick-on tabs can be converted into a bitewing film.

The film sensitivity, or speed, determines how much radiation for how long (e.g., milliampere seconds) is necessary to produce an image on the film. The speed of the film is determined mainly by the size of the silver halide crystals in the film emulsion.

Films are designated by American National Standards Institute (ANSI) categories, with category A film being the slowest and category F film being the fastest. At present, only category E and D films are available for use. The category E film speed is twice as fast as category D film and thus needs half the radiation exposure. Both films are equally diagnostic. The early objections to category E film based on decreased definition and lack of contrast have not been supported by studies in the literature. Thus, because it has the same diagnostic capability and results in 50% less radiation exposure than category D film, category E speed film generally should be used.

PARALLELING VERSUS THE BISECTING TECHNIQUE

In periodontal radiographic diagnosis, use of the **paralleling technique** with a 16-in. film focal distance for periapical radiographs is the method of choice. In this technique, the teeth and the film are parallel to each other, and the central ray of the x-ray beam is directed perpendicular (right angle) to both. With this technique, there will be no dimensional distortion or false and misleading indications of bone levels. The 16-in. focal distance, the so-called long cone, is used to compensate for the image enlargement caused by the increase in tooth-to-film distance necessary to achieve the parallelism between the teeth and the film.

In the bisecting technique, the film is placed as close to the tooth as possible, and the central ray of the x-ray beam is directed perpendicular to an imaginary line between the angle formed by the long axis of the tooth and the plane of the film. This technique is not recommended for periodontal diagnosis because it results in a distortion and exaggeration of the alveolar bone level. Excess vertical angulation (i.e., distortion of the length of the roots, either foreshortening or elongation) may lead to a perception of early furcation involvement when there is actually no interradicular bone loss (Fig. 7–3 ■).

CONVENTIONAL RADIOGRAPHS USED IN PERIODONTICS

Table 7–1 ■ reviews the different types of conventional intraoral and extraoral radiographs used in conjunction with clinical data to recognize and classify periodontal diseases (Hodges 1997). Many radiographs are available, but periapical, bitewing, and panoramic radiographs are used most commonly in periodontics to evaluate periodontal structures.

Conventional radiographs give a history of past periodontal disease destruction but do not provide information on current periodontal disease status. As mentioned earlier, radiographs represent a two-dimensional view of three-dimensional objects, so it is difficult to recognize the slight changes in alveolar bone that would

FIGURE 7–3

Diagnostic quality. (Courtesy of Procter & Gamble, Cincinnati, OH)

TABLE 7–1		
SELECTION CRITERIA OF CONVENTIONAL RADIOGRAPHS FOR PERIODONTICS		
TYPE OF FILM	**INDICATIONS**	**LIMITATION'S**
Periapical	Viewing the apex of the root for any pathology (i.e., periapical radiolucency)	Technique errors may reduce the ability to detect crestal bone loss.
	Determining morphology (shape) of roots and root length	Detection of incipient interproximal dental caries.
	Recognizing horizontal and vertical patterns of bone loss	Detection of pathologic lesions in the mandible and maxilla.
	Evaluating implants	Evaluation of other structures such as sinuses and the mandibular canal.
Bitewing	Viewing interproximal dental caries	
	Viewing the alveolar crest bone height (use vertical bitewings)	Cannot view the apical area of a tooth.
	Evaluation of defective restorations (i.e., overhang)	Evaluation of the morphology and length of roots.
Panoramic	Viewing the area of the maxilla and mandibular arches (i.e., impacted teeth, sinuses, and pathologic lesions)	Not used for recognizing periodontal diseases or dental caries.

TABLE 7–2
BENEFITS AND LIMITATIONS OF CONVENTIONAL RADIOGRAPHS

Radiographs *do* show
  crestal alveolar bone levels
  clinical crown-to-root ratio
  calculus on proximal tooth surfaces
  metallic restorations
  morphology of roots (i.e., root length, root shape)

Radiographs *do not* show
  periodontal pockets
  buccal and lingual plates of bone
  hard-to-soft-tissue relationship
  a successfully treated patient
  bone loss until about 30 to 50% of loss of mineralization occurs

indicate early or mild periodontal disease. Other limitations and benefits of radiographs are discussed in Table 7–2 ■. As a result, radiographs are used primarily in periodontics to determine the severity and pattern of bone loss, the morphology (i.e., length and shape) of roots, root proximity, pathologic lesions such as a cyst or an abscess, and the effects of occlusion.

Just as a single periodontal probing recording only provides information on past disease activity, it is important to compare several sets of full-mouth radiographs over a period of time to evaluate for periodontal disease progression (Hollender 1992; Jeffcoat and Reddy 1991). In addition, radiographic findings always should be correlated with the corresponding probing depth measurements.

PERIAPICAL RADIOGRAPHS

A periapical radiograph shows the entire area around a tooth, including the apex of the root. Periapical radiographs are part of the full-mouth survey and are taken

FIGURE 7–4

View selection—bitewing. (Courtesy of Procter & Gamble, Cincinnati, OH)

of anterior and posterior teeth. The number of periapical films taken for a full-mouth survey varies from 14 to 20.

Film technique errors occur quite often with periapical radiographs as a result of improper alignment of the film with the tooth and the x-ray beam with the film. Excessive vertical angulation causes foreshortening (roots appear shorter and the alveolar crest appears to be closer to the cementoenamel junction than it truly is) and occlusal surfaces to be cut off. This can result in inaccurate recording of the crestal alveolar bone level. Insufficient vertical angulation causes elongation and roots to be cut off from the x-ray. Overlapping of proximal tooth surfaces is caused by improper horizontal angulation of the radiographic beam.

BITEWING RADIOGRAPHS

The bitewing radiograph is by far the best radiograph to interpret posterior alveolar bone levels and bone loss with the least amount of distortion or technique error. Bitewing radiographs show the crowns of the maxillary and mandibular teeth and the alveolar crest. Identification of carious lesions is best with bitewing radiographs. Posterior bitewing radiographs are part of the full-mouth survey and can include up to four views. Bitewing films can be placed either horizontally or vertically (Fig. 7–4 ■). Vertical bitewing radiographs are especially useful in periodontal patients with moderate to severe bone loss (this is determined by periodontal probing and previous radiographs, if available) in order to evaluate crestal bone. Horizontal bitewing radiographs do not show the entire bone height. Two posterior vertical bitewing radiographs may be sufficient, however, for visualization of both maxillary and mandibular teeth. The radiographs are taken perpendicular to the alveolar crest so that the crestal bone is depicted accurately. Anterior vertical bitewing radiographs also can be taken.

PANORAMIC RADIOLOGY

The image on a panoramic film shows the entire dentition and supporting bone structure from condyle to condyle on one film (Fig. 7–5 ■). The resulting image, however, does not have the same degree of definition seen on an intraoral periapical

FIGURE 7–5

View selection—panoramic. (Courtesy of Procter & Gamble, Cincinnati, OH)

- Provides global view of oral structures
- Tomogram through arc of jaw
- Not appropriate for periodontal diagnosis

or bitewing radiograph. This shortcoming is inherent to the pantomographic process and is also caused by the use of intensifying screens.

Many diagnostic problems in dentistry require a high degree of radiographic definition. Early detection of such conditions as disruption of the periodontal ligament, loss of crestal alveolar bone, a thickened periodontal ligament, and ongoing caries requires the maximum amount of radiographic definition. Because of this, panoramic films have very limited value in the diagnosis of periodontal disease. If a panoramic film is used instead of a full-mouth survey, it must be augmented with both anterior and posterior bitewing radiographs and selected periapical films where indicated. Many technique errors can occur with panoramic radiographs, including improper patient positioning and operator errors.

PERIODONTAL STRUCTURES

In order to recognize disease, the normal anatomy must be understood. Periodontal anatomy identified on radiographs includes the supporting structures such as the alveolar bone, periodontal ligament space, and cementum (Fig. 7–6 ■). Since gingiva is a noncalcified soft tissue structure, the x-rays go completely through it and are not absorbed, and thus the gingiva is not seen as a radiopaque structure.

INTERDENTAL SEPTUM

The normal crest of interproximal bone runs parallel to a line drawn between the cementoenamel junctions on adjoining teeth at a level approximately 2.0 mm apical to the cementoenamel junction (Fig. 7–7 ■). The shape of the alveolar crest is determined primarily by the contact area of adjacent teeth and the shape of the cementoenamel junction. The alveolar crest is flatter in posterior areas and more convex and pointed anteriorly. The width of the interdental septum can be determined by viewing a radiograph. The interdental septum can be narrow in cases of

FIGURE 7–6

Radiograph of the periodontal structures (1 = lamina dura; 2 = periodontal ligament space; 3 = interproximal bone; 4 = Alveolar bone crest; 5 = trabecular bone; 6 = interradicular bone; 7 = pulp).

FIGURE 7–7

Radiograph showing the normal relationship of the crestal bone level being parallel with the cementoenamel junctions of adjacent teeth. No bone loss is depicted in this radiograph.

close root proximity. In some instances, the roots of adjacent teeth are so close that there may be little to no cancellous bone. Teeth that frequently show close root proximity include the distobuccal root of the maxillary first molar and the mesiobuccal root of the maxillary second molar and the mandibular anteriors.

Radiographically, a thin radiopaque line surrounds the entire tooth and is continuous with the alveolar crest (see Fig. 7–6). This is referred to as the *lamina dura.* Clinically, it represents the alveolar bone that lines the tooth socket.

PERIODONTAL LIGAMENT SPACE

The periodontal ligament fibers (or principal fibers) transverse from the cementum to the alveolar bone. Since these fibers are soft tissue, they are not evident on radiographs. Instead, the space where the fibers are located appears as a radiolucuent area surrounding the entire tooth (see Fig. 7–6). On one side of the space

FIGURE 7–8

The maxillary second premolar shows a widened periodontal ligament space due to an excessive occlusal load placed on it.

is the cementum, and the other border is the lamina dura. Evaluating the width of the periodontal ligament (space) is important during the occlusal examination. If a tooth has excessive occlusal loads placed on it, the periodontal ligament compensates for the resulting tooth mobility by becoming thicker. This shows up on a radiograph as a widened periodontal ligament (Fig. 7–8 ■).

PERIODONTAL INTERPRETATION

Using radiographs as an evaluation tool in the recognition of periodontitis has several limitations that are listed in Table 7–2. It is difficult to determine changes in bone simply by viewing radiographs. For this reason, clinical data must be incorporated with radiographic findings in an assessment of periodontal status. For example, a patient's radiographs may show moderate bone loss, but previously the patient may have had periodontal surgery for pocket reduction. Thus the radiographs still show bone loss, but the periodontal charting shows probing depths from 1 to 3 mm without bleeding on probing. At this time the patient does not have periodontitis. The radiographs show past disease activity, not what is occurring presently.

BONE LOSS

Conventional radiographs represent an insensitive technique in detecting early, small bony defects (bone loss). Before bone loss is identified on a radiograph, approximately 30 to 50% loss of mineralization must occur (Jeffcoat 1992; Jeffcoat and Reddy 1991). In addition, radiographically, the cortical bone plates may hide slight bone loss.

Radiographic evaluation of alveolar bone loss associated with periodontitis is based on the status of the interdental septum. Fuzziness or breaks in the continuity of the lamina dura have been described as the earliest radiographic signs of bone loss (Carranza 1996). However, the radiographic observation that the loss of crestal

FIGURE 7–9

(a) A periapical radiograph showing a horizontal pattern of bone loss. (b) Vertical or angular bone loss on the mesial surface of the first molar with furcation involvement.

(a)

(b)

lamina dura is a sign of periodontitis is not totally accurate (Armitage 1996). Clinical studies have shown that sites did not break down even though there was a break in the lamina dura. Moreover, absence of crestal lamina dura is a common radiographic finding in normal, nondiseased interproximal sites (Rams, Listgarten, and Slots 1994). Thus it is more accurate to state that the presence of an intact crestal lamina dura represents a stable site than that the absence of a crestal lamina dura indicates a disease site (Armitage 1996; Rams, Listgarten, and Slots 1994).

Patterns of bone loss

The severity, distribution, and pattern of bone loss can be determined from radiographs. Clinically, as measured with a periodontal probe, two types of bony pockets exist: suprabony and infrabony. A gingival pocket or pseudopocket is not associated with bone loss. These bony pockets are associated with two patterns of bone loss: horizontal and vertical. In horizontal bone loss, interdental bone is destroyed equally along the surfaces of adjacent teeth (Fig. 7–9a ■). Suprabony pockets, where the base of the pocket is coronal to the alveolar bone crest, are characterized by horizontal bone loss. In vertical (angular) bone loss, the resorption on one tooth sharing the septum is greater than on the other tooth (Fig. 7–9b ■). Infrabony pockets, where the base of the pocket is apical to the alveolar crest, are associated with vertical bone loss.

Severity of bone loss

The severity, or amount, of bone loss is classified as mild, moderate, or severe. One way to determine the amount of bone loss is to determine the percentage of bone loss. This is done by measuring the length from the cementoenamel junction

FIGURE 7–10

The area between the premolar and molar shows uneven crestal alveolar bone that parallels the uneven cementoenamel junctions. There is horizontal bone loss but not angular bone loss.

to the tip of the root and the distance from the cementoenamel junction to the alveolar crest. The percentage of bone loss is calculated by dividing this number by the root length and multiplying by 100 (Hodges 1997). Bone loss of less than 20% is usually classified as mild; bone loss between 20 and 50% is moderate; and bone loss of more than 50% is severe. It also should be remembered that 30 to 50% bone loss must be present before it is evident radiographically.

Determination of bone loss

The first step in determining if there is radiographic bone loss is to draw an imaginary line connecting the cementoenamel junction of adjacent teeth and then a line on the alveolar crest. If the alveolar crest is more than approximately 2 mm apical to the cementoenamel junction, there is bone loss. The next step is to determine if the pattern of bone loss is horizontal or vertical. In vertical bone loss, the bone level is not parallel to the cementoenamel junctions of adjacent teeth. In horizontal bone loss, the bone level is parallel to the cementoenamel junctions of adjacent teeth. If a tooth is not in the normal occlusal plane (e.g., extruded, intruded, or tipped), the bone level will not be in a straight line, but neither will the cementoenamel junctions, so the lines will still be parallel to each other (Fig. 7–10 ■).

Despite these limitations, conventional radiographs are still mandatory in the recognition and treatment of periodontal diseases. They provide an excellent measurement of the history of periodontal disease in a patient and provide important information about the interproximal bone changes that occur over time (Douglass et al. 1991). The detection of predisposing factors is one of the most important roles of radiography in periodontal diseases, and the detection and elimination of local irritants are essential steps in prevention or actual periodontal therapy.

CALCULUS

Early deposits, small and not fully calcified, are not seen radiographically. Even calcified supragingival calculus, which is seen most often on the lingual surfaces of lower anterior teeth and the buccal surfaces of upper molars, is not seen clearly

FIGURE 7–11

Calculus spurs evident on all tooth surfaces.

in its early stage because of superimposition of tooth structure (e.g., roots) and cortical plates. Subgingival calculus on the proximal surfaces is more easily detected in the early calcified stages. Calculus appears as an irregularly pointed radiographic projection from the proximal root surface (Fig. 7–11 ■).

RESTORATIONS

Metallic restorations, such as amalgam and gold, will appear radiopaque on radiographs, whereas synthetic restorations, such as composites, will appear radiolucent. Radiographs can reveal metallic restorations with open contacts, poor contours, overhanging and deficient margins, and caries, all of which are etiologic factors in periodontal diseases. Composite restorations are much more difficult to evaluate because of their radiolucent appearance.

ANATOMIC CONFIGURATIONS

Only through radiographic examination can information about the size, shape, and positions of the roots of periodontally involved teeth be obtained. It is important to document the lengths of the root trunks of multirooted teeth to ensure tooth survival. A tooth with a short root trunk has "higher" furcation entrances and longer roots. A tooth with a long root trunk has shorter roots, but the furcation entrance is more apical. Therefore, more bone has to be destroyed in the development of a furcation involvement.

Another important factor in the overall periodontal prognosis is the shape of the roots. The space between the roots is important. Roots of multirooted teeth can be diverging, converging, or conical. Diverging roots have a larger surface area for periodontal attachment including bone. Teeth with thicker, diverging, longer roots have a better prognosis than conical or converging roots. Roots also can be long and tapered or short, bulbous, and conical. These factors are important in evaluating the present condition and planning periodontal and restorative therapy.

In restorative case planning, the crown-to-root ratio is an important factor. This ratio is the relationship of the length of the root embedded in bone compared with the length of the rest of the tooth. The greater the length of the tooth embedded in bone, the better is the prognosis for support of a fixed or removable prosthesis. A 2:1 crown-to-root ratio is desirable. Teeth with bulbous roots have more area for attachment than those with fine tapered roots.

RADIOGRAPHICALLY DETECTABLE PERIODONTAL CHANGES

GINGIVITIS

Because gingivitis is a soft-tissue change, there are no radiographic findings other than the presence of predisposing or contributing factors (e.g., condition of restorations).

SLIGHT (MILD) PERIODONTITIS

This stage of periodontal disease is characterized radiographically by changes in the crest of the interproximal bone septum and triangulation of the periodontal ligament space (Fig. 7–12 ■). Triangulation is widening of the periodontal ligament space at the crest of the interproximal septum that gives the appearance of a radiolucent triangle to what is normally a radiolucent band. Fading of the density of the crest with cup-shaped defects appears in the early stages of periodontitis.

MODERATE PERIODONTITIS

In this stage, bone loss may be apparent in both horizontal and vertical planes. Radiolucencies appear in the furcations of multirooted teeth, indicating interradicular bone loss. This is a furcation involvement and is confirmed clinically using a Nabers probe. In this stage, horizontal bone loss on the buccal or lingual

FIGURE 7–12

Slight (mild) chronic periodontitis. Generalized slight horizontal bone loss of less than 25%.

surface may go undetected because of superimposition. Careful examination of the radiograph in most cases reveals a difference in density indicating different levels of bone on the buccal and lingual surfaces (Fig. 7–13 ■).

SEVERE PERIODONTITIS

This stage of periodontal disease is easily identified radiographically by the advanced vertical and horizontal patterns of bone loss, furcation involvement, thickened periodontal ligament, and indications of changes in tooth position (Fig. 7–14 ■).

PERIODONTAL ABSCESS

The radiographic signs of a periodontal abscess may vary greatly. Such a diagnosis is dictated by an acute clinical manifestation. Clinically, a deep periodontal pocket is usually found. The periodontal abscess is caused by the occlusion of an

FIGURE 7–13

Moderate chronic periodontitis. Localized furcation involvement on the mandibular molar.

FIGURE 7–14

Severe chronic periodontitis. Generalized extensive horizontal and vertical bone loss of more than 50% and numerous furcation involvements.

existing pocket; therefore, the radiograph of the acute episode may not vary greatly from previous radiographs of the existing condition that produced the pocket. In other instances, there may be signs of rapid and extensive bone destruction.

FREQUENCY OF RADIOGRAPHS (SELECTION CRITERIA)

Among the many methods of reducing a patient's radiation exposure (e.g., collimation, filtration, and fast film), selection criteria also are very important and are the responsibility of the dentist. Selection criteria are descriptions of clinical conditions and historical data that identify patients who are most likely to benefit from a particular radiographic examination. These guidelines help the practitioner select which patient needs radiographs and determine which radiographs are needed. The final decision rests with the individual dentist and is determined by professional judgment.

The practice of taking radiographs based on a time interval rather than patient needs, as determined by clinical examination and dental history, is not considered the appropriate way to practice dental radiology. In relation to periodontal care, there should never be a policy, for example, that mandates a new full-mouth survey every 2 years or bitewing radiographs every 6 months. The radiographic needs of each patient are different and should not be based on the calendar but rather on a complete clinical examination and the history of previous periodontal therapy or signs and symptoms of the disease.

An expert panel of dentists under the auspices of the Public Health Service (U.S. Department of Health and Human Services 1987) has developed guidelines for the prescription of dental radiographs. One of the patient categories is "Periodontal disease or a history of periodontal treatment." The recommendations call for a full-mouth survey for every new patient, comprised of periapical and bitewing films. For the recall examination, radiographs should be taken for evaluation of previous periodontal therapy, e.g., surgery, bone grafting, implants, or when there is a dramatic change in the probing depth measurement. In any patient, radiographs should never be taken before there is a complete clinical examination. Based on this examination, a radiographic prescription is formulated, the films are taken, and a final classification and treatment plan are determined.

DIGITAL IMAGING

Radiographic improvements are designed to reduce patient radiation exposure and to simplify identification and measurement of changes in alveolar bone height. The most recent addition to dental radiology is **direct digital radiography.** Presently, about fifteen systems are available on the market, each with its own variations. Many clinicians are converting from film to digital imaging. With digital imaging, there is an up to 90% reduction in radiation exposure compared with conventional radiographs (Jeffcoat 1998). Direct digital radiography replaces the film used in a conventional intraoral radiograph with an electronic sensor. This sensor, the approximate size of intraoral film, is placed in the patient's mouth in the same manner as one would place film. The exposure is made, and the sensor sends impulses based on the penetration of the object by the x-ray photons to a

FIGURE 7–15

An example of a direct digital radiograph. This radiograph was taken during implant surgery to guide in the placement of the implant. Digital images can be changed electronically to improve contrast and density and can magnify the image. The mandibular canal (arrows) is well visualized. (Courtesy of Procter & Gamble, Cincinnati, OH).

computer. These impulses are then digitized and formed into an image by the computer. The image can be stored, printed in hard copy, darkened or lightened, reversed, colorized, magnified, measured, or transmitted to a remote sight.

A computer monitor creates an image using pixels or tiny dots that become a recognizable form when projected on the screen. Viewing the digital radiograph allows the clinician to determine bone loss through the percentage of lightness and darkness of pixels. White, the lightest shade, indicates the maximum amount of bone mineral, whereas black, the darkest shade, indicates absence of bone mineral (Fig. 7–15 ■).

From a periodontal standpoint, all the diagnostic criteria mentioned previously in terms of conventional radiographs stay the same. The instant imaging is a time advantage and the substantial reduction in patient exposure is desirable, but the periodontal diagnostic capabilities, when compared with film, are about equal. There may be some advantage in determining bone levels by image reversal or colorization, but this varies among practitioners. These systems are available for commercial in-office use.

DIGITAL SUBTRACTION RADIOLOGY

Digital subtraction radiology (DSR) magnifies images, allowing detection of osseous changes (bone loss) that are too small to be seen in a visual examination of conventional film. As mentioned earlier, comparing radiographs from different time periods is important in detecting progressive bone loss. Because of the superimposition of cortical plates and roots of teeth, it is almost impossible to detect

FIGURE 7–16

Computerized digital radiography is used to quantify the change in bone mineral. A baseline radiograph was taken (left). The area of red shading indicates 0.84 mm of bone loss between examinations taken over a 6-month period (right radiograph). This shading allows the area of change to be readily seen. (Courtesy of Procter & Gamble, Cincinnati, OH)

changes in the bone level unless there was a dramatic loss of bone (Jeffcoat 1994). In digital subtraction radiology, two images taken at two different visits are compared, and all structures that do not change, such as cortical plates and roots of teeth, are not shown on (subtracted from) the image. Any changes in bone level are indicated by a color-shaded area; red is for bone loss, and green is for bone gain (see Fig. 7–16 ■). DSR has not been used much in clinical practice because it is a difficult technique to master, but it is used frequently in clinical research.

RADIOGRAPHS IN IMPLANTOLOGY

At the present time, the basic diagnostic radiographs used in screening implant patients are conventional radiographs such as periapical, occlusal, and panoramic films. In addition, computed tomographic (CT) scans are used for a three-dimensional view of the bone. It is most important to realize that to diagnose and plan for implant placement, one must be able to view the implant site in three dimensions or planes. As dental professionals, we are used to seeing objects in two planes, mesiodistal and incisoapically. We do not see objects, in a three-dimensional view except with occlusal films in the buccolingual plane, and this information is critical in implant planning. Of the techniques used, only CT images can supply this information.

PERIAPICAL/OCCLUSAL FILMS

If the film can be placed parallel to the ridge and the field size allows for visualization of the entire proposed alveolar area, then periapical films can be used. Unfortunately, there are very few patients who fit this criterion, and thus periapical views are of limited value. Occlusal films, if they can be positioned, can augment the periapical film to view the third dimension.

PANTOMOGRAMS (PANORAMIC FILMS)

The panoramic film is currently the most commonly used radiograph in treatment planning for an implant patient. Pantomograms are ideal for showing the structures of the mandible and maxilla, including the locations of nerves. Although the field size is large enough in panoramic films, there is still no cross-sectional visualization. There is also an uneven amount of magnification (27%) in different areas of the mouth, and this can be very misleading in interpreting the radiograph. The exact location of the mandibular canal is difficult to determine on a pantomogram. Thus pantomograms should not be used as the only method for evaluating osseous structures.

CONVENTIONAL TOMOGRAMS

Cross-sectional tomograms are an excellent way to obtain the necessary field visualization. Tomograms are cross-sectional images perpendicular to the edentulous ridge. Images are often blurry or indistinct, and this procedure is time-consuming. Since very few offices have tomographic units, referral to medical radiologists or hospitals is necessary. If one is to refer a patient to this type of facility, it is probably better to refer for CT imaging.

COMPUTED TOMOGRAPHY (CT SCANNING)

Three-dimensional **computed tomography (CT)** imaging is essentially digitized tomography that results in an enhanced image in all dimensions or planes that is much easier to read than a conventional tomogram. The CT scanner makes a 1.0 to 1.5 mm thick slice or cut of the edentulous area (Fig. 7–17 ■). The tomogram measures the amount of energy transmitted through the object. The information is tansmitted to a computer, which displays the image on a monitor.

CT scans are ideal for locating the amount and quality of bone available for implant placement above the mandibular canal (this is where the mandibular nerve is located) in the posterior area of the mandible. When maxillary areas are being used as implant sites, CT scans should be used to locate the sinuses and determine the amount and quality of available bone.

FIGURE 7–17

Axial CT at the level of the maxillary sinus.

POSTOPERATIVE IMPLANT EVALUATION

Baseline radiographs are taken to verify the fit of the abutment to the fixture head and document bone levels around an implant. After placement of implants, clinical and radiographic evaluations are necessary at continuing care or supportive periodontal therapy visits. Periapical and panoramic films are used for posttreatment evaluation. The primary reason for taking radiographs postoperatively is to help monitor the bone level around the implant. Periapical films are best for this purpose. For the edentulous patient, follow-up radiographs should be taken annually for 3 years and then once every other year. Pantomograms are also used to determine bone changes and the status of the abutment and fixture. Alveolar bone loss of less than 0.2 mm per year after the first year of placement is considered acceptable for a successful implant (Albrektsson et al. 1986). CT scans cannot be used because the metallic implants produce image "noise" that interferes with proper interpretation.

SUMMARY

Adequate radiographs and imaging systems are necessary for a complete periodontal and implant examination. Many techniques and systems are available. Conventional radiographs are adequate for visualizing the tooth and surrounding tissues. Conventional radiographs are also used to determine the amount and quality of bone available for implant placement in the anterior sextant of the mandible and maxilla. However, CT scans are necessary to evaluate the implant site in the maxilla and posterior areas of the mandible for its osseous status and proximity to vital structures (e.g., sinuses and mandibular canal).

KEY POINTS

❖ Radiographic interpretation is used to supplement clinical findings from the periodontal assessment (e.g., probing depths, clinical attachment levels).

❖ Posterior vertical bitewing radiographs are ideal for visualizing the level of the alveolar bone crest.

❖ Radiographs do not show gingival and periodontal pockets or mobile teeth.

❖ The CT scan is the most commonly used imaging system for visualizing implant sites in the maxilla and posterior areas of the mandible.

REFERENCES

Albrektsson, T. G., Zarb, P. Worthington, and A. R. Eriksson. 1986. The long-term efficacy of currently used dental implants: A review and proposed criteria of success. *Int. J. Oral Maxillofac. Implants* 1:11–25.

Armitage, G. C. 1996. Periodontal diseases: Diagnosis. *Ann. Periodontol.* 1:37–215.

Carranza, F. A., Jr. 1996. Radiographic and other aids in the diagnosis of periodontal disease. In: *Clinical periodontology,* F. A. Carranza, Jr., and M. G. Newman (eds.), 8th ed., 362–374. Philadelphia: W. B. Saunders.

Douglass, G. L., S. M. Levine, J. Otomo-Corgel, T. N. Sims, and E. J. Taggart. 1991. Periodontal examination, diagnosis and treatment. *Can. Dent. Assoc. J.* 19:16–30.

Hodges, K. O. 1997. Recommendations for radiographs. In *Concepts in nonsurgical periodontal therapy,* ed. K. O. Hodges, 1st ed., 118–149. Albany: Delmar Publishers.

Hollender, L. 1992. Decision making in radiographic imaging. *J. Dent. Educ.* 56:834–843.

Jeffcoat, M. K. 1992. Imaging techniques for the periodontium. In *Advances in periodontics,* eds. T. J. Wilson, K. S. Kornnan, and M. G. Newman, 47–57. Chicago: Qintessence Publishing.

Jeffcoat, M. K. 1994. Current concepts in periodontal disease testing. *J. Am. Dent. Assoc.* 125:1071–1078.

Jeffcoat, M. K. 1998. Periodontal diseases: Epidemiology and diagnosis. Consensus reports from the 1996 world workshop in periodontics. *J. Am. Dent. Assoc.* 129:9S–14S.

Jeffcoat, M., and M. S. Reddy. 1991. A comparison of probing and radiographic methods for detection of periodontal disease progression. *Curr. Opin. Dentistry* 1:45–51.

Rams, T. E., M. A. Listgarten, and J. Slots. 1994. Utility of radiographic crestal lamina dura for predicting periodontitis disease activity. *J. Clin. Periodontol.* 21:571–576.

U.S. Department of Health and Human Services. 1987. *The selection of patients for x-ray examinations* (HHS Publication FDA 88-8273). Washington: U.S. Government Printing Office.

SELF-QUIZ

1. The radiographic evaluation of alveolar bone loss associated with periodontitis is based on the status of which one of the following structures? (p. 244)

   a. interdental septum
   b. cementoenamel junction
   c. periapical bone
   d. periodontal ligament fibers

2. Which one of the following radiographic structures is described as a thin radiopaque line surrounding the entire tooth and is continuous with the alveolar crest? (p. 245)

   a. dentin
   b. cementum
   c. lamina dura
   d. periodontal ligament fibers
   e. gingival fibers

3. Which one of the following types of radiographs has nearly 90% reduction in radiation exposure? (p. 252)

   a. panoramic
   b. periapical
   c. computed tomography
   d. digital imaging
   e. vertical bitewing

4. Which one of the following types of radiographs is best to evaluate the alveolar bone crest for moderate to severe bone loss? (p. 243)

   a. periapical
   b. horizontal bitewing
   c. vertical bitewing
   d. panoramic
   e. computed tomography

5. Which one of the following predisposing factors of periodontal diseases can be seen on radiographs? (pp. 246–247)

   a. gingival recession
   b. periodontal pockets
   c. furcation involvement
   d. tooth mobility

6. All the following types of radiographs are currently used in the treatment planning of implants *except* one. Which one is the exception? (pp. 254–255)

   a. periapicals
   b. bitewings
   c. panoramic
   d. CT scan

7. Which one of the following features does the computed tomographic process provide? (p. 255)

   a. a three-dimensional view of the area of interest
   b. a two-dimensional view of the area of interest
   c. a global view of all oral structures
   d. a close-up view of the periapical structures

8. All the following are reasons for using radiographs in periodontics *except* one. Which one is the exception? (p. 242)

   a. identify predisposing factors
   b. detect early to moderate bone changes
   c. determine the shape and depth of periodontal pockets
   d. serve as baseline data and as a means of evaluating posttreatment results

9. The normal crest of interproximal bone is located at a level (p. 244)

   a. 2 mm apical to the cementoenamel junction.
   b. 3.0 mm coronal to the cementoenamel junction.
   c. 2.0 to 3.0 mm coronal to the cusp tip of the crown.
   d. 3.5 mm apical to the cusp tip of the crown.

10. Which one of the following types of radiographs is used primarily in clinical research rather than clinical practice? (p. 254)

    a. panoramic films
    b. direct digital radiography
    c. digital subtraction radiography
    d. computed tomography

ADVANCES IN DETECTING AND MONITORING PERIODONTAL DISEASES

Denise Estafan, D.D.S., M.S.

Outline:

Introduction
Gingival Crevicular Fluid Assays
Microbial Tests
Immunologic Assays
Enzyme-Based Assays
Genetic Assays
Clinical Applications
Summary
Key Points
References
Self-Quiz

Goal:

To teach the dental hygienist methods that can be used as a supplement to conventional periodontal assessments for recognizing and monitoring periodontal diseases.

Education Objectives:

Upon completion of this chapter, the reader should be able to:

Evaluate the role of using adjunctive diagnostic aids as a predictor for periodontal breakdown;

Describe the advantages and disadvantages of the various adjunctive diagnostic methods for detecting periodontal disease activity; and

Describe the type of patient that may require adjunctive diagnostic testing.

KEY WORDS

- periodontal diseases
- periodontal disease activity
- gingival crevicular fluid
- host-derived enzymes
- periodontal pathogens
- genetics

INTRODUCTION

Currently, identifying inflammatory **periodontal diseases** involves recognizing disease severity. Such traditional tests as visual inspection, probing depths, clinical attachment levels, and radiographs have not changed in the last 40 years and are considered the foundation for a periodontal examination. However, newer examination techniques may provide additional information beyond that which can be obtained from a clinical examination. Such information may offer predictions about the future of periodontal disease progression and patient evaluation. Approximately 30% of periodontal diseases are recurrent, so it is necessary to monitor the patient to identify problem sites before further tissue damage occurs. Research is ongoing to determine the overall plausibility and effectiveness of these tests. Ultimately, the screening of at-risk patients may allow for improved treatment and prevention of periodontal diseases.

The past decade has seen the evolution of several diagnostic methods designed to be used as an adjunct or in combination with the clinical examination. These methods help in identifying **periodontal disease activity** or patients at risk for an episode of active disease and are designed to help determine the most appropriate mode of treatment. The present standard for periodontal disease activity is a change in clinical attachment level of 2 to 3 mm. Various methods are used to analyze the products of the host response to dental plaque and to identify specific microbial (bacterial) species. The greatest value of diagnostic testing may lie in the ability to monitor patients after treatment, as well as those in the supportive periodontal therapy phase. Hopefully, appropriate testing will allow the practitioner to make therapeutic decisions before the onset of disease activity or at an early stage in its development. The initial determination of the need for active periodontal therapy still depends on use of a periodontal probe, gingival inspection, and radiographs (Bader 1995). Therefore, these new assessment methods shift the focus from determining disease severity to evaluating disease progression or the risk of future periodontal breakdown—in essence, quantifying ongoing disease activity.

Adjunctive tests for the evaluation of periodontal diseases are divided into three main groups: **gingival crevicular fluid** assays, microbial tests, and genetic assays (Table 8–1 ■). Only a few of the tests are available in the United States for in-office use. Table 8–2 ■ reviews the advantages and disadvantages of various tests.

TABLE 8–1

SUPPLEMENTAL DIAGNOSTIC TESTS IN PERIODONTICS

Methods of detecting bacteria:
  Culture and sensitivity techniques (an outside laboratory is used)
  DNA probes (DMDx®; MicroDenteX, Fort Meyers, FL)
  Dark-field or phase-contrast microscopy (available commercially)
  Immunologic assays (not available commercially)
  Enzyme-based assays (not available commercially)

Methods of detecting sites actively breaking down or at risk for future destruction:
  Gingival crevicular fluid assays (not commercially available)
    Collagenase
    Aspartate aminotransferase

Genetic susceptibility test:
  Interleukin-1 genotype (PST™; Medical Science Systems, Flagstaff, AZ)

Diagnosis of PD   *Know generally*

TABLE 8–2
ADVANTAGES AND LIMITATIONS OF SELECTIVE ADJUNCTIVE TESTS

TEST	ADVANTAGES	LIMITATIONS
Culture	• Identifies specific microorganisms • Only test available that determines antibiotic sensitivity	• Expensive and time-consuming • Technique sensitive; diverse data from different labs (use of different media, sampling, transport) • Cell vitality must be preserved during transportation to lab • Some organisms may be lost through sampling
DNA probe assays	• Highly sensitive and specific for targeted periodontal pathogens • Viable organisms not needed • Samples sent by mail after collection chairside • Rapid identification (18 hours)	• Need special disposal procedures for radioactive waste • Does not determine antibiotic sensitivity of the bacteria being tested • Certain bacterial species may not be detected due to highly sensitive nature of the test • Performed in a lab
Microscopic test (phase-contrast microscopy)	• Good for chairside patient awareness of the importance of bacteria in periodontal disease • Motivational tool for patient's plaque-control habits	• Does not specifically identify bacterial species, only shape, size, and mobility • Not suitable to monitor disease activity
GCF enzyme assays	• Rapid and inexpensive • Technique insensitive, so easy to perform chairside • Good for screening purposes • In-office use	• Cannot identify specific bacteria, but allows for rapid assessment of bacterial enzymatic activity • Need sufficient amount of enzymes

GINGIVAL CREVICULAR FLUID ASSAYS

Of the three most common fluids found within the oral cavity [gingival crevicular fluid (GCF), serum, and saliva], GCF has been the focus of most research in recent years. GCF is a fluid that originates from the gingival connective tissue (lamina propria) and flows into the gingival crevice. As a result of inflammation, GCF is formed when fluids leak from dilated blood vessels within the lamina propria. As this fluid flows through the inflamed connective tissue, it picks up tissue breakdown products, enzymes, and other substances involved in the immune response. In this regard, it is an "inflammatory soup" containing subgingival bacteria, inflammatory cells, and a vast array of other substances (mediators) produced by bacteria and host cells. GCF is relatively easy to collect by placing paper strips into selected pockets (Fig. 8–1 ■). It is these features that make GCF a good source of potential markers of periodontal destruction.

In areas affected by periodontal disease, GCF is an abundant source of substances (e.g., inflammatory mediators) that appear to play a central role in the tissue breakdown processes associated with periodontitis. This idea has led to the investigation of certain inflammatory mediators and their possible role as markers for active periodontitis (Armitage 1992). Although these investigations have, over the past 20 years, resulted in the evolution of many techniques for assessing

FIGURE 8–1

Collection of gingival crevicular fluid (GCF). Placement of filter paper strips into the gingival crevice. (Courtesy of Pro-Dentec™, Batesville, AR.)

various aspects of disease, currently none are commercially available. Among the mediators that have been looked at most closely are **host-derived enzymes** (enzymes produced by host cells), inflammatory mediators, and tissue breakdown products.

HOST-DERIVED ENZYMES

During the disease process, certain host cells found in the body, such as polymorphonuclear leukocytes (neutrophils), release certain enzymes, including β-glucuronidase and elastase. These host-derived enzymes are components of GCF and have been reported to be associated with an increased risk of clinical attachment loss and bone loss (Lamster et al. 1988, 1995). Elevated levels of these enzymes in the GCF, which can be used as markers for periodontitis, are most evident 6 months before the occurrence of disease (Palcanis et al. 1992).

Aspartate aminotransferase (AST) is an intracellular enzyme (e.g., it stays inside the cell) that indicates cell death when it is present extracelluarly (e.g., outside the cell). Cell death leads to the release of the contents of the cell into the extracellular fluid. When AST is present at elevated levels in GCF, it has been shown to predict clinical attachment loss (Persson, DeRouen, and Page 1990), but over a shorter period than β-glucuronidase and elastase. Evidence from studies on AST in the GCF of patients at risk for periodontal disease indicates that elevated levels of the enzyme can predict clinical attachment loss an average of 3 months in advance (Chambers et al. 1991). Currently, however, no test is available commercially.

Collagenase is an enzyme that breaks down collagen and is responsible for normal collagen remodeling. In the presence of inflammation, however, excessive amounts of collagenase are produced that cause periodontal tissue destruction during periodontal inflammation. Collagenase is produced by and released from host cells such as neutrophils (Overall et al. 1991). Fibroblasts also produce and release collagen and collagenase, but this occurs during the normal tissue remodeling. Currently, however no test is available commercially to detect "high" collagenase levels in the GCF.

PROSTAGLANDIN E₂

Prostaglandin E_2 (PGE_2) is a metabolite of arachidonic acid that is associated with many inflammatory effects, including bone loss. PGE_2 concentrations in the GCF of patients with clinical attachment loss of 3 mm or more have been shown to be significantly higher than in patients without this level of attachment loss (Offenbacher, Odler, and van Dyke 1986). Identification of high levels of PGE_2 in GCF can indicate an increased risk of periodontal disease up to 6 months prior to its appearance clinically. Currently, however, no test is available commercially in the United States.

MICROBIAL TESTS

Bacterial plaque is the primary cause of the initiation and progression of inflammatory periodontal diseases. Suggested **periodontal pathogens** include *Actinobacillus actinomycetemcomitans, Porphyromonas gingivalis, Bacteriodes forsythus, Prevotella intermedia, Campylobacter rectus, Eikinella corrodens, Fusobacterium nucleatum, Capnocytophaga sputigena, Peptostreptococcus mitis, Selenomonas* spp., *Eubacterium* spp., and *Haemophilus* spp. (Socransky and Haffajee 1991; Tanner 1992).

Over the past few decades, the understanding of periodontal diseases has changed dramatically. Currently, it is theorized that specific bacterial types cause specific periodontal diseases, including localized and generalized aggressive periodontitis, and refractory cases (Loesche 1976; Slots 1986). Treatment of these specific periodontal diseases is best aimed at identification of the periodontal pathogens responsible. While no single one of these pathogens has been indicated as the organism responsible for disease progression, all the preceding bacteria are considered potential periodontal pathogens when identified in subgingival plaque samples. Identification of these pathogens allows for faster and better treatment aimed at eliminating or reducing bacterial levels.

Since gingivitis and chronic periodontitis are not commonly associated with specific bacteria, identification of these diseases probably would not benefit from the use of microbial testing.

Many methods for bacterial testing are available for research and clinical use. These include culturing, microscopic DNA and probe, and immunologic techniques.

CULTURE TECHNIQUES

Culturing allows for the growth of certain microorganisms found in periodontal pockets. Specific in-office procedures must be followed. After removal of supragingival plaque, samples of subgingival bacteria are taken from the plaque with a curet and are placed in a transport fluid and sent to a licensed clinical laboratory within a day or two to maintain bacterial viability (bacteria must be alive on reaching the laboratory). The laboratory then disperses the sample, dilutes it, and plates it on selective and nonselective media. The most common pathogens are identified, and antibiotic susceptibility is determined. A detailed report of the findings is then sent back to the dental office, including the systemic antibiotics to which the cultured bacteria are sensitive. Knowing the susceptibility or resistance of specific microorganisms to these antibiotics provides important guidelines for antibiotic use in conjunction with periodontal therapy.

Cost and time constraints limit the use of such a process, so it is not appropriate for all patients. However, culture analysis may be useful for patients who do not respond to conventional therapy, especially if they have taken antibiotics previously (Armitage 1993). Culturing is the only test that can determine the antimicrobial sensitivity of cultured bacteria. In addition, culturing is limited in that it can only detect living bacteria; some bacteria may not survive transportation to the laboratory. Only a few dental schools offer this service, including the University of Pennsylvania and the University of Southern California.

Microscopic Techniques

Identification of subgingival flora also may be accomplished through various microscopic techniques such as phase-contrast and dark-field microscopy. Rather than identifying specific bacteria, phase-contrast microscopy categorizes bacteria by motility (motile), and dark-field microscopy identifies the morphology or shape (e.g., cocci, rods). Bacterial shifts from nonmotile to motile species often indicate a change from health to disease (Listgarten and Levin 1981). Genus and species determination, as well as antibiotic susceptibility, is not possible using these techniques. Many dental offices use microscopic techniques solely for patient education. Clinically, a digital camera and monitor are attached to the microscope.

Nucleic Acid (DNA) Probe Analysis

All living organisms contain DNA (deoxyribonucleic acid), which carries all genetic information needed for the coding for proteins, the basic building blocks of life (Papapanou, Engelbretson, and Lamster 1999). The DNA of each species consists of a specific sequence that is unique to that organism. Nucleic acid probe analysis identifies DNA sequences specific for certain subgingival periodontal pathogens. In the dental office, plaque samples are collected by inserting a special sterile paper point into the base of a pocket. This paper point is then placed in an air-filled vial and mailed to a testing service. Bacterial DNA is so stable that no special transport fluid is required before mailing the sample, and the bacteria do not have to be living. This is a key advantage to using DNA as a biochemical marker in the identification of periodontal pathogens. The microorganism's DNA is cut into single-strand fragments. The DNA probe is made in the laboratory and labeled with either a radioactive or enzyme marker. If binding of the labeled DNA probe strands occurs, the test organism is thus identified. DNA probe reports are rapid, relatively inexpensive, and can detect nonviable species (Sonnier 1996, Loesche 1992). This test (DMDx® Test) is available through a few laboratories, including MicroDenteX in Fort Meyers, Florida. In the future, more pathogenic bacteria may be identified with DNA probes.

Currently, there is no reason to use DNA probes routinely in every patient. Such tests are expensive, only limited numbers of pathogens are identified, and no antimicrobial sensitivity is determined. DNA probes should be reserved for refractory cases where previous treatments have failed to control disease progression.

IMMUNOLOGIC ASSAYS

The enzyme-linked immunosorbent assay (ELIZA) is based on the specific binding of an antibody to an antigen on the surface of a microorganism. The primary antibody is detected by labeling with a fluorescent secondary antibody. ELIZA is able to identify specific bacteria. It is an expensive test and currently used only in research.

ENZYME-BASED ASSAYS

The enzymatic approach is based on the ability to screen for the presence of an enzyme unique to one or more bacterial species. In this assay, a plaque sample is exposed to a substance that is degraded by the specific enzyme in question. For example, *Treponema denticola, Porphyromonas gingivalis,* and *Bacteroides forsythus* produce a trypsin-like enzyme that degrades a substance called BANA (benzoyldi-arginine-2-naphthylamide). A positive test indirectly indicates the presence of one or more of the three bacteria (Papapanou, Engelbretson, and Lamster 1999).

GENETIC ASSAYS

Numerous established and potential risk factors are associated with periodontal diseases, including smoking, smokeless tobacco, systemic diseases, age, medications, stress, and **genetics** (heredity). All these factors, except for genetics and age, are acquired or environmental and can be controlled or eliminated. Genetics is an innate risk factor that one is born with and cannot be altered or modified. Kornman et al. (1997) addressed the first association between genetics and periodontal diseases. Interleukin-1 (IL-1) is a cytokine produced and secreted by inflammatory cells such as macrophages as a result of accumulation of bacterial plaque. IL-1 is responsible for inflammation and bone loss. Some individuals produce too much IL-1 in response to bacterial challenge. These individuals are more susceptible to the onset and rapid progression of periodontal diseases than individuals who do not show an IL-1 genotype (gene). IL-1 does not cause periodontal disease directly, but it predisposes the patient to the disease process by increasing inflammation when bacteria are present (Newman 1998). This information allows the patient to be monitored more closely and helps dental practitioners recommend optimal preventive therapy and supportive care programs (Newman 1998).

Recently, a test has become available that determines if a patient has an IL-1 genotype in his or her blood. This test is called PST™ (Periodontal Susceptibility Testing; Medical Science Systems, Inc., Flagstaff, AZ). The test is performed by taking a finger-stick blood sample from the patient. The sample is analyzed in a licensed medical laboratory to determine if the patient is positive or negative for the IL-1 genotype. An IL-1 gene-positive patient is about seven times more likely to develop or have advanced periodontal disease than a gene-negative patient, and this genotype occurs in approximately 30% of the population.

Clinical Applications

Although at present a good clinical judgment as to the presence of periodontal disease can be made using existing diagnostic procedures, this decision may be very subjective and sometimes unreliable. Therefore, there is a need for more precise decision making, and care should be taken in evaluating and using these new systems. However, presently, there are no completely validated assessment procedures that can identify progressing or active periodontitis.

Since the etiology of and risk factors for periodontal diseases are multifaceted, the most important steps for patient evaluation include a comprehensive clinical and radiographic analysis and identification of modifying systemic risk factors, including cigarette smoking and diabetes mellitus. Additionally, the host response contributes to the development and progression of the disease. Therefore, no microbial or host response test will definitively determine the initiation or progression of disease.

It is without foundation to use these tests on all periodontal patients. A critical factor that needs to be considered when a practitioner chooses to introduce diagnostic testing as part of patient care is when to use the tests. At a time when there is great pressure to reduce health care cost, judicious application is critical (Lamster 1996).

Culture and sensitivity testing can provide guidelines for antibiotic selection in certain cases, including periodontitis patients who are refractory to previous treatment. Such patients probably have been treated previously with numerous antibiotics, and bacterial resistance could have developed. DNA probe analysis can be helpful in these patients, providing rapid results within 24 hours. However, determination of the antibiotic susceptibility of the bacteria identified is not possible with this method. Assessment of the genetic susceptibility of a patient or of children of parents with advanced periodontal disease may soon prove to be an important tool in the initiation of preventive measures.

Summary

Traditional clinical assessments usually will detect inflammatory lesions and direct practitioners to areas requiring therapy and possible additional testing (Greenstein and Rethman 1998). Presently, microbial assays and host-response diagnostic tests appear to have meager use and limited applicability in routine diagnosis in periodontics. These adjunctive diagnostic tests may improve clinical decision making but require further confirmation followed by controlled clinical studies. Additional testing may be beneficial at specific sites or for individual patients when there is diagnostic uncertainty regarding the absence or presence of diseases or when the medical or dental history suggests that a patient is at risk of developing periodontitis (Greenstein and Rethman 1998). Currently, however, few of these tests are available commercially, and no test is available that will definitively determine if a site is actively losing attachment and bone or will lose attachment in the future. There are no specific guidelines to follow, but some factors to consider include cost of testing, age of the patient, patient motivation, and systemic health of the patient.

KEY POINTS

✢ No clinical test is available that will currently determine if a site is actively breaking down or predict periodontal breakdown; more research is needed.

✢ A combination of traditional and new diagnostic testing can, in some cases, provide more complete information for treatment planning.

✢ Bacterial culturing identifies pathogens and determines their susceptibility to various antibiotics.

REFERENCES

Armitage, G. C. 1992. Diagnostic tests for periodontal diseases. *Curr. Opin. Dent.* 21(1): 53–62.

Armitage, G. C. 1993. Periodontal diagnostic aids. *Calif. Dent. Assoc. J.* 21(11):35–46.

Bader, H. I. 1995. Contemporary periodontics and a vision for the future: Diagnostics and monitoring the treated case. *Dentistry Today* 1:42–45.

Chambers, D. A., P. B. Imrey, R. L. Cohen, et al. 1991. A longitudinal study of aspartate aminotransferase in human gingival cervicular fluid. *J. Periodont. Res.* 26:65–74.

Greenstein, G. S., and M. P. Rethman. 1998. Diagnosing destructive periodontal diseases. In *Periodontal therapy: Clinical approaches and evidence of success,* Vol. 1, (eds.) M. Nevins and J. T. Mellonig, 1st ed. Chicago: Quintessence.

Kornman, K. S., A. Crane, H.-Y. Wang, et al. 1997. The interleukin-1 genotype as a severity factor in adult periodontal disease. *J. Clin. Periodontol.* 24:72–77.

Lamster, I. B. 1996. In-office diagnostic tests and their role in supportive periodontal treatment. *Periodontology 2000* 12:49–55.

Lamster, I. B., L. G. Holmes, K. M. Williams-Gross, et al. 1995. The relationship of β-glucuronidase activity in crevicular fluid to probing attachment loss in patients with adult periodontitis: Findings from a multicenter study. *J. Clin. Periodontol.* 22:36–44.

Lamster, I. B., R. L. Oshrain, D. S. Harper, et al. 1988. Enzyme activity in crevicular fluid for detection and prediction of clinical attachment loss in patients with chronic adult periodontitis: Six-month results. *J. Periodontol.* 59:516–523.

Listgarten, M. A., and S. Levin. 1981. Positive correlation between the proportions of subgingival spirochetes and motile bacteria and susceptibility of human subjects to periodontal deterioration. *J. Clin. Periodontol.* 8:122–138.

Loesche, W. J. 1992. DNA probe and enzyme analysis in periodontal diagnostics. *J. Periodontol.* 63:1102–1109.

Loesche, W. J. 1976. Chemotherapy of dental plaque infections. *Oral Sci. Rev.* 9:65–107.

Newman, M. 1998. Genetic, environmental, and behavioral influences on periodontal infections. *Compend. Contin. Educ.* (Special Issue) 19(1):25–31.

Offenbacher, S., B. M. Odle, and T. E. van Dyke. 1986. The use of crevicular fluid prostaglandin E_2 as a predictor of periodontol attachment loss. *J. Periodont. Res.* 21:101–112.

Overall, C. M., J. Sodek, C. A. G. McCulloch, and P. Birek. 1991. Evidence for polymophonuclear leukocyte collagenase and 92-kilodalton gelatinase in gingival crevicular fluid. *Infect. Immun.* 59:4687–4692.

Palcanis, K. G., I. K. Larjara, B. R. Wells, et al. 1992. Elastase as an indicator of periodontal disease progression. *J. Periodontol.* 63:237–242.

Papapanou, P. N., S. P. Engelbretson, and I. B. Lamster. 1999. Current and future approaches for diagnosis of periodontal diseases. *N.Y. State Dent. J.* (April):32–38.

Persson, G. R., T. A. DeRouen, and R. C. Page. 1990. Relationship between gingival crevicular fluid levels of aspartate aminotransferase and active tissue destruction in treated chronic periodontitis patients. *J. Periodont. Res.* 25:81–87.

Slots, J. 1986. Bacterial specificity in adult periodontitis. A summary of recent work. *J. Clin. Periodontol.* 13:912–917.

Socransky, S. S., and A. D. Haffajee. 1991. Microbial mechanisms in the pathogenesis of destructive periodontal diseases: A critical assessment. *J. Periodont. Res.* 26:195–212.

Sonnier, K. E. 1996. Microbial testing: Present and future. *Clin. Update* 18(4):7.

Tanner, A. 1992. Microbial etiology of periodontal diseases: Where are we? Where are we going? *Curr. Opin. Dent.* 2(1):12–24.

Self-Quiz

1. Which one of the following tests is used to determine the susceptibility of bacteria to certain antibiotics? (pp. 263-264)

   a. phase-contrast microscopy
   b. DNA probe
   c. culture
   d. temperature

2. All the following types of patients may require adjunctive periodontal diagnostic testing *except* one. Which one is the exception? (p. 266)

   a. new patients who have not received therapy previously
   b. treated patients who initially present with advanced periodontal disease
   c. patients not responding to periodontal treatment
   d. patients with previously treated gingivitis

3. Which one of the following is the role of genetics as a risk factor for periodontal diseases? (p. 265)

   a. destruction of bone early in life
   b. production of excessive amounts of interleukin-1
   c. demonstration of high levels of bacteria in childhood
   d. presentation with highly inflamed soft tissues

4. Which one of the following is a goal for using host-based diagnostic periodontal tests? (p. 260)

   a. determines the need for future maintenance care
   b. identifies periodontal sites that are bleeding
   c. evaluates the need for more aggressive periodontal treatment
   d. distinguishes between active and inactive disease sites

5. Which one of the following tests is highly sensitive for specific periodontal pathogens present in a subgingival sample of plaque? (p. 264)

   a. culture
   b. DNA probe
   c. GCF enzyme assay
   d. microscopic technique

6. In which one of the following secretions are high levels of host-derived enzymes found? (p. 261)

   a. whole saliva
   b. crevicular fluid
   c. sweat
   d. serum

7. Which one of the following statements is related to adjunctive periodontal tests. (p. 266)

   a. Eventually they will replace conventional periodontal assessment techniques.
   b. They are used on all periodontal patients presenting in the office.
   c. Established guidelines need to be determined.
   d. They are cost-effective and easy to perform.

8. Which one of the following tests identifies the motility of bacteria? (p. 264)

   a. enzyme-linked immunosorbent assay (ELIZA)
   b. phase-contrast microscopy
   c. DNA probe
   d. GCF enzyme
   e. Temperature

9. Which one of the following host cells synthesize and release β-glucuronidase and elastase? (p. 262)

   a. mast cells
   b. lymphocytes
   c. neutrophils
   d. eosinophils
   e. fibroblasts

10. All the following statements are correct concerning the use of DNA probe assays *except* one. Which one is the exception? (p. 264)

   a. They are highly sensitive and specific for targeted periodontal pathogens.
   b. Samples are sent to an outside laboratory.
   c. They require viable microorganisms.
   d. They provide rapid identification.

Cheryl Westphal, R.D.H., M.S.

MEDICAL HISTORY:
The patient is a 39-year-old woman. Blood pressure is 130/82 mmHg, pulse rate is 64, and respiration rate is 16. The patient weighs 145 lb (65.9 kg). She is not under the care of a physician and has not had any illnesses requiring hospitalization within the last 5 years.

CURRENT MEDICATIONS:
The patient is taking an oral contraceptive containing estrogen/progestin (Lo/Ovral®).

DENTAL HISTORY:
The patient states that she brushes with a hard-bristled toothbrush twice a day and flosses only occasionally because she was never taught the proper technique. A previous dentist prescribed chlorhexidine oral rinse, which she is using twice a day. She has not used the rinse continuously and still has a few bottles left. Since then, she has not seen a dentist, which has been about 9 months.

SOCIAL HISTORY:
The patient is married with two young children. She denies drinking. Although the patient has a secure job, she says she is under a lot of stress at home and work. The patient smokes low-tar cigarettes (10 pack/years) and has not attempted to stop.

CHIEF COMPLAINT:
The patient states that "my teeth are sensitive to cold, and I don't like the stains on my teeth. I want a cleaning."

DENTAL EXAM:
The patient has generalized gingival recession and localized tooth abrasion. The maxillary right first molar has an overhanging MOD amalgam.

ORAL HYGIENE STATUS:
Fair. Generalized supra/subgingival plaque and calculus. Generalized staining.

GINGIVAL EXAM:
The gingiva is red, edematous, enlarged, and shiny and smooth. The contour of the papillae is bulbous, and the margins are rolled. Generalized bleeding on probing.

PERIODONTAL EXAM:
Probing depths range from 1 to 8 mm. The mandibular first molars have 8 mm on the direct facial surface and 2mm of gingival recession. There is no tooth mobility. Radiographs show bone loss around the mandibular first molars and the maxillary right first molar.

INTERPRETATION

Patient Problem	Basis for Discussion	Questions (Q)/Answers (A)	Chapter Location
Wants teeth cleaned	Patient wants her teeth cleaned due to buildup of plaque, calculus, and stains—knows it has been 9 months since she last saw a dentist.	Q) Does accumulation of plaque and calculus affect the oral health of the patient? A) Dental plaque is the primary risk factor for periodontal diseases, and calculus is a secondary factor.	6.III.B
Teeth are stained	Patient needs to stop smoking.	Q) Does cigarette smoking affect the periodontium and periodontal treatment? A) Greater probing depths, clinical attachment loss, gingival tissue changes, and bone loss have been reported in smokers; thus periodontal therapy may be less effective.	6.III.C
	Patient needs teeth cleaned due to retention of stains.	Q) Do tooth stains from smoking and chlorhexidine adversely affect the teeth? A) Stains will not directly affect teeth, but the significance of stains is related to the rough surface they may create and the resulting plaque retention sites. Also, it may be unaesthetic to the patient and others.	6.III.B
Medication: Lo/Ovral®	Patient does not want to use an alternative birth control method.	Q) Do oral contraceptives affect the periodontium? A) Elevated hormonal levels (progesterone) aggravate the gingival response to local irritants—gingival inflammation. Good plaque control is important.	6.III.C
Gingival recession and tooth abrasion	Patient should change the type of toothbrush and method used.	Q) What is the etiology of the gingival recession in this patient? A) Faulty toothbrushing	6.III.D
		Q) What is the etiology of the tooth abrasion? A) Over zealous toothbrushing technique with a hard-bristled toothbrush	6.III.A

INTERPRETATION, *continued*

PATIENT PROBLEM	BASIS FOR DISCUSSION	QUESTIONS (Q)/ANSWERS (A)	CHAPTER LOCATION
Overhanging restoration on the maxillary right first molar	Patient experiences difficulty in flossing.	Q) Is an overhang of periodontal concern? A) Overhangs are plaque traps—could result in bone loss.	6.III.A
Generalized bleeding and edematous tissue Localized bone loss Localized furcation involvement	Patient has generalized moderate gingivitis and localized (severe) chronic periodontitis.	Q) What is the etiology of the gingivitis? A) Dental plaque—hormones exaggerate the tissue response to plaque.	6.III.C
		Q) What is the etiology of the bleeding? A) Bleeding indicates inflammation in the lamina propria.	6.III.C
		Q) What is the etiology of the bone loss in the furca? A) Same etiology as progressive periodontal disease—dental plaque. More difficult to control plaque in furcas.	6.III.D
		Q) Are the periodontitis sites active or inactive (e.g., losing attachment)? A) Difficult to determine by conventional assessment tools. Currently, between 2 and 3 mm change in clinical attachment level must occur before a site can be labeled disease-active.	6.III.D, 8
	It is difficult to see the alveolar crest on the periapicals and bitewings molar films.	Q) What technique can be used to allow visualization of the maxillary and manibular alveolar crest. A) Use vertical bitewings.	7

1. Which one of the following statements is considered objective data in this patient's history. (p. 147)

    a. Cold hurts my teeth.

    b. My teeth have a lot of stains on them.

    c. The gingiva is erythematous and edematous.

    d. A hard-bristled toothbrush seems to work best.

    e. I occasionally use the mouthrinse that was prescribed

2. Which one of the following assessment tests is *most* appropriate for this patient? (p. 195)

   a. genetic susceptibility testing
   b. gingival and periodontal
   c. culture and sensitivity
   d. DNA probe

3. The amount of clinical attachment loss on the facial surface of the mandibular right first molar is _____ mm. (p. 217)

   a. 2
   b. 6
   c. 8
   d. 10
   e. 12

4. Which one of the following treatment goals is *most* important to discuss with this patient? (p. 147)

   a. Work out a financially acceptable plan that is affordable.
   b. Refer to a physician for smoking cessation.
   c. Stress the importance of keeping all appointments.
   d. Reduce plaque levels and stop the progression of periodontal disease.

5. The medications this patient is taking mimic which of the following medical conditions? (p. 202)

   a. diabetes mellitus
   b. hyperthyroidism
   c. pregnancy
   d. cirrhosis

6. Which one of the following types of radiographs would *best* show the overhang on the restoration on the maxillary right first molar? (p. 242)

   a. panoramic
   b. computed tomography
   c. horizontal bitewing
   d. digital subtraction radiology

7. Which one of the following Glickman's classification of furcation involvement is evident on the mandibular first molars? (p. 224)

   a. I
   b. II
   c. III
   d. IV

8. Which one of the following types of stains are present in this patient? (p. 188)

   a. extrinsic, endogenous
   b. extrinsic, exogenous
   c. intrinsic, endogenous
   d. intrinsic, exogenous

9. Which one of the following conditions is a consequence of the exposed root surfaces in the furca area of the mandibular first molars? (p. 168)

   a. caries
   b. fracture
   c. hypoplasia
   d. hypocalcification

10. Which one of the following histologic features explains the consistency of the interdental papillae in this patient? (p. 199)

   a. ulceration of the epithelium
   b. destruction of the gingival fibers
   c. accumulation of fluid in the tissue
   d. engorgement of blood in the tissue

PERIODONTAL DISEASES: THE PREVENTION AND TREATMENT PHASE

Section III

EVIDENCE-BASED TREATMENT PLANNING

Jill Rethman, R.D.H., B.A.
Michael P. Rethman, D.D.S., M.S.

Outline:

Evidence-Based Approach to Treatment
Etiology and Treatment Planning
Referral to a Periodontist
Informed Consent
Treatment Guidelines
Adjunctive Treatment
Geriatric Patients
Summary
Key Points
References
Self-Quiz

Goals:

To provide the dental hygienist with an understanding of periodontal diseases and evidence-based periodontal treatment planning.

Educational Objectives:

Upon completion of this chapter, the reader should be able to:

Discuss the evidence-based approach to treatment planning;

Describe treatment guidelines for periodontal patients;

Explain when more aggressive forms of therapy are needed and thus appropriate times for referral to a periodontist;

Explain "informed consent";

Describe geriatric patient considerations in periodontal treatment planning; and

Discuss periodontal prognostic signs.

KEY WORDS

- treatment planning
- evidence-based
- informed consent
- prognosis

𝓘n contrast with the past, when "pyorrhea" or "gum disease" was regarded as incurable, it is now known that in most cases periodontal diseases can be treated successfully—and the periodontium restored to health and the teeth maintained for a lifetime. The therapies selected to accomplish this depend on a thorough knowledge of periodontal diseases, treatment procedures, and the individual patient. In combination with the dentist and patient, the dental hygienist plays an integral role in the team approach to periodontal therapy.

Controlling inflammation is the initial treatment objective of therapies aimed at the periodontal diseases. The key to controlling inflammation is to eliminate, reduce, or change the makeup of microbes residing in the mouth. Elimination of deeper periodontal pocket depths is not always necessary, but it is usually desirable to obtain probing depths that are shallow enough for the practitioner and the patient to keep free of pathogenic dental plaque. This is also the goal of many of the periodontal surgical procedures. Of course, once inflammation is brought under control, the prevention of recurrent periodontitis is essential (Hancock 1996).

In recent years, research findings have shown that plaque microbes are not entirely responsible for the initiation and progression of the periodontal diseases (Ismail et al. 1990). The host's immune response to infection also can play an important role by producing chemical modulators that actually accelerate periodontal destruction (Grossi et al. 1994, 1995). Therefore, comprehensive periodontal therapy may soon include tactics to modulate the host's immune response in addition to traditional efforts to suppress periodontal pathogens.

This chapter explores current concepts of periodontal **treatment planning** based on contemporary scientific evidence.

EVIDENCE-BASED APPROACH TO TREATMENT

The main goal of the 1996 World Workshop in Periodontics was to improve treatment decisions made by practitioners. Rather than making clinical decisions based solely on experience, the **evidence-based** approach attempts to improve treatment results by using information from the research literature (e.g., articles in dental/scientific journals; Newman 1998). The periodontal literature can help practitioners better determine and evaluate the pros and cons of various treatments in the context of individual patients. Better therapeutic decision making is the result (Tables 9–1 through 9–3 ■).

The American Academy of Periodontology has developed practice parameters on the diagnosis and treatment of periodontal diseases. These parameters of care (American Academy of Periodontology, 2000) are strategies to assist dental practitioners in making clinical decisions from a range of treatment options to achieve a desired outcome.

ETIOLOGY AND TREATMENT PLANNING

For many years, periodontitis was thought to be the inevitable result of poor oral hygiene along with uncontrolled dental plaque and calculus accumulation. This was termed the *nonspecific plaque hypothesis* (Loesche 1976). In recent decades, research has suggested instead that there are microbial species whose

TABLE 9–1
CONSENSUS FINDINGS: DIAGNOSIS OF PERIODONTITIS

TEST	APPLICATION	STRENGTHS	WEAKNESSES	TYPE OF EVIDENCE
Periodontal screening and recording	All patients in every practice	Cost-effective, quick, easy, detects patients with periodontal disease	Does not provide a tooth-by-tooth assessment for later comparison during maintenance therapy; a full periodontal examination is needed for this purpose	Epidemiologic studies
Probing pocket depths	All patients	Shallow probing depths associated with a lack of future disease progression	Moderate to deep pockets in a single probing depth examination will not distinguish with certainty which teeth will undergo progressive periodontal destruction	Longitudinal studies
Gingival inflammation assessment	All patients	Absence of inflammation is associated with a lack of future disease progression; in treated patients, bleeding on probing is associated with an increased risk of progressive loss of attachment	Presence of inflammation will not distinguish with certainty which teeth will undergo progressive periodontal destruction	Longitudinal studies
Radiographic evidence of bone loss	At-risk patients as determined by PSR screening or periodontal examination	Absence of bone loss is associated with a lower risk of future disease progression	Presence of bone loss on a single radiograph will not distinguish with certainty which teeth will undergo progressive periodontal destruction	Longitudinal studies
Microbial plaque tests	High-risk or refractory patients	Absence of supragingival plaque is associated with a lack of disease progression In compromised or refractory patients, may be useful in determining the presence of pathogens	Routine testing offers limited benefit in adult periodontitis	Cross-sectional and longitudinal studies Case reports
Biochemical profiles in gingival crevicular fluid	Not yet determined	A number of biochemical markers may identify individuals at risk	At present, there are no specific biochemical profiles that characterize specific periodontal diseases	Cross-sectional and longitudinal studies

Source: From M. K. Jeffcoat, M. McGuire, and M. G. Newman. 1997. Evidence-based periodontal treatment: Highlights from the 1996 World Workshop in Periodontics. J. Am. Dent. Assoc. 128:713–724. Copyright 1997 by the American Dental Association. Reprinted by permission of ADA Publishing Co., Inc.

281

TABLE 9–2

CONSENSUS FINDINGS: NONSURGICAL TREATMENT OF GINGIVITIS AND PERIODONTITIS

TREATMENT CATEGORY	TREATMENT	STRENGTHS	WEAKNESSES	TYPE OF EVIDENCE
Professional mechanical therapy—used in the treatment of gingivitis and periodontitis	Scaling and root planing with manual instrument	Decreases gingival inflammation by 40% to 60%; decreases probing depth; facilitates gain in clinical attachment level	Requires attention to detail	Many longitudinal, cohort and randomized clinical trials
	Ultrasonic and sonic scaling and root planing	Results are similar to those for manual scaling and root planing		Longitudinal, cohort and randomized clinical trials
Chemical plaque control with mouthrinses and toothpastes	Chlorhexidine; triclosan with copolymer or triclosan with zinc citrate; essential oils; stannous fluoride	Significant reduction in gingival inflammation	No clear evidence that there is a substantial long-term benefit in periodontitis except to control coexisting inflammation	Randomized, double-blind clinical trials
Irrigation	Supragingival and subgingival irrigation used as an adjunct to brushing	Aids in the reduction of gingivitis	No clear evidence that there is a substantial long-term benefit for periodontitis	Randomized, double-blind clinical trials
Sustained-release antimicrobials	Intrapocket resorbable or nonresorbable delivery systems containing a tetracycline antibiotic	When used as an adjunct to scaling and root planing, gains in clinical attachment level and decreases in probing depth and bleeding	A few reported side effects include transient discomfort, erythema, recession, allergy and, rarely, Candida	Randomized, double-blind clinical trials
Systemic antibiotics	Tetracyclines, metronidazole, spiramycin, clindamycin, and combinations such as metronidazole and amoxicillin	May be useful to treat aggressive, destructive periodontitis	Not indicated for gingivitis; not indicated for most adult patients with periodontitis	Assessment of risk-benefit ratio; randomized, double-blind clinical trials; longitudinal assessment of patients' conditions

Source: From M. K. Jeffcoat, M. McGuire, and M. G. Newman. 1997. Evidence-based periodontal treatment: Highlights from the 1996 World Workshop in Periodontics. *J. Am. Dent. Assoc.* 128:713–724. Copyright 1997 by the American Dental Association. Reprinted by permission of ADA Publishing Co., Inc.

TABLE 9-3

CONSENSUS FINDINGS: SURGICAL PERIODONTAL THERAPY—SELECTED PROCEDURES

CATEGORY AND GOAL	TREATMENT	STRENGTHS	WEAKNESSES	TYPE OF EVIDENCE
Pocket therapy provides access to root surfaces and bony defects, reduces probing depths, facilitates plaque control and enhances restorative and cosmetic dentistry	Modified Widman flap to provide access to roots and bony defects for débridement; apically repositioned flap with or without bony recontouring; gingivectomy	All procedures decrease pocket depth; with the exception of gingivectomy, all increase clinical attachment level; after 5 years, greatest reduction in probing depth with osseous recontouring; apically repositioned flap with or without bony recontouring used in crown-lengthening procedures to provide biologic width	Procedures designed to reduce probing depths may increase recession; lack of professional maintenance and patient compliance can be detrimental to the long-term success	Randomized clinical trials; longitudinal studies
Regenerative procedures to facilitate growth of new periodontal ligament, cementum and bone over previously diseased root surfaces	Extraoral autogenous bone grafts	High potential for bone growth	Second surgical site (such as iliac crest); root resorption may be associated with fresh grafts	Limited case report data
	Intraoral autogenous grafts (such as maxillary tuberosity, healing extraction sites, osseous coagulum)	Case reports indicate bone gain of more than 50%; controlled studies comparing grafts with nongrafted bone show improved clinical attachment levels and bone, but not as great as those in case reports		Case reports; comparative controlled clinical studies
	Allografts—tissues transferred from one person to another; freeze-dried bone allograft	Bone fill has been reported in a high proportion of defects involving freeze-dried bone allograft		
	Alloplasts—synthetic grafts • Absorbable: plaster; calcium carbonates, ceramics such as tricalcium phosphate and absorbable hydroxyapatite (HA) • Nonabsorbable: dense HA, porous HA, bioglass • Calcium-coated polymer polymethylmethacrylate and hydroxymethylmethacrylate	Improved probing depth and attachment level Some evidence of histologic regeneration in calcium-coated polymer polymethylmethacrylate and hydroxymethylmethacrylate	Osteogenic potential may vary from vial to vial; patient differences; clinician variability Histologic findings indicate that synthetic grafts primarily act as fillers, with little if any regeneration	Field test; controlled clinical trials Controlled clinical trials

Continued

283

TABLE 9–3, CONTINUED

CONSENSUS FINDINGS: SURGICAL PERIODONTAL THERAPY—SELECTED PROCEDURES

CATEGORY AND GOAL	TREATMENT	STRENGTHS	WEAKNESSES	TYPE OF EVIDENCE
Guided tissue regeneration—physical barriers are used to facilitate selective cell population of the root surface after periodontal surgery to promote regeneration	Nonresorbable membranes	Significant improvement in clinical attachment level compared with débridement alone; most favorable results are in Class II furcations in the mandible and infrabony defects; no need for second-stage surgery (resorbable only)	Less favorable results in maxillary molar and Class III defects; nonresorbable membrane requires a second surgery to remove the membrane	Randomized, controlled clinical trials; uncontrolled studies; and case reports
	Resorbable materials		Clinical results similar to those for nonresorbable membranes but less evidence available to allow a comparison of predictability with respect to nonresorbable membranes	
Gingival augmentation to promote root coverage	Pedicle grafts Free soft tissue grafts (epithelialized or connective-tissue graft) Combination grafts • Connective tissue or biodegradable membrane barrier plus pedicle graft • Coronally positioned, previously placed soft tissue graft • Nonbiodegradable membrane barrier plus pedicle graft	Improve aesthetics/cosmetic results; decrease root sensitivity; manage defects resulting from root caries removal or cervical abrasion; manage mucogingival defects		Case reports; comparison studies
Endosseous dental implants	Two-stage and one-stage implants; titanium; titanium alloy; hydroxyapatite-coated implants	Dental implants are predictable replacements for missing teeth in fully and partially edentulous patients	While there are few studies in the literature, the clinician should use caution in the following cases: smoking, untreated periodontal disease, poor oral hygiene, uncontrolled systemic disease, history of radiation therapy, active skeletal growth	Longitudinal studies

Source: From M. K. Jeffcoat, M. McGuire, and M. G. Newman. 1997. Evidence-based periodontal treatment: Highlights from the 1996 World Workshop in Periodontics. J. Am. Dent. Assoc. 128:713–724. Copyright 1997 by the American Dental Association. Reprinted by permission of ADA Publishing Co., Inc.

presence tends to signal a greater likelihood of progressive periodontal destruction (Haffajee et al. 1991). Furthermore, for most patients, evidence suggests that procedures aimed at suppressing these species will improve clinical outcomes. However, for adults, front-line periodontal therapy remains largely nonspecific in design—because conventional clinical and self-care procedures often succeed among this predominating group of periodontitis patients. For periodontal diseases in young people, for refractory disease in adults, and in special situations, periodontal therapy may include procedures aimed at specific putative periodontal pathogens.

GOALS OF PERIODONTAL THERAPY

The ideal goal of periodontal therapy is to restore the periodontium to an attractive, comfortable, and functional state of health for the balance of the patient's life. Therefore, most periodontal therapy aims to prevent the initiation, progression, or recurrence of periodontal diseases. This can be termed *arrestive* periodontal therapy. However, where periodontal destruction has occurred, regeneration of the specialized periodontal tissue is often worth pursuing when possible. This is termed *regenerative* periodontal therapy. Successful regenerative periodontal therapy usually includes an arrestive component. The first step in developing a treatment plan should be to determine individual treatment goals for each patient.

PERIODONTAL THERAPY: ONGOING CARE

The management of most periodontal patients demands continued reassessments and adjustments to ongoing care. This is so because periodontal care is not permanent in the sense that many other highly successful dental therapies are considered. For most cases of chronic periodontitis, the only permanent periodontal end point is tooth (or implant) loss. Furthermore, no single periodontal treatment produces ideal outcomes for all patients.

Once a patient is practicing thorough daily oral hygiene self-care, the ideal interval between patient appointments—even for patients in periodontal maintenance programs—may be as brief as every 2 to 3 months (Axelsson and Lindhe 1981). Frequent reexaminations, reevaluations, and adjustments to therapy often are necessary for many years. Given this context, practitioners need to comply with their ethical and medicolegal responsibilities to refer periodontitis patients to specialists, provide comparable periodontal care in the general practice, or partner with a specialist to share responsibilities for periodontal patients. Suggestions governing what, when, and why to refer are made where appropriate throughout this chapter.

TREATMENT PLANNING

Once the examination is completed, the data must be analyzed. Data include the patient's medical and dental history, complete radiographs, detailed periodontal data, tooth conditions (including vitality, caries, and morphologic abnormalities), and dental awareness.

In addition to developing a "best case" treatment plan, reasonable alternatives should be considered and presented to the patient. Flowcharts may help delineate the general route a patient takes during treatment (Figs. 9–1 through 9–6 ■).

| FIGURE 9–1 |

Periodontal health. Gingival tissues are healthy when there is no bleeding after gentle probing.

First appointment: 45 minutes to 1 hour

- Comprehensive oral evaluation (new patients) or periodic oral evaluation (existing patients)—consisting of a medical and dental history update, vital signs, head and neck examination, and oral cancer screening.
- Complete x-ray series, including vertical bitewings (new patients) or indicated radiographs (existing patients).
- Oral hygiene instruction.
- Oral prophylaxis.
- Selective polishing, if needed.
- Nutritional counseling for the control of dental caries.
- Fluoride treatment (caries control).
- Tobacco counseling for the control and prevention of oral disease, if indicated.
- Suitable maintenance interval established (3, 6, or more months).

| FIGURE 9–2 |

Gingivitis. Probing depths of less than 4 mm. Plaque and calculus present. No bone loss or mobility.

First appointment: 1 hour

- Comprehensive oral evaluation (new patients) or periodic oral evaluation (existing patients)—consisting of a medical and dental history update, head and neck examination, and oral cancer screening. Make referrals if necessary.
- Periodontal examination.
- Complete x-ray series, including vertical bitewings (new patients) or indicated radiographs (existing patients).
- Note and record sites that bleed on gentle probing.
- Oral hygiene instruction after staining for plaque and relating stained areas to bleeding sites.
- Full-mouth debridement.
- Nutritional counseling for the control of dental caries.
- Tobacco counseling for the control and prevention of oral disease, if indicated.

Second appointment: At least 45 minutes, scheduled 7 to 10 days after first appointment.

- Review medical and dental history.
- Stain for plaque.
- Note and record sites that bleed on gentle probing.
- Evaluate tissue response to previous treatment on a site-by-site basis. If inflammation persists, determine the cause. If plaque or calculus are present, debride the area(s) and reinforce oral hygiene. Adjunctive antimicrobial mouthrinses may be recommended.
- Reinforce plaque control instruction.
- Selective polishing, if indicated.
- Nutritional counseling for the control of dental caries, if needed.
- Fluoride treatment (caries control).
- Tobacco counseling for the control of oral disease, if needed.
- If gingival health has been achieved, a suitable maintenance interval is established (3 to 6 months), or after 7 to 10 days, a third appointment is scheduled if needed.
- Referral to periodontist if necessary with alternating maintenance visits planned.

FIGURE 9–3

Slight chronic periodontitis. Probing depths of 4 to 5 mm clinical attachment loss (CAL) of 1 to 2 mm. Slight horizontal bone loss (up to 20%). No mobility or furcation involvement. Supra- and subgingival deposits. Bleeding on probing.

First appointment: 1 hour
- Comprehensive oral evaluation (new patients) or periodic oral evaluation (existing patients)—consisting of a medical and a dental history update, head and neck examination, and oral cancer screening. Make referrals if necessary.
- Periodontal examination. Sites that bleed on probing should be recorded.
- Complete x-ray series, including vertical bitewings (new patients) or indicated radiographs (existing patients).
- Stain for plaque and relate stained areas to bleeding sites as part of oral hygiene instruction (patient learns cause and effect).
- Periodontal debridement by quadrant (use of local anesthesia is determined by the practitioner).
- Adjunctive antimicrobial irrigation or mouthrinse, if indicated.
- Nutritional counseling for the control of dental caries.
- Tobacco counseling for the control and prevention of oral disease, if indicated.
- Application of desensitizing medicaments, if needed.

Second, third, and fourth appointments: At least 45 minutes (each scheduled 7 to 10 days after previous appointment)

- Review medical and dental history.
- Evaluate tissue response from previous treatment.
- Stain for plaque.
- Chart sites that bleed on gentle probing.
- Relate stained areas to any bleeding sites as part of oral hygiene instruction (patient learns cause and effect).
- Reinforce plaque-control instruction.
- Continue debridement procedures by quadrant.
- Nutritional counseling for the control of dental caries.
- Tobacco counseling for the control and prevention of oral disease, if indicated.
- Sustained, slow-release, local-delivery antimicrobials may be used at sites not fully responsive to self-care and debridement. (Although long-term use is not yet scientifically validated, so long as clinical parameters are promptly reassessed and nonresponders are referred, this tactic should offer little or no risk.)
- Application of desensitizing medicaments, if needed.

Fifth appointment (reevaluation of therapy): At least 45 minutes (scheduled 4 to 6 weeks after previous appointment)

- Review medical and dental history.
- Evaluate tissue response from previous treatment.
- Oral and dental examination.
- Periodontal examination; record sites that bleed on probing.
- Stain for plaque and relate stained areas to any bleeding sites as part of oral hygiene instruction (patient learns cause and effect).
- Selective polishing, if indicated.
- Nutritional counseling, if needed.
- Tobacco counseling, if indicated.
- Application of desensitizing medicaments, if needed.

At this time, the patient may be put on a suitable maintenance interval of every 2 to 4 months if inflammation appears arrested (e.g., no bleeding on probing from deep pockets at sites that patient is maintaining plaque-free) and there is no other reason to refer to specialist (e.g., unresolved dentinal hypersensitivity, gingival recession, desire or need for periodontal plastic surgery). Over time, this interval can be increased in patients who remain inflammation-free.

If there are nonresponsive sites characterized by deep (>4 mm) probing depths that bleed on probing or at sites of previous attachment loss, referral to the periodontist is appropriate. Given the potential for rapid loss of attachment at any susceptible site, a decision to engage in "watchful waiting" is ethically and legally problematic.

If bleeding on probing persists at shallower sites (gingivitis), the practitioner should reevaluate the patient's self-care techniques and remove any subgingival calculus from suspect sites. Referral to the periodontist is an option for these patients as well.

Figure 9–4

Moderate chronic periodontitis. Probing depths of 6 to 7 mm clinical attachment loss (CAL) of 3 to 4 mm. Moderate horizontal/vertical bone loss (20 to 50%). Mobility and early furcation involvement. Supra- and subgingival deposits. Bleeding on probing.

First appointment: 1 hour

- Comprehensive oral evaluation (new patients) or periodic oral evaluation (existing patients)—consisting of a medical and dental history update, head and neck examination, and oral cancer screening. Make referrals if necessary.
- Complete x-ray series, including vertical bitewings (new patients) or indicated radiographs (existing patients). Referral to the periodontist depends on the type and amount of bone loss.
- Periodontal examination. Sites that bleed on probing should be recorded.
- Stain for plaque and relate stained areas to bleeding sites as part of oral hygiene instruction (patient learns cause and effect).
- Nutritional counseling for the control of dental caries.
- Tobacco counseling for the control and prevention of oral disease, if indicated.
- Application of desensitizing medicaments, if needed.

Second, third, and fourth appointments: 1 hour (each scheduled 7 to 10 days after previous appointment)

- Review medical and dental history.
- Evaluate tissue response from previous treatment.
- Chart sites that bleed on gentle probing.
- Stain for plaque and relate stained areas to any bleeding sites as part of oral hygiene instruction (patient learns cause and effect).
- Reinforce plaque-control instruction.
- Periodontal debridement by quadrant (local anesthesia may be indicated).
- Adjunctive antimicrobial irrigation or mouthrinse, if indicated.
- Nutritional counseling for the control of dental caries.
- Tobacco counseling for the control and prevention of oral disease, if indicated.
- Application of desensitizing medicaments, if needed.

Fifth appointment (reevaluation of therapy): 1 hour (scheduled 4 to 6 weeks after previous appointment):

- Review medical and dental history.
- Evaluate tissue response from previous treatment.
- Oral and dental examination.
- Periodontal examination; record sites that bleed on probing.
- Stain for plaque and relate stained areas to any bleeding sites as part of oral hygiene instruction (patient learns cause and effect).
- Periodontal debridement by quadrant (local anesthesia may be indicated).
- Adjunctive antimicrobial irrigation or mouth rinse, if indicated.
- Sustained, slow-release, local-delivery antimicrobials may be used at nonresponsive sites. [Long-term use (longer than 9 months) is not currently scientifically validated. However, if clinical parameters are promptly reassessed and nonresponders are referred, this tactic should offer little or no risk.]
- Selective polishing, if indicated.
- Nutritional counseling, if needed.
- Tobacco counseling, if indicated.
- Application of desensitizing medicaments, if needed.

At this time, the patient may be put on a suitable maintenance interval of 2 to 4 months if inflammation appears arrested (e.g., no bleeding on probing from deep pockets at sites that patient is maintaining plaque-free) and there is no other reason to refer to specialist (e.g., unresolved dentinal hypersensitivity, gingival recession, desire or need for periodontal plastic surgery).

However, if bleeding on probing persists at sites with deeper (>4 mm) probing depths or at sites of previous attachment loss, referral to the periodontist is indicated—probably for periodontal surgery at those sites.

If no bleeding on probing is present but deep pockets persist, referral to the periodontist may be considered. Research suggests that deep pockets will not break down further if they repeatedly fail over time to demonstrate bleeding on probing (Lang et al. 1990). However, this should be viewed in light of other research showing that deeper pockets are more likely than shallower pockets to experience additional attachment loss due to periodontitis (Haffajee et al. 1991; Grbic and Lamster 1992).

FIGURE 9–5

Severe chronic periodontitis. Probing depths of more than 8 mm clinical attachment loss (CAL) of ≥ 5 mm. Horizontal and vertical bone loss (>50%). Mobility and furcation involvement.

First appointment: 1 Hour

- Comprehensive oral evaluation (new patients) or periodic oral evaluation (existing patients)—consisting of a medical and dental history update, head and neck examination, and oral cancer screening. Make referrals if necessary. If the patient does not want to be referred to the periodontist, document the refusal in the patient's chart.
- Complete x-ray series, including vertical bitewings (new patients) or indicated radiographs (existing patients). If severe bone loss and heavy deposits exist, consider immediate referral to the periodontist for legal ramifications. If it is decided that initial therapy is to be done in the general practitioner's office, the following steps should be performed.
- Periodontal examination. Sites that bleed on probing should be recorded.
- Stain for plaque and relate stained areas to bleeding sites as part of oral hygiene instruction (patient learns cause and effect).
- Nutritional counseling for the control of dental caries.
- Tobacco counseling for the control and prevention of oral disease.
- Application of desensitizing medicaments, if needed.

Second appointment: 1 hour (scheduled as soon as possible after initial visit)

- Review medical and dental history.
- Stain for plaque and relate stained areas to bleeding sites as part of oral hygiene instruction (patient learns cause and effect).
- Reinforce plaque-control instruction.
- Periodontal debridement by quadrant (use of local anesthesia may be indicated).
- Adjunctive antimicrobial irrigation or mouthrinse, if indicated.
- Nutritional counseling for the control of dental caries.
- Tobacco counseling for the control and prevention of oral disease, if indicated.
- Application of desensitizing medicaments, if needed.

Third, fourth, and fifth appointments: 1 hour (scheduled every 7 to 10 days)

- Review medical and dental history.
- Evaluate tissue response from previous treatment.
- Stain for plaque and relate stained areas to bleeding sites as part of oral hygiene instruction (patient learns cause and effect).
- Reinforce plaque-control instruction.
- Continue debridement procedures by quadrant.
- Adjunctive antimicrobial irrigation or mouthrinse, if indicated.
- Sustained, slow-release, local-delivery antimicrobials may be used at nonresponsive sites. [Long-term use (longer than 9 months) is not currently scientifically validated. However, if clinical parameters are promptly reassessed and nonresponders are referred, this tactic should offer little or no risk.]
- Nutritional counseling for the control of dental caries.
- Tobacco counseling for the control and prevention of oral disease, if indicated.
- Application of desensitizing medicaments, if needed.

Sixth appointment (reevaluation of therapy): 1 hour (scheduled 4 to 6 weeks after previous appointment)

- Review medical and dental history.
- Evaluate tissue response from previous treatment.
- Periodontal examination; record sites that bleed on probing.
- Stain for plaque and relate stained areas to bleeding sites as part of oral hygiene instruction (patient learns cause and effect).
- Reinforce plaque-control instruction.
- Selective polishing, if indicated.
- Sustained, slow-release, local-delivery antimicrobials may be used at nonresponsive sites [Long-term use (longer than 9 months) is not currently scientifically validated. However, if clinical parameters are promptly reassessed and nonresponders are referred, this tactic should offer little or no risk.]
- Nutritional counseling for the control of dental caries.
- Fluoride treatment for root caries control, if indicated.
- Tobacco counseling for the control and prevention of oral disease, if indicated.
- Application of desensitizing medicaments, if needed.
- At this time, referral to the periodontist is necessary for legal ramifications.

Only rarely will the procedures outlined above result in resolution of inflammation in pockets of more than 8 mm. (If this occurs, treat as for moderate chronic periodontitis.) Therefore, these patients are often referred early on to a periodontist.

FIGURE 9–6

Refractory periodontitis (nonresponsive cases). The patient is biologically resistant to conventional therapy.

First appointment: 1 hour

- Comprehensive oral evaluation (new patients) or periodic oral evaluation (existing patients)—consisting of a medical and dental history update, head and neck examination, and oral cancer screening. If this is an existing patient and previous treatment in the office has been ineffective, immediate referral to the periodontist is appropriate.
- If the patient does not want to be referred to the periodontist and wants treatment in the general practitioner's office, document the patient's informed refusal in the chart.
- Complete x-ray series, including vertical bitewings (new patients) or indicated radiographs (existing patients). If severe bone loss and heavy deposits, consider immediate referral to a periodontist for legal ramifications. Even though referral is indicated, if it is decided that therapy is to be done in the general practitioner's office, the following steps should be performed.
- Periodontal examination. Sites that bleed on probing should be recorded.
- Stain for plaque and relate stained areas to bleeding sites as part of oral hygiene instruction (patient learns cause and effect).
- Periodontal debridement by quadrant (use of local anesthesia is determined by the practitioner) in conjunction with systemic antibiotics (4 to 5 appointments).
- Consider adjunctive diagnostic/bacteriologic tests (e.g., genetic test, culture, DNA probe).
- Nutritional counseling for the control of dental caries.
- Tobacco counseling for the control and prevention of oral disease, if indicated.
- Application of desensitizing medicaments, if needed.

Third, fourth, and fifth appointments: 1 hour (scheduled every 7 to 10 days)

- Review medical and dental history.
- Evaluate tissue response from previous treatment.
- Chart sites that bleed on gentle probing.
- Stain for plaque and relate stained areas to bleeding sites as part of oral hygiene instruction (patient learns cause and effect).
- Reinforce plaque-control instruction.
- Continue debridement procedures by quadrant.
- Nutritional counseling for the control of dental caries.
- Tobacco counseling for the control and prevention of oral disease, if indicated.
- Application of desensitizing medicaments, if needed.

These patients are best treated by a periodontist.

Phases of treatment

Ideal treatment planning incorporates a logical interplay between periodontal and nonperiodontal procedures. This is so because successful management of the periodontal diseases is a multifaceted discipline that can be affected by other dental conditions and treatments. Table 9–4 ■ depicts four sequential phases that are guidelines for overall case management.

Phase I: Nonsurgical/Initial Preparation   The goal of Phase I therapy is to reduce all etiologic and risk factors to the maximum extent possible—short of surgical intervention. Conditions associated with pain, such as a periodontal abscess, necrotizing ulcerative gingivitis, or traumatic injury, should be treated at this time. Nonrestorable teeth should be identified and extracted. Teeth needing endodontic therapy should be treated. *extraction of hopeless teeth*

TABLE 9–4
PHASES OF PERIODONTAL TREATMENT

Phase I or initial therapy: Disease control

- Emergency care; relief of acute symptoms*
- Oral hygiene instruction*
- Nutritional counseling*
- Correction of inadequate restorations (e.g., overhang or poorly contoured restorations,* open proximal contacts)
- Periodontal debridement*
- Antimicrobial therapy (oral rinses, oral irrigation, controlled-release products)*
- Systemic antibiotics, if indicated
- Fluoride application for caries control or desensitization, if indicated*
- Smoking cessation*
- Minor orthodontic movement
- Occlusal therapy (including night guards*)
- Extraction of hopeless teeth
- Reevaluation of initial therapy*

Phase II therapy: Surgical correction

Phase III therapy: Restorative/prosthetic care

- Final restorations fabricated

Phase IV therapy: Maintenance care

- Evaluation of patient's oral hygiene*
- Smoking cessation*
- Treatment depends on the condition of the periodontium

*Procedures that may be performed by dental hygienists in some jurisdictions. Check with individual state practice regulations.

Oral hygiene instruction and patient education are performed. *Patients need to learn that diligent self-care is the critical foundation for successful periodontal treatment.* Figures 9–1 through 9–6 emphasize self-care training, professional analyses, and technique refinement to a degree some may consider excessive. However, failure to provide compulsive clinical emphasis on patient motivation and self-care techniques invites many treatment failures that could be avoided.

Oral prophylaxis and periodontal debridement may be performed. The tissue responses to in-office and improved self-care may be assessed as soon as a week later.

Multiple appointments during this phase help the patient better understand his or her role as cotherapist. They also help build the key concept of a patient-hygienist-dentist team—organized to fight together against periodontitis on a site-by-site basis.

As this phase draws to a close, if signs of inflammation persist at deeper probing sites—especially those the patient is keeping free of supragingival plaque—the need for periodontal surgery is often obvious to everyone.

Phase II: Periodontal Surgery   Although evidence exists suggesting an approximate equivalence between arrestive outcomes of closed debridement procedures and open (surgical) procedures in many types of periodontal defects, practitioners need to know that the design of these nonsurgical studies (e.g., 20 minutes of root planing per tooth) is clinically unrealistic (Pihlstrom et al. 1983; Lindhe et al. 1984; Ramfjord et al. 1987).

Many periodontal surgical procedures are performed to provide the practitioner with better and faster access to deep periodontal pockets. These surgeries may be arrestive or regenerative. A single surgical procedure may incorporate both elements. For example, an osseous (bone) graft may be placed in a deep infrabony defect on one tooth, whereas bone in adjacent areas may be reduced to facilitate the placement of a pocket-eliminating apically positioned surgical flap that establishes a maintainable gingival form.

Other periodontal surgical procedures may be performed to address gingival recession. The indications for such surgery include dentinal sensitivity, aesthetic complaints, or continuing recession. Many times these procedures are both arrestive and regenerative in character.

Other periodontal surgical procedures may be performed to maximize the aesthetic results associated with new restorative dentistry. Examples include ridge augmentation and crown lengthening. Procedures performed for aesthetics alone are usually termed *periodontal plastic surgery*.

Phase III: Restorative Care   Restorative dentistry is performed in this phase. Ideally, periodontal and prosthetic dentists work together to design restorations that satisfy aesthetic, comfort, and functional needs without compromising future periodontal health.

Phase IV: Maintenance Care   Phase IV consists of periodontal maintenance (also termed *recall* or *continuing care*). The goal of periodontal maintenance is to prevent continued periodontal destruction. Maintenance care includes reexamination and assessment of the periodontal condition and patient self-care. It often includes an oral prophylaxis and may include periodontal debridement and other local therapies that target persistently inflamed sites.

The frequency of periodontal maintenance visits is individualized and depends on the patient's periodontal status, medical condition, and self-care motivation and effectiveness. For further information, see Chapter 18.

REFERRAL TO A PERIODONTIST

Although patients experiencing periodontal problems may be referred to a periodontist at any time, preliminary phases of periodontal therapy often are performed in the general practice. Sometimes, especially for mild cases, this is all that is necessary to achieve the goal of periodontal therapy. However, even for patients who are ultimately referred, the benefits of the self-care training, motivation, and emphasis on team building in the general practice increase the likelihood of treatment success by the periodontist and beyond. Hygienists, general practitioners, and periodontists who function as a team maximize the likelihood of optimal outcomes.

Although a licensed general practitioner legally may provide comprehensive periodontal therapy to any informed and consenting patient, he or she is ethically and legally required to meet the same standard of care for such therapy as a specialist. Therefore, with the welfare of periodontal patients in mind, the following referral guidelines are proposed—with the knowledge that exceptions occur.

GUIDELINES FOR REFERRAL

Any patient who has one or more periodontal sites that show persistent signs of inflammation should be considered for referral. Often these patients fit in one or more of the following categories:

1. Chronic periodontitis with deeper probing depths, furcation involvement, and/or problematic gingival recession
2. Aggressive (localized, generalized) periodontitis
3. Periodontitis associated with systemic diseases (such as diabetes mellitus)
4. Periodontitis with significant or increasing tooth mobility
5. Periodontal lesions adjacent to necrotic (or endodontically treated) teeth
6. Refractory (considered nonresponsive to treatment) or recurrent periodontitis (responsive, but still headed downhill)
7. Patients who have aesthetic concerns about the interplay between teeth, restorations, and the gingiva or alveolar arches
8. Patients with mucocutaneous disorders affecting the oral soft tissues (e.g., pemphigus, lichen planus)

INFORMED CONSENT

Before examination and treatment, the patient must give consent. For medicolegal reasons, **informed consent** is usually recorded using a document signed by the patient and the practitioner, because any treatment provided without consent legally may constitute a battery. Furthermore, a valid consent requires that the patient be made reasonably knowledgeable about the risks and benefits associated with the proposed treatments, alternative treatments, and no treatment. Minor children and the mentally incapacitated ordinarily cannot execute a valid consent.

For periodontal patients, the informed consent form should be clearly reflect that the patient understands and accepts the need for periodontal maintenance and oral hygiene self-care.

TREATMENT GUIDELINES

The following treatment guidelines were written for new patients but can be adapted for existing patients. Although treatment planning guidelines are helpful, it is important to remember that treatment must be tailored to each patient. Experience and the scientific literature have demonstrated that responses to therapy can vary from one patient to another or even in the same patient at different sites and at different times. Therefore, each patient may respond uniquely to the therapy provided.

This section contains guidelines for treating typical periodontal patients and patients with other periodontal conditions, including medication- and hormone-influenced gingivitis, gingivitis and periodontitis related to systemic conditions, aggressive periodontitis, and acute periodontal conditions.

As discussed previously, these guidelines include intensive and continual emphasis on self-care, self-care assessment (by the practitioner), and professional reassessments (of tissue status) on a site-by-site basis. For many patients, these are essential for long-term treatment success. Furthermore, the suggested time allowance for each appointment is subject to change based on the patient's response to care. Of course, these are only guidelines. The ultimate decision making and responsibility for how to treat a patient rests with the individual practitioner.

PERIODONTAL HEALTH

Patients presenting with no bleeding on gentle probing and light to no supragingival plaque and calculus only require an oral prophylaxis (see Fig. 9–1). Subgingival root debridement is contraindicated. Once oral hygiene efficacy is assured, a suitable periodontal maintenance schedule is determined, usually every 6 to 12 months.

The motivated and periodontally healthy patient is often "dentally aware." Indeed, past dental therapy may be responsible for the healthy state the patient now enjoys. Such patients generally enjoy discussing new advancements in dentistry. They usually welcome improvements in professional and self-care and may question the practitioner about new treatment concepts. Oral hygiene instruction time may be used to discuss new oral hygiene products and their applications. The patient must be reminded of the need for future examinations (since problems may occur even though the patient currently appears healthy).

GINGIVITIS

Plaque-induced gingivitis

Most cases of gingivitis are plaque-related and are best treated by periodontal debridement and oral hygiene instructions (see Fig. 9–2). The therapeutic goal is to establish gingival health by eliminating the etiologic factors. The ultimate objective is to prevent sites from progressing to periodontitis. Since we are unable to predict which sites will progress, the entire mouth must be treated. Patients need to be aware of the need for adequate toothbrushing and the use of interdental cleaning aids. Supplemental use of antimicrobial agents (e.g., mouthrinses) is recommended in certain patients, such as those with severe bleeding that interferes with debridement procedures or those with poor manual dexterity. Following initial therapy, the patient is placed on a well-monitored periodontal maintenance program.

For all types of gingivitis, initial periodontal debridement and oral hygiene instructions are the key to minimizing microbial plaque accumulation.

Sulcular sites that bleed on gentle probing should be noted and recorded and pointed out to the patient. Plaque staining will reveal areas of plaque accumulation. These should be recorded as well. Bleeding often occurs at these sites. The patient needs to understand this relationship. The patient also needs to appreciate that if a site bleeds as a result of self-care, that site usually needs more self-care attention, not less. This runs counter to the intuition of most patients, whose common response to bleeding is to "leave the area alone."

If the patient is taught to understand that the destructive process is at an early stage and that proper professional and self-care likely will return the tissues to health, treatment is more likely to succeed. Involve the patient as a "cotherapist."

Gingival enlargement

Gingival enlargement or overgrowth is sometimes seen in patients with orthodontic appliances or in patients taking certain drugs. Removal of dental plaque and calculus by meticulous oral hygiene and regular professional mechanical debridement may help to prevent or slow gingival overgrowth. Therefore, initial treatment should focus on improved self-care and professional plaque and calculus removal. Unfortunately, gingival enlargement still may occur, making it difficult to perform effective self-care and even interfering with chewing, speech, and appearance.

For orthodontic patients, surgical removal of fibrotic pseudopockets can be performed at any time, but recurrence is likely if orthodontic appliances remain. For patients with drug-induced gingival enlargement, overgrowth usually requires surgical intervention. Recurrence is common if the drug is continued. Therefore, it is important to inform the patient's physician about the oral condition and inquire if an alternative drug could be prescribed.

Hormone-associated gingivitis

Pregnancy, oral contraceptives, and puberty can contribute to gingivitis. Treatment of hormone-influenced gingivitis is aimed at lowering plaque levels by maintaining meticulous oral hygiene. Frequent periodontal maintenance also may help.

PERIODONTITIS

Chronic periodontitis (formerly termed adult periodontitis is by far the most common form of periodontitis seen in otherwise healthy patients. Aggressive periodontitis (formerly termed *early onset periodontitis*), refractory periodontitis, periodontitis associated with systemic conditions, and peri-implantitis are less common but are more difficult to treat and should be referred.

Chronic periodontitis

In general, the treatment of patients with chronic periodontitis begins with oral hygiene instructions and periodontal debridement, followed by surgical therapy if needed. Patients are then monitored, and treatment is modified as necessary as part of an ongoing periodontal maintenance program. Repeated surgeries sometimes are necessary.

Periodontal patients who demonstrate attachment loss and probing pocket depths of 4 to 5 mm (slight periodontitis) often respond adequately (e.g., elimination of bleeding on probing) to periodontal debridement and effective oral self-care (see Fig. 9–3). In moderate periodontitis (attachment loss with probing depths of 6 to 7 mm; see Fig. 9–4) and severe periodontitis (attachment loss with probing depths of more than 8 mm; see Fig. 9–5), periodontal debridement is less predictable (Stambaugh et al. 1981). Following oral hygiene instruction and periodontal debridement, such patients are usually referred to the periodontist—often for periodontal surgery at nonresponsive sites.

Patients with gingival recession should be evaluated. If the recession causes tooth pain, is progressing, or interferes with aesthetics, gingival grafting may be indicated.

It should be noted that chronic periodontitis is site-specific. Some patients demonstrate clinical attachment loss and/or probing depths that are normal at some sites, suggestive of slight periodontitis at other sites, and indicative of moderate or severe periodontitis at others. Therefore, periodontal debridement and improved self-care may be adequate at some sites but inadequate at others in the same patient. The most problematic sites guide ideal patient management. In other words, the persistence of even one diseased site is sufficient to justify referral for more aggressive therapy.

Refractory periodontal patients who do not respond to proper periodontal treatment (see Fig. 9–6) despite quality self-care and participation in a well-monitored periodontal maintenance program should be referred to a periodontist.

Aggressive periodontitis

Apparently healthy young people (younger than 30 years of age) can have underlying immune system irregularities that may manifest as periodontitis with rapid attachment loss and bone destruction (Tonetti and Mombelli 1999). Treatment of this type of periodontitis is similar to that for chronic forms of periodontitis except that surgical intervention and antibiotic therapy often are used early in therapy. Therefore, these patients should be referred promptly to a periodontist.

NECROTIZING PERIODONTAL DISEASES

Necrotizing ulcerative gingivitis (NUG) and necrotizing ulcerative periodontitis (NUP) are collectively referred to as *necrotizing periodontal diseases*. Necrotizing ulcerative gingivitis (NUG) is an infection localized to the gingiva. Contributory risk factors include emotional stress, poor oral hygiene, cigarette smoking, and HIV infections (Rowland 1999). NUP involves the attachment apparatus and is seen primarily in individuals with systemic conditions including, but not limited to, HIV infection, severe malnutrition, and immunosuppression (Novak 1999).

It is important to distinguish between NUG and primary herpetic gingivostomatitis. The latter is highly contagious, and both are seen most commonly in young adult populations. Both are painful and can occur simultaneously. Patients with primary herpetic gingivostomatitis usually have a fever and show small ulcerations on the hard palate and attached gingiva remote from the gingival margins. NUG patients are often afebrile and show oral ulcerations extending from the marginal and papillary gingiva.

NUG is treated by addressing its causes. At the first appointment, supragingival debridement with an ultrasonic or sonic scaler is recommended. (Note that if herpetic infection is suspected, aerosol-creating procedures are contraindicated.) Patients are instructed to rinse with a mixture of 1 tablespoon of 3% hydrogen peroxide in 1/2 glass of warm water and to gently brush with a soft or extrasoft toothbrush twice daily. Pain medication may be prescribed. The NUG patient is advised to avoid alcohol and tobacco, eat a balanced diet, and rest. The patient should be reevaluated a few days later. By then, the pain usually has diminished, and generalized periodontal debridement is performed. Oral hygiene instructions are reinforced. NUG patients should be reevaluated a few weeks later. Sometimes these patients show signs of periodontitis and need ongoing therapy.

If primary herpetic gingivostomatitis is suspected, refer such patients to a periodontist or physician.

In NUP patients, treatment is aimed at periodontal debridement, improved oral hygiene self-care, and frequent use of an antiplaque rinse or irrigant such as chlorhexidine gluconate. Oral fungal infections are sometimes seen, and these may require antifungal medication.

AIDS-related oral lesions may not fully respond to therapy. Periodontal debridement may expose necrotic bone that should be removed (Murray 1994). Local anesthesia, pain medication, and antibiotics may be necessary. Frequent periodontal maintenance visits are recommended. Oral care should be provided in collaboration with the patient's physician. Referral to a periodontist should be considered.

PERI-IMPLANTITIS

Treatment of peri-implant diseases may include mechanical debridement, oral hygiene instructions, mouthrinses, systemic antibiotics, arrestive and regenerative periodontal surgery, and/or implant removal. Referral to a periodontist is recommended.

PERIODONTAL EMERGENCIES

Gingival abscess

A gingival abscess is an acute infection characterized by a localized, painful edema at the free gingival margin (Fig. 9–7 ■). Usually there are no signs of periodontitis in the patient's mouth. Foreign objects such as popcorn kernels, fish bones, or seeds that become lodged in the gingival crevice are responsible for many gingival abscesses. Calculus is usually not the cause. Since the abscess develops fairly rapidly, the patient often will know the cause.

Treatment requires removal of the etiologic agent by periodontal debridement. Since the gingiva may be friable, careful tissue manipulation is advised. Local anesthesia may be helpful. Scaling establishes drainage through the gingival crevice. The patient can be placed on a warm saline rinse (rinse every 1 to 2 hours for several days). If treated adequately, the condition will resolve within a matter of days.

FIGURE 9–7

Gingival abscess involving the mandibular central incisor. (Courtesy Ann Goodwin, NYU College of Dentistry)

Periodontal abscess

A periodontal abscess, also called a *lateral abscess,* is a localized purulent nidus of acute inflammation within the periodontal tissues. A periodontal abscess develops as a result of a bacterial infection that eventually leads to the formation of pus (suppuration). Periodontal abscess formation is often seen in deep periodontal pockets and in furcation sites. Such patients often have a number of sites with chronic periodontitis. Periodontal abscesses can occur as a result of inadvertent embedding of a foreign body subgingivally (calculus fragment, popcorn husk, seeds, shellfish fragments, etc.) that obstructs the normal sulcular drainage of gingival crevicular fluid and inflammatory by-products of chronic periodontitis. To reestablish drainage, a fistula may form that drains pus through the otherwise intact surface of the gingiva or mucosa. Patients with diabetes mellitus are more susceptible to periodontal abscess formation. Periodontal abscesses sometimes are seen following scaling and root planing at sites with deeper probing pocket depths.

The periodontal abscess presents as a shiny, swollen, discolored mass on the gingiva or mucosa. Finger pressure may produce purulent drainage. The involved tooth is often tender to percussion, mobile, and may feel "high" to the patient. Patients usually complain of pain. Occasionally, patients may demonstrate localized lymphadenopathy and fever.

Practitioners often must be able to differentiate between a periodontal abscess and a periapical (endodontic) abscess. An endodontic abscess usually occurs adjacent to the apex of a necrotic tooth. It often heals following endodontic therapy. Table 9–5 ■ shows the usual characteristics of periapical and periodontal abscesses.

Treatment of a periodontal abscess consists of two phases. The first phase involves management of the acute signs and symptoms. This is done by establishing drainage and removing any foreign causative agent (if applicable). Block anesthesia is likely necessary.

In general, vigorous subgingival debridement will reestablish drainage and remove any foreign body. A soft diet, rest, analgesics, and warm salt water rinses are prescribed. Antibiotics may be prescribed if systemic involvement (e.g., fever and/or lymphadenopathy) is suspected. The successfully treated patient will notice improvement within 24 hours of treatment. If symptoms fail to improve promptly, emergency surgical access to the affected root surface may be necessary.

Once acute symptoms resolve, periodontal surgery to eliminate the deep periodontal pocket is performed.

TABLE 9–5	
DIFFERENCES BETWEEN A PERIODONTAL AND PERIAPICAL ABSCESS	
PERIODONTAL ABSCESS	**PERIAPICAL ABSCESS**
Vital tooth	Nonvital tooth
No tooth caries	Tooth caries present
Deep pocket	No pocket
Tooth mobility	No or minimal mobility
Draining fistula usually located at lateral aspect of tooth	Draining fistula usually located in apical area
Lateral radiolucency	Apical radiolucency

FIGURE 9–8
Pericoronitis. The third molar is partially covered by a "gingival flap." (Courtesy: Ann Goodwin, NYU College of Dentistry)

Pericoronal abscess

Pericoronal abscess, also referred to as *pericoronitis,* is a localized infection involving the gingiva adjacent to a partially erupted mandibular third molar (Fig. 9–8 ■). The gingival flap (or operculum) overlying the erupting tooth usually disappears once the tooth fully erupts, but many of these teeth remain partially erupted indefinitely because of inadequate arch space for complete eruption.

Patients usually complain of a dull ache and may demonstrate limited jaw opening (trismus). Food debris is often found under the operculum. Irrigation with saline, iodine solution, or water is common therapy. If the infection is severe or systemic involvement is suspected, antibiotics may be indicated. Ultimately, removal of the operculum or extraction of the erupting tooth may be necessary but is better performed when the patient no longer has acute local infection and trismus.

ADJUNCTIVE TREATMENT

ANTIMICROBIALS

Systemic antibiotics often are prescribed as part of the treatment of aggressive periodontitis or of periodontitis patients with systemic maladies. For example, administration of a systemic antibiotic, debridement, and surgery constitute an appropriate course of therapy for a patient with localized juvenile periodontitis.

In an otherwise healthy chronic periodontitis patient, antibiotics usually are reserved for a specific refractory infection or as an adjunct to certain periodontal surgical procedures. In the case of refractory periodontitis, specific antibiotics are selected based on identification of the suspected pathogens.

The guidelines governing the use of systemic antibiotics in patients with periodontitis are constantly changing. Therefore, practitioners who would use systemic antimicrobials to treat periodontitis must remain very up-to-date with the appropriate biomedical literature.

Controlled-release antimicrobial drug systems as a supplement to periodontal debridement may be indicated when clinical signs of inflammation (bleeding on probing) persist in pockets of 5 mm or greater. However, continuing reassessment is needed to determine if other therapies are indicated, since successful long-term use of these devices has yet to be validated clinically.

Antimicrobial rinses and toothpastes are widely advertised. Chlorhexidine gluconate rinses are prescribed routinely for specified periods when mechanical plaque control is not feasible (e.g., after surgery, after acute infection). Over-the-counter antimicrobial rinses are of limited value but may provide benefits for some patients. Use of mouthrinses should not be a substitute for mechanical self-care.

PROGNOSIS

Prognosis is a prediction of the future course of a malady with or without treatment. All aspects of the patient's history, data from the clinical examination, and the patient's healing capacity are factors.

Common clinical factors used in assigning a prognosis are reviewed in Table 9–6 ■ (McGuire and Nunn 1996). This checklist can be reviewed as part of developing a prognosis for each patient. The more unfavorable factors noted, the worse is the prognosis.

Prognosis is usually reported using a graded scale. This may be a simple scale such as good, guarded, or poor or a scale with more intervals such as good, fair, poor, questionable, or hopeless (Table 9–7 ■; McGuire and Nunn 1996).

Determination of prognosis is important in treatment planning so that the practitioner and patient can agree on a plan that best satisfies the patient's overall goals while minimizing disappointments if setbacks occur. Realistic prognoses are of amplified importance in complex cases that combine periodontal and restorative therapies. This is so because in these patients, the unexpected loss of a key abutment tooth may necessitate replacement of complicated and expensive crown and bridge prosthetics.

TABLE 9–6
COMMON CLINICAL FACTORS USED IN DETERMINING A PROGNOSIS

Factors affecting prognosis of individual teeth

- Amount of bone remaining
- Depth of pockets
- Pattern of bone loss, horizontal or vertical
- Tooth mobility
- Type of infrabony defect: one, two, or three walls
- Root anatomy, favorable or unfavorable
- Furcation involvement
- Crown-to-root ratio, favorable or unfavorable
- Caries or pulpal involvement, yes or no
- Missing teeth and restorative dentistry

Factors affecting overall prognosis

- Age
- Significant medical history (e.g., diabetes)
- Smoker, yes or no, past smoker
- Family history of periodontal diseases, yes or no
- Oral hygiene: good, fair, or poor
- Compliant with treatment and home care, yes or no

Source: Adapted from McGuire and Nunn, 1996.

TABLE 9–7
PROGNOSTIC CLASSIFICATION FOR INDIVIDUAL TEETH

- Good prognosis: Adequate periodontal support around the tooth and can be easily maintained by the practitioner and the patient.
- Fair prognosis: About 25% bone loss. Class I furcation involvement present and can be properly maintained.
- Poor prognosis: About 50% bone loss. Class II furcation involvement present and can be maintained but with difficulty.
- Questionable prognosis: Greater than 50% bone loss around the tooth. Class II and III furcation involvements present that cannot be maintained.
- Hopeless prognosis: Not enough bony support around the tooth to maintain it in its socket. Extraction of tooth recommended.

Source: Adapted from McGuire and Nunn, 1996.

GERIATRIC PATIENTS

Although the same general guidelines already provided for chronic periodontitis patients apply to the elderly, geriatric patients often have special needs. They may present with uncontrolled dental plaque and/or xerostomia. Other oral pathologies, including oral cancers, are more common among members of this age group.

PLAQUE CONTROL

Age-related factors may limit the ability of a patient to perform adequate oral self-care. Visual impairment can diminish an individual's ability to see oral structures and debris. Using a toothbrush or dental floss may be impossible for patients with arthritis or stroke-related impairments. Dementia may affect an individual's ability or motivation to perform daily oral hygiene procedures. Virtually any debilitating systemic illness may predispose patients to periodontitis—and many of these maladies are seen more commonly in aged populations. Most important, periodontal treatment may be complicated by multiple medical conditions.

XEROSTOMIA

Decreased saliva production occurs with advancing age. Furthermore, many of the hundreds of medications known to decrease salivary flow are used by older people. Antidepressants, antihistamines, antihypertensives, antipsychotics, diuretics, antiparkinsonians, and antianxiety agents all may contribute to xerostomia (Brangan 1994). Older patients, with decreased protective properties of saliva, are at increased risk for dental caries and periodontal diseases.

If a patient complains of xerostomia, or if dryness seems to be contributing to oral problems, relevant systemic medications should be identified and alternatives considered. Saliva substitutes may be recommended, but these have limited effectiveness and can be expensive.

ORAL CANCER

The best-documented avoidable oral cancer risk factors are tobacco use and alcohol consumption. Oral cancer occurs twice as often in men than in women. The incidence of lip cancer is related to exposure to sunlight. Smoking cessation reduces the odds of circumoral cancer in adult patients (National Oral Health Information Clearinghouse 1997).

TREATMENT CONSIDERATIONS

When treating geriatric patients, the practitioner must consider systemic concerns that may complicate the management of periodontal conditions. It may be important for the dentist and hygienist to consult with a patient's physician to review pertinent details of the patient's medical conditions.

Treatment goals for the elderly are the same as for the young, that is, the preservation (or restoration) of an aesthetic, comfortable, and functional dentition. This is not to suggest that age should not be a factor in planning how best to achieve these goals; indeed, conservative therapy may be more appropriate in older patients for a number of reasons. Whatever treatment is planned, it should be flexible and adapted to each patient's particular needs. As these needs change, so should the therapy.

Successful treatment of the elderly often requires a high degree of cooperation between the practitioner, patient, and other supporting caregivers. Modified self-care routines may be necessary, such as use of a toothpick instead of floss, a toothbrush with a modified handle such as a tennis ball, and the frequent use of antimicrobial agents (such as fluorides or chlorhexidine) along with mechanical plaque control. Automated oral hygiene devices may facilitate more effective plaque control.

SUMMARY

Research supports the majority of procedures routinely performed by the dental hygienist to prevent or arrest the progression of the common periodontal maladies. Science, combined with a century of clinical experience and inferential skills, has produced the periodontal parameters of care for today. As time passes, continued scientific testing of new and old therapeutic tactics along with clinical experience will continue to underpin future parameters for periodontal care.

At the beginning of the twenty-first century, periodontal treatment planning remains complicated. For now, ongoing periodontal care should be modulated based on the response of the patient to self-care and treatment rendered previously. If a desired and optimal response is not achieved, some other reasonable approach must be used and assessed. Critical analyses of outcomes will sometimes suggest that referral to a specialist is in the best interest of the patient.

Quality assessment has been defined as "a measure of care provided in a particular setting" (Burt and Eklund 1992). *Quality assurance* is a broader concept that encompasses assessment of care along with the "implementation of any necessary changes to either maintain or improve the quality of care rendered" (Burt and Eklund 1992).

Dental hygienists have the professional responsibility to promote the oral health of the public in the most effective ways possible. As excerpted from the American Dental Hygienists Association's (1998) Code of Ethics, "We acknowledge the following responsibilities to patients or clients:

- Provide oral health care utilizing high levels of professional knowledge, judgment, and skill.
- Serve as an advocate for the welfare of clients.
- Provide clients with the information necessary to make informed decisions about their oral health and encourage their full participation in treatment decisions and goals.
- Refer clients to other healthcare providers when their needs are beyond our ability or scope of practice.
- Educate clients about high-quality oral health care."

KEY POINTS

- ❖ Evidence-based periodontal treatment based on dental literature focuses on the recognition of risk, prognosis and treatment factors.
- ❖ The evidence-based approach is a good model for evaluating the results of periodontal therapy.
- ❖ The ideal goal of periodontal therapy is to restore the periodontium destroyed by disease to a comfortable and functional state of health.
- ❖ Periodontal treatment involves ongoing care and demands continued reassessments.

REFERENCES

American Academy of Periodontology. 1996. *Annals of periodontology: 1996 world workshop in periodontics.* Chicago: American Academy of Periodontology.

American Academy of Periodontology. 2000 Parameters of Care. J. Periodontol 71 (Supplement): 847–883.

American Dental Hygienist's Association. 1998. *1998–1999 Bylaws and code of ethics.* Chicago: ADHA.

Axelsson, P., and J. Lindhe. 1981. The significance of maintenance care in the treatment of periodontal disease. *J. Clin. Periodontol.* 8:281–294.

Burt, B., and S. Eklund. 1992. *Dentistry, dental practice and the community.* Philadelphia: W. B. Saunders.

Brangan, P. 1994. Dental hygiene care for the older adult. In: *Dental hygiene theory and practice,* M. L. Darby and M. Walsh (eds.), 873–912. Philadelphia: W. B. Saunders.

Grbic, J., and I. Lamster. 1992. Risk indicators for future periodontal attachment loss in adult periodontitis: Tooth and site variables. *J. Periodontol.* 63:262–269.

Grossi, S., J. Zambon, A. Ho, et al. 1994. Assessment of risk for periodontal disease: I. Risk indicators for attachment loss. *J. Periodontol.* 65:260–267.

Grossi, S., R. J. Genco, E. E. Machtei, et al. 1995. Assessment of risk for periodontal disease: II. Risk indicators for alveolar bone loss. *J. Periodontol.* 66:23–29.

Haffajee, A., S. Socransky, J. Lindhe, et al. 1991. Clinical risk indicators for periodontal attachment loss. *J. Clin. Periodontol.* 18:117–125.

Hancock, E. B. 1996. Prevention. *Ann. Periodontol.* 1:223–249.

Ismail, A., E. Morrison, B. Burt, et al. 1990. Natural history of periodontal disease in adults: Findings from the Tecumseh Periodontal Disease Study, 1959–1987. *J. Dent. Res.* 69:430–435.

Lang, K., R. Adler, A. Joss, and S. Nyman. 1990. Absence of bleeding on probing: An indicator of periodontal stability. *J. Clin. Periodontol.* 17:714–721.

Lindhe, J., E. Westfelt, S. Nyman, et al. 1984. Long-term effect of surgical/nonsurgical treatment of periodontal disease. *J. Clin. Periodontol.* 11:448–458.

Loesche, W. 1976. Chemotherapy of dental plaque infections. *Oral Sci. Rev.* 9:65–107.

McGuire, K. M., and M. E. Nunn. 1996. Prognosis versus actual outcome: II. The effectiveness of clinical parameters in developing an accurate prognosis. *J. Periodontol.* 67:658–665.

Murray, P. A. 1994. Periodontal diseases in patients infected by human immunodeficiency virus. *Periodontology 2000* 6:50–67.

National Oral Health Information Clearinghouse. 1997. *Detecting oral cancer.* Bethesda, MD: National Institute of Dental Research.

Newman, M. 1998. Improved clinical decision making using the evidence-based approach. *J. Am. Dent. Assoc.* 129:4S–8S.

Novak, M. J. 1999. Necrotizing ulcerative periodontitis. *Ann. Periodontol.* 4:74–77.

Pihlstrom, B., R. McHugh, T. Oliphant, and C. Ortiz-Campos. 1983. Comparison of surgical and nonsurgical treatment of periodontal disease: A review of current studies and additional results after 6½ years. *J. Clin. Periodontol.* 10:524–541.

Ramfjord, S., R. Caffesse, E. Morrison, et al. 1987. Four modalities of periodontal treatment compared over 5 years. *J. Clin. Periodontol.* 14:445–452.

Rowland, R. W. 1999. Necrotizing ulcerative gingivitis. *Ann. Periodontol.* 4:65–73.

Stambaugh, R. V., M. Dragoo, D. M. Smith, and L. Carasali. 1981. The limits of subgingival scaling. *Int. J. Periodont. Restor. Dent.* 1(5):31–41.

Tonetti, M. S., and A. Mombelli. 1999. Early-onset periodontitis. *Ann. Periodontol.* 4:39–52.

SELF-QUIZ

1. Which one of the following factors improves the treatment decisions made by dental/medical practitioners? (p. 280)

   a. clinical experience of the practitioner and use of scientific literature
   b. following the advice of fellow dental practitioners
   c. following the advice of fellow medical practitioners
   d. consulting with the dental companies

2. Which one of the following statements is the ideal goal of periodontal therapy? (p. 285)

   a. Control or eliminate and prevent the initiation, progression, or recurrence of periodontal diseases.
   b. Promote tissue healing by regeneration or replacement of the lost tissue with new bone, cementum, and periodontal ligament.
   c. Restore the periodontium to an attractive, comfortable, and functional state of health for the balance of the patient's life.

    d. Allow the attachment apparatus to relax.

    e. Remove all microbial plaque every day.

3. Which one of the following steps should be first in developing a plan to treat a patient? (p. 285)

    a. Teach proper use of oral hygiene aids.

    b. Determine the treatment goals.

    c. Discuss the case with the patient.

    d. Decide on the proper maintenance interval.

    e. Obtain informed consent for periodontal maintenance.

4. All the following are phases of treatment *except* one. Which one is the exception? (pp. 290–292)

    a. Phase I: disease control

    b. Phase II: surgical correction

    c. Phase III: restorative/prosthetic care

    d. Phase IV: maintenance care

    e. Phase V: implant care

5. In which one of the following phases of treatment is reevaluation of initial therapy completed? (p. 290)

    a. I

    b. II

    c. III

    d. IV

    e. V

6. Which one of the following treatment steps is *most* appropriate in controlling pregnancy-associated gingivitis? (p. 295)

    a. surgical intervention

    b. oral irrigation with chlorhexidine

    c. plaque control with toothbrushing and flossing

    d. systemic antibiotics

    e. estrogen supplements

7. Which one of the following treatments is *most* appropriate for patients with localized aggressive periodontitis (formerly termed localized juvenile periodentitis? (p. 296)

    a. periodontal debridement, systemic antibiotics, and surgery

    b. periodontal debridement and surgery

    c. oral rinsing and periodontal debridement

    d. oral irrigation and periodontal debridement

    e. improved oral hygiene and watchful waiting

8. Which one of the following sequences is the *best* initial treatment for a patient with gingival enlargement caused by phenytoin? (p. 295)

    a. oral hygiene instructions, periodontal debridement, systemic antibiotics, and surgery

    b. oral hygiene instructions and periodontal debridement

    c. periodontal debridement and systemic antibiotics

    d. periodontal debridement and surgery

    e. discontinuation of phenytoin

9. Which one of the following definitions *best* describes the term *prognosis?* (pp. 299–300)

    a. prediction of the future course of a condition with or without treatment

    b. prediction of the future course of a condition without treatment

    c. identification and naming of the type of condition present

    d. patient's healing capacity

10. Which one of the following is the *most* important consideration when treating geriatric patients? (pp. 301–302)

    a. Therapy may be complicated by multiple medical conditions.

    b. The ability to properly understand oral hygiene instructions may be impaired.

    c. Anxiety level is higher in this age group.

    d. Severe frailty inhibits normal maneuvering in the dental office.

    e. Physical impairments are possible.

ORAL HYGIENE SELF-CARE

Diana L. Mercado Galvis, R.D.H., M.S.
Judith Kreismann, R.D.H., B.S., M.A.

10

Outline:

Definition of Oral Hygiene Self-Care
Periodontal Disease Control
Self-Cleansing Mechanism
Patient Education
Preventive Measures
Oral Hygiene Self-Care Methods
Oral Irrigation
Home Care for Periodontal Patients
Advice to the Patient
Effects of Improper Use of Oral Hygiene Devices
Dentinal Hypersensitivity
Summary
Key Points
References
Self-Quiz

Goal:

To educate the dental hygienist in the fundamentals of counseling periodontal patients on oral hygiene self-care.

Educational Objectives:

Upon completion of this chapter, the reader should be able to:

Describe preventive measures taken to prevent and control the progression of periodontal diseases;

Discuss preventive care as it relates to private practice;

Discuss the various toothbrushing methods used to maintain gingival health;

Compare the effectiveness of a powered toothbrush versus a manual toothbrush;

Discuss the importance of interdental cleaning in maintaining periodontal health; and

Discuss an effective plaque-control regimen following periodontal surgery.

KEY WORDS

- plaque biofilms
- oral hygiene self-care
- patient education
- primary prevention
- secondary prevention
- patient motivation

*T*here is no alternative to well-performed oral hygiene self-care as a preventive measure. The willingness and ability of patients to keep dental plaque below the threshold for disease is essential. Preventive measures are important for a healthy periodontium as well as to achieve a successful outcome of periodontal therapy. Preventive measures in periodontics depend on the removal of supra- and subgingival dental **plaque biofilms.** The most common preventive methods involve both personal and professional mechanical plaque control. Preventive measures should address the control or elimination of etiologic factors as well as identified risk factors for inflammatory periodontal diseases (Hancock 1996). *The control of supragingival plaque in conjunction with professional tooth cleaning subgingivally forms the basis for the management of progressive periodontal diseases* (Corbet and Davies 1993). Supragingival plaque control contributes to preventing or moderating subgingival microbial recolonization, which can control progressive periodontal diseases. This chapter focuses on fundamental information related to oral hygiene self-care for the periodontal patient.

DEFINITION OF ORAL HYGIENE SELF-CARE

Oral hygiene self-care, also known as *oral physiotherapy* or *oral home care,* is defined as physical therapy for the mouth or oral cavity. It refers to daily oral health care practices employed by the patient to prevent dental and gingival diseases and maintain optimal oral health. The rationale for oral hygiene self-care as well as professional periodontal debridement is the elimination or suppression of harmful microorganisms found in supragingival biofilms. Consequently, plaque control prevents the potential detrimental effects of pathogenic microorganisms on the teeth and periodontium. The primary method of oral hygiene self-care is the use of such mechanical oral hygiene measures as a toothbrush and interdental cleaning devices. Since not all bacteria in biofilms are pathogenic (disease-producing), the objective of treatment is not total elimination of all bacteria but rather control of the bacteria.

PERIODONTAL DISEASE CONTROL

There is overwhelming evidence that the accumulation of supragingival dental plaque on tooth surfaces near the free gingival margin is associated with the development of gingivitis. Thus removal of dental plaque from tooth surfaces is a basic step in the prevention and treatment of gingivitis. Periodontitis, characterized by loss of connective tissue attachment and subsequent bone loss, is always preceded by gingivitis. The subgingival plaque bacteria play an important role in the progression of periodontal diseases. The subgingival bacteria are derived from the supragingival dental plaque. If supragingival plaque is not removed, subgingival plaque develops. Therefore, meticulous mechanical supragingival plaque control can reduce the risk for the development of periodontitis or for disease recurrence after periodontal therapy or prevent further loss of attachment if periodontitis is already present (Addy and Adriaens 1998; Westfelt 1996). Clinical trials have shown that professionally delivered and frequently repeated supragingival tooth cleaning, combined with optimal self-performed plaque control, has a marked effect in controlling subgingival microflora in moderate to deep periodontal pockets (Hellström et al. 1996).

SELF-CLEANSING MECHANISM

The oral cavity possesses a "self-cleansing mechanism" that acts as a natural method for removing oral debris. The teeth, their alignment, occlusion, gingiva, tongue, cheeks, and saliva work together to remove oral debris. This self-cleansing mechanism is limited, however, and does not prevent dental caries and periodontal diseases. Therefore, mechanical plaque control is the most widely accepted method of preventing dental caries and periodontal diseases.

PATIENT EDUCATION

Educating the periodontal patient about oral hygiene self-care is one of the most important roles of the dental hygienist. **Patient education** provides the patient with the necessary information and skills for the prevention of dental caries and periodontal diseases. A thorough knowledge of oral hygiene self-care is essential for dental hygienists to help plan successful preventive strategies related to a patient's individual plaque-control needs.

Studies have shown that the method used to educate patients about oral hygiene self-care techniques is not critical (Glavid et al. 1985). Therefore, instructions can be given personally by the hygienist, or the patient may be provided with a self-instruction manual, pamphlet, or videotape.

PREVENTIVE MEASURES

The primary goal of prevention is to achieve the lowest plaque level possible. Total elimination of bacteria is neither possible nor desirable, because a number of beneficial bacteria exist in the oral cavity that are necessary for a balanced oral environment.

Preventive measures are classified into two main groups depending on when mechanical plaque control is instituted during the disease process. **Primary prevention** describes preventive measures taken to prevent disease from occurring. It aims at reducing plaque in all individuals regardless of their susceptibility to disease. On the other hand, if periodontal disease is already present in an individual, the goal of treatment changes from preventing the occurrence of disease to preventing the disease from progressing further or preventing the recurrence of the disease after treatment. This is **secondary prevention** (Garmyn, van Steenberghe, and Quirynen 1998).

MECHANICAL PLAQUE CONTROL

Plaque control involves the regular removal of dental plaque from the teeth and adjacent oral tissues and the prevention of its accumulation (Darby and Walsh 1994). Removal of dental plaque and other deposits on the surface of the teeth can be accomplished by the self-cleansing mechanism or mechanical methods. Since dental plaque is not always visible to the naked eye, patients may be unaware of it until it is disclosed. For this reason, a disclosing agent is recommended for patient education and prior to the patient's daily oral hygiene self-care regimen.

EVALUATION

Disclosing solutions show only gross changes and the quantity of stainable material. They do not differentiate between food and plaque, nor do they reveal the presence of microorganisms. Nevertheless, exposure of plaque is a necessary first step in evaluation and can be accomplished with either disclosing tablets or liquid. The patient chews the tablet and passes the fragments along the teeth with the tongue. The liquid form is swabbed along the teeth and gingival margin with a cotton-tip applicator. With either method, once the disclosing solution has been placed on the teeth, the patient rinses lightly once with water. The dental plaque will appear the color of the dye in the disclosing agent. The dental hygienist can use this visual resource to demonstrate the appropriate techniques of oral hygiene self-care to the patient. It is important to show the patient areas where plaque accumulates in proximity to the gingiva. Patients can self-disclose dental plaque periodically to determine the effectiveness of their oral hygiene self-care techniques. However, merely teaching patients about the use of disclosing agents in their dental health education instruction frequently is not sufficient to motivate them to clean their teeth more effectively. Visual feedback may play an important part in health education, but it is just as important to show patients the results of their efforts by written methods or photography.

ORAL HYGIENE SELF-CARE METHODS

Proper oral hygiene self-care accomplishes plaque control, improves appearance, refreshes the breath, and provides a sense of oral cleanliness. The oral hygiene plan designed for the patient should be based on the patient's specific oral hygiene needs. Numerous mechanical cleansing devices, including toothbrushes and interdental aids, are available commercially in today's highly competitive product market. The dental hygienist should be familiar with the particular characteristics of each product in order to make the most appropriate selection for each patient.

TOOTHBRUSHES

Manual toothbrushes: Design

Clinical evaluation of the efficiency of toothbrushes and other oral hygiene devices is constrained by such factors as the time devoted to the method, the patient's hand pressure and dexterity, **patient motivation,** and the criteria used for measuring plaque (Yankell and Saxer 1999). Therefore, toothbrush recommendations should be based on the toothbrushing method prescribed, the patient's intraoral characteristics, patient motivation, the patient's manual dexterity, and product cost.

The standard manual toothbrush consists of a handle and head with bristles and/or filaments. Toothbrush designs vary greatly depending on the desired characteristics. The handle may be straight (conventional) or angled, have a double angulation of the neck, come with or without thumb rests, and/or have a wavelike contour. The shank may be conventional (straight), offset, twisted, or curved. The head may have any of the following features: diamond shaped, squared, rounded, and of variable sizes for infants, children, young adults, and adults. The bristles/filaments (bristles are made of individual filaments) are most often made from nylon. Compared with natural bristles, nylon bristles have shown certain superior qualities, such as bristle durability, cleanliness, and resistance to the accumulation of bacteria and fungi. Bristle stiffness is classified as soft, medium, and hard. Soft bristles are the most highly recommended. Hard bristles have been shown to cause gingival recession and excessive tooth wear, resulting in cervical abrasion (Fig. 10–1 ■). Toothbrush bristle planes vary greatly. The flat (conventional), dome, bilevel, rippled, and tuft profiles are unique to each toothbrush. Frandsen (1986) reported that daily brushing with a conventional flat-bristle brush removes only 50% of plaque from tooth surfaces, with removal of plaque from interproximal surfaces especially lacking. Newer brushes using more tapered and narrow bristles have been designed to more effectively reach interproximal areas, but more research and data evaluation must be done. Research on toothbrush bristles has focused much attention on end rounding of the bristles. End-rounded bristles aid in reducing damage to the gingival tissue. Despite manufacturers' attempts to fabricate toothbrushes with a high percentage of acceptable end-rounded bristles, studies have shown that poorly rounded, sharp and pointed, or flat bristle tips may be present in significant numbers even among brushes making claims of superior end rounding (Dellerman, Hughes, and Burkett 1994).

Alternatives to conventional toothbrushes have been studied. One example is a disposable polyester foam sponge on a stick impregnated with a nonfoaming dentifrice. These spongelike brushes have been used frequently in hospitals and nursing homes and are shown to possess plaque-preventive capabilities. The spongelike brush was found to be effective in retarding accumulation of plaque from a plaque-free baseline on both facial and lingual tooth surfaces (Lefkoff, Beck, and Horton 1995). It is especially useful after periodontal surgery.

FIGURE 10–1

Improper use of a toothbrush caused gingival recession and tooth abrasion, identified by a notching in the cervical area of the maxillary lateral incisors and canines.

Care of toothbrushes

The basic care of toothbrushes includes cleaning the brush after each use with a strong stream of warm water to force particles, toothpaste, and bacteria from the bristles. The toothbrush is then tapped against the edge of the sink to release excess particles and water. It is recommended that the brush be air dried in an upright position and have no contact with other toothbrushes. Portable toothbrush containers need to have air vents to prevent bacterial growth. The life of a toothbrush varies and is affected by the length of time in use, forcefulness of the toothbrushing stroke, amount of pressure exerted on the bristles as they are flexed, and bristle quality and design. Worn bristles are less effective in plaque removal than new ones. As a rule, once the bristles have lost their original shape (e.g., splayed or frayed), it is time to replace the toothbrush with a new one. The taper of the bristle tips may become worn as well and lose effectiveness. One manufacturer provides an indicator color strip within the toothbrush bristles. Once the color wears, the brush should be replaced.

Toothbrushing methods

Numerous toothbrushing methods have been described in the dental literature. These methods are classified according to the direction of toothbrush movement: (1) *horizontal—scrub method;* (2) *circular—Fones method;* (3) *roll—Rolling stroke technique; and* (4) *vibratory—Bass, Stillman, and Charters methods. Earlier studies on toothbrushing methods could not confirm clinically significant differences among various brushing methods, and no further research in this area has been done in recent years.* Thus it can be concluded that improvement in oral hygiene may not depend on the type of toothbrushing method used (Jepsen 1998). The correct method of brushing, for an individual, is that which best removes the plaque and does not cause damage to tooth or gingiva.

Horizontal Scrub Method   The horizontal scrub technique is probably the most commonly used method. The toothbrush bristles are placed perpendicular (90° angle) to the tooth, and the brush is moved back and forth in horizontal motions. For the anterior lingual and palatal tooth surfaces, the brush is held in a vertical position with the heel against the gingival margin, and the scrub stroke is performed in a vertical direction. This technique may be adequate for children with primary teeth, but long-term use in adults may result in gingival recession and cervical abrasion.

Fones Method   The Fones or circular toothbrushing method is performed by positioning the bristles perpendicular to the tooth and using a circular scrubbing stroke. Buccal surfaces are cleaned while the molars are in occlusion, and for cleaning the anterior facial surfaces, the teeth are placed edge to edge. The lingual and palatal tooth surfaces are brushed with an in-and-out stroke. This method is recommended as an easy-to-learn first technique for young children.

Rolling Stroke Technique   In the Rolling stroke technique, emphasis is placed on cleaning the facial and lingual tooth surfaces rather than the sulcular area. The bristles are placed at a 45° angle on the gingiva in an apical direction. The brush stroke is then activated by sweeping the bristles toward the occlusal or incisal surface in a rolling fashion. This stroke is repeated slowly three to four times for each facial and lingual area. The technique requires good manual dexterity and concentration.

Bass Method   Currently, the Bass method is the most widely used toothbrushing technique for adults presenting with or without periodontal diseases. It is also recommended for patients with dental implants. Other interchangeable names are *sulcular* or *intrasulcular brushing*. The Bass method is based on the use of a soft, multitufted toothbrush with rounded-end bristles guided at a 45° angle to the gingival margin (Fig. 10–2a,b ■). The sides of the bristles are against the tooth surface. A vibratory action of the bristles using 10 strokes for each area disrupts the dental plaque at the gingival margin. With proper technique, plaque approximately 1 m subgingivally also will be removed. The lingual and palatal surfaces of the anterior teeth are cleansed with the brush head placed vertically to the long axis of the tooth (Fig. 10–2c ■), and the occlusal surfaces are brushed with a back-and-forth motion. Cleansing of the interdental areas is limited. The modified Bass method also uses the Rolling stroke toward the incisal or occlusal surface.

Stillman Method   The Stillman method was used originally for gingival stimulation and maintenance of normal gingival contour. The toothbrush is placed at a 45° angle facing toward the gingival margin. The bristles are positioned partly on the gingival margin, causing the gingiva to blanch, and partly on the tooth and

---

FIGURE 10–2

(a) Diagram of toothbrush placement in the Bass method. (Copyright © 1997. Rylander H. and Lindhe J. Cause-related Periodontal Therapy. Munksgaard, Copenhagen. Eds. Lindhe J., Karring T., Lang N. P. *Clinical Periodontology and Implant Dentistry*.) (b) Clinically: bristles are placed at a 45° angle to the gingival margin and placed into the interdental areas and gingival sulci without excessive force. With the brush in this position, small vibratory movements or rotary movements can effectively remove plaque. (c) Placement of toothbrush for the palatal surface of anterior teeth.

(a)

(b)

(c)

FIGURE 10–3

Modified Stillman method. The sides of the bristles are placed partly on the teeth and gingiva. The brush is shimmied in a lateral direction as the brush is moved coronally.

then shimmied (vibratory movement) approximately 1 mm in a mesiodistal direction to the count of 10 (Fig. 10–3 ■). The brush is repositioned by rotating the wrist with care not to force the bristles over the gingival margin. In the anterior lingual regions, the brush is held in a vertical direction. In the modified Stillman technique, as the brush is shimmied, the bristles roll down toward and over the occlusal or incisal third of each tooth. This is an attempt to enhance brushing of the entire facial and lingual tooth surfaces. The anterior lingual and palatal tooth surfaces are cleansed using the brush in the vertical position.

Charters Method The Charters method is best indicated when the interdental papillae are missing, thus leaving interdental areas open. The original use of this method was for gingival stimulation or massage, but currently, there is no rationale for this purpose. The bristles are placed at a 45° angle toward the incisal or occlusal surface, with the sides of the bristles placed against the gingiva (Fig. 10–4 ■). The brush is then shimmied downward until the bristles engage the gingiva and interproximal area. The vibratory action extends the bristles into the proximal space. This is repeated four to six times in the same area. Occlusal surfaces are cleansed with a circular or rotary motion. This method should not be used when the contour of the interdental papillae is normal. The modified Charters method uses as Rolling stroke toward the occlusal or incisal surface.

Frequency of toothbrushing

Toothbrushing must be carried out on a regular basis. It is difficult to determine the number of times a day an individual must brush, since the frequency of brushing is tailored to meet individual needs. An individual should brush as many times a day as it takes to effectively remove dental plaque. Factors that affect the recom-

FIGURE 10–4

Diagram showing the Charters' method. The brush with the bristles is placed parallel to the long axis of the tooth pointing incisally. (Copyright © 1997. Rylander H. and Lindhe J. Cause-related Periodontal Therapy. Munksgaard, Copenhagen. Eds. Lindhe J., Jarring T., Lang N.P. *Clinical Peridontology and Implant Dentistry*).

45°

mendations for frequency of toothbrushing include rate of dental plaque formation, plaque visibility, state and susceptibility of oral disease, diet, and presence of contributory factors. Low-risk patients should be directed to brush at least twice a day. High-risk patients should brush more frequently, especially after meals. The use of disclosing agents is highly recommended because it allows meticulous removal of visible plaque from the teeth. The patient should individualize his or her own brushing technique to optimize plaque control. Current data on toothbrushing time suggests that people think they brush longer than they actually do. The average time spent brushing is between 24 and 60 seconds, but the recommended brushing time actually is about 3 minutes (Cancro and Fischman 1995).

POWERED TOOTHBRUSHES

Alternatives to manual toothbrushes include powered toothbrushes. A new generation of sonic and ultrasonic toothbrushes has become available. Powered toothbrushes were designed originally to simulate the action produced using a manual brush. However, effectiveness still depends on brush and bristle placement. Powered toothbrushes originally were recommended for patients lacking fine motor skills or patients with physical or mental impairments, but recent innovations in technology have increased their use for patients with periodontal disease, as well as patients with dental implants.

Mechanism of action

There are many types of powered sonic and ultrasonic toothbrushes on the market today. Variations in brush head, bristle design, and brush movement exist. The various mechanical motions occur in rapid short strokes in one or a combination of the following directions: reciprocating (in and out or up and down), rotational, counterrotational, oscillating (vibrational). A newer generation of powered toothbrushes work by sonic waves and ultrasonic action. Table 10–1 ■ describes a variety of commercially available powered toothbrushes and their respective modes of action. Despite all the advances in technology, no single powered toothbrush design completely removes plaque.

TABLE 10–1
COMMERCIALLY AVAILABLE POWERED TOOTHBRUSHES

PRODUCT	FEATURES AND MODE OF ACTION
Rotadent™ (Pro-Dentec, Batesville, AR)	This is the first of the new-generation powered toothbrushes that was designed differently from the conventional electric brush (rotary motion, no timer). This brush has three interchangeable brush heads that rotate similar to a prophy angle. One is shaped like a cut, with short bristles in the center, and is used on facial and lingual surfaces. The second is a single tuft of pointed bristles for the interproximal area. The third is a longer tuft of bristles for open embrasures.
Interplak® (Conair Corp., East Hanover, NJ)	Introduced into the market in the mid-1980s. Rectangular brushhead with six to eight bristle tufts that individually counterrotate; timer is available. Children's model is available. It consists of ten tufts of rotating bristles in a removable head. Each tuft rotates a turn and a half in one direction before changing direction to rotate a turn in a half in the opposite direction. The twisting action of the bristles accounts for facial, lingual, and interproximal effectiveness.
Braun Oral-B® 3D Plaque Remover (Braun, Oral-B, Belmont, CA)	Combines two distinct brushing motions: in-and-out high-frequency pulsations and side-to-side oscillations. Cup-shaped brushhead with FlexiSoft bristles that give with pressure. If the brush is pressed with too much force on the tooth, the brushing motion will stop. Interdental tips clean interproximal areas. The 3D neck is angled 3°, providing better maneuverability for posterior teeth. The brush is equipped with a memory timer that memorizes lapsed brushing time for when the brush may be briefly switched off.
Plaque Remover® Braun Oral-B (Belmont, CA)	Introduced into the market in 1996. Small round head oscillates 2800 times per minute. Movements are similar to a prophy angle, and the head rotates back and forth (oscillates). The small head allows the brush to be adapted to each tooth individually, reaching interproximally and subgingivally. Small head size necessitates longer than 2-minute brushing time for a complete dentition.
Sonicare® Plus with grip (Optiva Corp, Bellevue, WA)	Introduced in 1993. The brushhead is rectangular in shape. Moving at 31,000 strokes per minute, Sonicare's high-speed back-and-forth motion creates sonic (sound) waves that travel through toothpaste into difficult-to-clean areas. Attached plaque is removed by the effect of the vibrations carried through the dentifrice bubbles. The Smartimer® has a 2-minute automatic shutoff timer and the Quadpacer® quadrant timer beeps at 30-second intervals.
Plaque Control 3000™ Plaque Removal Instrument (Teledyne Water Pik, Fort Collins, CO)	2100 elliptical (circular) strokes per minute; no timer. This brush has a soft, compact, contoured brush head that moves in an elliptical motion similar to the motion of the manual Bass toothbrushing method. Ergonomically designed handle for comfort, control, and ease of use.
SenSonic® Plaque Removal Instrument (Teledyne Water Pik, Fort Collins, CO)	Sonic brushing with 30,000 brush strokes per minute and a soft, contoured, compact bristle design to remove plaque and reduce stains. The built-in electronic feedback system automatically adjusts speed for optimal performance, and the ergonomic handle is designed for comfort and brushing control. The SenSonic Advanced Plaque Removal Instrument has a timer, an automatic shutoff, and a battery indicator light.
Ultra Sonex® (Brewster, NY)	A manual toothbrush with a piezoelectric transducer embedded in the brushhead. Operates at 1.6 million cycles per second. A dentifrice is used to conduct the ultrasonic waves to the teeth and soft tissues.

Effectiveness

Various studies with conflicting results have examined the effectiveness of powered toothbrushes compared with conventional brushes in plaque removal. Since most studies in the 1960s and 1970s failed to show that powered toothbrushes remove plaque better than manual toothbrushes, they were not so popular. In the 1996 World Workshop in Periodontics it was concluded that limited evidence supports the fact that powered toothbrushes offer additional benefits compared with manual toothbrushes (Hancock 1996).

A few powered toothbrushes may be superior in removing plaque from interproximal areas than conventional manual toothbrushes (Bader 1992; Saxer and Yankell 1997). One study suggests that the sonic toothbrush (Sonicare®, Optiva Corp., Bellevue, WA) is more beneficial in resolving inflammation and reducing pocket depths in patients with moderate periodontal disease (O'Beirne et al. 1996). However, other randomized, controlled clinical studies have not proven conclusively any differences in the efficacy of plaque removal between manual and powered toothbrushes (Van der Weijden et al. 1993; Preber et al. 1991). A recent clinical study using 62 adult patients with significant amounts of plaque, calculus, and inflammation demonstrated that brushing with either a manual or ultrasonic toothbrush significantly reduced bleeding and gingival inflammation. Neither toothbrush showed superiority over the other in removing plaque (Forgas-Brockmann, Carter-Hanson, and Killoy 1998). The novelty of using a new device may in part increase self-care efforts, thus improving oral hygiene.

Powered toothbrushes have been found to be superior in removing tooth stains (Grossman et al. 1996). The Braun Oral-B® Plaque Remover (Braun, Oral-B, Belmont, CA) and Sonicare® have been shown to be superior to a manual toothbrush in removal of chlorhexidine stains (Moran and Addy 1995).

Recommending a powered toothbrush

Factors to consider when recommending a powered toothbrush include the toothbrush design, brushing motion, patient's interest and motivation, and the costs and benefits. Placement of bristles and the head of the toothbrush is important to avoid tissue trauma. The powered toothbrush should be moved slowly in sequence around the mouth using less pressure than with a manual toothbrush, thus producing less cervical abrasion and tissue trauma. Evaluation of a patient's ability to improve his or her plaque and gingival indices over time is the best method for determining the success of a specific powered toothbrush. Use of powered toothbrushes is safe on titanium dental implants.

The use of powered toothbrushes by patients with poor self-care compliance has shown some advantages (Hellstadius, Asman, and Gustafsson 1993). Use of a powered toothbrush (counterrotational) in periodontal patients in a periodontal maintenance program has proved to be helpful in reducing plaque levels and enhancing gingival conditions (Yukna and Shaklee 1993). Other patients that may benefit from the use of powered toothbrushes include those with limited manual dexterity, orthodontic patients, and children (parental brushing of children's teeth).

INTERDENTAL CARE

Interdental cleaning is a primary area of neglect. A major factor in disease initiation and control is the anatomy of the interdental area. Cleansing of these interproximal areas depends on tooth alignment and tissue configuration. Supplemental aids are necessary because, despite new toothbrush designs, brushing alone is ineffective in the removal of interproximal plaque.

Various considerations are appropriate when recommending interdental cleaning devices. These factors are as follows:

1. The presence or absence of interdental papillae
2. Alignment of teeth

FIGURE 10–5

Three types of gingival embrasures. Interdental cleaning devices are specific for each type of embrasure. (a) Type I embrasure is completely filled with interdental gingiva. (b) Type II embrasure has partial loss of interdental gingiva (mandibular anterior teeth). (c) Type III embrasure has complete loss of interdental gingiva.

(a)

(b)

(c)

3. Shape of teeth
4. Tissue contour
5. Condition of restorations
6. Tightness of contact area
7. Presence of bridges, dental implants, and orthodontic appliances
8. Patient motivation and interest in interproximal cleaning
9. Effectiveness of patient's self-care
10. Size of gingival embrasure

Types of gingival embrasures

There are three types of gingival embrasures (Fig. 10–5a,b,c ■): Type I, in which the embrasure is completely filled with gingiva; Type II, in which there is slight to moderate recession of the interdental papillae; and Type III, in which there is extensive or complete loss of interdental papillae (Darby and Walsh 1994).

Available interdental cleaning devices include dental floss, dental tape, interdental brushes, interdental stimulators, and oral irrigators (Table 10–2■). Determination of which interdental aid is to be used depends on the type of gingival embrasure.

TABLE 10–2		
CLINICAL FEATURES OF INTERDENTAL CLEANING DEVICES		
TYPE OF DENTAL DEVICE	**USE**	**LIMITATIONS**
Dental floss	Type I gingival embrasures.	Use caution not to cause tissue trauma. Not recommended for diastemas and Types II and III gingival embrasures.
Dental tape	Broad and flat for wider spaces and assists in polishing proximal surfaces.	Difficult to use for tight contact areas and Types II and III embrasures.
Dental floss threader	Floss is threaded through a plastic needle-like device. Best to use under pontics, around orthodontic wires, and where teeth are splinted or soldered.	Use caution not to injure the gingiva with the point of the threader.
Dental floss holder	Patients with limited manual dexterity or who do not want to place fingers in the mouth. For Type I embrasures.	Sometimes it is difficult to get the floss through the contact area; floss must be taut. Do not use in Types II or III embrasures.
Tufted floss	To clean beneath pontics, around orthodontic wires, and between splinted teeth. The yarn portion of the floss is used for actual cleaning where space permits.	Not intended for Type I gingival embrasures. Use caution with the tip of the floss.
Rubber-tip stimulator	Used for the removal of dental plaque along the gingival margin. Also can be used in an open embrasure.	To avoid tissue trauma, do not place tip subgingivally.
Wooden wedge	Use in Type II and III embrasures with shallow pockets.	Use caution not to cause tissue trauma. Difficult to adapt lingually.
Interdental brushes	Use in Type II and III embrasures and furcation involvement areas.	Do not use in Type I embrasures.
Implant floss	Use around implant posts or abutments	Avoid forcing floss into the gingiva.
Electric interdental cleaner	Good for patients with limited manual dexterity. Good for all types of embrasures, including around bridges and implants. Available with a filament and FlexiTip stimulator.	Follow manufacturer's instructions.

Dental Floss and Dental Tape   Numerous types of nylon dental floss are available: waxed, unwaxed, flat, round, colored, flavored, shred resistant, and impregnated with substances such as fluoride, baking soda, and tetrasodium pyrophospate. Floss is indicated for use in Type I gingival embrasures, where the embrasures are completely filled with interdental papillae. It is also effective

FIGURE 10–6

Floss holder. The floss is held tightly between two prongs. (Courtesy of John O. Butler Company, Chicago, IL)

around implants. Dental floss is 80% effective in removing interproximal dental plaque. Waxed dental floss may be more resistant to tearing or shredding but may be too bulky for tight contacts. Teflon-coated floss is made of polytetrafluoroethylene and is inserted easily into difficult access areas and resists fraying (Ciancio, Shilby, and Farber 1992). Unwaxed floss is thin and easily manipulated through tight contact areas. Even though patients prefer to use waxed floss rather than unwaxed floss (Beaumont 1990), there is actually no difference between the two flosses in efficacy in removing interproximal plaque (Hill, Levi, and Glickman 1973). Floss may fray and tear where teeth are crowded or in areas where restorations are defective. Dental tape is broad and flat and should be used in open interdental spaces or between teeth without tight contacts and for polishing proximal tooth surfaces. The major advantage of colored floss is patient appeal and the patient's ability to see what is removed by flossing. This factor may help motivate the patient to floss regularly.

A floss modification called *tufted dental floss,* made by many manufacturers, has a stiff straight end with a section of unwaxed floss and an area of thicker nylon meshwork. The stiff end allows the floss to be passed easily under bridges, around implant abutments, through exposed furcations, or between orthodontic appliances.

The floss holder is a yokelike device with a space between the two prongs of the yoke. The floss is secured tightly between the two prongs designed to facilitate movement of the floss interproximally, as shown in Fig. 10–6 ■. It is recommended for patients with limited manual dexterity.

The floss threader is a needle-like device (Fig. 10–7 ■) to facilitate floss use under pontics and splinted crowns, between orthodontic appliances, through a gingival embrasure, or between teeth with tight contacts. It is used by threading approximately 12 inches of floss through the loop and then drawing it through the interproximal space. The floss is then engaged against the tooth surface.

Caution is necessary in flossing to avoid injury to the gingiva. The floss may cut the gingiva if it is pulled too quickly past the contact and/or if it is positioned too forcefully beneath the gingiva. Damage to the junctional epithelium may occur, especially in healthy gingiva. The patient should be instructed to perform flossing procedures in a systematic fashion (hence all mandibular and maxillary

FIGURE 10–7

The floss threader is a needle-like device. Floss is placed through the loop for access underneath pontics, exposed furcations, orthodontic appliances, and splinted crowns. (Courtesy of John O. Butler Company, Chicago, IL)

FIGURE 10–8

Floss is not as effective as an interdental brush in removing interdental plaque from tooth concavities. (Courtesy of John O. Butler Company, Chicago, IL)

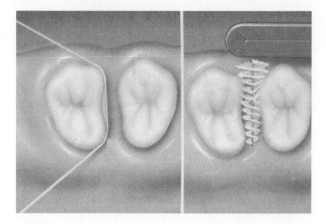

teeth are included). Mastering the flossing technique requires time and patience. Patients are discouraged and less motivated to incorporate the flossing regimen into their oral hygiene program when they have difficulties with manual dexterity or when they do not have the patience to do the job well.

Floss also has been designed specifically for cleaning implants. The denture is removed before cleaning the abutments. The floss is looped from facial to lingual around the abutment and gently placed subgingivally until resistance is met. It is then crisscrossed and used in a sliding back-and-forth, up-and-down motion. Implant floss is made of braided nylon filaments and can be washed off after each use.

Interdental and Single-Tuft Brushes   Exposed furcations, root concavities (e.g., mesial concavity on the maxillary first premolar), and type II and III gingival embrasures usually are best cleaned with an interdental or single-tuft brush (also called end-tuft brush) (Fig. 10–8 ■). Other uses for such brushes include the distal surface of the

FIGURE 10–9

(a) Variations in types of interdental brushes. Uses of an interdental brush (b) in a Type II embrasure and (c) around implant abutments. (Courtesy of John O. Butler Company, Chicago, IL)

(a)

(b)

(c)

terminal molar, around pontics and maligned teeth, and around orthodontic appliances or dental implant abutments. The premoistened brush is inserted interproximally and used in an in-and-out direction. However, such brushes should not be forced to fit into gingival embrasures.

Interdental brushes consist of nylon filaments twisted onto a metal wire or a nylon-coated plastic wire that does not scratch or cause tissue trauma. Interchangeable bristles come in a variety of sizes, such as cylindrical, tapered, and large cylindrical (Fig. 10–9a,b,c ■). A unique wireless soft foam insert is available for postoperative periodontal care, implant maintenance, and medicament applications.

The single-tuft brush, also called an *end-tuft brush,* consists of a group of small bristles or tufts that are flat or tapered on a straight or angled handle (Fig. 10–10a,b,c,d ■).

Rubber-Tip Stimulator   The rubber-tip stimulator consists of a flexible rubber tip attached to a handle or at the end of a toothbrush. It is not recommended for healthy gingiva that completely fills the gingival embrasure, but it can be useful in Type II or Type III embrasures. Generally, it is used for removing plaque at the gin-

FIGURE 10–10

(a) Variations in single-tufted brushes (tapered and nontapered). (Courtesy Oral-B Labs, Belmont, CA.) Use of a single-tufted brush (b) around orthodontic appliances, (c) dental implants, and (d) the distal surface of the terminal tooth. (Courtesy of John O. Butler Company, Chicago, IL)

(a)

(b)

(c)

(d)

gival margin, exposed furcation areas, concave surfaces, and open interdental areas. The tip is inserted gently into the interdental area and inclined approximately 45° toward the occlusal surface following the contour of the gingiva. It also can be placed interproximally at a 90° angle. A back-and-forth or rolling motion is used. It was thought originally that use of the rubber tip increased keratinization and vascular function through gingival stimulation, but there is no clinical evidence to support this (Rounds and Tilliss 1999).

Wooden Toothpicks Wooden toothpicks are available as either a toothpick-in-holder or a triangular balsa wood stimulator. These devices should be used where interdental papillae are missing (Type II and Type III embrasures). Since wooden toothpicks are difficult to use on lingual surfaces and they do not reach subgingivally, they are not as effective as dental floss.

The triangular stimulator should be moistened with saliva and then inserted interproximally, flat side toward the papilla, moving in an in-and-out burnishing stroke. Discard the wedge if it becomes splayed.

The toothpick-in-holder is a plastic-handled instrument with a tapered, conical opening at one end where the toothpick is inserted; the excess portion is broken off. It is used for plaque removal along the gingival margin, within the sulcus, in root concavities, in furcation areas, and around orthodontic appliances; it also can be used for the application of medicaments (e.g., fluoride or a desensitizing agent). The blunt point and sides of the toothpick are placed in the sulcus to engage, debride, and dislodge adherent plaque.

Electric Interdental Cleaning Devices One of the more recent advances in interdental cleaning is the Braun Oral-B Interclean® (Redwood City, CA), an electric interdental cleaning device that consists of a thin, flexible cleaning filament (Fig. 10–11a,b ■). The filament is placed into the interdental space and disrupts and sweeps away plaque by an elliptical movement using over 100 cleaning strokes per second. Individuals who are unable to floss or those who will not floss may find automated interproximal cleansing easier. This device has been shown to reduce plaque, gingivitis, and bleeding equal to or better than floss (Gordon, Frascella, and Reardon 1996). Other automated interdental cleaners are available and include sonic devices, filament tips, brush tips, and flossers.

Other Interdental Cleaning Devices Knitting yarn may be used in Type III embrasures. It is used on the mesial and distal surfaces of natural teeth and dental implant abutments and the distal surface of the last tooth in an arch. Nylon, cotton, and rayon are preferred over wool yarn, which may irritate the gingiva. Approximately 14 inches of yarn is used in the same fashion as regular floss.

Soft pipe cleaners can be purchased commercially and are recommended for cleansing if there is advanced bone loss and the papillae have receded, leaving open gingival embrasures and/or Class IV open furcation involvements, on the distal of the last tooth in the arch, and for malpositioned or separated teeth. Care must be taken, however, because the sharp wire center of the pipe cleaner may

FIGURE 10–11

(a) Braun Oral-B Interclean®. (b) Interproximal use of the device. (Courtesy of Oral-B Labs, Belmont, CA)

(a)   (b)

scratch the cementum or injure the gingiva. The pipe cleaner is moved in a facial-lingual direction, cleaning the proximal surfaces of the teeth.

Alternatively, a gauze strip can be formed from a folded gauze pad and used through a large opening in the furca, drawing it in a facial-lingual direction. It is another effective plaque remover for use on proximal surfaces of teeth that are adjacent to edentulous areas, teeth that have diastemas, and for dental implant abutments.

TONGUE CLEANSING

A number of tongue cleansing devices are available. These are used in a pull or forward motion. A soft bristle toothbrush also may be used for tongue cleansing. When using a toothbrush, a brushing stroke starting on the posterior-most aspect of the dorsum of the tongue is performed with a roll to the tip of the tongue. Tongue brushing will improve tongue appearance and halitosis by removing coatings associated with bacteria, food, and smoking.

ORAL IRRIGATION

Oral irrigation emerged in the late 1960s as an adjunct to brushing and flossing. Early studies indicated that mechanical water-pressure devices did not remove significant amounts of supragingival plaque but only loosened food debris and less adherent materials (Lobene 1969). However, regardless of the plaque index, reductions in gingivitis and calculus formation were evident as early as 1969 (Lobene 1969; Lobene and Soparkar 1970; Lainson, Bergquist, and Fraleigh 1970). Today, there is a preponderance of clinical studies that address the use of oral irrigation on gingivitis and periodontitis maintenance patients and show significant reductions in clinical parameters (e.g., bleeding on probing and gingival inflammation).

TABLE 10–3 HOME ORAL IRRIGATORS		
NAME	**MANUFACTURER**	**DESCRIPTION**
Water Pik® dental systems	Teledyne Water Pik, Fort Collins, CO	Two tips are available; standard jet tip for supragingival irrigation and the Pik Pocket® tip for subgingival irrigation.
Viajet®	Oratec Corporation, Herndon, VA	Two standard tips for supragingival irrigation, and two sulcus tips for marginal application are available. For office use: A cannula (stainless steel tube) adapter for subgingival application is available.
Braun Oral-B® Plaque Removal System	Oral-B, Belmont, CA	This device is only available with the powered brush (sold as one unit). Plastic tips are available for supragingival use only, and the tips cannot be removed.

The primary use of oral irrigation is to nonspecifically reduce bacteria and their byproducts that lead to the initiation or progression of periodontal diseases (Drisko 1996). The target area of irrigation is unattached or loosely attached microorganisms at the subgingival level. With our current understanding of the pathogenesis of periodontal infections and the role endotoxins play in the immune response, irrigation may have a more significant place in self-care routines, especially since the highest concentrations of endotoxins have been found within the loosely adherent subgingival plaque (Daly, Seymour, and Kieser 1980).

Supragingival irrigation dilutes (Ciancio 1990) and flushes away bacteria coronal to the gingiva, which helps to prevent or treat gingivitis (Drisko 1996) and also reduces subgingival bacteria. Subgingival irrigation attempts to directly reduce the pocket microflora in an effort to prevent initiation of periodontitis or to help its reduction (American Academy of Periodontology 1995). However, irrigation does not remove adherent dental plaque, calculus, or stains.

DEVICES

Oral irrigation devices generally are power-driven pulsating devices that deliver water or a medicament to the site. The pulsations create two zones of hydrokinetic activity. The *impact zone* is the area where the irrigant comes in contact with the tooth surface, and the *flushing zone* is the deflection of the irrigant subgingivally (Cobb, Rodgers, and Killoy 1988). A pulsating stream of water provides better flushing than a continuous stream because it incorporates a compression and decompression phase, which allows debris and bacteria to be displaced more efficiently (American Academy of Periodontology 1995). Products are available that are nonpulsating and non-power-driven, but to date, there is no evidence that they are clinically effective.

A Water Pik™ (Teledyne Water Pik, Fort Collins, CO; Fig. 10–12a ■) is one such home irrigation device (Table 10–3 ■). Water or a medicament is delivered to

---

FIGURE 10–12

(a) Water Pik® dental systems. (Courtesy of Teledyne Water Pik, Fort Collins, CO.) (b) Placement of standard jet tip. (Courtesy of Teledyne Water Pik, Fort Collins, CO.)

(a)

(b)

the gingival margin with a standard jet tip (Fig. 10–12b ■) placed at a 90° angle to the long axis of the tooth. The jet tip is positioned directly interproximally so that the stream of water or medicament reaches the target slightly subgingivally. The tip is passed along the gingival margin to the next proximal area and held in place for 5 to 6 seconds. The procedure is usually performed over a bathroom sink beginning with a low- pressure setting. Pressure may be increased as needed or according to patient comfort and gingival health. Eakle, Ford, and Boyd (1986) found that a standard jet tip delivered an irrigant 44 to 71% into the depth of pockets. In addition, use of a standard jet tip with a Water Pik® oral irrigator placed on medium pressure was found to have a positive effect on subgingival microorganisms at probing depths of up to 6 mm (Cobb, Rodgers, and Killoy 1988).

Some home irrigation devices have accessory delivery tips designed for targeted direct subgingival delivery. A Water Pik® oral irrigator using a Pik Pocket® subgingival irrigation tip (Fig. 10–13 ■) delivers an irrigant to approximately 90% of the depth of pockets ranging from 0 to 6 mm (Braun and Ciancio 1992). The Pik Pocket® tip is designed for controlled, targeted low-pressure delivery of a medicament or water.

EFFICACY

Studies repeatedly show statistically significant reductions in gingivitis, bleeding on probing, probing depth, and periodontal pathogens in gingivitis and periodontal maintenance patients with the use of oral irrigation over normal oral hygiene (Flemming et al. 1990; Newman et al. 1994; Chaves et al. 1994; Cobb, Rodgers, and Killoy 1988). Subgingival calculus must be removed before irrigation because it interferes with penetration of the agent (Pitcher, Newman, and Strahan 1980).

It appears that using a standard jet tip or a specialized delivery tip is effective with specific home irrigation devices. Caution must be taken when evaluating the research because not all products have been studied in clinical trials. Therefore, established efficacy with one product may not be true for another. It is always advisable to contact the manufacturer and request copies of the clinical trials that support product claims.

FIGURE 10–13

Pik Pocket® subgingival delivery tip placement in furcation of mandibular first molar. (Courtesy of Teledyne Water Pik, Fort Collins, CO.)

INDICATIONS

Adjunctive oral irrigation may not be necessary for all patients. However, Chaves et al. (1994) found an added benefit for patients with good oral hygiene. Oral irrigation is an ideal adjunct when supragingival mechanical aids (e.g., toothbrushes, floss, and interproximal brushes and devices) are not sufficient to keep the bacterial load below the threshold of disease. It is also ideal for delivering antimicrobial agents deeper into pockets. Patients with physical challenges, orthodontic appliances, or prosthodontic replacements such as implants and crowns or those who need an adjunctive method to reduce repopulation of bacteria between periodontal maintenance appointments are also ideal candidates for supplemental home oral irrigation. Subgingival irrigation may be better than rinsing in the maintenance of gingival health around dental implants (Felo et al. 1997).

Patients with plaque-induced gingivitis can benefit most from oral irrigation because the disease is in its early stage. Patients with slight and moderate chronic periodontitis also may benefit from oral irrigation. However, patients with severe chronic periodontitis and refractory periodontitis require more aggressive treatment and referral to a periodontist.

CAUTIONS

Controlled powered-driven home irrigation devices are safe for patients to use on a daily basis. Thorough patient evaluation is always necessary prior to recommending any device or aid to a patient. It is important to match the correct product with the patient's specific needs. Also, take the time to instruct patients on the proper use of their device.

Oral irrigation should not be used when a periodontal abscess or ulcerations are present. Once the problem has been resolved, it then may be appropriate to recommend irrigation therapy. Since the American Heart Association (AHA) has not established guidelines for patients requiring antibiotic prophylaxis and use of home oral irrigation, it is recommended that these patients do not use oral irrigation (Drisko 1996).

Irrigation versus toothbrushing

Controversy exists over whether irrigation provides an additional benefit over toothbrushing and flossing. Irrigation is not a substitute for toothbrushing or flossing. Toothbrushing plus irrigation may be better than toothbrushing alone in patients with poor oral home care (Flemming et al. 1990). Supragingival irrigation is adequate as an adjunctive therapy to decrease inflammation (e.g., redness and bleeding), but there is no significant reduction in probing depth or gain in clinical attachment. Irrigation distributes antimicrobial agents into interproximal areas better than rinsing. There may be no difference between irrigating with a medicament (chemical agent) or with water, however. In patients with good oral hygiene, daily brushing and flossing remain the most efficient methods for controlling gingivitis.

HOME CARE FOR PERIODONTAL PATIENTS

The important role of oral hygiene in controlling dental plaque growth and recolonization immediately after periodontal surgery cannot be overestimated (Sanz and Herrera 1998). The degree of oral hygiene maintained by the patient also influences the healing response after periodontal surgery (Flores-de-Jacoby and Mengel 1995; Palcanis 1996). Presently, it is unknown if the healing response results from the improvement in and maintenance of low plaque levels by the patient (Westfelt 1996) or is related to the increased frequency of periodontal maintenance visits after surgery (Ramfjord 1987).

Following periodontal surgery, patients should be cautious around the periodontal dressing. It is likely that they will be inclined to avoid brushing the area, but they should be instructed to lightly brush the exposed tooth surfaces and all other areas of the dentition with a soft or ultrasoft toothbrush. The Bass method should be avoided; other methods that do not place the bristles directly into the gingival crevice are recommended to prevent trauma to the healing tissue.

Periodontal patients frequently have localized or generalized blunted papillae due to the disease process or as a consequence of periodontal surgery. Because of the open interdental spaces, the use of interdental brushes and single-tuft brushes is recommended.

ADVICE TO THE PATIENT

Noncompliance with oral hygiene self-care is a major factor in the recurrence of periodontal diseases. One role of the dental hygienist is to determine the patient's enthusiasm and manual dexterity in performing plaque control (Baker 1995). This entails having good professional communications skills and patience, since it is not easy for patients to change their habits. Besides lack of motivation, other reasons for plaque control failure include poor technique, lack of knowledge, and inconsistent performance (Van Dyke et al. 1999).

Flossing can be done either before or after toothbrushing, but most patients floss before brushing. Patients often find flossing to be a difficult experience. Therefore, the dental hygienist must introduce flossing from an educational perspective and then gradually instruct the patient about technique. It is best not to have the patient start with too many plaque-control devices at one time. Rather, it may be advantageous to introduce effective toothbrushing at the first appointment and then reinforce it at subsequent visits. The patient's toothbrushing method should only be changed or modified if it is ineffective in removing plaque. Flossing or other methods of interdental cleaning can be introduced at a later time. By gradually having the patient master each technique separately, he or she will not be overwhelmed.

Oral hygiene self-care programs are based on a patient's individual needs. Keeping the program simple will increase patient compliance. Try to adapt the oral hygiene program to the patient's lifestyle. Establishing good oral hygiene habits involves having patients clean their teeth in a systematic pattern (e.g., starting on the maxillary right and ending on the mandibular right). However, strict adherence to one approach may not always be in the best interests of thorough plaque removal and improved gingival health.

Oral physiotherapeutic products have limitations. Brushing and flossing are effective in the mechanical removal of most supragingival plaque but are limited in removing subgingival plaque due to the design of the devices and the contour of the gingiva. A periodontal patient may be able to access the subgingiva only slightly. The techniques described in this chapter can be modified to permit cleansing of all accessible areas of the dentition. A different regimen is applied after periodontal surgery, and the patient must be familiar with the various cleaning aids needed. The dental hygienist must introduce these new aids to the patient.

The iatrogenic effects of dentistry need to be eliminated prior to setting expectations for plaque removal. For example, unpolished amalgam restorations retain more plaque than polished ones. Composite materials may accumulate plaque greater than amalgam. Ill-fitting margins, overhangs, and rough surfaces on restorations should be evaluated for replacement or finishing because of plaque-retentive possibilities.

Patients with gingival enlargement (drug-induced or hormonal) must be especially compliant with frequent maintenance visits and good oral hygiene self-care. Keeping plaque levels to a minimum has been shown to reduce the development of gingival enlargement in some patients. Since the gingiva is overgrown and pseudopockets result, it is difficult for such patients to practice optimal toothbrushing and flossing.

EFFECTS OF IMPROPER USE OF ORAL HYGIENE DEVICES

Once the importance of oral hygiene is explained to the patient and he or she begins to use numerous oral hygiene devices, the next step is to ensure that the patient is using each device correctly.

TOOTHBRUSHING

Factors that can cause acute or chronic tissue problems include incorrect bristle angulation or placement, heavy or long brushing strokes, a toothbrush with hard bristles, extremely abrasive toothpaste, and loss of concentration. Acute soft tissue lesions appear as small ulcers, red areas, or denuded gingiva. Chronic, long-standing gingival lesions present as gingival recession, rolled marginal gingiva, or gingival clefting (Fig. 10–14 ■). Gingival recession was found to occur mostly on the buccal surfaces of maxillary first molars, premolars, and canines (Björn, Andersson, and Olsson 1981). Hard tissue lesions present as toothbrush abrasions occurring at the cervical area of teeth (see Fig. 10–1). Tooth abrasion in most cases is due to the combined effect of toothbrushing and the use of dentifrices containing abrasives (Sangnes 1976). Cervical abrasion may occur once the root surface has been exposed by gingival recession. Thus, in order for cervical abrasions to occur, they must be preceded by gingival recession.

FIGURE 10–14

Soft tissue trauma caused by improper toothbrushing. Note rolled free gingival margins.

The Bass method is one of the more technique-sensitive toothbrushing methods. This method requires the patient to have good manual dexterity and concentration when applying the bristles to each area along both dental arches to minimize damage to soft tissue. The soft tissue needs to be evaluated at each maintenance visit for signs of improper brushing. Generally, powered toothbrushes do not cause soft or hard tissue damage.

INTERDENTAL DEVICES

Dental floss, interdental brushes, and single-tufted brushes can cause injury to the gingiva if improper techniques are used. Each device is indicated in different types of gingival embrasures. Gingival ulcers, cuts, and clefts can result from improper technique.

Floss should not be forced too deeply into the gingival crevices. When floss is used as part of the daily plaque-control routine, the junctional epithelial cells adhering to the enamel are in a continuous state of disruption and healing (Waerhaug 1981). Interdental brushes and single-tufted brushes should not be forced into a gingival embrasure that has an intact papilla.

Interdental cleaning is easy to master if the dental hygienist provides proper teaching and supervision to the patient.

DENTINAL HYPERSENSITIVITY

Maintaining plaque control is of utmost importance in reducing the sensitivity of exposed root surfaces. Often patients have difficulty complying with oral hygiene procedures because of the discomfort experienced during toothbrushing. Thus these areas are not cleaned and become more sensitive. Identification of a lesion is difficult, and frequently, toothbrushing is a major factor in localizing the sensitivity. Accordingly, root surfaces must be desensitized and an adequate oral hygiene self-care program maintained. In patients with good oral hygiene but with dentinal hypersensitivity, use of a desensitizing agent is recommended.

DESENSITIZATION

A number of treatments are available for sensitive teeth. The type of treatment depends on the severity of the problem and the history of prior intervention. The following steps are recommended for desensitization:

1. Use the air syringe to assess whether there is sensitivity. Write it down as a score of 0, 1, 2, or 3.
2. Recommend use of a desensitizing dentifrice for about 4 to 6 weeks. The patient is instructed to brush two times a day for 1 minute.
3. Instruct the patient on proper brushing so that the situation does not get worse. The patient's brushing technique must be corrected if treatment is to be successful.
4. Discuss the role of diet with the patient. Acidic and citrus foods should be limited in the patient's diet. If the patient frequently consumes acidic foods or juices, he or she should be instructed to rinse the mouth with sodium bicarbonate to help neutralize the acidity.

5. At the next examination, do the air syringe test again, and if the sensitivity is gone, the patient can go back to his or her regular dentifrice. If the sensitivity reappears later, the patient can use the desensitizing dentifrice again. If the sensitivity is still present, an in-office treatment should be tried.

PATIENT-APPLIED TREATMENT

Basically, potassium nitrate and stannous fluoride products are available for patient-applied treatments (Table 10–4 ■).

Dentifrices

Patient-applied medicaments are available as dentifrices, gels, and rinses. Dentifrices are helpful when many tooth surfaces are sensitive. For patients with mild sensitivity without loss of substantial tooth structure, a densensitizing dentifrice is recommended. Because it can take several weeks to see results, fluoride has been added to most dentifrices. It appears that a potassium nitrate–containing dentifrice works the fastest. A complete list of desensitizing dentifrices is found in Chapter 11.

The longer the dentifrice is in contact with the dentin surface, the greater is its success. Thus more frequent applications are advised. Instead of using a dentifrice in the usual manner, it may be more effective if the undiluted dentifrice is applied with a cotton applicator directly on the tooth surface.

Fluorides

Of all the fluorides, stannous fluoride shows the most promise for topical application in periodontal therapy as an antibacterial and desensitizing agent. Application of stannous fluoride (0.4%) on a daily basis, after some time, can be therapeutic in reducing dentinal hypersensitivity. However, it often stings the gingiva, and patients may not comply with treatment. In addition, stannous fluoride will stain dentin more than enamel because of its porous nature, making it unaesthetic. Because it is

TABLE 10–4		
PATIENT-APPLIED DESENSITIZING AGENTS		
PRODUCT	**ACTIVE INGREDIENT**	**METHOD OF USE**
Gel-Kam® gel (Colgate Oral Pharm., Canton, MA)	0.4% stannous fluoride	Apply to toothbrush and brush teeth. This product is available over-the-counter without a prescription. Available in 4.3-oz tubes or a pack with 2- to 3.5-oz tubes.
Gel-Kam® Oral Care Rinse (Colgate Oral Pharm., Canton, MA)	0.63% stannous fluoride	Patient places 1/8 fluid oz of concentrate in marked mixing vial (included in box) and adds water as directed to prepare a 0.1% stannous fluoride rinse. Rinse over a 3-week period.
STANIMAX™ Perio Rinse (SDI Labs, Glenview, IL)	0.63% stannous fluoride	1/8 fluid oz is diluted with warm water to make 1 oz of the rinse in a measuring cup that is provided.
STANIMAX™ Brush-on Gel (SDI Labs, Glenview, IL)	0.4% stannous fluoride	Apply gel to a toothbrush.

nonabrasive, extrinsic stains will build up if it is used instead of toothpaste. Stannous fluoride is also available in a 0.63% oral rinse that dilutes to a 0.1% solution.

IN-OFFICE TREATMENT

If therapeutic dentifrices are not successful, in-office application of medicaments is recommended. Several products are available, including ferric oxalate, fluoride (with or without iontophoresis), bonding agents, varnishes, and glass ionomers (Table 10–5 ■).

Oxalate salts

Most oxalates (ferric oxalate and potassium oxalate) are available as acidic solutions. Oxalates are capable of blocking the dentinal tubules when they are placed on an area of exposed dentin. Often the patient brushes the oxalate off. Thus the patient must be instructed not to brush too vigorously so that the dentin will not be removed. It is best to watch the patient brush in the office.

Fluorides

Most dental practitioners use fluoride for management of hypersensitivity. Stannous fluoride is applied topically on the exposed dentin, forming a sort of granular layer

TABLE 10–5
CHAIRSIDE DESENSITIZING PRODUCTS

PRODUCT	ACTIVE INGREDIENT	METHOD OF USE
Dentinbloc® (Colgate Oral Pharm., Canton, MA)	1.09% sodium fluoride, 0.40% stannous fluoride, 0.14% hydrogen fluoride	Saturate a cotton pellet and apply to dry exposed dentin. Do not burnish; use light pressure.
Sensodyne® Sealant (Block Drug Corp., Jersey City, NJ)	6% ferric oxalate	Saturate a cotton pellet and apply to dry exposed dentin. Do not burnish; use light pressure.
Protect® Drops (John O. Butler Comp., Chicago, IL, available in a dropper bottle or unit dose ampule)	2.7% potassium oxalate	Saturate a cotton pellet and apply to dry exposed dentin. Do not burnish; use light pressure.
Dentin conditioners	Aluminum oxalate	Saturate a cotton pellet and apply to dry exposed dentin. Use light pressure; do not burnish.
STANIMAX-PRO™ (SDI Labs, Glenview, IL)	3.28% stannous fluoride	Can be used as a gel or diluted one-to-one with water to form a 1.64% stannous fluoride rinse.
Duraflor® (Pharmascience Inc., Montréal, Canada)	50 mg sodium fluoride varnish	Apply to affected area with a cotton pellet.
Duraphat® (Colgate Oral Pharm., Canton, MA)	5% sodium fluoride varnish	Apply to affected area with a brush that comes with kit or with a cotton pellet.

over the dentin surface that does not come off with simple washing, so it seals or decreases dentin permeability.

Sodium fluoride is available as a paste (33% sodium fluoride, 33% kaolin, 33% glycerin). Sodium fluoride works best for about 7 to 14 days, and then its effects dissipate.

Various sodium fluoride solutions have been tried with limited success. When iontophoresis is used to allow the fluoride ion to penetrate into the dentinal tubules, longer-lasting effects, up to 3 to 4 months, are seen. A second application usually is necessary.

Restorative materials

Bonding agents are improving rapidly, but they are not used very much at this time. Use of such agents is a technique-sensitive procedure. Often the restoration is finished with a diamond bur, which may open up new tubules below the restoration, recreating sensitive dentin. Since the restoration is located at the cervical third of the tooth, overhangs or rough surfaces may create more problems.

If the sensitivity can be narrowed down to just one or two teeth, a glass ionomer can be used as a last resort.

SUMMARY

Supragingival and subgingival dental plaque biofilms play a major role in the initiation of periodontal diseases. Since the subgingival microflora is derived originally from supragingival plaque, it is necessary to disrupt both groups of bacteria. This is accomplished through mechanical supragingival plaque removal by the patient using toothbrushes and interdental devices and by the dental hygienist by removal of subgingival plaque.

It would seem that gingivitis should be treated easily with plaque removal. Unfortunately, many obstacles prevent the timely removal of plaque. Besides lack of motivation to learn and perform toothbrushing and flossing skills, many patients also perform inconsistently, lack knowledge, and employ poor technique.

KEY POINTS

❖ Plaque removal prevents gingivitis.
❖ Since periodontitis is usually preceded by gingivitis, the removal of supragingival plaque is important in controlling the development of subgingival plaque and periodontitis.
❖ The main goal of prevention is to achieve the lowest plaque level possible.
❖ Plaque-control measures by the patient and professional maintenance appointments are both important in maintaining gingival health and are essential parts of primary and secondary prevention of periodontitis.
❖ Dental floss is indicated for interproximal plaque removal in Type I gingival embrasures.
❖ There is no difference in efficacy of plaque removal with waxed or unwaxed dental floss.

REFERENCES

Addy, M., and P. Adriaens. 1998. Epidemiology and etiology of periodontal diseases and the role of plaque control in dental caries: Consensus report of group A. In *Proceedings of the European Workshop on Mechanical Plaque Control,* ed. N. P. Lang, R. Attström, and H. Löe, 99–101. Chicago: Quintessence Books.

American Academy of Periodontology. 1995. Position paper: The role of supra- and subgingival irrigation: I. The treatment of periodontal diseases. Chicago: Committee on Research, Science and Therapy.

Bader, H. J. 1992. Review of currently available battery operated toothbrushes. *Compend. Contin. Educ. Dent.* 13:1163–1169.

Baker, K. 1995. The role of dental professionals and the patient in plaque control. *Periodontology 2000* 8:108–113.

Beaumont, R. H. 1990. Patient preference for waxed or unwaxed dental floss. *J. Periodontol.* 61:123–125.

Björn, A. L., U. Andersson, and A. Olsson. 1981. Gingival recession in 15-year-old pupils. *Swed. Dent. J.* 5:141–146.

Braun, R., and S. Ciancio. 1992. Subgingival delivery by an oral irrigation device. *J. Periodontol.* 63:469–472.

Cancro, L. P., and S. L. Fischman. 1995. The expected effect on oral health of dental plaque control through mechanical removal. *Periodontology 2000* 8:60–74.

Chaves, E. S., K. S. Kornman, M. A. Manwell, A. A. Jones, D. A. Newbold, and R. C. Wood. 1994. Mechanism of irrigation effects on gingivitis. *J. Periodontol.* 65:1016–1021.

Ciancio, S. G. 1990. Powered oral irrigation and control of gingivitis. *Biol. Ther. Dent.* 5:21–24.

Ciancio, S. G., O. Shilby, G. A. Farber. 1992. Clinical evaluation of the effect of two types of dental floss on plaque and gingival health. *Clin. Prevent. Dent.* 14:14–18.

Cobb, C. M., R. L. Rodgers, and W. J. Killoy. 1988. Ultrastructural examination of human periodontal pockets following the use of an oral irrigation device in vivo. *J. Periodontol.* 59:155–163.

Corbet, E. F., and W. I. R. Davies. 1993. The flow of supragingival plaque in the control of progressive periodontal disease: A review. *J. Clin. Peridontol.* 20:307–313.

Daly, C., G. Seymour, and J. Kieser. 1980. Bacterial endotoxin: A role in chronic inflammatory periodontal disease? *J. Oral Pathol.* 9:1–15.

Darby, M., and M. Walsh. 1994. *Dental hygiene theory and practice,* 37. Philadelphia: W. B. Saunders.

Dellerman, P. A., T. J. Hughes, and T. A. Burkett. 1994. A comparative evaluation of the percent acceptable end-round bristles in the Crest Complete, the Improved Crest Complete and the Oral-B Advantage toothbrushes. *J. Clin. Dent.* 5:74–81.

Drisko, C. H. 1996. Non-surgical pocket therapy: Pharmacotherapeutics. *Ann. Periodontol.* 1:491–566.

Eakle, W. S., C. Ford, and R. L. Boyd. 1986. Depth of penetration in periodontal pockets with oral irrigation. *J. Clin. Periodontol.* 13:39–44.

Felo, A., O. Shibly, S. G. Ciancio, F. R. Lauciello, and A. Ho. 1997. Effects of subgingival chlorhexidine irrigation on peri-implant maintenance. *Am. J. Dent.* 10:107–110.

Flemming, T. F., M. G. Newman, F. M. Doherty, E. Grossman, A. H. Mechkel, and M. B. Bakdash. 1990. Supragingival irrigation with 0.06% chlorhexidine in naturally occurring gingivitis: I. Six-month clinical observations. *J. Periodontol.* 61:112–117.

Flores-de-Jacoby, L., and R. Mengel. 1995. Conventional surgical procedures. *Periodontology 2000* 9:38–54.

Forgas-Brockmann, L. B., C. Carter-Hanson, and W. J. Killoy. 1998. The effects of an ultrasonic toothbrush on plaque accumulation and gingival inflammation. *J. Clin. Periodontol.* 25:375–379.

Frandsen, A. 1986. Mechanical oral hygiene practices. In *Dental plaque control measures and oral hygiene practices,* ed. H. Löe and D. V. Kleinman, 93–116. Oxford, England: IRL Press.

Garmyn, P., D. van Steenberghe, and M. Quirynen. 1998. Efficacy of plaque control in the maintenance of gingival health: Plaque control in primary and secondary prevention. In *Proceedings of the European Workshop on Mechanical Plaque Control,* ed. N. P. Lang, R. Attström, and H. Löe, 107–120. Chicago: Quintessence Books.

Glavid, L., H. Christensen, E. Pedersen, H. Rosendahl, and R. Attström. 1985. Oral hygiene instruction in general dental practice by means of self-teaching manuals. *J. Clin. Periodontol.* 12:27–34.

Gordon, J. M., J. A. Frascella, and R. C. Reardon. 1996. A clinical study of the safety and efficacy of a novel electric interdental cleaning device. *J. Clin. Dent.* 7:70–73.

Grossman, E., M. Cronin, W. Dembling, and H. Proskin. 1996. A comparative study of extrinsic tooth stain removal with two electric toothbrushes and a manual brush. *Am. J. Dent.* 9:25–29.

Hancock, E. B. 1996. Prevention. *Ann. Periodontol.* 1:223–249.

Hellstadius, K., B. Asman, and A. Gustafsson. 1993. Improved maintenance of plaque control by electric tooth brushing in periodontitis patients with low compliance. *J. Clin. Periodontol.* 20:235–237.

Hellström, M. K., P. Ramberg, L. Krok, and J. Lindhe. 1996. The effect of supragingival plaque control on the microflora in human periodontitis. *J. Clin. Periodontol.* 23:934–940.

Hill, H. C., P. A. Levi, and I. Glickman. 1973. The effects of waxed and unwaxed dental floss on interdental plaque accumulation and interdental gingival health. *J. Periodontol.* 53:411–414.

Jepsen, S. 1998. The role of manual toothbrushes in effective plaque control: Advantages and limitations. In *Proceedings of the European Workshop on Mechanical Plaque Control,* ed. N. P. Lang, R. Attström, and H. Löe, 121–137. Chicago: Quintessence Books.

Lainson, P. A., J. Bergquist, and C. M. Fraleigh. 1970. Clinical evaluation of Pulsar, a new pulsating water pressure cleansing device. *J. Periodontol.* 41:401.

Lefkoff, M. H., F. M. Beck, and J. E. Horton. 1995. The effectiveness of a disposable tooth cleansing device on plaque. *J. Periodontol.* 66:218–221.

Lobene, R. R. 1969. The effect of a pulsed water pressure cleansing device on oral health. *J. Periodontol.* 40:51–54.

Lobene, R. R., and P. M. Soparkar. 1970. The effect of a pulsating water pressure device on gingivitis, plaque and calculus. In Program and Abstracts of the 48th General Meeting International Association for Dental Research, March 1970.

Moran, J. M., and M. Addy. 1995. A comparative study of stain removal with two electric toothbrushes and a manual brush. *J. Clin. Dent.* 6:188–193.

Newman, M., M. Cattabriga, D. Etienne, et al. 1994. Effectiveness of adjunctive irrigation in early periodontitis: Multicenter evaluation. *J. Periodontol.* 65:224–229.

O'Beirne, G. O., R. H. Johnson, G. Rutger Persson, and M. D. Spektor. 1996. Efficacy of a sonic toothbrush on inflammation and probing depth in adult periodontitis. *J. Periodontol.* 67:900–908.

Palcanis, K. G. 1996. Surgical pocket therapy. *Ann. Periodontol.* 1:589–617.

Pitcher, G. R., H. N. Newman, and J. D. Strahan. 1980. Access to subgingival plaque by disclosing agents using mouthrinsing and direct irrigation. *J. Clin. Periodontol.* 7:300–308.

Preber, H., V. Ylipaa, J. Bergström, and H. Ryden. 1991. A comparative study of plaque removing efficiency using rotary electric and manual toothbrushes. *Swed. Dent. J.* 15:229–234.

Ramfjord, S. P. 1987. Maintenance care for treated patients. *J. Clin. Periodontol.* 14:433–437.

Rounds, M. C., and T. S. I. Tilliss. 1999. Personal oral hygiene: Auxiliary measures to complement toothbrushing. In *Primary preventive dentistry,* ed. N. O. Harris, and F. Garcia-Godoy, 125–154. Norwalk, CT: Appleton & Lange.

Sangnes, G. 1976. Traumatization of teeth and gingiva related to habitual tooth cleaning procedures. *J. Clin. Periodontol.* 3:94–103.

Sanz, M., and D. Herrera. 1998. Role of oral hygiene during the healing phase of periodontal therapy. In *Proceedings of the European Workshop on Mechanical Plaque Control,* ed. N. P. Lang, R. Attström, and H. Löe, 248–267. Chicago: Quintessence Books.

Saxer, U. P., and S. L. Yankell. 1997. Impact of improved toothbrushes on dental diseases: II. *Quintessence Int.* 28:573–593.

Van der Weijden, G. A., M. M. Danser, A. Nijboer, M. F. Timmerman, and U. Van der Velden. 1993. The plaque-removing efficacy of an oscillating/rotation toothbrush: A short-term study. *J. Clin. Periodontol.* 20:273–278.

Van Dyke, T., S. Offenbacher, B. Pihlstrom, M. Putt, and C. Trummel. 1999. What is gingivitis? Current understanding of prevention, treatment, measurement, pathogenesis and relation to periodontitis. *J. Int. Acad. Periodontol.* 1:3–10.

Waerhaug, J. 1981. Healing of the dentoepithelial junction following the use of dental floss. *J. Clin. Periodontol.* 8:144–150.

Westfelt, E. 1996. Rationale of mechanical plaque control. *J. Clin. Periodontol.* 23:263–267.

Yankell, S. L., and U. P. Saxer. 1999. Toothbrushing and toothbrushing techniques. In *Primary preventive dentistry*, ed. N. O. Harris, and F. Garcia-Godoy, Norwalk, CT: Appleton & Lange. 77–102.

Yukna, R. A., and R. L. Shaklee. 1993. Evaluation of a counterrotational powered brush in patients in supportive periodontal therapy. *J. Periodontol.* 64:859–864.

SELF-QUIZ

1. Which one of the following statements describes the rationale for periodontal oral hygiene self-care? (p. 308)

   a. reduction in the risk for development of dental caries

   b. augmentation of the immune reaction to a bacterial insult

   c. elimination or suppression of harmful microorganisms found in supragingival plaque biofilms

   d. disruption of the number of subgingival microbial flora with a delay in the repopulation of pathogens

2. Which one of the following oral hygiene regimens is *best* for a patient after periodontal surgery? (p. 329)

   a. Resume regular brushing and flossing regimens.

   b. Use a soft toothbrush and an antimicrobial mouthrinse.

   c. Use powered toothbrush and floss.

   d. Use oral irrigation with chlorhexidine.

3. A patient says that he is doing the best he can with his home care, but he still has moderate to heavy supragingival deposits. Which one of the following advice should the dental hygienist give to this patient? (p. 310)

   a. Not to worry because everyone gets some accumulations.

   b. Use an antimicrobial mouthrinse.

   c. Improve or change method of home care.

   d. Refer to a specialist.

4. Waxed dental floss has proven to be more effective in interdental cleaning than unwaxed dental floss *because* it is easier for the patient to handle. (p. 320)

   a. Both the statement and the reason are correct and related.

   b. Both the statement and the reason are correct but *not* related.

   c. The statement is correct, but the reason is *not*.

   d. The statement is *not* correct, but the reason is correct.

   e. *Neither* the statement *nor* the reason is correct.

5. Various toothbrushing methods are described in the literature *because* some methods are superior in removing plaque than others. (pp. 312–314)

    a. Both the statement and the reason are correct and related.
    b. Both the statement and the reason are correct but *not* related.
    c. The statement is correct, but the reason is *not*.
    d. The statement is *not* correct, but the reason is correct.
    e. *Neither* the statement *nor* the reason is correct.

6. All the following factors need to be considered when recommending interdental cleansing devices *except* one. Which one is the exception? (pp. 317–318)

    a. amount of plaque
    b. manual dexterity
    c. prescence of a bridge
    d. type of gingival embrasure

7. Which one of the following methods *best* evaluates for effectiveness of a patient's oral hygiene? (p. 309)

    a. show and tell
    b. feedback
    c. disclosing agents
    d. self-documentation

8. Which one of the following oral hygiene aids is *best* to remove dental plaque on the proximal surface of a tooth that has a Type I gingival embrasure? (p. 319)

    a. toothbrush
    b. interdental brush
    c. rubber-tip stimulator
    d. wooden wedge
    e. dental floss

9. Which one of the following steps should be done *first* when treating a patient for dentinal hypersensitivity? (p. 331)

    a. Recommend a desensitizing dentifrice for 4 to 6 weeks.
    b. Instruct the patient on the proper toothbrushing method.
    c. Identify the tooth that is painful.
    d. Apply sodium fluoride.

10. Which one of the following types of dental plaque is the primary target for oral irrigation? (p. 326)

    a. subgingival unattached
    b. subgingival attached
    c. tooth associated
    d. tissue associated

PERIODONTAL PHARMACOLOGY 11

Mea A. Weinberg, D.M.D., M.S.D., R.Ph.
Ulana K. Cirincione, R.D.H., M.S.

Outline:

Selected Drug Information Resources
Rationale for Use of Chemical Agents
Delivery Systems
Dental Plaque as a Biofilm
Drug Actions
Topical Delivery Systems
Antiplaque/Antigingivitis Agents
Systemic Drug Delivery
Controlled-Release Drug Delivery
Antibiotic Resistance
Enzyme-Suppression Therapy
Summary
Key Points
References
Self-Quiz

Goal:

To provide the dental hygienist with current concepts about the adjunctive use of chemical agents in the prevention and treatment of the inflammatory periodontal diseases.

Educational Objectives:

Upon completion of this chapter, the reader should be able to:

Discuss the rationale for the use of chemical agents in the treatment of the inflammatory periodontal diseases;

List and discuss the various types of drug delivery systems;

Describe the newest types of controlled-release devices; and

Discuss enzyme suppression therapy.

KEY WORDS

- chemotherapeutic agents
- periodontal pathogens
- antibiotic resistance
- topical drug devices
- controlled-release drug devices
- systemic drug delivery
- biofilm
- substantivity

*P*eriodontal therapy can be divided into three types of treatment:

- *Mechanical therapy.* This deals with the removal of plaque through mechanical (periodontal) debridement and toothbrushing and flossing.
- *Chemical therapy.* This is the administration of chemical agents to aid in the removal/suppression of the bacterial load.
- *Enzyme suppression therapy.* The newest approach to the treatment of inflammatory periodontal diseases, this deals with inhibiting the enzyme collagenase which causes destruction of collagen, rather than focusing on bacterial reduction.

SELECTED DRUG INFORMATION RESOURCES

It is important for the dental hygienist to be aware of the generic names and trade names of drugs. The *generic name* is the official name of the drug as determined by the United States Adopted Names Council. The *trade name* of a drug is the registered property of a specific manufacturer and is protected for 17 years so that the manufacturer has the exclusive rights for that specific drug.

Numerous drug reference books are available. Selected resources include the following:

- *The Physicians' Desk Reference* (PDR®) (Medical Economics Company, Inc., Montvale, NJ). This is published once a year and is essentially a conglomerate of the patient package inserts that the manufacturers supply for each drug.
- *Delmar's Dental Drug Reference* (Delmar Thompson™ Learning, Albany, NY).
- *Mosby's Dental Drug Reference* (Mosby-Year Book, Inc., St. Louis, MO).
- *Drug Information Handbook for Dentistry* (Lexi-Comp, Inc., Hudson, OH).
- *ADA Guide to Dental Therapeutics* (ADA, Chicago, IL).

RATIONALE FOR USE OF CHEMICAL AGENTS

Although periodontal debridement and periodontal surgery are currently and will always be the foundation for controlling inflammatory periodontal diseases, several factors can substantiate the adjunctive use of chemical or **chemotherapeutic agents** (e.g., antiseptic mouthrinses and antibiotics). An *antiseptic* is a substance that prevents or inhibits the growth of microorganisms or kills microbes on contact. An *antibiotic* is a substance that is synthesized by microorgansims that prevents or inhibits the growth of bacteria by either stopping multiplication or killing the bacteria.

Instrumentation often leaves behind significant numbers of **periodontal pathogens** (Waerhaug 1978). Repopulation of these pathogens can occur within 60 days of periodontal debridement (Sbordone et al. 1990). In addition, certain periodontal pathogens such as *Actinobacillus actinomycetemcomitans* and *Por-*

phyromonas gingivalis invade the gingival epithelium and connective tissue and elude removal by periodontal debridement (Renvert et al. 1990; de Graaf, van Winkelhoff, and Goené 1989). Other periodontal pathogens, such as *Bacteroides forsythus, Prevotella intermedia,* and *Peptostreptococcus micros,* live in nonperiodontal sites such as the tongue, tonsils, saliva, and buccal mucosa (Asikainen, Alaluusua, and Saxén 1991). These sites are a source for reinfection and must be considered in the overall treatment process. Other factors influencing the use of chemical plaque-control agents include the manual dexterity of the patient.

A number of chemical agents have been studied clinically and shown to be successful in the further suppression of dental plaque in certain types of periodontal diseases when used in conjunction with periodontal debridement and surgery. The role of antimicrobial agents as part of the periodontal treatment plan in certain patients has gained significant importance in recent years since the acknowledgment that periodontal diseases are infectious diseases with specific bacteria as the cause (Loesche 1976). Based on the specific plaque hypothesis, treatment is geared toward the elimination or reduction of specific bacteria (e.g., *A. actinomycetemcomitans, P. gingivalis, P. intermedia,* and spirochetes). Thus antimicrobial agents can be instituted as a supplement, not a replacement, during nonsurgical and surgical therapy. Since there are also beneficial bacteria living in the mouth, it is not desirable nor a goal to eliminate all intraoral bacteria. Unfortunately, systemic antibiotics used indiscriminately can result in **antibiotic resistance,** in which an antibiotic is ineffective against certain bacteria. This is becoming a worldwide problem.

DELIVERY SYSTEMS

Currently, two systems are available for the delivery of chemotherapeutic agents: local and systemic systems. **Topical** and **controlled-release drug devices** are local delivery systems. Each delivery system has advantages and limitations (Table 11–1 ■).

Topical application delivers the agent or drug to an exposed surface such as the teeth and gingiva. The most common route for the supragingival topical delivery of antimicrobial agents is by a mouthrinse, a dentifrice, or an oral irrigator. Subgingival topical delivery of antimicrobial agents is by oral irrigation or the use of controlled-release devices.

Controlled-release delivery devices are placed directly into the periodontal pocket and are designed to release a drug slowly over 24 hours for prolonged drug action. Antimicrobials are delivered into the periodontal pocket by fibers, gels, chips, ointments, acrylic strips, or collagen films.

Systemic drug delivery involves taking a tablet or a capsule orally with subsequent distribution of the agent through the circulation to the subgingival pocket area.

Choice of the delivery system is based on the target site. For instance, if gingivitis were being treated, oral rinses or irrigation would be chosen for supragingival plaque control. If, on the other hand, a certain type of periodontitis is being treated, the target site is the base of the periodontal pocket. Since oral rinses do not reach subgingivally, the delivery system of choice would be either oral irrigation or systemic or controlled-release delivery.

TABLE 11–1

MAIN FEATURES OF DRUG DELIVERY SYSTEMS

DELIVERY SYSTEM	TARGET SITE	ADEQUATE CONCENTRATION AT TARGET SITE	STAYS AT TARGET SITE LONG ENOUGH	REACHES THE GCF	ADVANTAGES
Systemic: tablets, capsules	Periodontal pocket; epithelium and connective tissue; nonperiodontal sites (e.g., saliva, tongue, buccal mucosa, tonsils)	Fair concentrations reached due to some dilution by the time it reaches pocket area; frequent dosing is necessary to maintain therapeutic levels	No	Yes	Reaches all intraoral sites where bacterial reservoirs are found
Topical: oral rinses	Supragingival	Adequate concentrations, but therapeutic level dramatically declines by being washed out by saliva	No	No	No systemic adverse side effects; no antibiotic resistance develops
Topical: dentifrices	Supragingival	Adequate concentrations, but therapeutic level dramatically declines by being washed out by saliva	No	No	No systemic adverse effects; high patient compliance
Topical: subgingival irrigation	Periodontal pocket	Adequate concentrations, but therapeutic level dramatically declines by being washed out by GCF	No	No	No systemic adverse side effects
Controlled-release: fibers, gel, chips	Periodontal pocket	Adequate concentrations; therapeutic levels are relatively constant for several days	Yes	Yes	Maintains therapeutic levels in the GCF for several days; no systemic adverse side effects; concentrates in pocket without dilution through entire body; possible development of bacterial resistance to the antibiotic (more studies needed)

DENTAL PLAQUE AS A BIOFILM

As mentioned earlier, dental plaque exists as a **biofilm.** A plaque *biofilm* is defined as "matrix-enclosed bacterial populations adherent to each other and/or to surfaces or interfaces" (Costerton et al. 1994). Plaque biofilms are of varying thicknesses, and in order to penetrate the biofilm, antibiotic concentrations must be several times greater than that needed to kill bacteria in a test tube (laboratory conditions)(Kleinfelder, Müller, and Lange 1999). Subgingival biofilms cannot be removed by toothbrushing, flossing, or the use of antimicrobial agents. It is necessary to physically remove the biofilm by instrumentation, and then the antimicrobial agent can be administered. For this reason, administration of antimicrobial agents should never be the sole treatment and always should be as an adjunct to periodontal debridement and/or periodontal surgery. The biofilm structure also may account for the rapid rebound or repopulation of the pathogenic flora, which occurs frequently after the use of antimicrobial agents (Page et al. 1997).

DRUG ACTIONS

When considering the use of chemotherapeutic agents, the dental hygienist should be aware of the pharmacokinetics and pharmacodynamics of the drug. Pharmacokinetics involves knowledge of the drug's absorption, distribution, metabolism, and excretion. Pharmacodynamics relates to the drug's mechanism of action. In addition, any adverse side effects and drug-food interactions should be noted, and the patient should be informed.

TOPICAL DELIVERY SYSTEMS

Topically applied antimicrobial agents have been developed based on a need for treatment of gingival bleeding and inflammation in association with gingivitis. Mouthrinsing and oral irrigation are two approaches used for supragingival application of antiseptic solutions. Oral rinses are the most common form of topical delivery. Oral rinses are ideal vehicles for the delivery of topical antimicrobials because of their relative simplicity of formulation and ease of use for patients.

MOUTHRINSES

Mouthrinses generally are divided into two classifications: *therapeutic rinses,* used to treat diseases such as gingival diseases, and *cosmetic rinses,* used to freshen the breath. Indications for using oral rinses are as follows:

1. as an addition to home care regimens that have failed to achieve plaque-control goals by other means;
2. as an addition to periodontal instrumentation;
3. where oral hygiene may be inadequate or difficult to accomplish for many people, as in the physically or mentally compromised;

4. following surgical procedures, when brushing and flossing are generally not practical;
5. as a preprocedural rinse, to reduce aerosolized bacteria in the dental office (when masked, the clinician is protected; however, after the mask is removed, aerosols remain in the dental operatory);
6. as a preprocedural rinse, to reduce the incidence of bacteremia (bacteria in the bloodstream); and
7. for maintenance of dental implants.

Topical antimicrobial agents delivered by a rinse are effective only against supragingival bacteria. *No antimicrobial rinse has been shown to be effective against periodontitis because oral rinses do not reach the subgingival area.* Mouthrinses may be discontinued if oral health conditions can be maintained without their use.

Halitosis, or breath malodor (bad breath), is caused by the production of volatile sulfur compounds, primarily methylmercaptan and hydrogen sulfide, in the mouth. A thorough medical history is necessary to rule out a systemic disease as the cause. Oral risk factors include periodontal disease, inadequate oral hygiene, xerostomia, tongue coatings, oral cancer, gingivitis, periodontitis, and mouth infections. Nonoral risk factors include aging, alcohol and/or tobacco use, the consumption of strong foods (e.g., onions or garlic), and upper respiratory and gastrointestinal problems (Page 1997). Treatment to eliminate halitosis depends on its cause(s). Hiding the mouth odor by using mouthrinses is not recommended. In patients in whom oral factors are involved, dental care is indicated. In patients in whom nonoral or medical factors are suspected, referral to a physician is required.

ORAL IRRIGATION

An alternate route of topical drug delivery is through patient or professionally applied oral irrigation. As discussed in Chapter 10, home irrigation is an effective way to deliver an agent subgingivally. This is generally done on a daily basis by the patient using a recommended powered device. Home irrigation has been proven to reach farther into the pocket than rinsing (Braun and Ciancio 1992; Eakle, Ford, and Boyd 1986; Flotra et al. 1972; Mashimo et al. 1980). The addition of an antimicrobial agent has reduced clinical parameters in some studies. Fleming et al. (1990) demonstrated an enhanced effect on reducing gingivitis when a 0.06% solution of chlorhexidine was used as the irrigant compared with rinsing and water irrigation. Conversely, the addition of Listerine® (Warner-Lambert, Morris Plains, NJ) as an irrigant was as effective as placebo in reducing gingivitis and improving gingival health (Ciancio et al. 1989). However, the addition of Listerine® resulted in greater reductions in plaque and gingival bleeding and a moderate decrease in total bacteria counts, although it was not statistically significant. Subgingival irrigation with chlorhexidine has been shown to decrease subgingival microflora and inflammation around implants (Lavigne et al. 1994).

Target site of irrigation

The target of irrigation is the subgingival microflora, regardless of where the tip of the device is placed. It is a misconception that if the tip is placed at the gingival margin, it is only effective on supragingival plaque; it is effective against both supragingival and subgingival bacteria. Cobb, Rodgers, and Killoy (1988) found that supragingival irrigation had an effect on subgingival microorganisms at probing depths of up to 6 mm. Irrigation attempts to reduce the potential of developing gingivitis or decreases existing gingivitis and directly reduces pocket microflora in an attempt to control or prevent the initiation of periodontitis.

In-office irrigation

An antimicrobial agent also can be applied professionally in-office. This can be accomplished by using an air- or powered-driven device (e.g., Perio Pik™ Subgingival Irrigation Handpiece, Teledyne Water Pik®, Fort Collins, CO; Fig. 11–1 ■), ultrasonic unit (piezoelectric) scaler (Piezon Master 400, EMS, Richardson, TX; Fig. 11–2 ■), or handheld syringe. Caution must be taken when using a handheld syringe because the delivery pressure cannot be controlled and may exceed a safe pressure for delivery into a periodontal pocket. Control is also compromised because of the inability to fulcrum and may affect the delivery to the apical aspect of the pocket. Penetration of an irrigant with an ultrasonic unit may be limited due to little lateral dispersion of agents and inaccessibility of the tip to certain areas (Nosel et al. 1991).

At present, a single episode of in-office irrigation has been shown only to have limited or no beneficial effects by itself, but it may be of some advantage if patients perform subgingival irrigation at home between continuing-care appointments (Jolkovsky et al. 1990). Repeated irrigations over a period of time or longer exposure to an antibiotic has shown efficacy in some patients (Christersson, Norderyd, and Puchalsky 1993; Clark et al. 1989). The use of 2% chlorhexidine alone over a 15-week period was nearly as effective in reducing clinical parameters as periodontal debridement alone (Southard et al. 1989).

Many different chemical agents have been used as irrigants (Table 11–2 ■). Owing to differences in protocol, type of agent used, concentrations, and levels of disease, oral irrigation is inconclusive in terms of efficacy, and research is ongoing.

TABLE 11–2

CHEMICAL AGENTS USED AS IRRIGANTS

- Water
- Chlorhexidine
- Povidone-iodine
- Essential oils
- Hydrogen peroxide
- Fluoride
- Tetracycline

FIGURE 11–1

Perio Pik™ (Teledyne Water Pik™, Fort Collins, CO) subgingival irrigation handpiece for in-office subgingival irrigation fits into a standard handpiece holder. (Courtesy Teledyne Water Pik®, Fort Collins, CO.)

Ultrasonic scaler (Piezon Master 400, EMS, Richardson, TX) for professional in-office subgingival irrigation of solutions during ultrasonic scaling. There is a built-in reservoir for the irrigant.

ANTIPLAQUE/ANTIGINGIVITIS AGENTS

Antimicrobial agents ideally should inhibit microbial colonization on tooth surfaces and prevent the subsequent formation of plaque. They also should eliminate or suppress the pathogenicity of existing plaque. Antiseptics have a greater potential to prevent the formation of plaque than to resolve established plaque and gingivitis.

An antimicrobial agent relies on two factors for efficacy. Success depends on the amount of time the agent stays in contact with the target site and how well the agent gains access to the target site. A major requirement for the success of antimicrobial therapy is **substantivity,** which is the ability of the drug to adsorb or bind to intraoral surfaces such as teeth and soft tissues with subsequent release of the drug in its active form (Stabholz et al. 1993). Substantivity involves the ability of the drug to stay at the target site for longer periods of time, thus maintaining therapeutic levels. It is ideal to have a drug with high substantivity that will be bound in the oral cavity and released over a period of hours in order to prolong the effects. Lack of substantivity can be overcome by more frequent use of the agent, but this would likely result in noncompliance and undesirable side effects.

CLASSIFICATION OF ORAL RINSES

Topical antimicrobial oral rinses can be classified as either first- or second-generation agents. First-generation agents have antibacterial properties with low substantivity and limited therapeutic value in reducing plaque and gingivitis. Examples include phenolic compounds, quaternary ammonium compounds, peroxide, and sanguinarine. Second-generation agents have antibacterial properties in addition to substantivity. Chlorhexidine gluconate is an example of a second-generation agent and is currently the only second-generation agent proven to prevent and control gingivitis. It is available in the United States only by a prescription. All first-generation mouthrinses are available over the counter (OTC) without a prescription.

In 1986, the American Dental Association (ADA) established guidelines for evaluation of the therapeutic effectiveness of products against gingivitis. For example, studies should be conducted over a minimum of 6 months, two studies with independent investigators should be conducted, and the active product should be used as part of a normal regimen and compared with a placebo or control product.

Most mouthrinses contain alcohol as a flavor enhancer and as a vehicle for the active ingredients. There has been some concern about the association of alcohol in mouthrinses with oral cancer. Various studies have shown inconsistent findings. Some studies document that there is no reason for patients to refrain from use of alcohol-containing mouthrinses (Ciancio 1993), while research from the National Cancer Institute has drawn an association between alcoholic mouthrinse to mouth and throat cancers (Winn, Blot, McLaughlin et al. 1991).

Bisbiguanides

Description and Mechanism of Action Chlorhexidine gluconate (Peridex®, Zila Pharmaceuticals, Cincinnati, OH; PerioGard®, Colgate Oral Pharmaceuticals, Canton, MA) is a cationic (positively charged) molecule. Originally, chlorhexidine was used in medicine as an antiseptic cream for wounds, as a preoperative skin cleanser, and as a surgical scrub. In 1970, the first study on the ability of chlorhexidine to inhibit the formation of plaque and maintain soft tissue health was released (Löe and Schiott 1970). It was not until 1986 that chlorhexidine became available in the United States by prescription at a 0.12% concentration with an alcohol concentration of 11.6%. It has the ADA seal of acceptance for the treatment of gingivitis.

After rinsing, chlorhexidine (positively charged) is attracted to and attaches onto the negatively charged bacterial cell walls, causing lysis or breakage of the cell wall and the contents of the cells leak out. Chlorhexidine enters the cell through the opening, resulting in death of the bacteria. By binding to the pellicle on the tooth surface, chlorhexidine inhibits plaque attachment. Chlorhexidine exhibits substantivity, with approximately 30% of the drug binding to oral tissues and the plaque on the teeth (Rölla, Löe, and Schiott 1971) and showing antimicrobial activity for 8 to 12 hours afterwards (Addy and Wright 1978; Schiott et al. 1970).

Indications Rinsing with chlorhexidine is indicated before, during, and after periodontal debridement to reduce plaque levels and gingival inflammation. Chlorhexidine rinses can improve wound healing and provide better plaque control after periodontal surgery when brushing and flossing is not feasible (Sanz et al. 1987). In the office, before using dental devices that produce an aerosol, such as power-assisted instruments or air polishing, it has been shown that a preoperative rinse with chlorhexidine markedly reduces contamination of the dental office (Warrall, Knibbs, and Glenwright 1987). Rinsing with chlorhexidine has been shown to decrease the severity of mucositis in patients receiving chemotherapy. Since peri-implantitis is similar to gingivitis, rinsing with chlorhexidine may be effective in implant plaque control.

Usage It is recommended to rinse twice a day for 30 seconds. The positive charge of chlorhexidine causes it to bind to the negatively charged molecules in toothpastes such as fluorides and sodium lauryl sulfate (a detergent) and thus inactivates them. Therefore, it is best to rinse either 30 minutes before or after toothbrushing or rinse very well with water after toothbrushing. Because of this inactivation by anionic compounds, chlorhexidine is not available in toothpaste form. Chlorhexidine can be used as an irrigant, but it is usually diluted with water to reduce the incidence of staining.

Adverse Side Effects Chlorhexidine is a relatively safe drug because it is poorly absorbed from the oral membranes and systemic circulation if swallowed. The most common adverse side effect is a yellow, brownish extrinsic staining of the teeth, tongue, and restorations within the first few days of use. Staining is more frequent with chlorhexidine than with other agents because of its affinity for oral surfaces. The staining may be associated with food dyes found within certain foods and beverages. This staining is not permanent and can be removed mechanically during professional prophylaxis. If the patient is compliant with oral home care, the staining is more likely on proximal tooth surfaces than facial or lingual surfaces. Other adverse side effects include a temporarily impaired taste perception and increased supragingival calculus formation.

Herbal extract: Sanguinarine

Sanguinarine is an extract of the bloodroot plant *Sanguinaria canadensis*. Viadent™ (Colgate Oral Pharmaceuticals, Canton, MA) contains sanguinarine and zinc chloride, which enhances the antiplaque effect. Its mechanism of action is the reduction of bacterial attachment to the cell wall. Numerous studies have been conducted and show mixed findings. Sanguinarine has moderate antiplaque and antigingivitis effects. Viadent is available as a mouthrinse with an alcohol concentration of 10% and as a dentifrice. When both are combined, more significant reductions in plaque and gingivitis are seen than using either one alone (Harper et al. 1990). Results may be due to the increased dose from the combination of the two formulations. There are no 6-month studies showing the efficacy of sanguinarine when the rinse and toothpaste are used separately. Adverse side effects from sanguinarine use are a burning sensation and slight staining of teeth.

Phenolic compounds

Listerine® (Warner-Lambert, Morris Plains, NJ) is a combination of phenolic compounds or essential oils, including thymol, eucalyptol, menthol, and methyl salicylate, in an alcohol vehicle. The mechanism of action is cell wall disruption, resulting in leakage of intracellular components and lysis of the cell. The original-formula Listerine contains 26.9% alcohol, whereas the Cool Mint and Fresh Burst Listerine contain 21.6% alcohol.

Because of low substantivity, effectiveness is strongly related to the duration of tooth contact. Clinical studies have shown it to significantly reduce plaque development in patients with minimal plaque levels (Gordon, Lamster, and Sieger 1985). A 6-month study comparing Listerine with a control product found that Listerine reduced plaque and gingivitis from 20 to 34%. The subjects had preexisting plaque and gingivitis, and no prophylaxis was performed at the beginning of the study (Lamster et al. 1983). In-office preprocedure rinsing with Listerine reduced the level of bacteria in the aerosol generated during ultrasonic scaling (Fine et al. 1992).

Recommendations are to rinse for 30 seconds with 2/3 oz once in the morning and once at night. Possible adverse side effects include a burning sensation and bitter taste.

Quaternary ammonium compounds

Quaternary ammonium compounds are positively charged (cationic) compounds similar to chlorhexidine, except that after rinsing they readily bind to oral surfaces and are released more rapidly or lose their activity on binding to the surface (Moran and Addy 1984). Substantivity is only approximately 3 hours (Roberts and Addy 1981). An increase in bacterial cell wall permeability leads to cell lysis and decreased attachment of bacteria to tooth surfaces. Cetylpyridinium chloride is the active ingredient in Scope® Original (Procter & Gamble, Cincinnati, OH) and Cepacol® (J. B. Williams, Glen Rock, NJ). The alcohol concentration is 14% for Cepacol and 18.9% for Scope Original.

Clinical data on plaque reduction and gingivitis control have been relatively inconclusive because of the variability in results between studies. Following an initial professional prophylaxis and suspension of all oral hygiene, chlorhexidine was found to be superior to cetylpyridinium in the reduction of plaque (Renton-Harper et al. 1996). Cetylpyridinium chloride may have some antiplaque action but less effect on gingivitis when used as an adjunct to conventional oral home care. Lack of substantivity limits clinical efficacy. As with chlorhexidine, to obtain the maximum effect, the patient should rinse very well or wait 30 minutes after brushing with a dentifrice before using the rinse. Adverse side effects are similar to those of chlorhexidine, including some staining, calculus formation, and mucosal ulceration.

The active ingredient in the newest formulation of Viadent™ is cetylpyridinium chloride (Viadent™ Oral Rinse Advanced Care, Colgate Oral Pharmaceuticals, Canton, MA). This product contains 0.05% cetylpyridinium chloride in a 6% alcohol base for the control of supragingival plaque and gingivitis.

Oxygenating agents

Oxygenating agents such as peroxides and perborates have been used in a mouthrinse formulations primarily for acute necrotizing ulcerative gingivitis and pericoronitis. Since hydrogen peroxide liberates gaseous oxygen, it provides a cleansing action and gentle effervescence for oral wounds. Its antimicrobial effect is directed at anaerobic microorganisms that cannot live in the presence of oxygen, and it has a physical effect on plaque through the bubbling of oxygen as it is released from the peroxide (Marshall, Cancro, and Fischman 1995). The Food and Drug Administration has approved its use as a temporary debriding agent in the oral cavity. However, antiplaque/antigingivitis claims are not well supported.

The safety of hydrogen peroxide has been disputed. Long-term use of 3% hydrogen peroxide has resulted in gingival irritation (Marshall, Cancro, and Fischman 1995; Rees and Orth 1986) and delayed tissue healing, and it may serve as a cocarcinogen in animals (Weitzman et al. 1986). A *cocarcinogen* is a compound that when administered with a low dose of a known carcinogen results in increased incidence of tumors. On the other hand, other studies found that adverse effects from exposure to 3% or less hydrogen peroxide were rare. It was concluded that exposure to less than 3% hydrogen peroxide was safe (Marshall, Cancro, and Fischman 1995). Long-term studies do not demonstrate any additional benefit over regular home care, however. Since many patients use hydrogen peroxide on a regular basis, the dental hygienist should question patients about their oral home-care practices.

Povidone-Iodine

Povidone-iodine is antibacterial and antiseptic. Its primary use is in the prevention and treatment of surface infections. Often povidone-iodine is combined with hydrogen peroxide as a subgingival irrigant for the reduction of gram-negative microorganisms. Most studies confirm that iodine may be a beneficial adjunctive treatment for the prevention and control of gingivitis when used with optimal oral hygiene self-care procedures (Clark et al. 1989). Iodine can stain teeth, clothing, skin, and restorations, however.

Fluorides

Fluorides have been used in dentistry primarily for dental caries prevention by reducing demineralization and enhancing remineralization. Fluoride rinses have not been proven clinically to prevent root caries (Paine, Slots, and Rich 1998). Its role as an antiplaque/antigingivitis agent is less well documented and shows controversial results.

Stannous fluoride (SnF_2) has been documented to exhibit antimicrobial properties in the control of gingival inflammation and bacterial repopulation. The tin molecule supposedly prevents bacterial adhesion to the tooth surface. Another indication for stannous fluoride is for dentinal hypersensitivity. Stannous fluoride is available as a dentifrice, a gel, and a concentrated oral rinse that is diluted with water. For home rinsing, available products include Gel-Kam® (available over the counter; Colgate Oral Pharmaceuticals, Canton, MA) and Stanimax™ (0.63% SnF_2). For in-office rinsing or irrigation, Stanimax-Pro™ (3.28% SnF_2; SDI Laboratories, Glenview IL) is available.

Extrinsic tooth staining occurs with extended use. Sodium fluoride is indicated for caries prevention and has not been documented to have any antiplaque/antigingivitis action.

Prebrushing rinses

A prebrushing rinse (Plax®, Pfizer, New York) that contains surfactants such as sodium lauryl sulfate (which functions as a detergent to help loosen and remove plaque), sodium benzoate (a preservative), and tetrasodium pyrophosphate (an anticalculus agent) is intended to be used before brushing. Studies have shown limited beneficial effects of this agent over rinsing with water alone (Grossman 1988).

Alcohol-free mouthrinses

Most mouthrinses contain alcohol as a vehicle to carry other ingredients and as a flavor enhancer. The form of alcohol in the rinse is either ethanol (ethyl alcohol) or a specially denatured (SD) alcohol that is made synthetically. Alcohol can cause drying of the oral mucosal tissues, especially when the agent is used for extended periods of time. Indications for a nonalcoholic mouthrinse include pregnant women, former alcoholics, patients who are taking medications that would additionally dry the mouth, patients taking metronidazole (an antibiotic), and patients who prefer to avoid alcohol. Table 11–3 ■ lists some nonalcoholic antimicrobial mouthrinses.

DENTIFRICES

A dentifrice is a toothpowder, toothpaste, or gel used in conjunction with a toothbrush to help remove plaque, materia alba, and stain from teeth. The word is derived from the Latin words *dens* ("teeth") and *fricare* ("to rub"). Although the mechanical action of brushing and flossing is the primary means of plaque removal, a dentifrice facilitates the oral hygiene process.

Currently, dentifrices are considered to be either cosmetic or therapeutic. Cosmetically, they function in cleaning and polishing teeth, removing extrinsic stains, and freshening the oral cavity. There is a continuing effort to obtain additional dental benefits from dentifrices through the inclusion of agents designed to have a therapeutic action. This includes caries reduction; control of gingivitis, plaque, and calculus formation; and reduction of dentinal hypersensitivity (Tables 11–4 ■ and 11–5 ■).

The main limitation of dentifrices as a therapeutic agent is the issue of patient compliance. Dental hygienists cannot control the frequency of use or amount or type of dentifrice used by a patient. Dentifrice selection is based most often on cosmetic qualities such as flavor, texture, appearance, and dispensability rather than on its therapeutic value. The public looks to dental professionals for specific recommendations. The dental hygienist must be up to date with product information and be able to recommend a dentifrice that will provide oral health benefits yet appeal to the patient for continued use. Dentifrices should be chemically stable, effective, and nontoxic (Cummins 1997). Products with the ADA seal of acceptance have sustained scrutiny and testing and can be safely recommended by dental hygienists.

TABLE 11–3
ALCOHOL-FREE ANTIMICROBIAL MOUTHRINSES

Rembrandt®, DenMat, Santa Maria, CA
Oral B® Plaque Rinse, Redwood City, CA
Listermint®, Warner-Lambert, Morris Plains, NJ
BreathRX®, Discus Dental, Culver City, CA

TABLE 11–4

DENTIFRICES WITH THERAPEUTIC BENEFITS (ADA SEAL OF ACCEPTANCE)

PRODUCT NAME	ACTIVE INGREDIENTS
Anticavity/antiplaque/antigingivitis	
Total™ Toothpaste (Colgate-Palmolive Co., New York, NY)	0.30% triclosan 0.24% sodium fluoride
Prevention of calculus	
Colgate® Tarter Control Gel (Colgate-Palmolive Co, New York, NY)	Tetrasodium pyrophosphate, 0.15% sodium fluoride
Colgate® Tartar Control Toothpaste (Colgate-Palmolive Co.)	Tetrasodium pyrophosphate, 0.15% sodium fluoride
Aquafresh® Tartar Control Toothpaste (SmithKline Beecham Consumer Brands, Pittsburgh, PA)	Tetrapotassium pyrophosphate, tetrasodium pyrophosphate, 0.221% sodium fluoride
Crest® Tartar Protection Fluoride Gel (Procter & Gamble, Cincinnati, OH)	Tetrapotassium pyrophosphate, disodium pyrophosphate, tetrasodium pyrophosphate, 0.15% sodium fluoride
Crest® Tartar Protection Fluoride Toothpaste (Procter & Gamble, Cincinnati, OH)	Tetrapotassium pyrophosphate, disodium pyrophosphate, tetrasodium pyrophosphate, 0.15% sodium fluoride

Source: Adapted from Mariotti, A. J. Mouthrinses and dentifrices. In *ADA Guide to Dental Therapeutics*, 1st ed., 210–212. Chicago: ADA Publishing Co.

TABLE 11–5

PATIENT-APPLIED DENTIFRICES FOR THE TREATMENT OF DENTINAL HYPERSENSITIVITY (ADA SEAL OF ACCEPTANCE)

ACTIVE INGREDIENT	PRODUCT NAME
5% potassium nitrate 0.15% sodium fluoride	• Crest Sensitivity Protection® (Procter & Gamble, Cincinnati, OH) • Protect Sensitive Teeth Gel® (John O. Butler Comp., Chicago, IL)
5% potassium nitrate sodium monoflurophosphate	Fresh Mint Sensodyne® Toothpaste (Block Drug, Jersey City, NJ)
0.4% stannous fluoride	Gel-Kam® Gel (Colgate Oral Pharmaceuticals, Canton, MA)

Dentifrice components

Dentifrices contain basic components along with an active ingredient for its intended use. The active agent provides the therapeutic benefit and can include fluoride for anticaries effect, potassium nitrate or strontium chloride for desensitization (reducing or eliminating dentin sensitivity), sodium pyrophosphate for calculus inhibition, or triclosan for plaque and gingivitis control. Recent formulations have incorporated a combination of these active ingredients for maximal patient benefits.

A typical dentifrice contains, besides water (15 to 50%), an abrasive (20 to 60%). Abrasives clean or polish tooth surfaces, allowing them to resist bacterial reaccumulation. The powders and pastes contain abrasives such as silicon oxides, chalk, hydrated aluminum oxide, and sodium bicarbonate. Generally speaking, commercial dentifrice powders are more abrasive than pastes. Abrasives usually do not damage the enamel, but they may dull tooth luster. Therefore, a polishing agent is incorporated into most dentifrices, forming an abrasive system (Fischman and Yankell 1999). Although abrasives can result in tooth wear, other factors such as brushing habits, including technique, pressure, direction, and frequency of brushing, and toothbrush bristle stiffness can influence the incidence of tooth abrasion. The more abrasive the dentifrice, the more likely it is to cause tooth wear in the cervical area. This area is more prone to abrasion because enamel is approximately 20 times harder than dentin or cementum (Fischman and Yankell 1999). There is no valid reason to use a dentifrice with a greater abrasiveness or polishing effect than necessary to prevent deposits, including stains on the teeth.

Humectants (20 to 40%) are a vehicle into which agents are incorporated to prevent hardening of the dentifrice when exposed to air. Common humectants are glycerin, sorbitol, mannitol, and polyethylene glycol. Surfactants (1 to 2%) act as detergents by contributing to the foaming action, lowering surface tension, and loosening deposits from the teeth. Sodium lauryl sulfate is the most commonly used detergent. Binders (1 to 2%; cellulose products, gums, alginates) prevent the separation of the solids and liquids in the dentifrice, maintain firmness and thickness, and ensure stability. Gels contain more binders to give the product a thicker quality. Flavoring and sweetening agents mask the poor-tasting ingredients and provide a pleasant flavor to the dentifrice. These include essential oils (peppermint, cinnamon, and wintergreen) and sodium saccharin. Colorants (1%) are dyes added to the dentifrice to enhance its attractiveness without staining or discoloring teeth or oral tissues or causing harm on ingestion.

Fluoride dentifrices

Dentifrices are the most widely used form of self-applied fluoride. Recommended for both children and adults, fluoride dentifrices can reduce caries by 20 to 30% when used twice daily on a regular basis. First introduced in the 1950s, fluoride dentifrices contained stannous fluoride as the anticaries agent. Current fluoride dentifrices contain sodium fluoride (0.24%) or sodium monofluorophosphate (0.76%). The anticaries efficacy of these two fluoride agents continues to be evaluated (Proskin and Volpe 1995). Although some analyses indicate that there is no statistically or clinically significant difference between the two fluoride agents (Volpe et al. 1995), it has been shown that the therapeutic benefit of fluoride depends on a dose-response relationship (Stephen 1994). Sodium fluoride dentifrices appear to be retained longer, however, when compared with dentifrices containing sodium monofluorophosphate (Shellis and Duckworth 1994) and thus may be more effective clinically (Duckworth et al. 1994).

Indications for fluoride gels include rampant caries, patients susceptible to caries, root caries, orthodontic appliances, dentinal hypersensitivity, and patients undergoing radiation therapy. Since over 95% of dentifrices contain fluoride and the benefits have been shown clinically for decades, issues of safety are of minor concern. Numerous studies have evaluated fluoride therapies for their impact on dental fluorosis (Stookey 1994). Dentifrices have been identified as a causative factor in the increased prevalence of mild enamel fluorosis. For this reason, young children must be monitored for inadvertent dentifrice ingestion.

The mechanism of fluoride's anticaries effect in root caries is not well understood. Fluoride gels may have a beneficial effect in the prevention of caries on exposed root surfaces. An example of a home-applied gel prescription product is

1.1% sodium fluoride (Prevident® 5000 Plus Gel, Colgate Oral Pharmaceuticals, Canton, MA; Neutracare®, Oral-B, Belmont, CA). These gels should be applied daily after home-care procedures. The gel is applied either by brushing it on the root surface for 1 minute or using a custom-made or disposable tray for 4 minutes (Low 1996).

Clinical studies report that the daily use of a fluoride paste reduces root surface caries by more than 65% (Jensen and Kohout 1988). More research is needed to truly confirm fluoride's role in the prevention of root caries. Therefore, fluoride dentifrices are recommended primarily for their antidental caries effects.

Stannous fluoride dentifrices

Initially, before the introduction of sodium fluoride and sodium monofluorophosphate, stannous fluoride was incorporated into dentifrices. Stannous fluoride (SnF_2) has made a comeback because of its effect on periodontal health. Stannous fluoride, in concentrations of greater than 0.3%, has been the most widely studied fluoride in controlling plaque and gingivitis. Clinical studies show mixed results, and stannous fluoride does not have the ADA seal of acceptance.

Used twice daily, a stannous fluoride dentifrice (Crest® Gum Care, 0.454% SnF_2, Procter & Gamble, Cincinnati, OH; Fig. 11–3 ■) has been reported to reduce gingivitis and gingival bleeding by 33.4 and 20.5% respectively (Perlich et al. 1995). On the other hand, when compared with a sodium fluoride dentifrice, stannous fluoride did not demonstrate significant effects on supragingival plaque (Beiswanger, Doyle, and Jackson 1995). Stannous fluoride dentifrices are substantive up to 5 hours when compared with comparable dentifrices without stannous fluoride (Elworthy et al. 1996).

Commonly reported adverse side effects include extrinsic tooth staining caused by the tin molecule and a metallic, bitter taste. Recent dentifrice formulations contain flavoring agents that mask the taste. Removal of stains caused by stannous fluoride is no more difficult than stain removal resulting from other product use (Beiswanger, Doyle, and Jackson 1995). Stannous fluoride is available as a brush-on gel, a mouthrinse, and a dentifrice.

FIGURE 11–3

The active ingredient in Crest Gum Care® (Procter & Gamble, Cincinnati, OH) is stannous fluoride. It has a broad-spectrum antimicrobial effect.

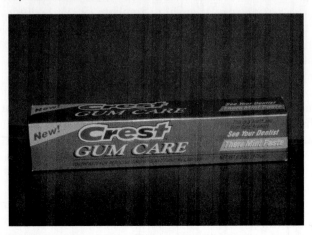

Triclosan-containing dentifrices

Triclosan is another type of therapeutic dentifrice. Triclosan is a phenolic compound with antiplaque/antigingivitis properties. It is a broad-spectrum antibacterial agent effective against Gram-positive and Gram-negative bacteria. Used as an antibacterial agent in soaps, deodorants, and cosmetics, triclosan recently has become available in the United States in a dentifrice formulation (Total™, Colgate Oral Pharmaceuticals, Canton, MA).

This product contains 0.3% triclosan and 2.0% polyvinylmethylether maleic acid (PVM/MA), which enhances its retention (substantivity) onto hard and soft oral surfaces and adds anticalculus properties (Ciancio 1997). Triclosan binds to plaque, resulting in a sustained impact on bacteria for over 12 hours after brushing (Volpe et al. 1996). Triclosan affects the quality of existing plaque (Lindhe et al. 1993) and plaque regrowth (Binney et al. 1996). When compared with other dentifrices, triclosan is as effective as stannous fluoride (Binney et al. 1997) and sodium fluoride dentifrices (Binney et al. 1995) in inhibiting plaque. In addition, this product is also claimed to prevent caries. No adverse side effects have been reported, and it is safe for oral use. Anionic agents, which are also present in most dentifrices, do not alter their antibacterial effectiveness. Triclosan has the ADA seal of acceptance.

Sodium bicarbonate/hydrogen peroxide dentifrices

Sodium bicarbonate (baking soda) has been used as a cleansing agent for many years and has been the primary abrasive agent in dentifrices (Fig. 11–4 ■). The therapeutic benefit of sodium bicarbonate dentifrices results from reduction of plaque and gingivitis and stain removal (Zambon, Mather, and Gonzales 1996; Koertge 1996). The mechanism of action is disruption of the bacterial cell membrane (Drake et al. 1995). Even though baking soda disintegrates quickly during brushing (so that its abrasive action is not sustained), it still removes stains (Koertge 1996). An additional benefit of baking soda dentifrices is their control of oral malodor (Brunette 1996).

FIGURE 11–4

Examples of dentifrices containing baking soda and peroxide. The low level of hydrogen peroxide does not seem to cause any adverse side effects. (Courtesy of Dr. Kirk Noraian, Northwestern University.)

Hydrogen peroxide is added to dentifrices for its antigingivitis properties. Some manufacturers claim that hydrogen peroxide–containing dentifrices were developed to whiten teeth by decolorizing stains. Others claim that hydrogen peroxide freshens the mouth because of its bubbling action. Consumers often view these agents as more "natural." The concept of combining sodium bicarbonate with hydrogen peroxide is based on the regimen supported by the Keyes technique. Most dentifrices contain a low level of hydrogen peroxide (<1%) that causes no harm to tissues (Marshall, Cancro, and Fischman 1995).

The Keyes technique has received much attention in the lay press for the treatment of periodontal disease without surgical intervention. The Keyes technique, originally developed by Dr. Paul Keyes in the late 1970s, is based on monitoring of the disease with phase-contrast microscopy and treatment. The first phase of treatment involves mechanical therapy, and this is followed by local antimicrobial therapy, in which the patient uses a toothpaste composed of 3% hydrogen peroxide, salt, and sodium bicarbonate. Oral irrigation at home and in the office is also done. In the last phase of treatment, patients are administered systemic antibiotics such as tetracycline. This type of treatment was found not to be any more effective than conventional periodontal therapy (Pihlstrom et al. 1987). In addition, oral ulcerations have been reported to result from short-term use of 3% hydrogen peroxide in combination with a salt solution (Levine 1987).

Research findings on the efficacy of these dentifrices are mixed. A 52% reduction in bleeding sites was found after a 3-month test (Fischman et al. 1992). Dentifrices containing hydrogen peroxide may decrease plaque and gingivitis, but mechanical access to submarginal sites is required for them to deliver a therapeutic effect (Marshall, Cancro, and Fischman 1995). When applied with a sulcular brush and an interproximal toothpick, sodium bicarbonate/hydrogen peroxide had no benefit in reducing the microbial flora in 4- to 7-mm pockets (Cerra and Killoy 1982). No antimicrobial benefits were exhibited when compared with conventional dentifrices (sodium fluoride, stannous fluoride) and mouthrinses (essential oils) (Bacca et al. 1997).

Given these mixed findings, dental hygienists should educate their patients about the limited benefits of these dentifrices. These products have the ADA seal of acceptance on the basis of their anticaries benefit, not antiplaque/antigingivitis claims.

Most home bleaching products contain as the active ingredient 0.75 to 10% hydrogen peroxide or 10 to 15% carbamide peroxide. Carbamide peroxide breaks down into hydrogen peroxide. Another component is urea, which helps in plaque removal. High levels (35%) of peroxide can penetrate the dentin and cause toxicity to the pulp. Broken down, leaky restorations near the cemento-enamel junction are major routes of entrance of peroxide (Marshall, Cancro, and Fischman 1995).

Tartar-control dentifrices

Calculus, although not a primary causative factor for periodontal disease, does play a role in dental plaque retention. Any attempt by patients to reduce calculus by home-care practices and preventive product use aids in improved oral health and cosmetic appearance. The introduction of soluble pyrophosphates into dentifrices provides a chemical means of reducing supragingival calculus formation. Calcium and phosphorous from saliva are prevented from incorporating into the plaque matrix to form calculus.

Pyrophosphates act as crystal growth inhibitors, especially large, organized crystals. This may delay mineralization of the plaque and make it more susceptible to mechanical removal. Once calculus has formed into an organized matrix, pyrophosphates are ineffective. Their effectiveness is limited to new supragingival calculus. For this reason, recommendations for use are appropriate after prophylaxis or scaling/root planing.

Many studies have evaluated the effectiveness of pyrophosphates on calculus formation (Gaengler, Kurbad, and Weinert 1993; Addy and Koltai 1994). Not only is there a reduction in new calculus formation, but also *the number of sites in the mouth that are calculus-free is increased* (Lobene 1989). Results after 3 and 6 months indicated significant reductions in supragingival deposits (Schiff 1987) by 35.5 and 45.9% respectively. Calculus inhibitors cause the newly formed deposits to be softer and easier for the clinician to remove. The amount of force and number of strokes by the dental hygienist are reduced (White et al. 1996). The addition of a copolymer (methoxyethylene and maleic acid) to a pyrophosphate dentifrice enhances the anticalculus effect (Singh et al. 1990).

Besides the effect on hard deposits, anticalculus dentifrices also may exhibit antimicrobial activity by killing or inhibiting bacterial growth (Drake, Grigsby, and Drotz-Dieleman 1994). Pyrophosphates have been found to reduce chlorhexidine-induced extrinsic stain (Bollmer et al. 1995).

True allergic reactions and mucosal (tissue) irritation are rare and most likely due to flavoring agents rather than the pyrophosphates. Tissue irritation has been reported in the form of tissue sloughing (peeling) and tooth surface sensitivity. Pyrophosphates in dentifrices also have been thought to interact with the fluoride compounds and interfere with the remineralization process. Fluoride uptake is not altered by pyrophosphates, however. The anticaries benefits are similar for regular-formula and tartar-control dentifrices. The ADA seal of acceptance has been given to tartar control dentifrices based on their anticaries properties. Because calculus inhibition is of cosmetic rather than therapeutic value, pyrophosphate dentifrices are not evaluated on the basis of their primary mode of action.

Desensitizing dentifrices

Gingival recession as a result of disease processes (inflammation and attachment loss), tooth malposition, faulty toothbrushing, or periodontal surgery can result in exposed dentin. This can result in hypersensitivity near the cervical area of the tooth. Usually, movement of fluid within the dentinal tubules causes discomfort in the exposed areas.

Treatment of dentin hypersensitivity focuses on blocking the opened dentinal tubules to prevent transmission of the noxious external stimuli and decreasing the intradental nerve excitability. Therapeutic products can be applied either professionally or by the patient. Most of the patient-applied OTC products must be used for a prolonged period of time for greatest effect. Since it takes many weeks for efficacy, manufacturers have added fluoride to the formula for its anticaries effect. It must be stressed to patients that optimal plaque control also will help to reduce the sensitivity.

Table 11–5 lists the more commonly used dentifrices for dentinal hypersensitivity. Potassium nitrate is effective in reducing cold and tactile sensitivity as compared with regular toothpaste (Silverman et al. 1996). Potassium nitrate acts quickly and directly on the pulpal nerves.

Other agents in dentifrices include dibasic sodium citrate and 0.4% stannous fluoride. Stinging and extrinsic staining may contribute to patient noncompliance with stannous fluoride. These dentifrices are ADA approved for the relief of dentin sensitivity. Since these products are dentifrices (pastes and gels), application is by means of a soft bristle toothbrush, brushing for at least 1 minute and making sure that all surfaces are brushed and then expectorating.

Strontium chloride is no longer used in dentifrices because fluoride could not be incorporated into the formulation. It used to be marketed as Sensodyne-SC® (Block Drug, Jersey City, NJ).

Minimal research has been done to evaluate the duration of the sensitivity decrease following cessation of use of desensitizing dentifrices. Some sensitivity may return within 6 to 12 weeks following use of such a dentifrice for 6 to 8 weeks.

Sanguinarine-containing dentifrice

Sanguinarine has been used in mouthrinses and now is also incorporated into a dentifrice. Long-term evaluations have been conducted on the effect of sanguinarine on plaque and gingivitis, and the benefits appear mixed. The antiplaque/antigingivitis effects have been reported to be greater with the combined use of the oral rinse and the dentifrice than with the oral rinse alone (Harper et al. 1990).

Zinc citrate–containing dentrifices

A new formulation called Viadent™ Advanced Care (Colgate Oral Pharmaceuticals, Canton, MA) has as its active ingredients 2% zinc citrate trihydrate, which is an antibacterial agent, and 0.8% sodium monofluorophosphate, which has anticaries properties. Sanguinarine is not in this new formulation.

Other dentifrice categories

Herbal-based and "natural" dentifrices are attractive alternatives to some patients interested in maintaining oral hygiene. Although these products have been documented to perhaps be as effective as conventional dentifrices in their ability to control plaque and gingivitis (Mullaby, James, Coulter et al. 1995), their efficacy remains questionable. As long as these "natural" toothpastes contain fluoride, patients receive anticaries benefit. Patients must be educated on the limitations of their choice of dentifrice. The primary benefit of some of these alternatives is motivational, in that patients may be encouraged to brush more regularly with their chosen dentifrice.

A relatively new toothpaste containing essential oils in its formulation relies on support of data from studies evaluating the antiseptic mouthrinse (Listerine®, Warner-Lambert, Morris Plains, NJ). Product acceptance is based on fluoride content, not on plaque and gingivitis benefits.

Dentifrices containing a lactoperoxidase system (Biotene®, Laclede Professional Products, Rancho Dominguez, CA) may be beneficial for special patient groups. Patients with xerostomia were relieved of their symptoms after a 4-week daily use of a lactoperoxidase dentifrice and mouthrinse (Kirstila et al. 1996).

SUMMARY

Antiseptics deserve continued evaluation, and their importance should not be underestimated. Currently, the most valuable application of antiplaque/antigingivitis agents is as an adjunct to conventional mechanical debridement and oral home care for short- to medium-term usage. Few advances in chemical plaque control have been achieved in recent years, except for the introduction of triclosan.

An important factor in the efficacy of any antiplaque/antigingivitis agent is an adequate contact time with the target site. Accordingly, the well-proven success of chlorhexidine is related to its substantivity more than to any unique action on the microflora (bacteria).

Fluorides have successfully decreased the rate of dental caries. Tartar-control dentifrices offer a cosmetic benefit. Desensitizing toothpastes may aid in the alleviation of dentinal hypersensitivity. Baking soda/hydrogen peroxide and sanguinaria dentifrices have not been shown to consistently elicit antiplaque/antigingivitis effects. Triclosan is the first chemical agent used in dentifrices that can claim benefits to periodontal health.

It is the function of the dental hygienist to advise patients on the role of oral rinses and dentifrices in the hygienic phase of treatment. The hygienist should use her or his knowledge of clinical studies to decide on the appropriate product for each patient.

SYSTEMIC DRUG DELIVERY

INDICATIONS

Systemic drug delivery through oral administration has several advantages and disadvantages (see Table 11–1). Antibiotics generally are unnecessary and inappropriate for reducing plaque levels and treating gingivitis, with the exception of necrotizing ulcerative gingivitis (NUG). Bacterial invasion (spirochetes) of periodontal tissues seen in NUG eludes mechanical removal with instruments.

Systemic antibiotics are useful as adjuncts in periodontal treatment for patients with aggressive periodontitis, refractory periodontitis, and immunodeficiency diseases. Patients with refractory periodontal diseases usually harbor persistent subgingival pathogens that are likely to be resistant to conventional treatment. In localized aggressive periodontitis patients, *A. actinomycetemcomitans* invades the gingival connective tissue and thus evades removal by mechanical instrumentation. Antibiotics will benefit patients with a periodontal abscess when there is accompanied systemic signs such as fever or lymphadenopathy.

SELECTION

Adjunctive systemic antibiotics may be used during initial and/or surgical therapy. It may be advantageous to perform microbiologic testing to determine the presence of specific bacteria to reduce the possibility of antibiotic resistance. Reevaluation with microbiologic testing 1 to 3 months after antimicrobial therapy may

TABLE 11–6
CLASSIFICATION OF SYSTEMIC ANTIBIOTICS USED IN PERIODONTICS

Tetracyclines
  Tetracycline HCl
  Doxycycline hyclate
  Minocycline HCl
Beta-lactam
  Penicillin VK
  Amoxicillin trihydrate
  Amoxicillin
  + clavulanic acid
Nitroimadazoles
  Metronidazole
Azalides (derivative of
  erythromycin)
  Azithromycin dihydrate
Lincomycins
  Clindamycin HCl
Fluoroquinolones
  Ciprofloxacin HCl

be done to verify elimination or suppression of the pathogens. However, the expense of this procedure may preclude its generalized use. Long-term use (1 to 2 months or longer) of systemic antibiotics is considered to be without foundation.

Proper selection and dosing of the appropriate antibiotic are necessary to avoid untoward reactions and antibiotic resistance. Many categories of antibiotics are available, and several are indicated in periodontal infections (Table 11–6■). The dental hygienist *must* be familiar with both the generic and brand or trade names of each drug. If the generic name of the drug is not listed in the PDR™, use another drug reference book. Not all drug names are found in the PDR. For example, Sumycin is a trade name for tetracycline HCl and is manufactured by a specific company.

Good oral hygiene is still mandatory and will favor a positive clinical response when patients are prescribed systemic antibiotics. As mentioned earlier, periodontal debridement must be performed before the administration of any antimicrobial agent. This will remove the biofilm that protects subgingival microorganisms, except in cases where the bacteria have invaded the soft tissue. Systemic antibiotics are given in certain situations and are always used as a supplement or adjunct to conventional periodontal debridement and oral hygiene self-care. Antibiotics should never be given as the only treatment regimen. Antibiotics are classified as being either bacteriostatic, which means they suppress the multiplication of the bacteria, or bactericidal, which means they kill the bacteria.

ADVERSE DRUG EVENTS

Heightened public interest in adverse drug events has motivated the government to require pharmaceutical companies to provide adverse drug reaction (ADR) information (Smith 1999). The requirement is to provide information on the percentage of adverse drug reactions caused by antibiotics in both hospital and nonhospital settings.

ADRs can range from mild reactions that disappear when the antibiotic is discontinued to severe reactions that are life-threatening, disabling, or result in hospitalization (Smith 1999). Table 11–7■ lists common adverse effects associated with antimicrobial agents.

SYSTEMIC ANTIBIOTICS

Tetracyclines

Tetracyclines as a group are bacteriostatic, inhibiting bacterial growth and multiplication by inhibiting protein synthesis. Two semisynthetic analogues of tetracycline, doxycycline hyclate and minocycline HCl, are broad-spectrum antibiotics, affecting both gram-positive and gram-negative microorganisms. Doxycycline and minocycline have been used in the treatment of *A. actinomycetemcomitans* infections in localized aggressive periodontitis (formerly known as localized juvenile periodontitis) and refractory periodontitis. Mandell et al. (1986) reported that while surgery and treatment with tetracycline were superior in localized aggressive periodontitis patients, it appeared that there was a possibility of reinfection with or incomplete elimination of *A. actinomycetemcomitans*.

TABLE 11–7

CLASSIFICATION OF ADVERSE EFFECTS OF SYSTEMIC ANTIMICROBIAL AGENTS

ADVERSE EFFECT	FEATURES
Hypersensitivity reactions	Involves allergic reactions to the antibiotic (e.g., rashes).
Gastrointestinal disturbances	Very common; includes nausea, vomiting, and diarrhea. Pseudomembranous colitis is the most severe gastrointestinal complication that requires immediate discontinuation of the antibiotic. Although initially believed to be a complication associated primarily with clindamycin, most oral and injectable antibiotics may produce this side effect.
Hepatotoxicity	Liver disease can occur with commonly administered antibiotics such as erythromycin, amoxicillin-clavulanic acid, and quinolones.
Photosensitivity reactions	Occurs with fluoroquinolones and tetracyclines (less with minocycline). Seen as an exaggerated sunburn. Patients should not be exposed to sun when taking these antibiotics.
Fungal infection	Fungal infections can occur especially with use of broad-spectrum antibiotics, which destroy bacteria, allowing fungi (*Candida albicans*) to overgrow, which may produce gastrointestinal irritation, stomatitis, and vaginal infection. Acidophilus (available in a soft gel tablet) or yogurt taken in conjunction with the antibiotic (except tetracycline) will replace some of the bacteria, thereby possibly preventing a fungal infection.

Anticollagenase Feature   Tetracyclines have both antibacterial and nonantibacterial properties. Besides affecting bacterial growth, they also affect the host response by inhibiting the production and secretion of collagenase by cells in the body such as polymorphonuclear leukocytes (PMNs) (Golub et al. 1984). Collagenase is an enzyme responsible for the destruction of collagen, which makes up the connective tissue of the periodontium. Tetracyclines also were found to inhibit bone resorption by affecting osteoclast function (Rifkin, Vernillo, and Golub 1993). This anticollagenase property does not depend on the drug's antibacterial actions.

Concentration in Gingival Crevicular Fluid   Another property of tetracyclines is their ability to concentrate in the gingival crevicular fluid (GCF) at two to four times blood levels following multiple doses (Gordon et al. 1981). Doxycycline (Pascale et al. 1986) and minocycline also concentrate in higher levels in the GCF than in serum. Tetracyclines exhibit higher substantivity than other antibiotics (Baker et al. 1983; Stabholz et al. 1993), which allows binding to root surfaces with a slow release into the GCF. The binding of tetracyclines to calcium ions in the GCF enhances their substantivity. These properties allow the drug to maintain high therapeutic levels in the GCF. It is advantageous for a drug to concentrate in high levels in the GCF because the GCF bathes the subgingival pocket area where the periodontal pathogens live.

Adverse Side Effects and Drug-Drug and Drug-Food Interactions   Common adverse side effects of tetracyclines include nausea, vomiting, and diarrhea. Gastrointestinal (stomach) upset is much less with the semisynthetic drugs because they are more highly absorbed from the gastrointestinal tract. Tetracyclines stain newly formed teeth during enamel deposition and should not be used during the last half of pregnancy or in children up to 8 years of age. A complex is formed with calcium orthophosphate that produces a yellow-gray fluorescent discoloration. Photosensitivity is another adverse side effect, resulting in exaggerated sunburn when patients are exposed to the sun.

Tetracyclines, except doxycycline and minocycline, should not be taken concomitantly with dairy products because tetracycline binds to calcium inhibiting its absorption. Tetracycline should be taken on an empty stomach (1 hour before or 2 hours after meals) because food delays its absorption. Doxycycline and minocycline can be taken without regard to meals. Absorption of all tetracyclines into the bloodstream is delayed with antacids. Tetracyclines, as well as other antibiotics, interfere with the metabolism of oral contraceptives. Estrogens, a component in oral contraceptives, must be metabolized (broken down) to its active form in the stomach by bacteria. Most antibiotics kill or stop the growth of these bacteria, inhibiting estrogen breakdown. Patients must use other forms of birth control if they are taking antibiotics concomitantly. Tetracyclines or any other bacteriostatic drug should not be given together with bactericidal antibiotics such as penicillin, metronidazole, or ciprofloxacin that would interfere with the bactericidal action of that drug. In order for a bactericidal drug to work, the bacteria need to be multiplying.

How Supplied   Tetracycline HCl (Sumycin): 100- and 250-mg capsules. Doxycycline hyclate (Vibramycin®, Pfizer, New York, NY, Vibra-Tabs®, Pfizer, New York, NY, Doryx®, Warner Chilcott Prof. Prod., Rockaway, NJ): 100-mg tablets and 50- and 100-mg capsules.

Penicillins (beta-lactams)

Penicillins as a group are bactericidal, and their mechanism of action is to inhibit bacterial cell wall synthesis. Penicillin VK has limited activity against gram-negative periodontal pathogens. It is indicated primarily in certain acute periodontal infections such as abscesses. Amoxicillin, a broad-spectrum penicillin, is used frequently in periodontics. Some bacteria produce enzymes called *beta-lactamases* that inactivate the penicillin molecule. To overcome this vulnerability, a beta-lactamase inhibitor such as clavulanic acid is combined with amoxicillin (Augmentin®, SmithKline Beecham, Philadelphia, PA).

Adverse Side Effects and Drug-Drug and Drug-Food Interactions   Approximately 5 to 10% of individuals are allergic to penicillin. It is best to take Augmentin® with food to decrease gastrointestinal upset. Severe gastrointestinal upset (e.g., nausea, vomiting, and diarrhea) occurs as a result of the acid component. Food does not interfere with absorption of amoxicillin into the bloodstream. Penicillins should not be taken together with bacteriostatic antibiotics because for a bactericidal antibiotic to work, the bacteria need to be multiplying, and this would be inhibited if a bacteriostatic antibiotic were administered concomitantly with penicillin.

How Supplied   Penicillin VK (Pen-Vee K, Penicillin VK): 250- and 500-mg tablets. Amoxicillin trihydrate (Polymox, Trimox, Amoxil): 250-mg capsules and 125-mg chewable tablets. Augmentin®, SmithKline Beecham, Philadelphia, PA: A "250" tablet contains: 250 mg amoxicillin and 125 mg potassium clavulanate; a "500" tablet contains 500 mg amoxicillin and 125 mg potassium clavulanate.

Cephalosporins *not useful in dental infections*

Cephalosporins are not considered to be the drug of choice for most types of dental infections, including periodontal diseases. These antibiotics do not provide an advantage over amoxicillin or penicillin. The predominant bacteria associated with periodontal diseases are not sensitive to cephalosporins.

Nitroimadazoles: *NUG*

Mechanism of Action and Indications   Metronidazole is specifically effective against obligate or strict anaerobic (live in a pure nonoxygen environment) microorganisms. Metronidazole penetrates well into the GCF, but not as high as the tetracyclines. Metronidazole is bactericidal, and its mechanism of action is to inhibit bacterial DNA synthesis.

Metronidazole is indicated in the treatment of acute nectrotizing gingivitis (ANUG). Metronidazole is also indicated when barrier membranes are used during guided tissue regeneration surgery. *P. gingivalis,* a strict anaerobe, is the primary bacteria that colonize on porous membrane material. It has been reported in both professional journals and in the lay press that periodontal debridement in conjunction with metronidazole may reduce the need for periodontal surgery (Loesche et al. 1996), but this remains controversial. Metronidazole in combination with amoxicillin or Augmentin may be effective against refactory and aggressive forms of periodontitis associated with *A. actinomycetemcomitans* and *P. gingivalis* infection. However, a recent study of 21 patients with moderate, untreated periodontal diseases evaluated the benefits of amoxicillin and Augmentin® after initial therapy. Patients received periodontal debridement twice during the study. After the second debridement, patients were assigned randomly to either the group that received the drug combination or the placebo group. Results indicated no added benefit when amoxicillin and Augmentin were taken after initial therapy (Winkel et al. 1999).

Adverse Side Effects and Drug-Drug Interactions   Antibiotic resistance to *altered taste perception* metronidazole is rare, but there are numerous adverse side effects. Gastrointestinal upset is seen frequently, especially nausea. A metallic taste in the mouth has been reported, as well as darkened urine. Consumption of alcohol beverages, including use of alcohol-containing mouthrinses, while taking metronidazole results in a disulfiram-like reaction. Disulfiram is a drug given to wean alcoholics off alcohol by acting to deter further ingestion of alcohol. It works by inhibition of the enzyme aldehyde dehydrogenase, causing a buildup of acetaldehyde, a toxic by-product of ethanol metabolism (Garey and Rodvold 1999). Within 5 to 10 minutes after metronidazole is taken with alcohol, serious non-life-threatening adverse side effects occur including headache, flushing, nausea, vomiting, and cramps. The reaction usually lasts for up to 1 hour; however, it may continue for a few days after discontinuation of the medication (Walker 1996). Alcohol should not be consumed during metronidazole therapy and for at least 3 days after discontinuing the drug. Metronidazole is contraindicated in patients taking anticoagulants (e.g., warfarin), lithium (a drug used for manic depression), and cimetadine (an antiulcer drug).

How Supplied   Metronidazole (Flagyl®, Searle, Chicago, IL): 375-mg capsules and 250- and 500-mg tablets.

Macrolides

Erythromycin, a macrolide antibiotic, is not used in the treatment of periodontal diseases because it is primarily effective against Gram-positive microorganisms and does not penetrate gram-negative bacterial cells. Erythromycin also does not penetrate the GCF to effective levels. Erythromycins are bacteriostatic and inhibit bacterial protein synthesis. Adverse side effects include severe gastrointestinal disturbances, including nausea, vomiting, and diarrhea.

Second-Generation Drugs: Azalides The newer second-generation erythromycins, referred to as *azilides,* have a broader spectrum of action with fewer adverse side effects. Azithromycin dihydrate shows promising results in periodontics. Azithromycin has several unique advantages. Azithromycin concentrates in phagocytes such as PMNs and macrophages, which contributes to its distribution into inflamed periodontal tissues (gingival connective tissue) in greater amounts than in plasma (Malizia et al. 1997). In addition, a postantibiotic effect is seen, whereby high antibiotic levels remain after the drug is discontinued (Malizia et al. 1997).

Adverse Side Effects and Drug-Drug and Drug-Interactions Erythromycins, except for azithromycin, should not be taken with nonsedating antihistamines such as astemizole (Hismanal®, Janssen Pharmaceuticals,Titusville, NJ). Erythromycin inhibits the metabolism or breakdown of these drugs, causing high blood levels, which can lead to cardiotoxicity. There are no contraindications to the use of fexofenadine (Allegra®, Hoescht Marion Roussel, Kansas City, MO) or loratadine (Claritin®, Schering Corporation, Kenilworth, NJ). Concurrent use of erythromycins and theophylline (an antiasthma drug) increases blood levels of theophylline. Capsules of azithromycin should be taken on an empty stomach, but tablets can be taken with food.

How Supplied Azithromycin (Zithromax®, Pfizer, New York, NY): 250-mg capsules and 600-mg tablets.

Lincomycins

Clindamycin HCl penetrates well into the GCF and is active against most periodontal pathogens except A. *actinomycetemcomitans* and *Eikenella corrodens* and is especially useful in treating refractory periodontitis. Clindamycin HCl inhibits bacterial protein synthesis and is bacteriostatic. Although the development of pseudomembranous colitis has been associated with the use of Clindamycin, it can occur with any antibiotic; however, its occurrence is usually hospital based. Suppression of normal intestinal bacteria allows the overgrowth of *Clostridium difficile,* which produces a toxin that causes severe watery diarrhea and fever. The antibiotic should be discontinued as soon as such signs appear. Clindamycin can be taken with food.

How Supplied Clindamycin HCl (Cleocin®, Pharmacia & Upjohn, Bridgewater, NJ): 75-, 150-, and 300-mg capsules.

Quinolones (fluoroquinolone)

Fluoroquinolones are bactericidal because they inhibit bacterial DNA replication. Quinolones are not actually an antibiotic, however, because they are totally synthetic. Nevertheless, they are frequently referred to as broad-spectrum antimicrobials with good activity against facultative gram-negative anaerobes. Adverse side effects include dizziness, convulsions, headache, hallucinations, and joint and cartilage damage (do not give to athletes). Ciprofloxacin should not be given to children younger than 18 years of age because of its effect on cell growth. Ciprofloxacin should not be administered with theophylline or caffeine because it inhibits their metabolism, resulting in increased blood levels. Dairy products and antacids delay absorption. Food does not slow absorption.

How Supplied   Ciprofloxacin HCl (Cipro®, Bayer, New Haven, CT): 100-, 250-, 500-, and 750-mg tablets.

CONTROLLED-RELEASE DRUG DELIVERY

The development of site-specific, controlled-release delivery systems has provided a further option for antimicrobial therapy by allowing therapeutic levels of a drug to be maintained in the periodontal pocket for prolonged periods of time. Many devices are available in the United States and Europe that incorporate an antimicrobial agent into a specific material (a polymer) that is placed into the periodontal pocket. The active ingredient is then released from the material, which subsequently exerts its antibacterial activity on subgingival bacteria over several days. Then the material is either removed from the pocket or is absorbed (dissolves). Types of materials used to incorporate antimicrobial drugs include fibers, gels, chips, collagen film, and acrylic strips. Controlled-release drug therapy is used as an adjunct to periodontal debridement and should not replace conventional mechanical therapy. They are indicated for use in recurrent pockets of 5 mm or greater that continue to bleed on probing. The intended results with these devices are gains in clinical attachment levels and reductions in probing depths and bleeding on probing.

Currently in the United States, Actiste® (Alza, Palo Alto, CA), PerioChip® (Perio Products, Ltd., Jerusalem, Israel, Cincinnati, OH), and Atridox® (Block Drug, Jersey City, NJ) are available commercially. Other controlled-release systems are available in Europe that have not been approved for use in the United States.

NONRESORBABLE CONTROLLED-RELEASE DEVICES

Tetracycline HCl fibers

The first controlled-release device approved in the United States in the early 1990s was Actisite®. Actisite® is an ethylene vinyl acetate flexible fiber impregnated with 12.7 mg of tetracycline HCl. It is placed subgingivally into the periodontal pocket, where the tetracycline is released slowly over 7 to 10 days. Substantivity is not a requirement. Actisite® is indicated for use in maintenance patients with recurrent pockets of 5 mm or greater that bleed and are resistant to treatment. While tetracycline was found to penetrate gingival epithelium (Ciancio, Cobb, and Leung 1992), serum levels of tetracycline following 10 days of therapy were less than 0.1 µg/ml (Rapley et al. 1992). Thus systemic adverse side effects are not seen with tetracycline fiber therapy.

Disadvantages in using tetracycline fibers include difficulty in placing and keeping the fiber in the pocket, bacterial resistance to tetracycline, and the inaccessibility of the drug to the adjacent gingival connective tissue and nondental sites such as the tongue, tonsils, and buccal mucosa, where bacteria also live.

Long-term studies demonstrate that tetracycline fiber treatment and periodontal debridement in patients in a maintenance program resulted in significant decreases in probing depths, increases in attachment level, and a decrease in the percentage of sites with bleeding on probing than fiber therapy or scaling alone (Newman, Kornman, and Doherty 1994; Michalowicz et al. 1995).

In another clinical study, Drisko et al. (1995) found that clinical changes following one or two applications of tetracycline fiber were no different than after mechanical debridement alone or fiber plus debridement. All treatments (fiber alone, debridement alone, and one or two fiber applications plus debridement) showed significant attachment level gains and reductions in probing depth and bleeding on probing.

Placement of the fiber in a periodontal pocket is technique-sensitive and takes about 5 to 15 minutes per tooth, similar to placement of a retraction cord. The fiber is placed around the entire tooth to the depth of the pocket, completely filling the pocket (Fig. 11–5 ■). Cyanoacrylate glue is placed on the opening of the pocket to keep the fiber in the pocket.

RESORBABLE CONTROLLED-RELEASE DEVICES

Chlorhexidine gluconate chip

The PerioChip® (Perio Products, Ltd., Jerusalem, Israel, Cincinnati, OH) is a gelatin maxtrix (bovine origin) containing 2.5 mg of chlorhexidine gluconate. This product received Food and Drug Administration approval in June 1998. PerioChip® is indicated for use as an adjunct to instrumentation in maintenance patients with pockets 5 mm or larger that bleed recurrently on probing (Jeffcoat et al. 1998). A recent clinical study comparing the efficacy of periodontal debridement alone with that of periodontal debridement plus PerioChip® revealed statistically significant reductions in probing depth and gains in clinical attachment in the periodontal debridement plus PerioChip® group. However, the

FIGURE 11–5

Actisite® (Alza, Palo Alto, CA) fiber placement. The fiber is placed in the deepest part of the pocket first, and then the rest of the pocket is completely filled. The fiber must be removed at 10 days.

magnitude of these changes was small (0.3 mm), so the results are not clinically significant (Jeffcoat et al. 1998). In this study, mechanical debridement was limited to only 1 hour in patients with moderately advanced peridontitis (5- to 8-mm pockets), which does not seem realistic.

After periodontal debridement, the chip is placed into the periodontal pocket (Fig. 11–6 ■). In contact with subgingival fluids it becomes sticky and binds to the epithelium lining the pocket, so no periodontal dressing is indicated. Its antibacterial action occurs when chlorhexidine is released over 7 to 10 days, after which it resorbs and does not have to be removed. Up to eight chips can be inserted into pockets in one visit. Another round of treatment can be done at 3 months.

Doxycycline hyclate gel

Atridox® is composed of 10% (42.5 mg) doxycycline hyclate in a gel formulation that is biodegradable and subsequently will resorb. The ingredients are available in two syringes (powder and liquid) that are mixed together (Fig. 11–7 ■) and injected into the pocket around the entire tooth (Fig. 11–8 ■). Atridox® is indicated for use in the treatment of chronic periodontitis to promote attachment level gain, to reduce pocket depths, and to reduce bleeding on probing. Atridox® may be used in patients who refuse to have periodontal debridement or periodontal surgery, and who are medically, physically, or emotionally compromised. Atridox® is also indicated as a supplement to periodontal debridement.

A randomized, controlled clinical study (Garrett, Johnson, and Stoller 1998) comparing Atridox® alone (all patients had a history of periodontal debridement at least 2 months before the study) and periodontal debridement alone reported that Atridox® produced clinical results comparable with periodontal debridement alone. Both groups showed a statistically significant reduction in pocket depths (an average of 1.3 mm) and gains in attachment levels (average of 0.8 mm).

FIGURE 11–6

PerioChip® is a film or chip containing the antimicrobial chlorhexidine gluconate. After a periodontal maintenance visit, PerioChip® is placed subgingivally in pockets 5 mm or greater in depth and bleed on probing.

FIGURE 11–7

Atridox® is prepared by joining/interlocking the two syringes. (Courtesy of Block Drug Corp., Jersey City, NJ)

FIGURE 11–8

Atridox® (Block Drug Corp., Jersey City, NJ). After pumping the materials between the two joined syringes, a cannula is connected to the syringe to apply into the pocket. (Courtesy of Block Drug Corp., Jersey City, NJ)

Levels of doxycycline in the pocket (GCF) peaked at 2 hours after placement into the pocket, and effective drug levels were maintained at 28 days (Stoller et al. 1998).

OTHER PRODUCTS

Some controlled-release products are available in other countries. Elyzol® (Dumex, Copenhagen, Denmark) is a 25% metronidazole gel that is injected into the pocket. Periocline® (Sunstar Corp., Osaka, Japan) and Dentomycin® (Cyanamid International, Wayne, NJ) are a 2% minocycline gel.

ANTIBIOTIC RESISTANCE

Bacterial resistance to antibiotics raises serious questions for health care providers. The danger is that an antibiotic will not be effective if administered later on for a truly life-threatening bacterial infection because the bacterial flora have become resistant to that antibiotic. Thus antibiotic resistance can lead to an increase in the incidence of disease. Patterns of antibiotic use in the United States also contribute significantly to the global problem. Patients often stop their antibiotic treatment prematurely, believing that if they feel better, it is not necessary to take the full course. Patients also self-medicate with leftover antibiotics from a previous infection. Patients may request antibiotics or other medications because they believe they will be beneficial. Many practitioners comply with such patient requests without evaluating the situation clinically, and many practitioners simply overprescribe antibiotics.

Therefore, it is extremely important to use antibiotics and antimicrobials conservatively, only when indicated, and with the narrowest possible spectrum of activity. Prolonged or repetitive courses of antibiotic treatment should be avoided. Antibiotics are an adjunct to treatment.

ENZYME-SUPPRESSION THERAPY

Although bacteria are the culprits in initiating inflammatory periodontal diseases, the inflammatory mediators, including cytokines and prostaglandins produced by the host (body) cells in response to the bacteria, are partly responsible for periodontal tissue breakdown. When produced in excess, inflammatory mediators induce destruction of healthy periodontal tissues. For example, prostaglandins facilitate bone resorption by stimulating the activity of osteoclasts.

MATRIX METALLOPROTEINASES

Host cells, including PMNs and fibroblasts, also respond to bacterial products by synthesizing and secreting matrix metalloproteinases (MMPs) in the host connective tissue. The MMPs are a family of enzymes that work together to break down connective tissue proteins, including collagen. MMPs that cause the breakdown of the periodontium include collagenase and gelatinase.

In healthy oral tissues, as part of the normal turnover of connective tissue, fibroblasts synthesize and secrete collagenase, which removes "old" collagen while new collagen is laid down. However, in the presence of disease (bacterial infection), PMNs produce collagenase in excessive amounts, which destroys periodontal tissues. Thus the third approach to therapy is to inhibit the collagenase synthesized and released by PMNs. Antibiotics are aimed at reducing or eliminating the periodontal pathogens but do not target the enzyme-producing cells.

SUBANTIMICROBIAL-DOSE DOXYCYCLINE

Golub et al. (1984) found that tetracyclines, especially doxycycline, have anticollagenase properties and inhibit collagenase activity. This group of investigators discovered that by using only 20-mg capsules of doxycycline, instead of the customary 50- or 100-mg capsules, collagenase would be inhibited. At these subantimicrobial doses, doxycycline only has anticollagenase activity and no antibacterial action. This subantimicrobial or low-dose doxycycline (SDD) formulation is available under the trade name Periostat® (CollaGenex, Newton, PA). Periostat® is indicated as an adjunct to periodontal debridement to promote attachment level gain and to reduce pocket depths in patients with chronic periodontitis. It is intended to improve the clinical outcome of periodontal debridement. Periostat® capsules are taken twice daily. Efficacy beyond 9 months of continuous dosing and safety beyond 12 months of continuous dosing have not been established.

In a large-scale clinical study, patients received debridement and either Periostat® or a placebo twice a day for 9 months. The results of the study showed that after 3 months of daily use, reductions in probing depth and improvements in attachment levels were statistically greater with SDD and debridement than with placebo and debridement (Ciancio and Ashley 1998). Reductions in probing depth from baseline were up to 38% greater with SDD in tooth sites with mild to moderate periodontitis (probing depths of 4 to 6 mm) and severe periodontitis (probing depths of 7 mm or more). Improvements in attachment from baseline were up to 54% greater with the SDD than with placebo in severely diseased sites. Although treatment differences in the per-patient mean change in probing depth and clinical attachment level were statistically significant, these differences were relatively small. However, the frequency of probing depth reduction of 2 mm or more was greater in the Periostat group than in the placebo group.

SUMMARY

The multifaceted approach to treating periodontal diseases uses mechanical instrumentation, which reduces the bacterial load, and locally and systemically administered antibiotics and host-modulating pharmacotherapies as treatment adjuncts.

Treatment of patients with gingivitis or chronic periodontitis is related to reducing the number of bacteria to a level conducive to health (Loesche 1976). This involves periodontal debridement, periodontal surgery, and if needed, oral rinses and oral irrigation. Frequently, these patients are overtreated using systemic antibiotics, which can lead to the development of bacteria that become resistant to antibiotics. Systemic antibiotics are contraindicated in these patients.

In a small percentage (around 20%) of patients with periodontitis, (Loesche 1976) specific bacteria (e.g., *A. actinomycetemcomitans, P. gingivalis, P. intermedia,* and spirochetes) can be implicated in the diseases (Loesche 1976; Slots 1986). Since these bacteria invade the soft tissues, treatment may include systemic antibiotics to eliminate the bacteria in the tissues. It is more difficult to recognize these types of patients. Examples include patients with localized aggressive periodontitis, necrotizing periodontal diseases, and refractory forms of periodontal diseases. In addition, patients with a compromised immune system, such as AIDS patients, can benefit from the use of antimicrobial agents.

Controlled-release antibiotics may be recommended as adjuncts to nonsurgical and surgical therapy, but convincing data have not been provided for their use as a single mode of therapy.

Antibiotic resistance of bacteria has enormous clinical and societal implications. In essence, when bacteria become resistant to an antibiotic, that antibiotic becomes ineffective. Although the prudent use of antibiotics will continue to be a valuable treatment option for certain forms of periodontal disease, the abuse and misuse of antibiotics must be addressed and monitored to prevent antibiotic resistance.

As advances are made in the development of new antimicrobial and antibiotic agents, the oral health care team will continue to play an integral part in ensuring that these agents are used appropriately. No data are available to support the long-term effectiveness of the newly approved controlled-release devices. Although many studies on site-specific drug therapy and submicrobial-dose doxycycline report statistically significant reductions in probing depths and improvements in attachment levels, the clinical benefit may not be significant. Further clinical studies are needed to determine clinical significance.

KEY POINTS

✣ Oral rinses are only effective supragingivally and do not have any effect on subgingival plaque.

✣ Oral irrigation may be useful between maintenance appointments to reduce bacterial reinfection (repopulation).

✣ Systemic antibiotics are indicated in certain inflammatory periodontal diseases such as localized or generalized aggressive periodontitis, and refractory forms of periodontal diseases.

✣ Controlled-release drug devices that slowly release antimicrobial agents are used in site-specific (recurrent) areas in chronic periodontitis.

✣ Enzyme-suppression therapy involves the inhibition of collagenase that is synthesized and released by neutrophils.

✣ Dental practitioners should contribute to limiting antibiotic resistance.

REFERENCES

Addy, M., and R. Koltai. 1994. Control of supragingival calculus. Scaling and polishing and anticalculus toothpastes: An opinion. *J. Clin. Periodontol.* 21:342–346.

Addy, M., and R. Wright. 1978. Comparison of the in vivo and in vitro antibacterial properties of povidone-iodine and chlorhexidine gluconate mouthrinses. *J. Clin. Periodontol.* 5:198–205.

Asikainen, S., S. Alaluusua, and L. Saxén. 1991. Recovery of *A. actinomycetemcomitans* from teeth, tongue, and saliva. *J. Periodontol.* 62:203–206.

Bacca, L. A., M. Leusch, A. C. Lanzalaco, et al. 1997. A comparison of intraoral antimicrobial effects of stabilized fluoride dentifrice, baking soda/hydrogen peroxide dentifrice, conventional NaF dentifrice and essential oil mouthrinse. *J. Clin. Dent.* 8:54–61.

Baker, P., T. Evans, R. Coburn, and R. Genco. 1983. Tetracycline and its derivatives strongly bind to and are released from the tooth surface in active form. *J. Periodontol.* 54:580–585.

Beiswanger, B. B., P. M. Doyle, and R. D. Jackson. 1995. The clinical effect of dentifrices containing stabilized stannous fluoride on plaque formation and gingivitis: A six-month study with ad libitum brushing. *J. Clin. Dent.* 6:46–53.

Binney, A., M. Addy, J. Owens, and J. Faulkner. 1997. A comparison of triclosan and stannous fluoride toothpastes for inhibition of plaque regrowth: A crossover study designed to assess carryover. *J. Clin. Periodontol.* 24(3):166–170.

Binney, A., M. Addy, S. McKeowns, and L. Everatt. 1995. The effect of commercially available triclosan-containing toothpaste compared to a sodium-fluoride containing toothpaste and a chlorhexidine rinse on 4-day plaque regrowth. *J. Clin. Periodontol.* 22(1): 830–834.

Binney, A., M. Addy, S. McKeowns, and L. Everatt. 1996. The choice of controls in toothpaste studies: The effect of a number of commercially available toothpastes compared to water on a 4-day plaque regrowth. *J. Clin. Periodontol.* 23(5):456–459.

Bollmer, B. L. V., O. P. Sturzenberger, V. Vick, and E. Grossman. 1995. Reduction of calculus and Peridex stain with Tarter Control Crest. *J. Clin. Dent.* 6(4):185–187.

Braun, R. E., and S. G. Ciancio. 1992. Subgingival delivery by an oral irrigation device. *J. Periodontol.* 63:469–472.

Brunette, D. M. 1996. Effects of baking soda–containing dentifrices on oral malodor. *Compend. Contin. Educ. Dent.* 17(Suppl. 19):22–31.

Cerra, M. B., and W. J. Killoy. 1982. The effect of sodium bicarbonate and hydrogen peroxide on the microbial flora of periodontal pockets: A preliminary report. *J. Periodontol.* 53:599–603.

Christersson, L. A., O. M. Norderyd, and C. S. Puchalsky. 1993. Topical application of tetracycline-HCl in human periodontitis. *J. Clin. Periodontol.* 20:88–95.

Ciancio, S. G. 1993. Alcohol in mouthrinse: Lack of association with cancer. *Biol. Ther. Dent.* 9(1):2–3.

Ciancio, S. G. 1997. Triclosan: A new antigingivitis agent. *Biol. Ther. Dent.* 13:23–26.

Ciancio, S. G., and R. Ashley. 1998. Safety and efficacy of subantimicrobial-dose doxycycline therapy in patients with adult periodontitis. *Adv. Dent. Res.* 12:27–31.

Ciancio, S. G., C. M. Cobb, and M. Leung. 1992. Tissue concentration and localization of tetracycline following site-specific tetracycline fiber therapy. *J. Periodontol.* 63:849–853.

Ciancio, S. G., M. L. Mather, J. J. Zambon, and H. S. Reynolds. 1989. Effect of a chemotherapeutic agent delivered by an oral irrigation device on plaque, gingivitis, and subgingival microflora. *J. Periodontol.* 60:310–315.

Clark, W. B., I. Magnusson, C. B. Walker, and R. G. Marks. 1989. Efficacy of Perimed antibacterial system on established gingivitis I. Clinical results. *J. Clin. Periodontol.* 16:630–635.

Cobb, C. M., R. I. Rodgers, and W. J. Killoy. 1988. Ultrastructural examination of human periodontal pockets following the use of an oral irrigation device in vitro. *J. Periodontol.* 59:155–159.

Costerton, J. W., Z. Lewandowski, D. DeBeer, D. Caldwell, D. Korber, and G. James. 1994. Biofilms, the customized microniche. *J. Bacteriol.* 176:2137–2142.

Cummins, D. 1997. Vehicles: How to deliver the goods. *Periodontology 2000* 15:84–99.

De Graaf, J., A. J. van Winkelhoff, and R. J. Goené. 1989. The role of *Actinobacillus actinomycetemcomitans* in periodontal disease. *Infection* 17:269–271.

Drake, D. R., B. Grigsby, and D. Drotz-Dieleman. 1994. Growth-inhibitory effect of pyrophosphate on oral bacteria. *Oral Micro. Immunol.* 9(1):25–28.

Drake, D., K. Vargas, A. Cardenzana, and R. Srikantha. 1995. Enhanced bacterial activity of Arm and Hammer Dental Care. *Am. J. Dent.* 8(6):308–312.

Drisko, C. L., C. M. Cobb, W. J. Killoy, et al. 1995. Evaluation of periodontal treatments using controlled-release tetracycline fibers: Clinical response. *J. Periodontol.* 66:692–699.

Duckworth, R. M., Y. Jones, J. Nicholson, A. P. Jacobson, and I. G. Chestnutt. 1994. Studies on plaque fluoride after use of F-containing dentifrices. *Adv. Dent. Res.* 8(2):202–207.

Eakle, W. S., C. Ford, and R. L. Boyd. 1986. Depth of penetration in periodontal pockets with oral irrigation. *J. Clin. Periodontol.* 13:39–44.

Elworthy, A., J. Greenman, F. M. Doherty, R. G. Newcombe, and M. Addy. 1996. The substantivity of a number of oral hygiene products determined by the duration of effects on salivary bacteria. *J. Periodontol.* 67:572–576.

Fine, D., C. Mendieta, M. Barnett, et al. 1992. Efficacy of preprocedural rinsing with an antiseptic in reducing viable bacteria in dental aerosols. *J. Periodontol.* 63:821–824.

Fischman, S. L., G. Kugel, R. B. Truelove, B. J. Nelson, and L. P. Cancro. 1992. Motivational benefits of a dentifrice containing baking soda and hydrogen peroxide. *J. Clin. Dent.* 3:88–94.

Fishman, S. L., and S. Yankell. 1999. Dentifrices, mouth rinses, and tooth whiteners. In *Primary preventive dentistry,* 5th ed., ed. N. O. Harris and F. García-Godoy, 103–125. Stamford, CT: Appleton and Lange.

Fleming, T. F., M. G. Newman, F. M. Doherty, E. Grossman, A. H. Meckel, and M. B. Bakdash. 1990. Supragingival irrigation with 0.06% chlorhexidine in naturally occurring gingivitis: I. Six-month clinical observations. *J. Periodontol.* 61:112–117.

Flotra, L., P. Gjermo, G. Rölla, et al. 1972. A 4-month study on the effect of chlorhexidine mouthrinses on 50 soldiers. *Can. J. Dent. Res.* 80:10–16.

Gaengler, P., A. Kurbad, and W. Weinert. 1993. Evaluation of anti-calculus efficacy: An SEM method of evaluating the effectiveness of pyrophosphate dentifrice on calculus formation. *J. Clin. Periodontol.* 20:144–146.

Garrett, S., L. Johnson, and N. Stoller. 1998. The influence of subgingival calculus levels on outcomes following treatment of periodontitis with subgingivally delivered doxycycline or periodontal debridement. *J. Dent. Res.* 77:923 (Abstract 2336).

Garey, K. W., and K. A. Rodvold. 1999. Disulfiram reactions and anti-infective agents. *Infect Med.* 16(11):741–744.

Golub, L. M., N. Ramamurthy, T. F. McNamara, et al. 1984. Tetracyclines inhibit tissue collagenase activity: A new mechanism in the treatment of periodontal diseases. *J. Periodont. Res.* 19:651–655.

Gordon, J. M., C. B. Walker, J. C. Murphy, J. M. Goodson, and S. S. Socransky. 1981. Tetracycline: Levels achievable in gingival crevice fluid and in vitro effect on subgingival organisms: 1. Concentrations in crevicular fluid after repeated doses. *J. Periodontol.* 52:609–612.

Gordon, J. M., I. B. Lamster, and M. C. Sieger. 1985. Efficacy of Listerine antiseptic in inhibiting the development of plaque and gingivitis. *J. Clin. Periodontol.* 12:697–704.

Grossman, E. 1988. Effectiveness of a prebrushing mouthrinse under single-trial and home-use conditions. *Clin. Prev. Dent.* 10:3–9.

Harper, D. S., L. J. Mueller, J. Fine, J. Gordon, and L. L. Laster. 1990. Clinical efficacy of a dentifrice and oral rinse containing sanguinaria extract and zinc chloride during six months of use. *J. Periodontol.* 61:352–358.

Jeffcoat, M. K., K. S. Bray, S. G. Ciancio, et al. 1998. Adjunctive use of a subgingival controlled-release chlorhexidine chip reduces probing depth and improves attachment level compared with periodontal debridement alone. *J. Periodontol.* 69:989–997.

Jensen, M. E., and F. J. Kohout. 1988. The effect of a fluoridated dentifrice on root and coronal caries in an older adult population. *J. Am. Dent. Assoc.* 117:829–832.

Jolkovsky, D. L., M. Y. Waki, M. G. Newman, et al. 1990. Clinical and microbiological effects of subgingival and gingival marginal irrigation with chlorhexidine gluconate. *J. Periodontol.* 61:663–669.

Kirstila, V., M. Lenander-Lumikari, E. Soderling, and J. Tenovuo. 1996. Effects of oral hygiene products containing lactoperoxidase, lysozyme, and lactoferrin on the composition of whole saliva and on subjective oral symptoms in patients with xerostomia. *Acta Odontol. Scand.* 54:391–397.

Kleinfelder, J., R. Müller, and D. Lange. 1999. Antibiotic susceptibility of putative periodontal pathogens in advanced periodontitis patients. *J. Clin. Periodontol.* 26:347–352.

Koertge, T. E. 1996. Management of dental staining: Can low-abrasive dentifrices play a role? *Compend. Contin. Educ. Dent.* 17(Suppl 19):33–38.

Lamster, I. B., M. C. Alfano, M. C. Sieger, J. M. Gordon. 1983. The effect of Listerine antiseptic on existing plaque and gingivitis. *J. Clin. Prev. Dent.* 5:12–16.

Lavigne, S. E., K. S. Drust-Bay, K. B. Williams, W. J. Killoy, and F. Theisen. 1994. Effects of chlorhexidine on the periodontal status of patients with HA-coated integral dental implants. *Int. J. Oral Maxillofax. Implants* 9:156–162.

Levine, R. A. 1987. The Keyes technique as a cofactor in self-inflicted gingival lesions: A case report. *Compend. Contin. Educ. Dent.* 8:266–269.

Lindhe, J., B. Rosling, S. S. Socransky, and A. R. Volpe. 1993. The effect of a triclosan containing dentifrice on established plaque and gingivitis. *J. Clin. Periodontol.* 20:327–334.

Lobene, R. R. 1989. A study to compare the effects of two dentifrices on adult dental calculus formation. *Clin. Dent.* 1:67–69.

Löe, H., and C. R. Schiott. 1970. The effect of mouthrinses and topical application of chlorhexidine on the development of dental plaque and gingivitis in man. *J. Periodont. Res.* 5:79–83

Loesche, W. 1976. Chemotherapy of dental plaque infections. *Oral Sci. Rev.* 9:65–107.

Loesche, W. J., J. Giordano, S. Soehren, et al. 1996. Nonsurgical treatment of patients with periodontal disease. *Oral Surg. Oral Med. Oral Pathol.* 81:533–543.

Low, M. L. 1996. Prevention and maintenance in periodontology: Supportive periodontal therapy. In *Periodontology for the Dental Hygienist,* ed. D. A. Perry, P. L. Beemsterboer, and E. J. Taggart, 298–299. Philadelphia: W.B. Saunders.

Malizia, T., M. R. Tejada, E. Ghelardi, et al. 1997. Periodontal tissue disposition of azithromycin. *J. Periodontol.* 68:1206–1209.

Mandell, R. L., L. S. Tripodi, E. Savitt, J. M. Goodson, S. S. Socransky. 1986. The effect of treatment on *Aa* in local juvenile periodontitis. *J. Periodontol.* 57:94–97.

Mariotti, A. J. 1998. Mouthrinses and dentifrices. In *ADA Guide to Dental Therapeutics,* 1st ed. 210–212. Chicago: ADA Publishing Co.

Marshall, M. V., L. P. O. Cancro, and S. F. Fischman. 1995. Hydrogen peroxide: A review of its use in dentistry. *J. Periodontol.* 66:786–796.

Mashimo, P. A., T. Umemoto, J. Slots, et al. 1980. Pathogenicity testing of *Macaca arctoides* subgingival plaque following chlorhexidine treatment. *J. Periodontol.* 51:190–199.

Michalowicz, B. S., B. L. Pihlstrom, C. L. Drisko, et al. 1995. Evaluation of periodontal treatments using controlled-release tetracycline fiber: Maintenance response. *J. Periodontol.* 66:708–715.

Moran, J., and M. Addy. 1984. The effect of surface adsorption and staining reactions on the antimicrobial properties of some cationic antiseptic mouthrinse. *J. Periodontol.* 55:278–282.

Mullaby, B. H., J. A. James, W. A. Coulter, and G. H. Linden. 1995. The efficacy of a herbal-based toothpaste on the control of plaque and gingivitis. *J. Clin. Periodontol.* 22:686–689.

Newman, M. G., K. S. Kornman, and F. M. Doherty. 1994. A 6-month multicenter evaluation of adjunctive tetracycline fiber therapy used in conjunction with periodontal debridement in maintenance patients. *J. Periodontol.* 65:685–691.

Nosel, G., M. Scheidt, R. O'Neal, and T. Van Dyke. 1991. The penetration of lavage solution into the periodontal pocket during ultrasonic instrumentation. *J. Periodontol.* 62:554–557.

Page, R. C. 1997. Causes of halitosis. *Oral Care Rep.* 7(4):7–8.

Page, R. C., S. Offenbacher, H. E. Schroeder, G. J. Seymour, and K. S. Kornman. 1997. Advances in the pathogenesis of periodontitis: Summary of developments, clinical implications and future directions. *Periodontology 2000* 14:216–248.

Paine, M., J. Slots, and S. Rich. 1998. Fluoride use in periodontal therapy: A review of the literature. *J. Am. Dent. Assoc.* 129:69–77.

Pascale, D., J. Gordon, I. Lamster, P. Mann, M. Seiger, and W. Arndt. 1986. Concentration of doxycycline in human gingival fluid. *J. Clin. Periodontol.* 13:841–844.

Perlich, M. A., L. A. Bacca, B. W. Bollmer, et al. 1995. The clinical effect of a stabilized stannous fluoride dentifrice on plaque formation, gingivitis and gingival bleeding: A six-month study. *J. Clin. Dent.* 6:54–58.

Pihlstrom, B. L., L. F. Wolff, M. B. Bakdash, E. M. Schaffer, J. R. Jensen, D. M. Aeppli, and C. L. Bandt. 1987. Salt and peroxide compared with conventional oral hygiene: I. Clinical results. *J. Periodontol.* 58:291–300.

Proskin, H. M., and A. R. Volpe. 1995. Comparison of the anticaries efficacy of dentifrices containing fluoride as sodium fluoride or sodium monofluorophosphate. *Am. J. Dent.* 8:51–58.

Rapley, J. W., C. M. Cobb, W. J. Killoy, and D. R. Williams. 1992. Serum levels of tetracycline during treatment with tetracycline-containing fibers. *J. Periodontol.* 63:817–820.

Rees, T. D., and C. E. Orth. 1986. Oral ulcerations with use of hydrogen peroxide. *J. Periodontol.* 57:689–692.

Renton-Harper, P., M. Addy, J. Moran, R. M. Doherty, and R. G. Newcombe. 1996. A comparison of chlorhexidine, cetylpyridium chloride, triclosan, and C3LG mouthrinse products for plaque inhibition. *J. Periodontol.* 67:486–489.

Renvert, S., M. Wikström, G. Dahlén, J. Slots, and J. Egelberg. 1990. On the inability of root debridement and periodontal surgery to eliminate *Actinobacillus actinomycemtemcomitans* from periodontal pockets. *J. Clin. Periodontol.* 17:351–355.

Rifkin, B. R., A. T. Vernillo, and L. M. Golub. 1993. Blocking periodontal disease progression by inhibiting tissue destructive enzymes: A potential therapeutic role of tetracyclines and their chemically modified analogs. *J. Periodontol.* 64:819–827.

Roberts, W. R., and M. Addy. 1981. Comparison of in vitro and in vivo antibacterial properties of antiseptic mouthrinses containing chlorhexidine, alexidine, CPC and hexetidine: Relevance to mode of action. *J. Clin. Periodontol.* 8:295–310.

Rölla, G., H. Löe, and R. C. Schiott. 1971. Retention of chlorhexidine in the human oral cavity. *Arch. Oral Biol.* 16:1109–1116.

Sanz, M., M. G. Newman, L. Anderson, and W. Motaska. 1987. A comparison of the effect of a 0.12 percent chlorhexidine gluconate mouthrinse and placebo on postperiodontal surgical therapy. *J. Dent. Res.* 66:280 (Abstract).

Sbordone, L., L. Ramaglia, E. Gulletta, and V. Iacono. 1990. Recolonization of the subgingival microflora after periodontal debridement in human periodontitis. *J. Periodontol.* 61:579–584.

Schiff, T. G. 1987. The effect of a dentifrice containing soluble pyrophosphate and sodium fluoride on calculus deposits. *Clin. Prev. Dent.* 9:13–16.

Schiott, C. R., H. Löe, S. B. Jensen, M. Kilian, R. M. Davies, and L. Glavid. 1970. The effect of chlorhexidine mouthrinses on the human oral flora. *J. Periodont. Res.* 5:84–89.

Shellis, R. P., and R. M. Duckworth. 1994. Studies on the cariostatic mechanisms of fluoride. *Int. Dent. J.* 44(3 Suppl 1):263–273.

Silverman, G., E. Berman, C. B. Hanna, et al. 1996. Assessing the efficacy of three dentifrices in the treatment of dentinal hypersensitivity. *J. Am. Dent. Assoc.* 127:191–201.

Singh, S. M., M. E. Petrone, A. R. Volpe, K. N. Rustogi, and J. Norfleet. 1990. Comparison of the anticalculus effect of two soluble pyrophosphate dentifrices with and without a copolymer. *J. Clin. Dent.* 2:53–55.

Smith, C. 1999. Adverse effects of antibiotics. *U.S. Pharmacist* (May):46–60.

Slots, J. 1986. Bacterial specificity in adult periodontitis: A summary of recent work. *J. Clin. Periodontol.* 13:912–917.

Southard, S. R., C. L. Drisko, W. J. Killoy, C. M. Cobb, and D. E. Tira. 1989. The effect of 2 percent chlorhexidine digluconate irrigation on clinical parameters and the level of *Bacteroides gingivalis* in periodontal pockets. *J. Periodontol.* 60:302–309.

Stabholz, A., J. Kettering, R. Aprecio, G. Zimmerman, P. J. Baker, and U. M. E. Wikesjo. 1993. Antimicrobial properties of human dentin impregnated with tetracycline HCl or chlorhexidine: An in vitro study. *J. Clin. Periodontol.* 20:557–562.

Stephen, K. W. 1994. Fluoride toothpastes, rinses and tablets. *Adv. Dent. Res.* 8:185–189.

Stoller, N., L. Johnson, S. Trapnell, C. Harrold, and S. Garrett. 1998. The pharmacokinetic profile of a biodegradable controlled-release delivery system containing doxycycline compared to systemically delivered doxycycline in gingival crevicular fluid, saliva, and serum. *J. Periodontol.* 69:1085–1091.

Stookey, O. K. 1994. Review of fluorosis risk of self-applied topical fluorides, dentifrices, mouthrinses and gels. *Comm. Dent. Oral Epidemiol.* 22(3):181–186.

Volpe, A. R., M. E. Petrone, R. Davies, and H. M. Proskin. 1995. Clinical anticaries efficacy of NaF and SMFP dentifrices: Overview and resolution of the scientific controversy. *J. Clin. Dent.* 6:1–28.

Volpe, A. R., M. E. Petrone, W. DeVizio, and R. M. Davies. 1996. A review of plaque, gingivitis, calculus and caries clinical efficacy studies with a fluoride dentifrice containing triclosan and PVM/MA copolymer *J. Clin. Dent.* 7(Suppl):1–14.

Waerhaug, J. 1978. Healing of the dentoepithelial junction following subgingival plaque control: II. As observed on extracted teeth. *J. Periodontol.* 49:119–134.

Walker, C. B. 1996. Selected antimicrobial agents: Mechanism of action, side effects and drug interactions. *Periodontology 2000* 10:12–28.

Warrall, S. F., P. J. Knibbs, and H. D. Glenwright. 1987. Methods of reducing contamination of the atmosphere from use of an air polisher. *Br. Dent. J.* 163:118–119.

Weitzman, S. A., A. B. Weitberg, T. P. Stossel, J. Schwartz, and G. Shklar. 1986. Effects of hydrogen peroxide on oral carcinogenesis in hamsters. *J. Periodontol.* 57:685–688.

White, D. J., B. W. Bollmer, R. A. Baker, et al. 1996. Quanticale assessment of the clinical scaling benefits provided by phyrophosphate dentifrices with and without triclosan. *J. Clin. Dent.* 7(spec. issue):46–49.

Winkel, E., A. van Winkelhoff, D. Barendregt, G. van der Weijden, M. Timmerman, and U. van der Velden. 1999. Clinical and microbiological effects of initial periodontal therapy in conjunction with amoxicillin and clavulanic acid in patient with adult periodontitis. *J. Clin. Periodontol.* 26:461–468.

Winn, D., W. Blot, J. McLaughlin, et al. 1991. Mouthwash use and oral conditions in the risk of oral and pharyngeal cancer. *Cancer Res.* 51:3044–3047.

Zambon, J. J., M. L. Mather, and Y. Gonzales. 1996. A microbiological and clinical study of the safety and efficacy of baking-soda dentifrices. *Compend. Contin. Educ. Dent. Suppl.* 17:39–44.

SELF-QUIZ

1. All the following results are possible after site-specific chemotherapy *except* one. Which one is the exception? (p. 365)

    a. reduction in probing depth

    b. gain in clinical attachment

    c. reduction in bleeding

    d. formation of alveolar bone

2. Which one of the following procedures *most* effectively removes supra/subgingival plaque biofilms? (p. 343)

    a. oral rinsing

    b. oral irrigation

    c. systemic antibiotics

    d. periodontal debridement

    e. controlled-release drugs

3. All the following are indications for the use of mouthrinses in periodontics *except* one. Which one is the exception? (pp. 343–344)

    a. limited manual dexterity

    b. gingivitis

    c. periodontitis

    d. peri-implantitis

4. Which one of the following antimicrobial agents possesses high substantivity to the root surface? (p. 361)

   a. cetylpyrimidium
   b. sanguinarine
   c. tetracycline
   d. erythromycin
   e. chlorhexidine

5. Which one of the following instructions should be given to a patient rinsing with chlorhexidine? (pp. 347–348)

   a. Rinse immediately after brushing.
   b. Rinse immediately before brushing.
   c. Wait about 30 minutes after brushing.
   d. Wait about 1 hour after brushing.

6. Which one of the following antimicrobial mouthrinses contains the highest concentration of alcohol? (p. 348)

   a. Listerine®
   b. PerioGard®
   c. Scope®
   d. Viadent®

7. All the following are ways a dental practitioner can contribute to limiting antibiotic resistance *except* one. Which one is the exception? (p. 369)

   a. Prescribe drug at the first sign of infection.
   b. Avoid prolonged course of the medication.
   c. Instruct the patient on proper use.
   d. Prescribe an antibiotic with the narrowest possible spectrum of activity.

8. Which one of the following is the primary function of fluorides in dentifrices? (p. 354)

   a. desensitizing
   b. flavoring
   c. anticaries
   d. abrasive
   e. whitening

9. All the following properties of tetracyclines favor its use in periodontics *except* one. Which one is the exception? (pp. 360–362)

   a. substantivity
   b. antifungal
   c. antibacterial
   d. anticollagenase

10. Which one of the following indications is for site-specific drug delivery? (p. 365)

    a. probing depths of less than 4 mm
    b. pockets with suppuration and bleeding
    c. nonresponding bleeding sites with probing depths of 5 mm or more*
    d. sites with bone loss, suppuration, bleeding, and probing depths of less than 5 mm

PERIODONTAL INSTRUMENTATION

Outline:

I. HAND-ACTIVATED INSTRUMENTATION

Diana L. Mercado Galvis, R.D.H., M.S.
Judith Kreismann, R.D.H., M.S.

Goal:

To provide the dental hygienist with objectives and therapeutic outcomes of hand-activated instrumentation.

Educational Objectives:

Upon completion of this chapter subsection, the reader should be able to:

Discuss the rationale for periodontal debridement;

Explain the clinical outcomes of periodontal debridement;

Discuss the effects of nonsurgical treatment on the subgingival microflora;

Describe the effects of combined oral hygiene self-care with subgingival periodontal debridement on clinical attachment loss; and

Describe the healing response in gingivitis and periodontitis after periodontal debridement.

*B*ecause periodontal disease activity is site-specific within the same mouth and differs between individuals, choice of treatment is determined on a site-to-site basis and/or on a patient-to-patient basis. The critical factor in the success of periodontal therapy is not only the thoroughness of the professional debridement but rather the achievement of a high standard of oral hygiene self-care.

NONSURGICAL PERIODONTAL THERAPY

The traditional emphasis of the initial phase of **periodontal therapy** or nonsurgical therapy is control of the supragingival microbial plaque and disruption or removal of subgingival gram-negative microflora, thus delaying the repopulation of pathogenic microorganisms (Magnusson et al. 1984). Subgingival plaque originates either from an apical extension of growing supragingival plaque (Waerhaug 1978) and/or from incomplete subgingival instrumentation. In either case, it is essential to control the supragingival microbial activity through oral hygiene self-care and subgingival plaque removal by professional mechanical instrumentation

(Cobb 1996; Katsanoulas, Renee, and Attström 1992; Dahlen et al. 1992; Sbordone et al. 1990). Subgingival debridement decreases the number of periodontal pathogens such as *Porphyromonas gingivalis* and *Prevotella intermedia* in subgingival plaque and shifts the plaque composition to a predominately gram-positive aerobic species associated with periodontal health.

Thus nonsurgical therapy is based on returning the gingival tissue to a healthy, noninflamed state that can be maintained easily by the patient and the practitioner.

TERMINOLOGY

The traditional therapy for removing supragingival and subgingival plaque, its byproducts and toxins, and calculus has been scaling and root planing. *Scaling* is defined as the mechanical removal of supragingival and subgingival dental plaque, calculus, and stains (tooth-accumulated materials) from the crown and root surfaces. Thus scaling is performed both supragingivally and subgingivally. Subgingival scaling removes the adherent plaque and calculus attached to the root surface. Subgingival calculus is mineralized plaque that often adheres tenaciously to root surfaces and thus is very difficult to remove. *Root planing* is defined as a "definitive treatment procedure designed to remove cementum or surface dentin that is rough, impregnated with calculus, or contaminated with toxins or microorganisms" (Ciancio 1989). The rationale for root planing is to smooth the root surface so as to decrease the surface area to which calculus and plaque attach. Another aim is to obtain a smooth root surface by removing cementum (including some dentin) that is impregnated with bacterial toxins.

Over the past few years, the term **periodontal debridement** has emerged in the literature, and it is defined as the removal of any foreign material, including dental plaque, its by-products and toxins, calculus, and diseased or dead tissue, from the coronal tooth surfaces, root surfaces, sulcus or pocket, and periodontium (e.g., supporting bone). Thus the difference between periodontal debridement and scaling and root planing is that it encompasses more than just the root surfaces. It includes the pocket space, the pocket wall, and the underlying tissues (O'Hehir 1999). Rather than total removal of cementum and the attainment of smooth root surfaces, conservation of cementum and the achievement of a good tissue healing response through control of bacterial infection are the objectives of periodontal debridement (O'Hehir 1999). **Supragingival debridement** is the mechanical removal of dental plaque and calculus from tooth surfaces above the gingival margin. **Subgingival debridement** is the mechanical removal of dental plaque and calculus from tooth surfaces below the gingival margin. Even though periodontal debridement encompasses many procedures and currently is the newest terminology for instrumentation, the terms *scaling* and *root planing* should not be completely eliminated from the periodontal vocabulary.

Deplaquing describes the mechanical disruption of nonattached, free-floating subgingival plaque and its by-products from the sulcus or pocket. Deplaquing is recommended at reevaluation and maintenance appointments.

The term *prophylaxis* has multiple meanings. One interpretation is that a prophylaxis is a complete scaling and polishing. For others, it means a supragingival debridement or a coronal polish. According to *Current Dental Terminology*, a reference guide of the American Dental Association (ADA), a prophylaxis refers to "a scaling and polishing procedure to remove coronal plaque, calculus, and stains" (American Dental Association 1995). This definition may need to be redefined. Use of the term *coronal* in this definition implies that the dental hygienist does not provide subgingival instrumentation, but prevention requires subgingival consideration. A prophylaxis is a preventive procedure performed for patients presenting with a healthy periodontium. Polishing is performed to remove stains from the teeth and has not been shown to have any therapeutic benefits. For this reason, the American Dental Hygienist's Association's position on polishing is that it is a procedure that should be performed selectively when teeth have stains (American Dental Hygienist's Association 1995).

In some states, dental hygienists are permitted to perform closed gingival curettage or soft tissue curettage. Curettage involves removal of the diseased lining of the soft tissue pocket wall (soft tissue debridement), including the junctional epithelium and the underlying inflamed connective tissue. The goal of gingival curettage is to reduce or eliminate periodontal inflammation. Indications for performing curettage include the presence of inflamed gingival tissues and shallow suprabony pockets. However, the benefits of soft tissue curettage are questionable, and as a separate procedure, it has no justifiable application during active therapy for chronic periodontitis (Ciancio 1989). Kalkwarf (1989) demonstrated that the healing effects of curettage were not any better than scaling and root planing alone. It is noteworthy, however, that some inadvertent gingival curettage does occur as a result of scaling and root planing procedures.

PERIODONTAL DEBRIDEMENT

Treatment of **inflammatory periodontal diseases** has evolved significantly during the past decades. It was once thought that a primary goal of traditional scaling and root planing was the achievement of smooth root surfaces that were free of deposits. This intent was based on the assumption that bacteria would attach to rough surfaces (e.g., calculus and irregular root topography) and interfere with soft tissue healing. It is now known that bacteria adhere to *any* surface, rough or smooth. Therefore, *evaluation of successful periodontal debridement depends primarily on the soft tissue response.* The clinical significance of root surface roughness or smoothness is still undetermined (Jacobson, Blomlöf, and Lindskog 1994), but the dental hygienist nevertheless should strive to remove as much subgingival calculus as possible and to achieve root smoothness because they *may* affect plaque accumulation. Oberholzer and Rateitschak (1996) concluded that striving for total root smoothness during periodontal surgery seems to be unnecessary; however, the value of a cleaned tooth surface cannot be minimized in periodontal tissue healing response.

Mechanical nonsurgical therapy consisting of oral hygiene self-care and periodontal instrumentation is intended to prevent, arrest, control, or eliminate periodontal diseases in order to ultimately maintain the teeth in a functional state of health (Cobb 1996). Periodontal debridement remains the current basis of nonsurgical periodontal therapy.

COMBINED PERSONAL AND PROFESSIONAL DEBRIDEMENT

Periodontal instrumentation is performed during the initial or preliminary phase of periodontal therapy. The beneficial effects of periodontal debridement combined with oral hygiene self-care in the treatment and prevention of periodontal diseases have been well documented. These include reduction of clinical inflammation, establishment of more beneficial microorganisms and less pathogenic microorganisms, reduction in probing depths, and a gain in attachment (American Academy of Periodontology 1997; Kaldahl et al. 1996).

One clinical study reported that in the presence of supragingival plaque, a subgingival microflora containing greater than 5% spirochetes and motile rods was reestablished in 4 to 8 weeks after mechanical instrumentation. Sites devoid of supragingival plaque following supervised oral hygiene and mechanical instrumentation had less than 5% gram-negative bacteria (Magnusson et al. 1984). A more recent investigation studied the effects of supragingival plaque control alone and plaque control combined with subgingival debridement on clinical attachment loss over a 3-year period (Westfelt et al. 1998). Results showed a reduction in bleeding scores following the combined treatment of plaque control and subgingival debridement. Plaque scores were reduced in both groups. Increased attachment loss of 2 mm or more was low in the combined treatment group. This study demonstrated that supragingival plaque control is not enough to prevent further attachment loss in periodontitis patients.

RATIONALE AND INDICATIONS FOR PERIODONTAL DEBRIDEMENT

The purpose of periodontal debridement is to treat and resolve inflammation in the periodontal soft tissues by removing the irritants, which are the supragingival and subgingival plaque and calculus. In conjunction with oral hygiene self-care, which also decreases supragingival plaque accumulation, repopulation of subgingival pathogenic microflora is delayed and shifts the composition of pocket material from a pathogenic gram-negative microflora to gram-positive species, which are more conducive to periodontal health.

Periodontal debridement is indicated at sites showing (1) signs of gingival inflammation, (2) elevated levels of bacterial pathogens, and (3) progressive attachment or alveolar bone loss (Cobb 1996). Various forms of instrumentation are used, including hand-activated instrumentation and powered-driven instrumentation (e.g., sonic and ultrasonic instrumentation).

OUTCOMES OF PERIODONTAL DEBRIDEMENT

The ultimate long-term outcome or end point for mechanical nonsurgical therapy is preservation of the form and function of the dentition (Cobb 1996). Determining the effects of nonsurgical periodontal treatment requires the use of measurable clinical end points. Most clinical studies, as well as private practices, measure the probing depths, gain or loss of clinical attachment (measuring the clinical attachment levels), and alveolar bone height and document bleeding on probing, visual signs of gingival inflammation, and changes in subgingingival microflora (Cobb 1996).

Reduction of the fluid and cellular components of an inflammatory lesion in the lamina propria should result in an increased proportion of collagen fibers, which when combined with reattachment of the junctional epithelium or the formation of a long junctional epithelium will produce increased resistance to passage of the probe tip. This results in a gain in clinical attachment.

Probing depths/clinical attachment level

Subgingival root debridement is contraindicated in sites that do not have periodontal pockets. A landmark clinical study showed that subgingival root debridement of teeth with initially shallow probing depths of less than 3 mm slightly decreased or did not alter probing depths, but loss of clinical attachment did occur (Lindhe et al. 1982). Taking into consideration a number of clinical studies over the past years, Cobb (1996) determined that thorough debridement of moderately deep pockets (4 to 6 mm) usually results in a mean reduction in probing depth of 1.29 mm and a mean gain in clinical attachment of 0.55 mm, whereas sites with deeper probing depth (7 mm or more) showed a mean reduction in probing depth of 2.16 mm and a gain in clinical attachment of 1.29 mm. Care in selecting sites that will benefit from subgingival debridement is essential in the prevention of clinical attachment loss.

Subgingival microflora

Periodontal debridement of pockets causes profound shifts in the composition of the subgingival microflora. After subgingival debridement, the number of gram-negative microorganisms decreases, especially spirochetes, and the number of gram-positive rods and cocci increases. However, this therapy may be ineffective in eliminating *Actinobacillus actinomycetemcomitans* from affected subgingival sites (Cobb 1996) because it invades soft tissue (Renvert et al. 1990).

Unfortunately, shifts in microfloral composition are transient, and usually the pocket area becomes repopulated with subgingival microorganisms within days to months. Since the subgingival microflora originate in supragingival areas (Waerhaug 1978), regular and effective plaque control and professional subgingival therapy are absolutely critical for long-term control of inflammatory periodontal diseases (Cobb 1996).

Bleeding on probing

Periodontal debridement has predictably reduced the levels of inflammation. A vast number of clinical studies conducted over recent years have shown that periodontal debridement has reduced bleeding in approximately 57% of sites (Cobb 1996).

TREATMENT SEQUENCE

The treatment sequence for periodontal debridement varies depending on clinical findings and diagnosis. The first step, after the disease is classified and a treatment plan is developed, is oral hygiene self-care instructions specifically designed for the patient's needs. Instrumentation procedures should be performed in a logical and orderly manner and usually are done to completion by quadrant.

Some patients with severe inflammation due to heavy plaque and calculus deposits may require initial debridement followed by a waiting period of a few weeks to allow the inflammation in the lamina propria to subside. The tissues will then be more resistant to penetration by instruments, and more definitive treatment can then be given.

Most patients undergoing subgingival debridement require topical and/or local anesthesia (Palmer and Floyd 1995). However, the patient must not have any allergy or sensitivity to the agent used. Two types of topical anesthetics are available: amide types, such as 5 or 10% lidocaine, and ester types, such as benzocaine (varied concentrations are available, but usually it is 20%). The possibility of allergic reactions is greater with lidocaine because it shows greater absorption into the systemic circulation than benzocaine. When a topical anesthetic is used, best results are obtained when a small amount is applied on a cotton-tip applicator, the tissues are dried prior to application of the agent, and the applicator is held in contact with the mucous membranes for 1 to 2 minutes. Alternatives include the use of an anesthetic patch, an anesthetic rinse, or electronic anesthesia. Topical anesthetic sprays should not be used because high doses of the agent can be absorbed into the circulatory system.

Local anesthesia is best applied by quadrant. It is recommended to treat one or two quadrants during a single visit depending on the number of teeth present as well as the degree of difficulty of the intervention. When two quadrants are treated during the same appointment, usual practice is to treat the upper and lower quadrants on either the right or the left side of the face. Both mandibular quadrants should not be treated during the same appointment so as to avoid patient discomfort and to prevent an inability on the part of the patient to control his or her mandible with both sides anesthetized.

Posttreatment care focuses on the prevention of dental plaque formation. A long-term plaque-free dentition is an unrealistic goal, and for this reason, periodic periodontal maintenance visits are required to monitor and identify disease recurrence (Westfelt 1996).

PERIODONTAL DEBRIDEMENT PROCEDURES

Before debridement procedures are started, it is necessary to obtain a written informed consent from the patient. The procedure and its expected outcomes are explained to the patient. It is important for the patient to understand that the decreased probing depths primarily due to gingival shrinkage may cause gingival recession and "longer looking" teeth and that teeth may respond with hypersensitivity to cold, toothbrushing, or sweets. Such hypersensitivity is usually not permanent, but it may cause pain and discomfort that lasts for a few weeks to months.

Subgingival debridement

Calculus Removal   As periodontal debridement is started on a patient, the primary goal is to remove gross deposits from supragingival and subgingival tooth surfaces. The ultimate goal of subgingival debridement is to render a root surface free of plaque, calculus, and endotoxins to enable soft tissue healing. Complete calculus removal is essentially not attainable (Kepic, O'Leary, and Kafrawy 1990), and total root smoothness is not necessary for adequate tissue healing. Clinical studies have shown that practitioners who spent an average of 12 to 15 minutes to complete the debridement of each tooth with hand and ultrasonic instruments fail to remove calculus from all surfaces. After debridement, about 47% of all nonfurcated surfaces and 63% of 6 mm or larger pockets showed residual calculus. Surgical access reduced the frequency of residual calculus to 20 and 38%, respectively. Teeth with furcations had a higher frequency of residual calculus, and surgical access did not provide any additional benefit (Caffesse, Sweeney, and Smith 1986; Buchanan and Robertson 1987; Fleischer et al. 1989).

While total elimination of causative factors is an appropriate treatment goal, reduction of dental plaque and calculus below threshold levels appears to control the disease process and improve clinical signs of inflammation (Robertson 1990), producing significant reductions in gingivitis, tooth loss, attachment loss, severity of disease, and probing depths (American Academy of Periodontology 1997). Thus, if periodontal debridement can achieve elimination of inflammation and disease progression, then no further treatment is necessary. If periodontal debridement fails to achieve these objectives, then periodontal surgery may be necessary.

Root Surface Characteristics With the development of a gram-negative bacterial flora in the gingival crevice, events occur that eventually cause breakdown of the attachment apparatus. If elimination or disruption of the subgingival bacteria is not accomplished, rapid growth and maturation occur. During growth and after the death of subgingival gram-negative microorganisms, endotoxins or lipooligosaccharides are released from their cell walls. Endotoxins are highly toxic compounds that are capable of penetrating the junctional epithelium and entering the connective tissue, resulting in destruction of periodontal tissues. This causes loss of connective tissue attachment from the root surface, apical migration of the junctional epithelium, and bone loss. A periodontal pocket forms, and the root surface (cementum) becomes contaminated when exposed to this new subgingival pocket environment. The cementum is sufficiently porous to allow binding of endotoxins and colonization of dental plaque and calculus onto the altered root surfaces. Cementum that is rough and impregnated with calculus or contaminated with toxins or microorganisms and dentin is referred to as *contaminated, altered,* or *necrotic cementum.*

Cementum Removal The periodontal literature offers no firm conclusions about either the feasibility of or the need for removal of all contaminated cementum. In the past it was thought that the presence of cementum-bound endotoxins inhibited tissue healing after periodontal debridement. Much investigation has been directed toward the elimination of this contaminated or necrotic cementum. It is the consensus that endotoxins found on diseased root surfaces are weakly and superficially bound and that 99% may be removed by brushing (Nakib et al. 1982; Moore, Wilson, and Kieser 1986). The primary reason for removing the superficial layer of cementum by subgingival debridement is to remove plaque and calculus from the irregularities on the root surface. Extensive subgingival debridement for a prolonged amount of time is unnecessary (Cheetham, Wilson, and Kieser 1988), and total removal of cementum is not the goal because the attachment of new soft tissue to the root surface is enhanced by the presence of cementum (Somerman et al. 1987). O'Leary and Kafrawy (1983) concluded that total removal of cementum under routine clinical conditions is not a realistic objective of therapy. Smart et al. (1990), using ultrasonic instrumentation, showed that contaminated root surfaces could be rendered comparable to healthy teeth. Therefore, the key to periodontal therapy is the removal of plaque and calculus in order to reduce the number of oral bacteria below the threshold level capable of initiating inflammation (American Academy of Periodontology 1997). Precisely how much cementum is removed as a result of root planing is uncertain.

Therefore, it is important to attain relatively smooth root surfaces only for the purpose of reducing plaque retention without excessive and unnecessary removal of cementum and dentin. *The therapeutic goal of debridement therapy is to control bacterial infection as opposed to simply removing deposits from root surfaces.*

ADVERSE EFFECTS OF PERIODONTAL DEBRIDEMENT

Subgingival debridement may cause dentinal hypersensitivity as a result of removal of the thin outer layer of cementum and exposure of the underlying dentin. Usually, teeth are not sensitive immediately after the periodontal debridement; hypersensitivity may take about 3 to 4 days to appear. Treatment of dentinal hypersensitivity is discussed in Chapters 10 and 11.

LIMITATIONS OF PERIODONTAL DEBRIDEMENT

Pocket depth

The effectiveness of periodontal debridement depends on the effectiveness of the mechanical removal of dental plaque and calculus. Root debridement does not always remove all plaque and calculus from subgingival tooth surfaces. Studies have shown that considerable amounts (54 to 57%) of calculus remain on the root surfaces of teeth with moderate or advanced pockets and that more residual calculus is found on tooth surfaces with increasing probing depths (Wylam et al. 1993). There was no significant difference whether an anterior or a posterior tooth was debrided (Sherman et al. 1990).

Current conclusions about the effectiveness of periodontal debridement in deeper pockets are conflicting, and there is as yet no agreement on whether nonsurgical instrumentation is effective in advanced periodontal lesions (Forabosco et al. 1996). The most frequently lost teeth in patients receiving comprehensive periodontal treatment are the molars. Explanations for this relate to the difficulty in achieving adequate daily plaque removal and the difficulty in properly debriding molars. Stambaugh et al. (1981) found that the average probing depth for "efficient" removal of plaque, calculus, and necrotic cementum was 3.73 mm. Rateitschak et al. (1992) found that surfaces where curets could reach usually were free of plaque and calculus, but in deep pockets the curet did not reach the base of the pocket. Consequently, modified curets with longer shanks were developed to increase treatment effectiveness in deeper pockets.

Furcations and root anatomy

Access for adequate instrumentation in the furcation area is often difficult, if not impossible, given the special anatomic characteristics of multirooted teeth (Greene 1995; Fleischer et al. 1989). Pathogenic microbial flora frequently persist in furcation lesions (Loos, Claffey, and Egelberg 1988). Narrow furcation openings make periodontal debridement a challenge. Fifty-eight percent of molars have furcation entrance diameters that are smaller than the smallest diameter of a relatively new curet, which is 0.75 mm (Bower 1979a; Parashis, Anagnon-Vareltzides, and Demetriou 1990).

Knowledge about the morphology of the furcation area and the variations in root form and structure is important for effective instrumentation. Root concavities, which are depressions found on the proximal root surfaces, are plaque and calculus traps, making instrumentation extremely difficult. For instance, a deep mesial concavity is found on the maxillary first premolar. On the maxillary first molars, the mesiobuccal root has the greatest incidence of concavities, whereas both the mesio- and distobuccal roots of the mandibular first molars have concavities (Bower 1979b; Fig. 12–1 ■). Mandibular incisors and the mesial root of the maxillary first premolar also have proximal concavities. Moreover, any other root also may have root concavities.

Time spent and clinician skill

Controversy exists over how much time should be spent on subgingival debridement. Subgingival debridement is sensitive to both technique and operator skill. Since endotoxins are just weakly bound to the root surface (Moore, Wilson, and Kieser 1986),

FIGURE 12–1

Root morphology. Root concavities in the maxillary molar decrease the effectiveness of debridement.

it is not necessary to spend a great deal of time debriding. However, a considerable amount of time still should be spent in effectively removing subgingival plaque, calculus, and necrotic cementum. If this procedure is done incorrectly, root gouging may occur, resulting in the production of grooves and pits in the root surface.

A clinical study (Anderson et al. 1996) evaluating single versus multiple episodes of subgingival instrumentation to determine effectiveness concluded that there was no significant difference between the two treatments. It was suggested that calculus remaining after one thorough episode of instrumentation is not likely to be removed by repeated instrumentation. How much time is enough? Most researchers suggest that periodontal debridement should take at least 10 minutes per tooth (Lowenguth and Greenstein 1995). Coldiron et al. (1990) found that cementum removal was generally achieved on periodontally healthy roots with 20 strokes of a curet, but residual calculus remained.

The results of a clinical study assessing periodontal debridement forces in periodontally involved molars show a broad range of forces being applied by the practitioner (Zappa et al. 1993). Additionally, the quality of periodontal debridement done on a molar may be primarily determined by the attitude of the practitioner, who subjectively treats the tooth according to his or her habits, rather than according to the characteristics of the root surfaces being treated (Zappa et al. 1993).

Most studies confirm that the more experienced the clinician, the more calculus-free the root surfaces were in deeper pockets and in hard-to-reach areas such as furcations (Brayer et al. 1989).

HEALING RESPONSE AND THE OUTCOME OF THERAPY

An expected outcome of debridement is tissue healing. Healing results in tissue repair, shrinkage of gingival tissue, and the renewal of epithelial cells in contact with tooth surfaces (Caton, Nyman, and Zander 1980; Caffesse, Mota, and Morrison 1995).

Generally, the same healing features of periodontal tissues are seen following debridement of any chronically inflamed site. Initially, following debridement, there is an acute inflammatory reaction due to the traumatic nature of the therapy. This inflammation subsides within 24 to 48 hours. Over the next week, there is a gradual reduction of inflammatory cells, epithelial tissue healing, and finally, connective tissue maturation with collagen deposition.

Gingivitis: Healing after periodontal debridement

Histologically, in gingivitis, once dental plaque and calculus are removed, the pocket epithelium will re-form into junctional epithelium and reattach to the adjacent tooth surface as it was in health. The inflammatory cells in the gingival connective tissue are replaced by collagen; this improvement results in an apparent "gain in clinical attachment".

Clinically, there is a reduction in or elimination of inflammation (e.g., bleeding) and the elimination of edema, both of which result in tissue shrinkage and occasionally gingival recession. Gingiva that is fibrotic will not shrink, as does edematous tissue. The gingiva often returns to its salmon pink color. The greatest reduction in probing depths occurs after 4 to 6 weeks and is primarily due to (1) tissue shrinkage, which may result in gingival recession, and (2) re-formation of collagen, which results in greater resistance to probing (Fig. 12–2a■). The reductions obtained in probing depths as a result of nonsurgical therapy are in the range of 1 to 2 mm.

Periodontitis: Healing after periodontal debridement

Histologically, in periodontitis, after the removal of dental plaque, calculus, and necrotic cementum, some healing will occur. In most patients, healing occurs by repair rather than regeneration (e.g., formation of new bone, cementum, and periodontal ligament). Histologically, repair of the root epithelial interface has been described as a long junctional epithelial attachment that prevents the formation of a new connective tissue attachment (Cobb 1996). Research has shown, however, that the presence of a long junctional epithelium does not represent an area of less resistance to infection (Caffesse, Sweeney, and Smith 1986; Beaumont, O'Leary, and Kafrawy 1983). However, patients who are erratic in their compliance with oral hygiene self-care do not do as well with a long junctional epithelium as patients with complete compliance (Wilson, Schoen, and Fallon 1989).

The pocket epithelium transforms back into junctional epithelium, which begins to reattach along the root surface between the gingival connective tissue and the root (see Fig. 12–2b■). The formation of a long junctional epithelium results in closure of the pocket. This reestablishment of the junctional epithelium most likely occurs within 1 (Caton and Zander 1979) or 2 (Waerhaug 1978) weeks. The inflammatory cells in the gingival connective tissue are replaced by collagen, but a long junctional epithelium prevents the formation of a gingival connective tissue attachment (gingival fibers). The greatest reduction in probing depths and gain in clinical attachment level can be measured after 4 to 6 weeks (Barrington 1981), although true gains in clinical attachment are seen primarily after periodontal surgery, if at all. Gains in clinical attachment level after treatment do not necessarily mean that new gingival connective tissue attachment has been achieved (Armitage 1996). It may simply indicate that the probe is more resistant to penetration once the gingival collagen has re-formed. This gives the appearance of a gain in clinical attachment when it actually may

FIGURE 12–2

Healing of the gingival tissues after subgingival debridement. (a) In gingivitis, the tissues will heal, with the junctional epithelium reattaching to the clean tooth surface. (b) In periodontitis, after root planing, the tissues heal by formation of a long junctional epithelial attachment to the root surface.

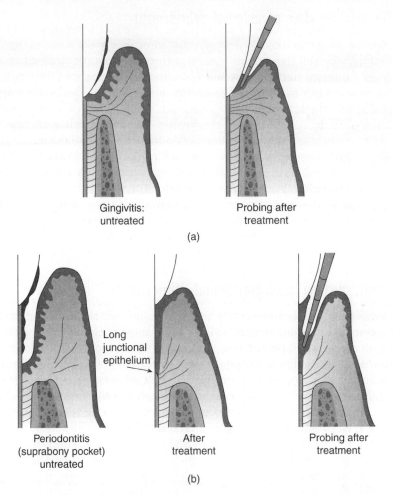

Gingivitis: Probing after
untreated   treatment

(a)

Long
junctional
epithelium

Periodontitis   After   Probing after
(suprabony pocket)   treatment   treatment
untreated

(b)

not be. It is the distance between the base of the periodontal pocket (before treatment) and the tip of the periodontal probe when placed into the crevice (after treatment). A true gain in clinical attachment after periodontal treatment indicates that a new connective tissue attachment (collagen fibers inserting) to the root has occurred.

Residual or undetected calculus that instrumentation has failed to remove is often present. Despite incomplete calculus removal, Sherman et al. (1990) showed that sites still could respond favorably. Haffajee et al. (1997) found that periodontal debridement demonstrated clinical improvement in subjects with chronic periodontitis even though only modest changes in subgingival microflora were seen. This suggests potential targets for therapy and indicates that radical alterations in subgingival microflora may not be necessary.

REEVALUATION OF INITIAL THERAPY: TISSUE RESPONSE

After appropriate initial therapy, a planned reevaluation should assess the current state of health or disease. The treatment sequence for the reevaluation appointment consists of a medical history update, a soft tissue examination, a plaque index, determination of the presence of bleeding, an oral hygiene self-care evaluation, and periodontal probing. Pretreatment findings are compared with the current status of the patient. It is important to evaluate and emphasize the patient's oral hygiene self-care techniques. Controversy exists regarding the recommended time interval between the initial therapy and the reevaluation appointment. Recommendations range from a minimum of 2 weeks to a maximum of 6 weeks after periodontal debridement to allow for tissue healing, although waiting longer than 6 weeks may augment the healing response. A shorter time period may be indicated if the patient has been classified as a potential surgical patient. If results of initial therapy show improvement, but with some residual 5-mm probing depths, the patient should be placed on periodontal maintenance and reevaluated in a few months. Reevaluation at regular intervals is essential to alert the dental hygienist to areas where plaque control has failed and inflammation has returned. Unstable sites should be retreated or monitored closely for signs of attachment loss. At the reevaluation appointment, a decision is made regarding whether the patient qualifies for surgical intervention, continues with initial therapy, or is placed on a periodontal maintenance schedule. Factors that may influence this decision include the overall treatment plan, including restorative procedures, as well as the desires of the patient.

Reevaluation includes an examination of the gingival tissues. If inflammation persists, which is apparent clinically as bleeding on probing and redness, the cause needs to be determined. Persistent inflammation may result from incomplete debridement, patient noncompliance with home care, or a systemic disease. The desired microbial response is a change in the composition of the bacteria found within the pocket from a pathogenic Gram-negative species (e.g., spirochetes, *P. gingivalis*, *P. intermedia*) to a more beneficial Gram-positive species such as cocci or nonmotile bacteria (Mousques, Listgarten, and Phillips 1980).

SUMMARY

The philosophy of periodontal therapy has changed over the past decade as a result of further understanding of the disease process. Therapy is based on up-to-date clinical and microbial studies. The decision to perform periodontal debridement as a definitive treatment should depend on the severity of periodontal disease, the inflammatory status of the gingiva, treatment objectives of the dental hygienist, treatment time, and the skill of the operator (Lowenguth and Greenstein 1995).

Selection of the proper instrument involves considering the following factors: the amount of calculus, the type of tissue tone (e.g., firm, edematous, or hard and fibrotic), probing depths (or type of disease present), root morphology, and location of the calculus. Root smoothness is no longer the main criterion for periodontal instrumentation, although all detectable deposits should be removed so as to achieve a successful soft tissue response. The primary goal of periodontal debridement is to make the root and the soft tissue biologically compatible (Wilson, Schoen, and Fallon 1989). In most cases, periodontal debridement improves clinical parameters, decreasing both gingival inflammation (evidenced by less bleeding) and probing depths. Improvements in microbial parameters are transient, and the microflora soon return to pretreatment levels. Therefore, the patient requires continuous maintenance or plaque control. Both periodontal debridement and daily plaque removal by the patient are equally important for the maintenance of periodontal health and will continue to be the standard of periodontal therapy.

KEY POINTS

✤ Successful periodontal treatment, maintenance of periodontal health, and the regeneration of periodontal tissues depend on the removal of supra- and subgingival deposits.

✤ Oral hygiene self-care and mechanical subgingival instrumentation are indicated in the treatment of inflammatory periodontal diseases to reduce inflammation and microbial levels. The clinical end point to periodontal debridement is a good tissue healing response.

✤ Periodontal debridement has been shown to disrupt or alter the subgingival microflora, thus slowing down repopulation.

✤ Although meticulous debridement may remove some cementum, the intentional, aggressive removal of diseased cementum does not seem to be necessary; endotoxins are loosely attached to the root surface and can be removed easily.

✤ The type of healing occurring after subgingival debridement is a long junctional epithelium attachment to the root surface, which is considered to be a type of repair.

REFERENCES

American Academy of Periodontology. 1997. Treatment of gingivitis and periodontitis. *J. Periodontol.* 68:1246–1253.

American Dental Association. 1995. *Current dental terminology.* Chicago: ADA.

American Dental Hygienist's Association. 1995. *A position paper on selective tooth polishing.* Chicago: ADHA.

Anderson, G. B., J. Palmer, F. Bye, B. Smith, and R. Caffesse. 1996. Effectiveness of subgingival scaling and root planing: Single versus multiple episodes of instrumentation. *J. Periodontol.* 67:367–373.

Armitage, G. C. 1996. Periodontal diseases: Diagnosis. *Ann. Periodontol.* 1:37–215.

Barrington, E. P. 1981. An overview of periodontal surgical procedures. *J. Periodontol.* 52:697–702.

Beaumont, R., T. O'Leary, and A. Kafrawy. 1984. Relative resistance of long junctional epithelial adhesions and connective tissue attachments to plaque-induced inflammation. *J. Periodontol.* 55:213–223.

Bower, R. C. 1979a. Furcation morphology relative to periodontal treatment: Furcation entrance architecture. *J. Periodontol.* 50:23–27.

Bower, R. C. 1979b. Furcation morphology relative to periodontal treatment: Furcation root surface anatomy. *J. Periodontol.* 50:366–374.

Brayer, W. K., J. T. Mellonig, R. M. Dunlap, K. W. Marinak, and R. E. Carson. 1989. Scaling and root planing effectiveness: The effect of root surface access and operator experience. *J. Periodontol.* 60:67–72.

Buchanan, S. A., and P. S. Robertson. 1987. Calculus removal by scaling and root planing with and without surgical access. *J. Periodontol.* 58:159–163.

Caffesse, R. G., L. F. Mota, and E. D. Morrison. 1995. The rationale for periodontal therapy. *Periodontology 2000* 9:7–13.

Caffesse, R. G., P. L. Sweeney, and B. A. Smith. 1986. Scaling and root planing with and without periodontal flap surgery. *J. Clin. Periodontol.* 13:205–210.

Caton, J., S. Nyman, and H. Zander. 1980. Histometric evaluation of periodontal surgery: II. Connective tissue attachment after four regenerative procedures. *J. Clin. Periodontol.* 7:224–231.

Caton, J., and H. Zander. 1979. The attachment between tooth and gingival tissues after periodontic root planing and soft tissue curettage. *J. Periodontol.* 50:462–466.

Cheetham, W. A., M. Wilson, and J. B. Kieser. 1988. Root surface debridement: An in vitro assessment. *J. Clin. Periodontol.* 15:288–292.

Ciancio, S. G. 1989. Non-surgical periodontal treatment. In: *Proceedings of the world workshop in clinical periodontics,* Vol. 2, ed. M. Nevins, W. Becker, and K. Kornman, 1–22. Chicago: American Academy of Periodontology.

Cobb, C. M. 1996. Non-surgical pocket therapy: Mechanical. *Ann. Periodontol.* 1:443–490.

Coldiron, N. B., R. A. Yukna, J. Weir, and R. F. Caudill. 1990. A quantitative study of cementum removal with hand curettes. *J. Periodontol.* 61:293–299.

Dahlen, G., J. Lindhe, K. Sato, H. Hanamura, and H. Okamoto. 1992. The effect of supragingival plaque control on the subgingival microbiota in subjects with periodontal disease. *J. Clin. Periodontol.* 19:802–809.

Fleischer, H. C., J. T. Mellonig, W. K. Brayer, J. L. Gray, and J. D. Barnett. 1989. Scaling and root planing efficacy in multirooted teeth. *J. Periodontol.* 60:402–409.

Forabosco, A., R. Galetti, S. Spinato, P. Colao, and C. Casolari. 1996. A comparative study of a surgical method and scaling and root planing using Odontoson. *J. Clin. Periodontol.* 23:611–614.

Greene, P. R. 1995. Non-surgical periodontal therapy: Essential and adjunctive methods. *Br. Dent. J.* 179:28–34.

Haffajee, A. D., M. A. Cugini, S. Dibart, C. Smith, L. R. Kent, Jr., and S. S. Socransky. 1997. The effect of scaling and root planing on the clinical and microbiological parameters of periodontal diseases. *J. Clin. Periodontol.* 24:324–334.

Jacobson, L., J. Blomlöf, and S. Lindskog. 1994. Root surface texture after different scaling modalities. *Scand. J. Dent. Res.* 102:156–160.

Kaldahl, W. B., K. L. Kalkwarf, D. Kashinath, D. Patil, M. P. Molvar, and J. K. Dyer. 1996. Long-term evaluation of periodontal therapy: I. Response to four therapeutic modalities. *J. Periodontol.* 67:93–102.

Kalkwarf, K. L. 1989. Tissue attachment. In: *Proceedings of the world workshop in clinical periodontics,* Vol. 5, ed. M. Nevins, W. Becker, and K. Kornman, 1–21. Chicago: American Academy of Periodontology.

Katsanoulas, T., I. Renee, and R. Attström. 1992. The effect of supragingival plaque control on the composition of the subgingival flora in periodontal pockets. *J. Clin. Periodontol.* 19:760–765.

Kepic, T. J., T. J. O'Leary, A. H. Kafrawy. 1990. Total calculus removal: An attainable objective? *J. Periodontol.* 61:16–20.

Lindhe, J., S. S. Socransky, S. Nyman, and A. Haffajee. 1982. Critical probing depth. *J. Clin. Periodontol.* 9:323–336.

Loos, B., N. Claffey, and J. Egelberg. 1988. Clinical and microbiological effects of subgingival debridement in periodontal furcation pockets. *J. Clin. Periodontol.* 15:453–463.

Lowenguth, R. A., and G. Greenstein. 1995. Clinical and microbiological response to nonsurgical mechanical periodontal therapy. *Periodontology 2000* 9:14–22.

Magnusson, I., J. Lindhe, T. Yoneyama, and B. Liljenberg. 1984. Recolonization of a subgingival microbiota following scaling in deep pockets. *J. Clin. Periodontol.* 11:193–207.

Moore, J., M. Wilson, and J. B. Kieser. 1986. The distribution of bacterial lipopolysaccharide (endotoxins) in relation to periodontal involved root surfaces. *J. Clin. Periodontol.* 13:748–751.

Mousques, T., M. A. Listgarten, R. W. Phillips. 1980. Effect of scaling and root planing on the composition of the human subgingival microbial flora. *J. Periodont. Res.* 15:144–151.

Nakib, N. M., N. F. Bissada, J. W. Simmelink, and S. N. Goldstine. 1982. Endotoxin penetration into root cementum of periodontally healthy and diseased human teeth. *J. Periodontol.* 53:368–378.

Oberholzer, R., and K. H. Rateitschak. 1996. Root cleaning or root smoothing: An in vivo study. *J. Clin. Periodontol.* 23:326–330.

O'Hehir, T. E. 1999. Debridement = scaling and root planing plus. RDH May:14, 62.

O'Leary, T. J., and A. D. Kafrawy. 1983. Total cementum removal: A realistic objective. *J. Periodontol.* 54:221–226.

Palmer, R. M., and F. D. Floyd. 1995. Periodontology: A clinical approach: 3. Non-surgical treatment and maintenance. *Br. Dent. J.* 178:263–268.

Parashis, A. O., A. Anagnou-Vareltzides, and N. Demetriou. 1990. Calculus removal from multirooted teeth with and without surgical access: II. Comparison between external and furcation surfaces and effect of furcation entrance width. *J. Clin. Periodontol.* 20:294–298.

Rateitschak, P., J. Schwarz, R. Guggenheim, M. Duggelin, and K. Rateitschak. 1992. Nonsurgical periodontal treatment: Where are the limits? An SEM study. *J. Clin. Periodontol.* 19:240–244.

Renvert, S., M. Wikström, G. Dahlen, J. Slots, and J. Egelberg. 1990. Effect of subgingival debridement on the elimination of *Actinobacillus actinomycetemcomitans* and *Bacteroides gingivalis* from periodontal pockets. *J. Clin. Periodontol.* 17:345–350.

Robertson, P. B. 1990. The residual calculus paradox. *J. Periodontol.* 61:65–66.

Sbordone, L., L. Ramaglia, E. Gulletta, and V. Iacono. 1990. Recolonization of the subgingival microflora after scaling and root planing in human periodontitis. *J. Periodontol.* 61:579–584.

Sherman, P. R., L. H. Hutchens, Jr., L. G. Jewson, J. M. Moriarty, G. W. Greco, and W. T. McFall, Jr. 1990. The effectiveness of subgingival scaling and root planing: I. Clinical detection of residual calculus. *J. Periodontol.* 61:3–8.

Smart, G. J., M. Wilson, E. H. Davies, and J. B. Kieser. 1990. The assessment of ultrasonic root surface debridement by determination of residual endotoxins levels. *J. Clin. Periodontol.* 17:174–178.

Somerman, M. J., S. Y. Archer, A. Shteyer, et al. 1987. Protein production by human gingival fibroblasts is enhanced by guanidine EDTA extracts of cementum. *J. Periodont. Res.* 22:75–77.

Stambaugh, R. V., M. Dragoo, D. M. Smith, and L. Carasali. 1981. The limits of subgingival scaling. *Int. J. Periodont. Restor. Dent.* 1(5):31–41.

Waerhaug, J. 1978. Healing of the dentoepithelial junction following subgingival plaque control: II. As observed on extracted teeth. *J. Periodontol.* 49:119–134.

Westfelt, E. 1996. Rationale of mechanical plaque control. *J. Clin. Periodontol.* 23:263–267.

Westfelt, E., H. Rylander, G. Dahlén, and J. Lindhe. 1998. The effect of supragingival plaque control on the progression of advanced periodontal disease. *J. Clin. Periodontol.* 25:536–541.

Wilson, T. G., Jr., J. Schoen, and P. Fallon. 1989. Removing tooth-borne dental deposits: Mechanical means by the professional. In: *Dental maintenance for patients with periodontal diseases,* ed. T. G. Wilson, Jr., 67–96. Chicago: Quintessence Books.

Wylam, J. M., B. L. Mealey, M. P. Mills, T. C. Waldrop, and D. C. Moskowicz. 1993. The clinical effectiveness of open versus closed scaling and root planing on multirooted teeth. *J. Periodontol.* 64:1023–1028.

Zappa, U., J. P. Röthlisberger, C. Simona, and D. Case. 1993. In vivo scaling and root planing forces in molars. *J. Periodontol.* 64:349–354.

SELF-QUIZ

1. Which one of the following healing responses is seen in gingivitis after periodontal debridement? (p. 389)

   a. formation of new bone, cementum, and periodontal ligament

   b. formation of new cementum and periodontal ligament

   c. reattachment of the junctional epithelium

   d. reattachment of the alveolar mucosa

2. Which one of the following healing responses is seen in periodontitis after periodontal debridement? (p. 389)

   a. reattachment of the sulculuar epithelium

   b. reattachment of the desmosomes

   c. formation of new bone, cementum, and periodontal ligament

   d. formation of a long junctional epithelium

3. Which one of the following definitions describes a gain in clinical attachment after periodontal debridement? (p. 389)

   a. bone fill and formation of new cementum

   b. improved gingival tone and reattachment of the junctional epithelium

   c. improved gingival tone and increased mature collagen fibers

   d. gingival recession, bone fill, and establishment of a new periodontal ligament attachment

4. After periodontal debridement, on which one of the following does clinical success depend? (pp. 390–391)

   a. amount of time spent on the procedure

   b. number of quadrants completed

   c. total removal of calculus

   d. tissue response

5. Which one of the following benefits is seen after subgingival debridement? (pp. 382–383)

    a. disruption of the Gram-negative microbial flora
    b. repopulation of Gram-negative anaerobic flora
    c. removal of Gram-positive facultative flora
    d. interference with attachment of Gram-positive anaerobic flora to root surfaces

II. POWER-DRIVEN SCALERS

Cynthia Fong, R.D.H., M.S.

Goal:

To provide the dental hygienist with the fundamental principles of power-driven scalers.

Educational Objectives:

Upon completion of the chapter subsection, the reader should be able to:

Explain the rationale for using power-driven scalers;

List and discuss the different types of power-driven scalers;

Discuss the history of power-driven scalers, including the development of the new modified ultrasonic inserts;

List and discuss examples of commercially available sonic and ultrasonic devices;

Discuss the effectiveness of power-driven scaling over standard hand-activated instrumentation;

Describe the technique and use of periodontal ultrasonic inserts; and

Discuss the care and maintenance of ultrasonic units and inserts.

Over the last four decades, the literature has changed considerably in what it has documented as the chief etiologic agent of periodontal diseases. Concomitantly, the primary purpose of periodontal instrumentation also has changed. In the 1960s, research supported a nonspecific plaque hypothesis that was based on a causal relationship between plaque and disease. The *quantity* of plaque was of particular concern, not necessarily the *quality* of plaque. Calculus was viewed as the primary cause of periodontal inflammation, and if the deposits were removed through the process of scaling, the disease could be controlled. Although a clear relationship was established between calculus and soft tissue response by the 1970s, the literature began to deviate away from focusing solely on the removal of calculus. Removing dental plaque, endotoxins (lipoòligosaccharides), and cementum through definitive scaling and root planing also was required to treat the disease. Research documented a specific plaque hypothesis, and a differentiation was made between loosely adherent plaque and adherent plaque. It also was established that endotoxins could be removed through gentle dental procedures such as brushing, suggesting that effective root surface debridement could

KEY WORDS
- power-driven scalers
- ultrasonic devices
- sonic device

be achieved by methods other than traditional hand instrumentation (Moore, Wilson, and Kieser 1986). By the 1980s it was well established that the *quality* of plaque played a greater role in contributing to periodontal disease than the *quantity* of plaque. Periodontal inflammation was directly correlated with number and types of invasive microorganisms, and antimicrobial usage began. Clinicians began to focus on periodontal debridement and the disruption of bacterial colonies during instrumentation in order to treat the disease. Woodall (1993) defined periodontal debridement as the "treatment of gingival and periodontal inflammation through mechanical removal of tooth and root surface irritants to the extent that the adjacent soft tissues maintain or return to a healthy non-inflamed state." Instrumentation emphasized disrupting microorganisms, as supported by a critical-mass theory, which was defined at the 1989 World Workshop on Clinical Periodontics as "the reduction of the quantity (mass) of pathogenic microflora below the level (critical) where the host can defend itself." In the 1990s, research showed periodontal disease to be a definite disease process in which an interaction occurs between microbes and the host response. It also was established that complete removal of diseased cementum is neither attainable nor desirable, regardless of the device used (Corbet, Vaughan, and Kieser 1993; Fukazawa and Nishimura 1994; Eschler and Rapley 1991). Currently, clinicians concentrate on treatment to stimulate the host's immune response. *Tissue response is stressed as an end point of therapy rather than root smoothness*. The diagnosis and treatment of specific sites rather than full mouth treatment are emphasized in order to achieve the current objectives of periodontal therapy.

The paradigm shifts that have occurred in periodontal therapy have led clinicians to broaden the scope and increase their use of **power-driven scalers** (the term *power scaler* is also used in this book) for the purposes of full-mouth periodontal debridement. Historically, since power scalers were first introduced in 1955, their use has been restricted to removing heavy supragingival deposits of calculus. However, a current review of the literature reveals that this premise is no longer true as a result of changes in the physical design (size and shape of the tip) of power scaling instruments and documentation of the effects that ultrasonics have on microorganisms. Consequently, modified power scaling instruments can now be used subgingivally, are indicated for the removal of light deposits and for deplaquing, and should be considered to have a primary role in root debridement.

This chapter subsection provides the reader with a review of the literature as it relates to power scalers, their mechanisms of action, types, special characteristics, commercial examples of units and inserts, insert sterilization and replacement, clinical recommendations, clinical technique, and treatment evaluation.

EFFICACY OF POWER-DRIVEN SCALERS

The efficacy of ultrasonic devices was first documented in 1957 by Johnson and Wilson. This classic study demonstrated not only that ultrasonic devices were capable of removing calculus but also that only light pressure was needed. Stains were removed effectively and cementum was unharmed if the working end of the device was flat instead of sharp. Little hemorrhaging was associated with such devices. In addition, ultrasonic devices were faster than hand instruments, and clinicians preferred them to hand instrumentation.

The current literature continues to document the ability of power scalers to remove calculus efficiently and also demonstrates that similar levels of gingival health are attained, as well as histologic repair rates, when compared with the use of hand instruments (Copulos et al. 1993; Torfason et al. 1979; Oosterwaal et al. 1987; Chiew et al. 1991; Hou et al. 1987; Biagini et al. 1988). Copulos et al. (1993) treated selected sites of patients diagnosed with periodontal disease with either a modified slim-diameter ultrasonic insert or a Gracey curet. Clinical parameters were evaluated using a plaque index, a gingival index, and bleeding on probing. Results showed that the modified insert was as effective as the curet, and the insert was significantly quicker.

The suggestion that root planing with hand instruments does not always have to follow ultrasonic instrumentation was made as early as 1979 (Torfason et al. 1979). This study provided the validity to this suggestion by showing that there were no clinically significant differences on the effect of gingival healing or in subgingival root surface roughness and cementum removal after treatment with hand instruments or ultrasonic devices.

Traditionally, one universal type of power scaling insert, which is large in diameter, enabled clinicians to remove gross deposits of supragingival calculus. However, with the advent of modified slim-diameter inserts, changes occurred with regard to when, where, why, and how power scalers could be used for periodontal debridement. The research has well documented the expanded role of modified ultrasonic inserts in comparison with unmodified universal inserts or hand instruments (Dragoo 1992; Drisko 1993; Leon and Vogel 1987). It has been demonstrated consistently that modified inserts provide better access to subgingival areas (in particular furcations), cause less damage, remove deposits better, require less time, and produce less operator fatigue than unmodified inserts or hand instruments (Bower 1979). Thirty-three papers were reviewed by Drisko (1993), who concluded that root debridement could be achieved without overinstrumentation using power scalers.

Several studies also have documented that ultrasonic devices are capable of easily altering or lysing (breaking up) and removing endotoxins that were present on tooth and root surfaces (Olsen and Socransky 1981; Thilo and Baehni 1987; Walmsley et al. 1990; Smart et al. 1990). In particular, gram-negative pathogens were found to be more susceptible to ultrasonic sonification than gram-positive pathogens. The ability of ultrasonic devices to eliminate microflora is related to their effects of acoustical streaming, acoustical turbulence, and cavitation. In general, acoustics are the energy associated with sound waves. *Acoustical streaming* is the unidirectional fluid flow caused by ultrasound waves and occurs at lower acoustical pressures than cavitation. *Acoustical turbulence* is created when movement of the device tip causes the coolant to accelerate, producing an intensified swirling effect that disrupts the bacterial matrix. Turbulence is increased as the power knob is adjusted to higher power settings. *Cavitation* is the formation of bubbles in liquids as a result of rapid changes, such as those induced by ultrasound. When the bubbles implode, they produce shock waves in the liquid. All these ultrasonic effects were documented in a study that used ultrasonic devices and concluded that "cavitational activity within the cooling water supply of the ultrasonic scaler results in a superficial removal of root surface constituents" (Walmsley et al. 1990). These effects also support expansion in the use of ultrasonic devices beyond the traditional removal of heavy supragingival calculus deposits to include the more current objectives of periodontal therapy, which are to disrupt bacterial colonies and stimulate the host immune response.

LIMITATIONS

Although, the literature has clearly documented the advantages of using ultrasonic devices for periodontal therapy, there are also limitations (Table 12–1 ■). Increased access and adaptability are realized only if a slim-diameter ultrasonic insert is used for debridement. Access and adaptability are not enhanced if an unmodified insert is used. Patient comfort can be classified as both an advantage and a limitation because comfort depends on an individual's pain response, acceptance of treatment, and operator technique. Some patients may claim that treatment with ultrasonic devices is more comfortable than treatment with hand instrumentation because it is more efficient and requires less treatment time. However, other patients may find the aerosols and sounds produced by an ultrasonic device disagreeable, resulting in the perception of discomfort. Unlike Gracey curets that possess only one lower cutting blade for debridement, power scaling inserts have a minimum of two and a maximum of four surfaces that can be used for removing deposits. The lavage of a power scaler not only contributes to the bactericidal effect of ultrasonics but also serves to enhance the field of vision by flushing and removing the debris from the area after removal.

Of the limitations cited in Table 12–1, less tactile sense on the part of the technician is absolute when compared with hand instruments. However, adaptation of an inactivated insert will provide the clinician with a gross evaluation of the amount of deposit remaining before a final assessment of the debridement is made with an explorer. As a result of the aerosols that are generated by a power scaler, preprocedural rinses, proper placement of a high-volume evacuator tip or saliva ejector, and use of protective barriers for both the patient and the clinician are highly recommended.

MECHANISM OF ACTION

The ability of a power-driven scaler to efficiently remove deposits is related to its clinical power. Clinical power is based on the device's frequency, stroke, type of motion, and angulation of that motion against the tooth surface.

TABLE 12–1	
ADVANTAGES AND LIMITATIONS OF ULTRASONIC DEBRIDEMENT	
ADVANTAGES	**LIMITATIONS**
Less time	Heat production
Less fatiguing	Requires water and suction
Sharpening is eliminated	Less tactile sense
Increased access and adaptability	Noise level
Patient comfort	Patient comfort
Multiple sides of the insert are active	Aerosol production
Promotes faster healing of the treated periodontal wound	Impeded visibility
Lavage	
Bactericidal effect	

Frequency is defined as the number of times per second the insert tip moves back and forth during one cycle. A 30-kHz frequency means that the insert tip is vibrating 30,000 times per second; a 25-kHz insert tip vibrates at 25,000 times per second. Forgas et al. (1991) conducted a study to determine if differing frequencies, 25 versus 30 kHz, differed significantly in their ability to remove calculus. Results showed no significant difference with regard to clinical efficacy of either frequency. However, the 30-kHz frequency was preferred by 71.43% of the clinicians participating in the study. Reasons cited were ease of operation, maneuverability of the handpiece, perceived effectiveness, efficiency, and vibration of the handpiece.

Frequency directly affects the portion of the insert tip that is active. During debridment, only the active area of the insert tip is capable of efficiently removing deposits. Higher frequencies reduce the amount of active tip area. A 25-kHz frequency enables the clinician to adapt the anterior 4.3 mm of the insert tip, whereas a 30-kHz frequency possesses an active area of 4.2 mm and a 50-kHz frequency has an active area of 2.3 mm. The upper part of Fig. 12–3 ■ depicts a 30-kHz insert in which approximately the anterior third of the insert can be adapted for debridement, whereas the lower part depicts a 42-kHz insert in which only the anterior sixth of the insert can be adapted for the efficient removal of the deposit.

Stroke is the second mechanism of action. *Stroke* defines the maximum distance the insert tip moves during one cycle. The power knob on the unit adjusts the stroke length. As the adjustment of the power knob is increased from low to high, the length of the stroke, or distance the insert tip moves, increased without a change in the frequency. The power knob also defines the amount of electrical energy that is provided to the handpiece used to generate movement of the insert tip. Frequently, the term *amplitude* is also used when referring to stroke. Amplitude is equal to one-half the distance of a single stroke.

A power scaler's type of motion, also referred to as *stroke pattern,* can be either linear or elliptical to orbital. The type of motion has an impact on the clinical technique used during instrumentation and will be discussed later in this chapter.

A characteristic associated only with ultrasonic devices and not with sonic devices is tuning. An ultrasonic device is tuned either automatically or manually. Tuning affects the frequency of the device. First-generation ultrasonic devices were tuned manually. Automatically tuned devices have two control knobs

---

FIGURE 12–3

Active tip area in relation to frequency. (Reprinted with permission from Dentsply Preventive Care, York, PA)

FIGURE 12–4

Front view of an auto-tuned device. (Reprinted with permission from Dentsply Preventive Care, York, PA)

FIGURE 12–5

Front view of a manually tuned device. (Reprinted with permission from Dentsply Preventive Care, York, PA)

(Fig. 12–4 ■), a power control knob and a water-control knob, whereas a manually tuned device generally has a third knob that controls the tuning of the device (Fig. 12–5 ■). With both devices, the water-control knob enables the clinician to control the amount of water delivered to the insert. As discussed previously, the power knob for both devices controls the length of the stroke. Many clinicians erroneously believe that adjusting the power knob controls the frequency of the insert. In fact, the unit, through motional feedback, controls the frequency of an automatically tuned device. The feedback is a constant self-adjustment of energy to ensure that the insert is vibrating at its set frequency. This ensures that the insert will efficiently remove the deposit regardless of its location or quantity. The frequency of a manually tuned device is not constant.

FIGURE 12–6

Cavitron SPS. (Reprinted with permission from Dentsply Preventive Care, York, PA)

It fluctuates during debridement and must be readjusted by the clinician through sight and sound to ensure that the insert is vibrating at its peak efficiency. As a result of the frequent readjustments required when using a manually tuned device, most clinicians currently use an automatically tuned device. Clinicians who elect to use a manually tuned device say that by adjusting both the power and tuning knobs to low, patient comfort can be increased during instrumentation. This premise has not been substantiated in the scientific literature. However, the use of low power and low tuning, regardless of the quantity of deposit requiring removal, will compromise the device's ability to efficiently remove the deposit. Essentially, the decision to use an automatically tuned device versus a manually tuned device should be based on the type of patient population typically treated, objective of instrumentation, and the importance placed on controlling the variables associated with each device. An example of a unit that offers sustained scaling performance at all power controls, including an extended low-low power control that is ideal for deplaquing, is presented in Fig. 12–6 ■.

DISTINGUISHING FEATURES OF POWER-DRIVEN SCALERS

There are two distinct types of power-driven scalers, ultrasonic or sonic, based on operating frequencies (Table 12–2 ■). **Ultrasonic devices** are further classified as either magnetostrictive or piezoelectric. Ultrasonic instruments convert high-frequency electric current into mechanical vibrations. A **sonic device** uses compressed air as its energy source to move a rotor system that produces vibrations of the sonic tip. The tip is attached to a high- or slow-speed handpiece to which water is supplied through the tubing (Fig. 12–7 ■). Sonic devices operate at a much lower frequency than ultrasonic devices. Lower frequencies result in an audible sound during activation. The type of motion or stroke pattern associated with a sonic tip is elliptical to orbital. This enables the clinician to adapt all surfaces of the sonic tip, including the two lateral borders, the back, and the face for debridement.

		TABLE 12–2	
TYPES AND CHARACTERISTICS OF POWER-DRIVEN SCALERS			
CHARACTERISTIC	**SONIC**	**MAGNETOSTRICTIVE ULTRASONIC**	**PIEZOELECTRIC ULTRASONIC**
Soundwave level	Audible	Inaudible	Inaudible
Energy source	Compressed air	Electrical energy applied to metal stacks or rod	Electrical energy applied to crystals
Frequency (cycles per second, Hz)	3000–8000	18,000–42,000	24,000–45,000
Active tip surfaces	All (back, face, and lateral borders)	All (back, face, and lateral borders)	Two (lateral borders)
Type of insert motion (stroke pattern)	Elliptical to orbital	Elliptical to orbital	Linear

Source: Adapted with permission from K. Jankowski. (Dentsply, York, PA)

	FIGURE 12–7

Sonic device attached to slow-speed handpiece. (Reprinted with permission from Dentsply Preventive Care, York, PA)

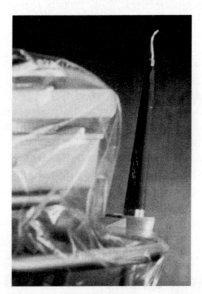

Both magnetostrictive and piezoelectric ultrasonic devices use high levels of electrical energy that is converted to mechanical energy. As the electrical energy is applied to a magnetostrictive insert, it magnetically changes its dimension to produce vibrations. Both ultrasonic and sonic scalers use, in part, mechanical vibrations to dislodge calculus deposits from tooth surfaces.

The constant elongation and contraction of a magnetostrictive insert produces heat that necessitates the supply of water to serve as a coolant. Magnetostrictive technology uses inserts consisting of a working tip, connecting body, and either a metal stack (Fig. 12–8 ■) or a single ferromagnetic rod. The connecting body is housed within either a metal or plastic grip. The decision to select an

Magnetostrictive insert with stacks. (Reprinted with permission from Dentsply Preventive Care, York, PA)

insert with a plastic versus metal grip is entirely up to clinician preference. All magnetostrictive devices have an elliptical to orbital stroke pattern.

Piezoelectric technology uses a tip instead of an insert that is screwed into a permanently sealed handpiece, similar to a sonic device. Ceramic crystals are housed within the handpiece, and these also change dimensions as electrical energy is applied to produce vibrations. Less heat is generated with a piezoelectric versus a magnetostrictive device, although water is still required to counterbalance the frictional heat generated by the movement of the insert and to enhance visibility by flushing debris away from the site following removal.

EXAMPLES OF POWER-DRIVEN SCALERS

Table 12–3 ■ lists the current commercially available ultrasonic devices, and Table 12–4 ■ provides a list of sonic devices. Prices and features of power scalers, such as autoclavable handpieces, autoclavable water lines, built-in lavage dispensers, and dual handpieces, vary widely. Therefore, it is recommended that clinicians contact the manufacturer directly for specific information. An excellent resource that will provide clinicians with an independent evaluation of power scalers is the June 1998 *Newsletter of the Clinical Research Associates,* which is devoted in its entirety to the analysis of sonic and ultrasonic devices (Clinical Research Associates 1998)

EXAMPLES OF POWER SCALING INSERTS AND TIPS

Sonic devices use tips that are screwed into a handpiece with a special wrench. The tips available for sonic scalers are basically limited to a sickle-shaped tip, a universal tip, and a periodontal-type tip (Table 12–5 ■). Essentially, all the tips are straight-shanked and large in diameter. The shank of the periodontal tip is longer in length than the sickle-shaped or universal tip. Two of the sonic tips, SofTip™ (Dentsply Midwest, York, PA) and VersaTip™ (MicroMotors, Inc., Santa Ana, CA), consist of an autoclavable base and a disposable tip, and they are designed specifically for the maintenance of titanium implants.

Ultrasonic devices offer a wider variety of inserts and tips than sonic devices (Tables 12–6 ■ and 12–7 ■). All piezoelectric tips possess an internal water delivery system. When selecting an insert, clinicians should first consider the patient's

TABLE 12–3
COMMERCIALLY AVAILABLE ULTRASONIC DEVICES

MANUFACTURER	MODEL	FREQUENCY(HZ)	TYPE
Amadent	P-5 Booster	30,000	Piezoelectric
	P-Max-Lux	27,000–33,000	Piezoelectric
Biotrol International	Amdent 830	25,000	Piezoelectric
Dentsply Preventive Care	Cavitron SPS	30,000	Magnetostrictive
	Cavitron Jet with SPS	30,000	Magnetostrictive
	Bobcat	25,000	Magnetostrictive
	Cavitron Endo	25,000	Magnetostrictive
EMS Systems	Piezon Master 400	28,000–32,000	Piezoelectric
	Mini Piezon	28,000–32,000	Piezoelectric
Engler Engineering	Sonus V	18,000	Magnetostrictive
Parkell	Perio Select 25-30	25,000 or 30,000	Magnetostrictive
	Turbo 25-20	25,000 or 30,000	Magnetostrictive
	Auto/Manual Tune	25,000	Magnetostrictive
	Clean Machine	25,000	Magnetostrictive
Periogiene	Odontoson	42,000	Magnetostrictive
Pro-Dentec	Pro-Select	45,000	Piezoelectric
	Sensor Sc/RP	45,000	Piezoelectric
South East Instruments	Autoscaler 25K	25,000	Magnetostrictive
	Autoscaler 30K	30,000	Magnetostrictive
Spartan USA	J-A18	40,000	Piezoelectric
Star-Tec	Star-Tec	40,000	Piezoelectric
Tony Riso	Multifunction 2530	25,000 or 30,000	Magnetostrictive
USI	25 MPLC	25,000	Magnetostrictive
	30 MPLC	30,000	Magnetostrictive
Young Dental Manufacturing	Young Piezo	40,000	Piezoelectric

Source: Adapted with permission from J. Schmidt. (Dentsply, York, PA)

TABLE 12–4
COMMERCIALLY AVAILABLE SONIC DEVICES

MANUFACTURER	MODEL	FREQUENCY (HZ)
A-Dec/W & H	Corsair II	6000
DentalEZ Group	Titan SW	7000
Dentsply Midwest	Quixsonic	6650
Kavo	Sonicflex 2000L	6000
	Sonicflex Lux	6000
Mar-a-Mar	K-2 Auto-Scaler	7000
Medidenta	ScaleRite	3000
Micromotors	Micro ICS Scaler	6000

TABLE 12–5
EXAMPLES OF COMMERCIALLY AVAILABLE SONIC TIPS

MANUFACTURER	TRADE NAME
A-Dec/W & H	1/2/3
DentalEZ Group	Universal Perio Sickle
Dentsply Midwest	Universal Perio Sickle SofTip
Kavo	1/2/3/4/5/6/7
Mar-a-Mar	Universal Perio
Medidenta	A/B/C
Micromotors	Universal Perio VersaTip

TABLE 12–6
EXAMPLES OF COMMERCIALLY AVAILABLE MAGNETOSTRICTIVE INSERTS

MANUFACTURER	TRADE NAME	SHANK DESIGN	WATER DELIVERY
Dentsply Cavitron	Focused Spray Slimline Slimline Focused Spray 10 Thru Flow Classic P	Straight/right/left Straight/right/left Straight Straight Straight/right/left	Internal External Internal Internal External
Engler Engineering Corporation	Marathon K Marathon K-P M Series	Straight Straight Straight	Internal Internal Internal
Hufriedy	Streamline Prophy Style/ Plus After Five/Plus Furcation/ Plus	Straight Straight Straight/right/left Straight/right/left	Internal External External External
Parkell Electronics Division	Perio Perio Beavertail Universal	Straight Right/left Straight Straight	Internal or External Internal Internal Internal or External
Periogene	Periodontal Probe Thin Line	Straight Straight/right/left	Internal External
Tony Riso	P-50 Standard P-100 Universal P-100 R/L	Straight Straight right/left	External External External
Ultrasonic Scaler Inserts, Inc.	Universal No. 3 Interproximal No. 4 Flat No. 10 Perio	Straight Straight Straight Straight/right/left	Internal Internal Internal Internal
Ultrasonic Services, Inc.	USI 10 USI H USI UH	Straight Straight/right/left Straight/right/left	External External External

TABLE 12–7		
EXAMPLES OF COMMERCIALLY AVAILABLE PIEZOELECTRIC TIPS		
MANUFACTURER	**TRADE NAME**	**SHANK DESIGN**
Amadent	1/2/3 Scaling	Straight
	10 P Scaling	Straight
	H Perio	Straight/right/left
Biotrol International	31/32/33/37/39	Straight
EMS Systems	Sub-10 Perio	Straight
	Supragingival Power	Straight
	Furcation	Right/left
Pro-Dentec	UltraSlim	Straight/right/left
Spartan USA	1/4/6/7	Straight
	2/3	Right/left
	5 Perio	Straight
Star-Tec	1/4/7/40	Straight
	5 Perio	Straight
	1/6/7	Straight
	5 Perio	Straight
Young Dental Manufacturing	8/9	Contra-angle straight

FIGURE 12–9

Inserts for the removal of heavy supragingival deposits. (Reprinted with permission from Dentsply Preventive Care, York, PA)

oral conditions and match the appropriate insert to the needs of the patient. In addition, the site of an insert's water delivery should be evaluated.

Assessment of the patient's oral conditions should include a determination of the severity or absence of disease, as well as the quantity and location of the deposits requiring removal. These factors will have a direct influence on the size and design of the insert used for debridement. If a patient presents with easily accessible heavy supragingival deposits, then a large straight-shank universal insert should be used. Several inserts are designed for this purpose (Fig. 12–9 ■). Although these inserts are used primarily supragingivally, if gingival consistency permits, they also can be used to remove subgingival deposits. Conversely, if light deposits require removal, then a thin, small-diameter insert should be used.

FIGURE 12–10

(a) Right, left, and straight small-diameter inserts with external water delivery. (b) Right, left, and straight small-diameter inserts with internal water delivery. (Reprinted with permission from Dentsply Preventive Care, York, PA)

(a)

(b)

FIGURE 12–11

Ball-tipped small-diameter inserts (right/left/straight). (Reprinted with permission from Dentsply Preventive Care, York, PA.)

Small-diameter inserts are available in a straight-shank design, as well as in contra-angled right and left designs, with either internal or external water delivery systems (Fig. 12–10a,b ■). Some small-diameter inserts are also available with a ball tip (Fig. 12–11 ■). The rationale behind straight, right, and left inserts is the same as for the various configurations of subgingival scaling hand instruments such as Gracey curets. Contra-angled inserts enable proper adaptation and decrease the likelihood of traumatizing the hard or soft tissues. Since these inserts are smaller in diameter than a universal insert, they provide better access subgingivally and produce less tissue distension, resulting in increased patient comfort.

FIGURE 12–12

External water tube. (Reprinted with permission from Dentsply Preventive Care, York, PA)

FIGURE 12–13

Internal water delivery at base. (Reprinted with permission from Dentsply Preventive Care, York, PA)

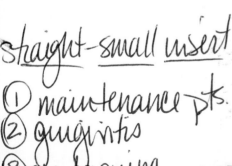

Handwritten notes:

right/left inserts
① periodontitis
② access furcations
③ pockets more than 4mm

straight-small insert
① maintenance pts.
② gingivitis
③ deplaquing
④ pocket no more than 4mm.

The indications for use of a straight small-diameter insert are for maintenance patients, for patients with gingivitis, for deplaquing, and when attachment levels are less than 4 mm. The right and left inserts are used as a complementary pair, similar to a double-ended hand instrument, such as a Gracey 11/12, for treating patients with periodontitis, to access furcations, and when attachment levels are greater than 4 mm.

Evaluating the site of an insert's water delivery is critical because it affects a clinician's ability to manage aerosols produced by ultrasonic devices. Historically, inserts have been manufactured with an external water tube (Fig. 12–12 ■), or water is delivered at the base of the insert (Fig. 12–13 ■). The greater the distance of water delivery, the greater is the difficulty in managing aerosols, which also contributes to impeding the clinician's visibility. If water is delivered at or near the working portion of the insert tip, this facilitates water management. A comparison of the water spray pattern that results from an insert whose water exits at the base versus an insert whose water exits at the anterior third is shown in Fig. 12–14 ■.

FIGURE 12–14

Examples of water spray patterns. (Reprinted with permission from Dentsply Preventive Care, York, PA)

FIGURE 12–15

Site of water delivery for the Focused Spray™ insert. (Reprinted with permission from Dentsply Preventive Care, York, PA)

Inserts by Dentsply Preventive Care (York, PA) with patented water designs are the Focused Spray™ insert (Fig. 12–15■) and the FSI® Slimline® insert (Fig. 12–16■). These uniquely designed inserts have water exiting at the anterior third of the insert for the Focused Spray™ insert and at the middle third for the FSI® Slimline® insert, which significantly reduce aerosol production.

INSERT STERILIZATION AND REPLACEMENT

When preparing an insert for sterilization, it should not be placed in cold sterilization or disinfectant solutions. These solutions may attack the plastic grip and alter the metal components of the insert, resulting in a shorter life span of the insert. The recommended sterilization procedure is to rinse the insert in water, dry it thoroughly, and then sterilize it in an all-paper or combination paper and

FIGURE 12–16

Site of water delivery for the focused-spray slim-line insert. (Reprinted with permission from Dentsply Preventive Care, York, PA)

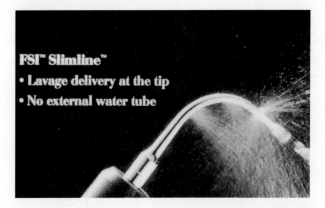

FIGURE 12–17

Efficiency indicator. (Reprinted with permission from Dentsply Preventive Care, York, PA)

plastic sterilization bag. Use of an all-plastic sterilization bag may cause the heat to be held in the bag for a prolonged period of time, which also could contribute to shortening the life span of the insert.

According to most manufacturers, ultrasonic inserts should be replaced, at a minimum, on a yearly basis. However, in actuality, replacement of an individual insert depends on its frequency of use. Factors to monitor that will determine if an individual insert requires replacement are degree of wear of the insert tip and, if applicable, condition of the stacks. These factors, in combination with an insert that is burnishing the deposit rather than removing it efficiently, will prescribe replacement.

On use, an insert tip will show wear and become shorter, which decreases its efficacy. To evaluate the degree of wear sustained by an insert, one of two methods can be used. Either a new insert can be used to serve as a control to determine the degree of wear, or a commercially available efficiency indicator can be used (Fig. 12–17 ■). If a new insert is used as a control, when more than 2 mm of the insert tip has worn, the tip should be replaced. When an efficiency indicator is used, if the insert being evaluated does not reach the red line on the indicator, then the insert requires replacement.

FIGURE 12–18

Splayed stacks. (Reprinted with permission from Dentsply Preventive Care, York, PA)

The metal stacks of a magnetostrictive insert also should be evaluated to determine replacement. The stacks of a new insert are straight and closely adapted. Through frequent use and repeated processing through sterilization cycles, coupled with mishandling, the stacks may become bent and permanently splayed, which affects the efficacy of the insert (Fig. 12–18■). A simple but effective test to determine if the degree of splaying will affect the efficacy of the insert adversely is to employ an insert "slip" test. This test requires that the insert be slipped into the handpiece until the rubber O-ring contacts the handpiece. If the insert slides into the handpiece smoothly, even if minor splaying is observed, then replacement is not necessary. However, if the insert binds before contacting the O-ring, then the insert needs to be replaced. If the clinician continues to use an insert in this condition, not only will excessive force be required to fully seat the insert, but it also increases the likelihood that the splayed stacks will come into contact with the internal borders of the handpiece on activation. This could further dampen the effectiveness of the insert in removing deposits.

CLINICAL RECOMMENDATIONS

Patient

Power scalers should not be used on all patients. A thorough review of the patient's medical history should be conducted to determine if an existing medical or dental condition would contraindicate the use of a power scaler or if prophylactic antibiotics are required. Table 12–8■ shows several considerations that should be addressed prior to treatment. If any type of potentially compromising medical condition exists, it would be prudent to consult with the patient's physician. However, consultation becomes essential if the patient is predisposed to infection or has an existing respiratory disease or an infectious disease transmitted by aerosols, since aerosol production is customary with power scalers.

TABLE 12–8
PATIENT CONSIDERATIONS

	CONDITION
Medical	Predisposition to infection
	Infectious disease transmitted by aerosols
	Respiratory diseases
	Pacemakers
	Children
Dental	Areas of demineralization
	Margins of restorations
	Extreme sensitivity
	Dental implants

Currently, there appears to be some uncertainty about the use of ultrasonic devices on patients with cardiac pacemakers. In 1973, the American Dental Association Council on Dental Materials and Devices cited the possible electromagnetic interference of ultrasonic devices on pacemakers (American Dental Association 1973). Although earlier studies recommended absolute avoidance of ultrasonic devices, the recent literature suggests that electromagnetic hazards may no longer exist because all pacemakers manufactured since the mid-1980s are shielded electrically, which would reduce or eliminate any external interferences (Adams et al. 1982; Toivone et al. 1991; Simon et al. 1975). However, the research is still not conclusive, and this has resulted in indecisive recommendations regarding the use of ultrasonic devices for patients with cardiac pacemakers. Therefore, until there is a consensus, clinicians should consult with the patient's cardiologist to determine the type and age of the pacemaker worn by the patient and if the cardiologist consents to the use of an ultrasonic device for periodontal debridement.

Using ultrasonic devices on pediatric patients for the removal of gross calculus is permissible, but such devices should be used with caution for fine debridement and deplaquing. Because deciduous teeth possess extremely large pulpal horns, the heat produced by an ultrasonic device may lead to active hyperemia or increased patient discomfort if the insert is allowed to contact the tooth or root surfaces for an extended period of time.

Dental considerations also warrant discussion. Areas of demineralization should be avoided because of the potential for perforating the intact surface enamel during ultrasonic debridement. In addition, prolonged exposure of ultrasonic inserts to the margins of amalgams, composites, and porcelain crowns should be avoided because it may have a negative impact on the integrity of the restoration. However, the use of ultrasonic devices for margination is acceptable, provided the clinician uses an insert that is broad and flat (Fig. 12–19■). Using a small-diameter insert (designed to remove calculus) to remove excess amalgam and overhangs not only will have a negative impact on the restoration but also may lead to fracture of the insert.

Patient comfort and acceptance of the treatment will be increased by the use of light pressure and the lowest effective power setting. In addition, adequate water supply, correct adaptation of the insert, and the use of short, controlled, intermittent, overlapping strokes also will minimize patient discomfort.

Providing the patient with protective eyewear and protective apparel may be indicated, especially if aerosol management is not adequate. Patient positioning,

FIGURE 12-19

Margination insert. (Reprinted with permission from Dentsply Preventive Care, York, PA)

preferably supine, also should be used to ensure an adequate field of vision and for proper evacuation of aerosols. If the patient exhibits extreme sensitivity, use of a topical or local anesthetic may be necessary. However, if anesthetics are used, extreme care must be taken to ensure that the insert tip is kept active and in constant motion to eliminate any unnecessary pulpal trauma.

Patient preparation also includes a thorough explanation of the procedure. The noise, heat, and aerosols produced by power scalers can be intimidating to some patients. In addition, patients need to understand that even though less time is required with power scalers, complete treatment is rendered.

Unit

The unit should be placed in a convenient location that enables easy access to the control knobs. The unit should be flushed for several minutes prior to the start of treatment to minimize contaminants that may have accumulated in the water line while the unit was dormant (American Dental Association 1996). Prior to insert attachment, the empty handpiece should be held in an upright position, and with the rheostat activated, the chamber of the handpiece should be allowed to fill with water. Doing this will eliminate the possibility of entrapping air bubbles within the handpiece that may cause the handpiece to overheat. It also will ensure that adequate water is being delivered to the insert.

To decrease the back drag of the handpiece line during use, it could be supported using one of the methods demonstrated in Figs. 12–20■ and 12–21■. Not only will this increase operator comfort, but it also will maintain the original integrity of the handpiece line.

The water control knob should be adjusted to ensure that adequate water comes in contact with the active area of the insert, with an approximate flow rate

FIGURE 12–20

Handpiece line supported by pinky finger. (Reprinted with permission from Dentsply Preventive Care, York, PA)

FIGURE 12–21

Handpiece line supported by draping on forearm. (Reprinted with permission from Dentsply Preventive Care, York, PA)

of 15 to 35 cc/min, depending on the insert used. Insufficient water may lead to pulpal damage and may contribute to patient discomfort. Although a small spray of water and a rapid drip are desirable, they are not essential for proper use of the device. Recommendations for the proper power and tuning settings were given earlier in this chapter.

TABLE 12–9
BASIC ULTRASONIC INSTRUMENTATION CRITERIA

1. Select the appropriate insert to match the needs of the patient.
2. Use the lowest effective power setting.
3. Adjust the water control to ensure that adequate water is in contact with the active portion of the insert or until a rapid drip or small spray is achieved.
4. Use a very light grasp.
5. Use a light but stable intraoral or extraoral fulcrum.
6. Adapt the insert so the point is not directed into the root or tooth surface.
7. Use a light, smooth, gentle touch.
8. Keep the insert tip in motion at all times, using overlapping horizontal, vertical, or oblique brush-like strokes.

Source: Adapted with permission from Dentsply Preventive Care. (York, PA)

Operator

Appropriate operator barriers, including protective eyewear, a facemask, or a facemask and shield and gloves, should be worn as mandated by the guidelines from the Centers for Disease Prevention and Control. When using power scalers, clinicians should select a facemask with a high bacterial filtration efficiency. One study revealed that a facemask worn during treatment in an aerosol environment should be rated at least 98% bacterial filtration efficient. It should effectively filter particles of at least 3 μm or larger, and the mask should be changed frequently (as often as every 20 minutes) if required (Christensen et al. 1991). It is recommended that clinicians consult the March 1989 newsletter of Clinical Research Associates, in which an evaluation of the efficacy of 42 different brands is presented (Clinical Research Associates 1989).

In addition, preprocedural rinses should be administered to all patients prior to ultrasonic debridement as a precautionary measure for the operator. Use of preprocedural rinses has been shown to significantly reduce the number of viable bacteria in dental aerosols typically associated with ultrasonics (Fine et al. 1993).

Clinical technique

Proper ultrasonic instrumentation can be achieved by using either a modified pen or pen grasp. However, during active instrumentation, the grasp and pressure used should be light, similar to an exploratory stroke, to enable the device to work efficiently. A finger rest, either intraoral or extraoral, is essential.

Table 12–9■ provides the basic ultrasonic instrumentation criteria. Correct adaptation of a power-scaling insert can be achieved through the use of either a traditional technique, which applies the basic principles of periodontal hand instrumentation, or a modified technique. Table 12–10■ defines the principles of the modified technique of ultrasonic debridement.

When a universal-type insert is used for removing heavy deposits, application of either the traditional (Fig. 12–22■) or the modified technique is acceptable. Similarly, if attachment levels are 4 mm or less, either technique can be employed with a small-diameter insert (Figs. 12–23■ and 12–24■). However, if attachment levels are greater than 4 mm, which would necessitate the use of contra-angled right and left inserts, then only a modified technique should be used. Table 12–11■ provides the correct selection of the right and left inserts, by quadrant, for the modified technique.

TABLE 12–10
MODIFIED ULTRASONIC INSTRUMENTATION CRITERIA

1. Place the convex back of the insert against the tooth.
2. The terminal shank should be parallel to the long axis of the tooth.
3. Direct the point away from the tooth and toward the tissue.
4. The point or tip of the insert should be directed apically, similar to the adaptation of a periodontal probe.
5. Never place the tip or point of the insert in contact with tooth or root surfaces.
6. Correct adaptation during activation is achieved by using the back or lateral borders of the insert.

FIGURE 12–22

Adaptation of universal insert to remove heavy supragingival deposits (traditional technique). (Reprinted with permission from Dentsply Preventive Care, York, PA)

FIGURE 12–23

Adaptation of straight small-diameter insert (traditional technique). (Reprinted with permission from Dentsply Preventive Care, York, PA)

FIGURE 12–24

Adaptation of straight small-diameter insert (modified technique). (Reprinted with permission from Dentsply Preventive Care, York, PA)

TABLE 12–11

CORRECT SELECTION OF RIGHT AND LEFT INSERTS BY QUADRANT

QUADRANT	INSERT
Maxillary right buccal	Left
Maxillary right lingual	Right
Maxillary left buccal	Right
Maxillary left lingual	Left
Mandibular left buccal	Left
Mandibular left lingual	Right
Mandibular right buccal	Right
Mandibular left lingual	Left

In lieu of using the information provided in Table 12–11■, the following visual cues may assist the clinician in ensuring that the correct contra-angled insert is used with the modified technique. Begin by placing the point of the insert on the occlusal surface of a molar (Fig. 12–25■); ensure that the insert grip extends over the anterior teeth of the arch to be instrumented. Next, observe the back of the insert (convex surface), and then place the tip of the insert on the buccal surface of the molar (Fig. 12–26■) and then on the lingual surface of the molar (Fig. 12–27■). If the tip of the insert flares toward the tooth surface as depicted in Fig. 12–27, then it is the incorrect insert. However, if the tip of the insert flares away from the tooth surface as depicted in Fig. 12–26, then the correct insert has been selected for debridement of the quadrant.

As the insert is activated, the length of the stroke should be short, with a controlled motion; the direction of the stroke can be multidirectional; and the pressure applied should be light and intermittent. Similar to hand instruments, it is crucial to keep the insert well adapted to the tooth surface, especially at the line angles of the tooth, in order to avoid trauma to the soft tissues.

The objectives of ultrasonic instrumentation are to remove calculus and to disrupt bacterial colonies. Calculus removal is achieved in a different manner with

FIGURE 12–25

Visual cue with insert tip on occlusal surface. (Reprinted with permission from Dentsply Preventive Care, York, PA)

FIGURE 12–26

Visual cue with insert flared away from the tooth. (Reprinted with permission from Dentsply Preventive Care, York, PA)

ultrasonic devices than with hand instruments. Deposits generally are removed by hand instruments in an apical-to-coronal fashion, requiring the instrument's cutting blade to be positioned at the most apical border of the deposit. However, with power scalers, the deposit can be removed in a coronal-to-apical fashion. Tactile sense must be developed with these power tips in order to feel the calculus deposits and position the tip properly. Continual movement is important, but movement should be controlled and deliberate rather than rapid and haphazard.

When subgingival deposits are few, as in a supportive periodontal patient (continuing-care or maintenance patient), a deplaquing stroke can be used. Deplaquing requires a series of sweeping strokes over the entire root surface. The tip of the insert is touched lightly to the root surface. Although cavitational action of the fluid lavage will create a halo effect around the instrument tip, limited lateral dispersion of the lavage solution is attained subgingivally. Therefore, every square millimeter of the root surface must be accessed with the tip of the insert (Nosal et al. 1991; O'Hehir 1995).

FIGURE 12–27

Visual cue with insert flared toward the tooth. (Reprinted with permission from Dentsply Preventive Care, York, PA)

Treatment evaluation

The ultimate determinant of treatment success is observation of the response of the tissues. However, during ultrasonic debridement, preliminary evaluations should be made by concentrating on the process of instrumentation and using both tactile and visual cues, similar to the process with hand instrumentation. Subsequently, posttreatment evaluation consists of monitoring the soft tissue response and determining the critical levels of periodontal pathogenic organisms present within the sulcus. If inflammation is not resolved, then the clinician may consider using a chemotherapeutic agent as the source of lavage. Several studies have documented positive responses with 0.12% chlorhexidine gluconate or 0.05% povodine-iodine (Reynolds 1992; Shiloah and Hovious 1993).

ULTRASONIC VERSUS HAND-ACTIVATED INSTRUMENTATION

Studies comparing hand- and power-driven scalers are difficult to assess because of the wide variety of study designs. With the advent of modified periodontal inserts, subgingival root debridement became possible. Most studies have had comparable results with hand- and power-driven scalers when considering residual plaque and calculus.

It has been documented that ultrasonic scalers with modified tips produced smoother roots with less damage, better access to the base of the pocket, and superior plaque and calculus removal than hand-activated instruments and also required less time (Dragoo 1992; Kocher and Plagmann 1997).

SUMMARY

Clearly, research supports the efficacy of power scalers in achieving the current objectives of periodontal therapy. However, it is imperative that clinicians comprehend all the variables that influence the use of such devices, including frequency, stroke, tunability, and water delivery, to ensure that they are used properly and efficiently. In addition, an understanding of the rationale for and appropriate sequencing of the variety of insert tips available not only will further contribute to efficient use of such devices but also will ensure that patient comfort and safety are not compromised.

KEY POINTS

✢ Ultrasonic and sonic instruments are used for removing dental plaque, supra- and subgingival calculus, and endotoxins from root surfaces.

✢ Review the patient's medical/dental history for contraindications.

✢ The patient should rinse with an antimicrobial mouthrinse before the procedure.

✢ Tactile sense must be developed with the tips of ultrasonic and sonic instruments.

✢ Powered-driven instruments may produce bacteremias, so the guidelines for patients at risk for infective endocarditis should be followed.

✢ Margins of bonded veneers and cemented restorations should be avoided when using powered-driven scalers.

REFERENCES

Adams, D., N. Fulford, N. Beechy, J. MacCarthy, and M. Stephens. 1982. The cardiac pacemaker and ultrasonic scalers. *Br. Dent. J.* 152:171.

American Dental Association Council on Dental Materials and Devices. 1973. Possible electromagnetic interference with cardiac pacemakers from dental casting induction machines and electrosurgical devices. *J. Am. Dent. Assoc.* (February):86.

American Dental Association Council on Scientific Affairs and American Dental Association Council on Dental Practice. 1996. Infection control recommendations for the dental office and the dental laboratory. *J. Am. Dent. Assoc.* 127:672–680.

Biagini, G., L. Checchi, M. Miccoli, V. Vasi, and C. Castaldini. 1988. Root curettage and gingival repair in periodontitits. *J. Periodontol.* 59:124–129.

Bower, R. C. 1979. Furcation morphology relative to periodontal treatment: Furcation root surface anatomy. *J. Periodontol.* 50:366–374.

Chiew, S. Y., M. Wilson, E. H. Davies, and J. B. Kieser. 1991. Assessment of ultrasonic debridement of calculus-associated periodontally involved root surfaces by the limulus amoebocyte lysate assay: An in vitro study. *J. Clin. Periodontol.* 18:240–244.

Christensen, R. P., R. A. Robinson, D. R. Robinson, B. J. Poleger, and R. W. Leavitt. 1991. Efficiency of 42 brands of face masks and 2 face shields in preventing inhalation of air borne debris. *Gen. Dent.* 39:414–421.

Corbet, E. F., A. J. Vaughan, and J. B. Kieser. 1993. The periodontally involved root surface. *J. Clin. Periodontol.* 20:402–410.

Clinical Research Associates. 1989. Face masks, dental clinical. *Clinical Research Associates Newsletter* 13(3):1–3.

Clinical Research Associates. 1998. Ultrasonic and sonic scalers. *Clinical Research Associates Newsletter* 22(6):1–3.

Copulos, T. A., S. B. Low, C. B. Walker, Y. Y. Trebilcock, and A. F. Hefti. 1993. Comparative analysis between a modified ultrasonic tip and hand instruments on clinical parameters of periodontal disease. *J. Periodontol.* 64:694–700.

Dragoo, M. R. 1992. A clinical evaluation of hand and ultrasonic instruments on subgingival debridement: I. With unmodified and modified ultrasonic scalers. *Int. J. Periodont. Rest. Dent.* 12:310–323.

Drisko, C. L. 1993. Scaling and root planing without over instrumentation: Hand versus power driven scalers. *Curr. Opin. Periodontol.* 78–88.

Eschler, B. M., and J. W. Rapley. 1991. Mechanical and chemical root preparation in vitro. *J. Periodontol.* 65:755–760.

Fine, D. H., J. Yip, D. Furgang, M. L. Barnett, A. M. Olshan, and J. Vincent. 1993. Reducing bacteria in dental aerosols: Preprocedural use of antiseptic mouthrinse. *J. Am. Dent. Assoc.* 124:56–68.

Forgas, L., C. Harter, J. Rapley, and W. Killoy. 1991. Comparison of two ultrasonic scalers: In vitro calculus removal. *Practical Hygiene.* March/April:36–40.

Fukazawa, E., and K. Nishimura. 1994. Superficial cemental curettage: Its efficacy in promoting improved cellular attachment on human root surfaces previously damaged by periodontitis. *J. Periodontol.* 65:168–176.

Hou, G., Y. Wu, M. Liou, and C. Tsai. 1987. The efficacy of nonsurgical periodontal therapy by ultrasonic scaling and root planing: I. Clinical evaluation of probing pocket depth. *Koahshing J. Med. Sci.* 3:723–733.

Johnson, W. N., and J. R. Wilson. 1957. The application of ultrasonic dental unit to scaling procedures. *J. Periodontol.* 28:264–271.

Kocher, T., and H. C. Plagmann. 1997. The diamond-coated sonic scaler tip: Part II: Loss of substance and alteration of root surface texture after different scaling modalities. *Int. J. Periodontics Restorative Dent.* 17(5):484–493.

Leon, L., and R. Vogel. 1987. A comparison of the effectiveness of hand scaling and ultrasonic debridement in furcations as evaluated by differential darkfield microscopy. *J. Periodontol.* 58:86–94.

Moore, J., M. Wilson, J. B. Kieser. 1986. The distribution of bacterial lipopolysaccharide (endotoxin) in relation to periodontally involved root surfaces. *J. Clin. Periodontol.* 13:748–751.

Nosal, G., M. J. Scheidt, R. O'Neil, and T. E. Van Dyke. 1991. The penetration of lavage solution into the periodontal pocket during ultrasonic instrumentation. *J. Periodontol.* 62:554–557.

O'Hehir, T. E. 1995. Periodontal debridement therapy. *Access* (May–June):49–53.

Olsen, I., and S. S. Socransky. 1981. Ultrasonic dispersion of pure cultures of plaque bacteria and plaque. *Scand. J. Dent. Res.* 89:307–312.

Oosterwaal, P. J., M. Matee, F. M. Mikx, M. A. Van't Hof, and H. H. Renggli. 1987. The effect of subgingival debridement with hand and ultrasonic instruments on the subgingival microflora. *J. Clin. Periodontol.* 14:528–533.

Reynolds, M. A. 1992. Clinical effects of simultaneous ultrasonic scaling and subgingival irrigation with chlorhexidine: Mediating influence of periodontal pocket depth. *J. Clin. Periodontol.* 19:595–600.

Shiloah, J., and L. A. Hovious. 1993. The role of subgingival irrigation in the treatment of periodontitis. *J. Periodontol.* 64:835–843.

Simon, A. B., H. Lindhe, G. H. Bonnette, and R. J. Schlentz. 1975. The individual with a pacemaker in the dental environment. *J. Am. Dent. Assoc.* 91:6.

Smart, G. J., M. Wilson, E. Davies, and J. Kieser. 1990. The assessment of ultrasonic root surface debridement by determination of residual endotoxin levels. *J. Clin. Periodontol.* 17:174–178.

Thilo, B. E., and P. C. Baehni. 1987. Effect of ultrasonic instrumentation on dental plaque microflora in vitro. *J. Periodont. Res.* 22:518–521.

Toivone, L., J. Valjus, M. Hongisto, and R. Mesto. 1991. The influence of elevated 50-Hz electric and magnetic fields of implanted cardiac pacemakers. *Pacing Electrophysiol* 14:12.

Torfason, T., R. Kiger, K. A. Selvig, and J. Egelberg. 1979. Clinical improvement of gingival conditions following ultrasonic versus hand instrumentation of periodontal pockets. *J. Clin. Periodontol.* 6:165–176.

Walmsley, A. D., T. F. Walsh, W. R. E. Laird, and A. R. Williams. 1990. Effects of cavitational activity on the root surface of teeth during ultrasonic scaling. *J. Clin. Periodontol.* 17:306–312.

Woodall, I. R. 1993. *Comprehensive dental hygiene care,* 4th ed., 533–570. St. Louis: C. V. Mosby.

SELF-QUIZ

1. Which one of the following is an advantage of modified ultrasonic inserts? (p. 399)

    a. better access to subgingival areas
    b. does not require a lot of water spray
    c. better control of the instrument
    d. eliminates the need for hand instrumentation

2. Which one of the following features explains how ultrasonic devices affect dental plaque matrix? (p. 399)

    a. directly inhibits gram-negative microbial growth
    b. slows down the formation of calculus
    c. alters and removes endotoxins
    d. dilutes the bacterial load

3. An ultrasonic insert used with a higher frequency removes calculus better than a lower-frequency insert *because* higher frequencies reduce the amount of active tip area on the tooth. (pp. 400–401)

    a. Both the statement and the reason are correct and related.
    b. Both the statement and the reason are correct but *not* related.
    c. The statement is correct, but the reason is *not*.
    d. The statement is *not* correct, but the reason is correct.
    e. *Neither* the statement *nor* the reason is correct.

4. Which one of the following features distinguishes an ultrasonic from a sonic scaler? (p. 403)

    a. Sonic devices operate at a much higher frequency than ultrasonic devices.
    b. Ultrasonic devices are further classified as either magnetostrictive or piezoelectric.
    c. Sonic instruments convert high-frequency electric current into mechanical vibrations.
    d. Ultrasonic instruments use compressed air as their energy source to move a rotor system that produces vibrations of the sonic tip.

5. Which one of the following actions of an ultrasonic instrument removes calculus from the tooth surface? (p. 401)

    a. biochemical changes
    b. physical movement
    c. sonic sensation
    d. mechanical vibrations

III. PROCEDURES FOR EXTRINSIC STAIN REMOVAL

Cynthia Fong, R.D.H., M.S.

Goal:

To provide the dental hygienist with knowledge of the different procedures for removing extrinsic tooth stains in the periodental patient.

Educational Objectives:

Upon completion of this chapter subsection, the reader should be able to:

Discuss the objectives of coronal polishing in periodontal patients;

Explain the rationale for using selective polishing;

Cite and compare research on power-driven polishing versus air-powder polishing for stain removal;

List and discuss the armamentarium required for performing porte polishing, power-driven polishing, and air-powder polishing;

List and discuss the patient considerations and patient preparation procedures required for air-powder polishing; and

Describe the clinical technique for porte, power-driven, and air-powder polishing.

*T*raditionally, polishing of teeth was performed as a routine procedure following periodontal debridement. However, since the literature no longer supports the idea that completely clean and smooth teeth inhibit the accumulation of new deposits and stains, major paradigm shifts have occurred with regard to polishing. Practitioners now should view polishing as "a selective procedure, and not every patient needs to have the teeth polished, especially on a routine basis" (Wilkens 1986). Furthermore, research now demonstrates that brushing and flossing performed by the patient produces similar results as professional polishing (Waring et al. 1988). In addition, previous ideas about the need for polishing teeth prior to fluoride treatment and sealant applications also have changed, since several studies now reveal that other methods of plaque control are equally efficient as plaque removal rendered by polishing (Tinanoff, Wei, and Parkins 1974; Steele, Waltner, and Bawden 1982; Houpt and Shey 1983; Donnan and Ball 1988; Brocklehurst, Joshi, and Northeast 1992). As a result of these changes, the dental profession has adopted a philosophy of **selective polishing** to signify the judicious application of polishing treatment (American Dental Hygienists' Association 1996;

KEY WORDS
• selective polishing
• oral prophylaxis
• coronal polishing
• air-powder polishing

Nunn 1997). Unfortunately, not all practitioners have chosen to embrace this philosophy (Rohleder and Slim 1985; Wilkens 1986; Nield and Houseman 1988). Resistance to change appears to be the cause of the attitudes of both practitioners and patients who continue to hold true to the idea that an **oral prophylaxis** is not complete until teeth are polished. However, the literature is conclusive on the facts that polishing has minimal therapuetic benefits, is not essential for the treatment of periodontal diseases, and should be rendered only for cosmetic purposes (Walsh et al. 1985; Woodall 1993). Routine polishing has been shown to have such detrimental side effects as an increased incidence of bacteremia, loss of enamel, trauma to the pulp and soft tissues, creation of aerosols, and heat production, only serving to provide additional reasons for such practitioners to reconsider their current practice habits (Swan 1979; Christensen and Christensen 1986; Woodall 1993). A practitioner's decision to polish teeth should be based on the evidence presented in the literature and the individual patient's oral conditions, not on long-standing tradition.

This chapter will discuss **coronal polishing** for the objective of removing extrinsic stains, from smoking or use of chlorhexidine mouthrinses in periodontal patients and in preparation for the application of preventive agents. The use of such devices as a porte polisher, rubber cup, and **air-powder polishing** devices will be described. Indications, contraindications, clinical technique, and preparation recommendations for the systems also will be highlighted.

DEVICES AND TECHNIQUES

Prior to initiating a procedure to remove stains, practitioners first should evaluate the stains to determine if they can be removed successfully. Only extrinsic stains that adhere directly to the teeth can be removed adequately with coronal polishing. If the stain is intrinsic or is contained within hard deposits found on the tooth, then alternative methods of removal must be employed. In addition, the locations and severity of the stains, as well as a review of the patient's medical history, must be assessed in order to select an appropriate device for stain removal.

PORTE POLISHER

The simplest device for stain removal is the porte polisher. This hand polishing instrument consists of a wooden point inserted into a single- or double-ended sterilizable handle. Wooden points, which typically are made of orangewood, are available in wedge-shaped and cone-shaped designs, which enhance access and proper adaptation to tooth surfaces. Stain removal is achieved through manual pressure of the point on the tooth in combination with the application of a moist abrasive agent. When using a porte polisher, a modified pen or palm grasp is recommended, with a secure finger rest. Slow, deliberate circular and linear strokes are executed with moderate to firm pressure to remove the stain. Although there are several advantages to using a porte polisher, such as portability, elimination of aerosol and heat production, easy maintenance, and minimal trauma to the hard and soft tissues, the time required to use this device effectively has deterred practitioners from using it routinely in practice. However, for high-risk patients, especially those who are susceptible to infections transmitted by aerosols, the porte polisher may be the only instrument of choice for stain removal.

POWER-DRIVEN POLISHING

Power-driven polishers are used by most practitioners for stain removal. A prophylaxis angle, which is attached to a slow handpiece, is used in conjunction with a rubber cup or brush and a polishing agent (Fig. 12–28 ■). Prophylaxis angles can be either sterilizable or disposable (Fig. 12–29 ■) right-angled or contra-angled. Rubber cups may either be webbed or nonwebbed and are available in either a soft flexible cup or a firm cup (Rethman 1997). Although bristled brushes are used primarily on occlusal surfaces, they also can be used on other coronal surfaces, if used with extreme caution. The stiffness of the bristles may cause trauma to exposed cementum and surrounding soft tissues. The cup or brush may attach to the sterilizable prophylaxis angle by a snap-on, screw-type, or latch-type mechanism. Disposable angles generally have a cup or brush attached to the angle by the manufacturer.

FIGURE 12–28

Rubber cup and brushes.

FIGURE 12–29

Disposable prophylaxis angle prevents cross-contamination.

Selection of a polishing or abrasive agent for stain removal depends on the type of stain present. An agent's abrasivity is determined by its particle size and shape; the larger and more irregular the particles, the more abrasive is the agent (Steele 1975; Wilkens 1989; Perry, Beemsterboer, and Carranza 1990). The degree of abrasion also can be affected by the rotational speed of the rubber cup and the pressure applied during treatment (Perry, Beemsterboer, and Carranza 1990). Slight stains require the use of a fine-grit agent, whereas heavier deposits require the use of a coarse-grit agent. Polishing agents should be used judiciously to minimize the adverse effects of polishing (Schoen and Dean 1996). Self-prepared agents, such as pumice and tin oxide, require mixing with water to assist in stain removal and reduce frictional heat (Wilkens 1989). Commercial polishing agents, which require no preparation and typically are supplied in single-dose units, are available in a wide variety of grits, flavors, and consistencies (Rethman 1997). In addition, many manufacturers offer polishing agents with fluoride additives, which may enhance the therapeutic value of the procedure.

Figures 12–30 ■ and 12–31 ■ illustrate the proper technique and procedures required for rubber cup polishing of natural teeth and dental implants.

Air-Powder Polishing

Devices used for air-powder polishing, which is also referred to as *air polishing*, have been in existence since the 1980s. Air polishers are available commercially as dedicated devices (Fig. 12–32 ■) or as combination devices, in which both ultrasonic scaling and air polishing devices are contained in one unit (Fig. 12–33 ■).

Efficacy

Despite extensive research documenting the efficacy and safety of air polishing, widespread use of such devices has not occurred (Willmann, Norling, and Johnson 1980; Atkinson, Cobb, and Killoy 1984; Weaks et al. 1984; Mishkin et al. 1986; Orton 1987; Horning, Cobb, and Killoy 1987; Strand and Raadal 1988; Hosoya and Johnston 1989). Lack of acceptance of air polishing is evidenced by a survey in which only 30% of the respondents indicated they use an air polisher, and only 22% reported using the system on a routine basis (White and Hoffman 1991). An independent evaluation of a commercially available air polishing device conducted by Clinical Research Associates revealed that "air polishers remove extrinsic stain more rapidly and thoroughly than scalers, abrasives in rubber cups, strips, etc. without significant changes in surface appearance of enamel or dentin" (Clinical Research Associates 1981). Clinical Research Associates also documented that an overwhelming majority of patients surveyed (94%) prefer air polishing over traditional rubber-cup polishing (Clinical Research Associates 1981). Patients indicated that their preference for air polishing was based on its ability to remove stains more thoroughly and that it required less chair time and was more comfortable than rubber-cup polishing.

It appears that the reason why practitioners are not using air polishers routinely in practice may be a lack of education in the proper use of the device, as well as several misconceptions about the device. Many practitioners are unsure of the safety and efficacy of air polishers, believing that they are more abrasive than prophylaxis paste, are messy, require an extensive amount of maintenance, and are limited in use solely for the purposes of removing extrinsic stains. However,

FIGURE 12–30

Clinical technique and procedures for rubber-cup polishing of natural teeth. [Copyrighted 1997, Montage Media Corporation; reproduced with permission from *The Journal of Practical Hygiene* 6(2).]

CLINICAL TECHNIQUE AND PROCEDURES FOR RUBBER CUP POLISHING OF NATURAL TEETH

PROCEDURE

As part of the patient education process, explain the importance of the daily elimination of plaque through proper patient self-care regimens. Debridement therapy prior to rubber cup polishing may have eliminated some stain. Therefore, select the surfaces to be polished based on the presence of any remaining extrinsic stain. The abrasiveness of the polishing agent selected should be based on the degree of stain present.

After rinsing, floss is used to remove any abrasive particles not flushed away. Many patients are not aware that the polishing procedure is cosmetic-based and not therapy-based. Open discussions with patients explaining the benefits and indications for polishing will help dismiss misconceptions about the polishing procedure's proper role in dental hygiene care.

- Use a preprocedural rinse.
- Use protective eyewear (patient and clinician).
- Use fine pastes whenever possible.
- Keep cup filled and moist.
- Use high velocity suction.
- Use a modified pen grasp with finger rest (*Figure 1*).
- Divide the facial and lingual surfaces into five segments: mesiocervical, central cervical, distocervical, mesial upper crown, and distal upper crown; then polish the occlusal surface, if needed (*Figure 2*).
- Use a steady, even speed.
- Use light, intermittent pressure.
- Use brushes on occlusal surface only (*Figure 3*).
- Irrigate or flush away residual paste (*Figure 4*).

TECHNIQUE HINTS

Update the medical history at each maintenance appointment to avoid polishing when contraindicated.

Use appropriate polishing agents based on the level of stain on tooth surfaces.

Choose suitable agents to be used with resins, acrylics, and composites to prevent surface alteration.

Follow an established, comfortable sequence to ensure all surfaces to be polished are completed.

Always use universal precautions, and personal protective equipment as needed, to limit the exposure to aerosols.

Modified pen grasp

Figure 1

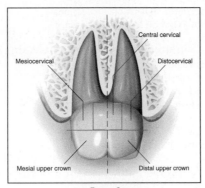

Central cervical
Mesiocervical
Distocervical
Mesial upper crown
Distal upper crown

Figure 2

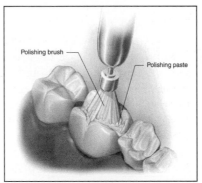

Polishing brush
Polishing paste

Figure 3

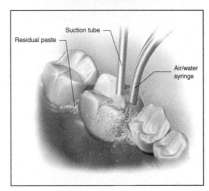

Suction tube
Residual paste
Air/water syringe

Figure 4

FIGURE 12–31

Clinical technique and procedures for rubber cup polishing of implants. [Copyrighted 1997, Montage Media Corporation; reproduced with permission from *The Journal of Practical Hygiene* 6(2).]

CLINICAL TECHNIQUE AND PROCEDURES FOR RUBBER CUP POLISHING OF IMPLANTS

PROCEDURE

Prior to the polishing procedure, remove any calcified deposits with implant-specific instruments. Metal instruments, sonic scalers, and ultrasonic scalers should not be used, as they will mar the titanium implant surface.

Based on individual implant health, antimicrobial agents may be applied after the polishing procedure is completed. End-tufted brushes, interproximal brushes, or specially designed floss dipped into the agent facilitates application. Professional application through subgingival irrigation may be indicated, if administered cautiously.

- A rubber cup and nonabrasive polishing paste are used for coronal polishing of the prosthesis and abutments (*Figure 1*).
- A rubber point is used with nonabrasive polishing paste to remove soft deposits and polish difficult access areas, such as the underside of the prosthesis (*Figure 2*).
- A unitufted rotary brush dipped into a nonabrasive polishing paste can also be used to polish implant abutments.
- In areas difficult to access, such as interproximal areas, where stain cannot be removed with a polishing cup, the use of an interdental brush (with a nonwire core) may be helpful.
- Nonabrasive polishing paste can be applied with a cloth-like floss.
- Select the appropriate floss to accommodate the superstructure and floss accordingly. Floss around the replacement teeth and the abutments, including copings and tissue bars. Limited access areas may require flossing cords with a narrow diameter or tufted floss (*Figure 3*).
- Rinse the mouth thoroughly to remove excess paste.

Figure 1

Figure 2

TECHNIQUE HINTS

Air-abrasive polishing is contraindicated to prevent marring the implant surface.

During the flossing portion of the polishing procedure, have the patient observe the motions of the clinician with a hand-held mirror. The patient can later emulate the technique during his or her self-care.

In general, implant patients should be seen for professional monitoring every 3 to 6 months. The first year after replacement requires more frequent monitoring.

Assess and document all plaque and calculus deposits regularly, informing the patient where more conscientious self-care is needed.

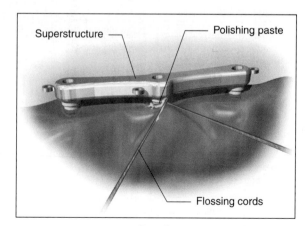

Figure 3

FIGURE 12–32

Cavitron® Prophy-Jet® 30. (Reproduced with permission from Dentsply Preventive Care, York, PA)

FIGURE 12–33

Cavitron® Jet with SPS™ Technology. (Reproduced with permission from Dentsply Preventive Care, York, PA)

none of these beliefs are supported in the current scientific literature. In fact, air polishing consistently has been shown to be a safe and efficient method for removing deposits (Gutmann 1998).

Tooth structure

Air-polishing systems use air, water, and sodium bicarbonate to create a slurry that is used as the abrasive agent for stain removal. It has been well documented that sodium bicarbonate is less abrasive on enamel than hand instruments and equivalent to rubber-cup polishing (Lehne and Winston 1983; Berkstein et al.

JetShield™ aerosol reduction device (close-up). (Reproduced with permission from Dentsply Preventive Care, York, PA)

1987; Kee-Nichol 1990). In addition, the average amount of tooth structure removed by an air polisher is significantly less (10.68 μm) than the amount removed with a hand curet (27.09 μm). In addition, stains are removed 3.15 times faster with an air polisher than with a hand curet (Berkstein et al. 1987).

Aerosols

Because air polishers produce aerosols, practitioners must take precautions to effectively manage the aerosols to avoid the possibility of atmospheric cross-contamination (Glenwright, Knibbs, and Burdon 1985; Worrall, Knibbs, and Glenwright 1987; Logothetis et al. 1988). Research has documented that high-volume evacuation provides the best preventive measure in reducing bacterial contamination (Worrall, Knibbs, and Glenwright 1987). Use of a preprocedural rinse, such as 0.2% chlorhexidine, also has proven useful in reducing contamination but has not been shown to be as effective as high-volume evacuation (Worrall, Knibbs, and Glenwright 1987). Use of a commercial product specifically designed to control air-polisher aerosols, such as JetShield™ (Dentsply Preventive Care, York, PA), also assists in significantly reducing the amount of air-polishing splatter (Fig. 12–34■). Harrel (1998) conducted a study to determine the efficacy of the Jet-Shield and found that it reduced spatter by more than 97%. One end of the shield contains a disposable cup and clear extension tube that is attached to the nozzle of the polisher. The other end consists of tubing that attaches to a saliva ejector or high-volume evacuator (Fig. 12–35■). Proper adaptation and use of this device also has been shown to minimize the potential for soft tissue abrasion (Fig. 12–36■; Harrel 1998). During activation, light pressure should be applied so that the cup flares slightly. The air-polishing nozzle should be pivoted inside the cup to ensure removal of deposits on all surfaces. The clear tubing and cup should be disposed of after each procedure, and the remaining gray tubing should be disinfected properly prior to reuse on future patients.

FIGURE 12–35

JetShield™ aerosol reduction device (view of tubing with connection to nozzle and suction). (Reproduced with permission from Dentsply Preventive Care, York, PA)

FIGURE 12–36

Clinical technique of JetShield™ aerosol reduction device. (Reproduced with permission from Dentsply Preventive Care, York, PA)

Aerosols also can be contained through proper clinical technique, as provided in Table 12–12 ■. Insert angulation, distance of the nozzle from the tooth surface, intermittent delivery of the slurry, manipulation of soft tissues, and adequate rinsing all serve to facilitate aerosol management and reduce splatter (Kee-Nichol 1990; Barnes 1991; Tolle-Watts and Thomson-Lakey 1992).

Precautions

Several precautions must be taken with air-polishing devices to ensure the safety of the patient and to minimize the potential for trauma to the soft or hard tissues. One precaution is to avoid prolonged exposure of the slurry on dentin and cementum.

TABLE 12–12
CLINICAL TECHNIQUE FOR AIR POLISHING

1. Review the medical history.
2. Have patient rinse with an antimicrobial mouthrinse.
3. Use standard operator preparation (i.e., wear face mask, protective eyewear or face shield, gloves, and protective gown).
4. Provide patient with protective eyewear and lubricate lips with non-petroleum-based lubricant.
5. Position the patient at a 45-degree angle.
6. Turn the patient's head toward you; use direct vision and external soft tissue fulcrums.
7. Place a 2 × 2 gauze square on lip and position saliva ejector.

8. Place nozzle tip as follows using a circular motion, interproximal to interproximal (sweeping motion).
9. Polish one or two teeth for 1 to 2 seconds and rinse.
10. Use your hand and patient's cheek and lips to contain aerosols.
11. Rinse excess slurry from the patient's mouth frequently.

Significant losses have been documented, although no adverse effects have been shown on sound enamel (Newman, Silverwood, and Dolby 1985; Galloway and Pashley 1987; Dederich, Gulevich, and Reid 1989). Therefore, loss of tooth structure can be minimized by avoiding prolonged exposure on root surfaces during treatment and by ensuring that a tooth is exposed to the slurry for no more than 10 seconds (Galloway and Pashley 1987). Localized gingival abrasion also can be prevented if the slurry is directed away from soft tissues, although any localized gingival abrasion resulting from use of an air polisher is virtually undetectable after 2 days (Kontturi-Narhi, Markkanen, and Markkanen 1989; Brown 1995). One final precaution is to avoid any technique that may cause a subcutaneous air emphysema. This condition can occur if the compressed air, water, and sodium bicarbonate slurry is introduced subgingivally (Liebenberg and Crawford 1997).

Varied uses

Although air-polishing devices are used by practitioners primarily for removing extrinsic stains from smoking or use of chlorhexidine mouth rinse, their scope of use can be broader (Table 12–13 ■). The literature clearly establishes the positive results that can be achieved with an air polisher during periodontal surgery (Gilman and Maxey 1986; Lavigne et al. 1988; Pippin et al. 1988). Surface preparation with an air polisher prior to sealant placement also has been documented to produce superior results when compared with the use of a rubber cup and pumice (Donnan and Ball 1988; Scott and Greer 1987; Scott et al. 1988; Brockmann, Scott, and Eick 1989, 1990; Huennekens, Daniel, and Bayne 1991). In addition, extensive research has confirmed the efficiency of using air polishers on orthodontic appliances without causing breakage or compromising the integrity of the bond (Barnes et al. 1990; Shultz et al. 1993; Gerbo, Barnes, and Leinfelder 1993). Use of air polishers on implants has shown the device to be efficient at removing plaque, calculus, and stain with minimal alteration of the implant, but

TABLE 12–13		
CLINICAL GUIDELINES FOR USE OF AN AIR POLISHER		
CONDITION	**SAFE FOR AIR POLISHING?**	**COMMENTS**
I. SYSTEMIC DISEASE		
Renal disease	No	Acid/base balance may be disrupted
Metabolic disorders	No	Acid/base balance may be disrupted
Patients on diuretics	No	Acid/base balance may be disrupted
Respiratory diseases	No	Aerosols may complicate breathing
Known infectious diseases	No	Danger of airborne contaminants
General population	Yes	Use recommended personal protective equipment and high BFE masks
II. DENTAL MATERIALS		
Orthodontic appliances	Yes	Most efficient cleaning method
Sealants	Yes	Safe for preparation and cleansing
Composite resins	No	Minimal contact advised
Amalgam restorations	Yes	Careful around margins; matte finish results
Porcelain	No	Margins may erode
Implants	?	More research needed
III. PROCEDURES		
Routine prophylaxis	Yes	Absolutely, unless medically contraindicated
Acid etching	Yes	Ideal preparation method
Orthodontic bonding	Yes	Excellent surface cleansing
Micro-abrasion prior to restoration placement	Yes	Follow manufacturers' guidelines
Periodontal surgery	Yes	Open flap, thorough root detoxification
Primary enamel prophy	?	Pilot research promising, more needed

Source: Copyrighted 1995, Montage Media Corporation; reproduced with permission from *The Journal of Practical Hygiene* 4(6).

there still appears to be concern about the possible long-term effects on fixtures and surrounding tissues (Parham et al. 1989; Bergnedal et al. 1990; Homiak, Cook, and DeBoer 1992; McCollum et al. 1992; Meschenmoser et al. 1998; Brookshire et al. 1997; Augthun, Tinschert, and Huber 1998). It has been suggested that additional research and more conclusive evidence are needed before guidelines for implant maintenance are established (Brown and Barnhart 1995).

Other restorations that require consideration when using an air polisher are composite resins, porcelain crowns, amalgams, and gold-alloy restorations. Some researchers have shown no significant differences in the surface texture of composite resins following air polishing, whereas others have suggested that the resins are vulnerable to the air-polishing slurry when exposed for long periods of time, warranting practitioners to use caution around these restorations (Cooley, Lubow, and Patrissi 1986; Barnes, Hayes, and Leinfelder 1987; Reel et al. 1989; Gorfil et al. 1989; Eliades, Tzoutzas, and Vongiouklakis 1991; Gutman, Marker, and Gutman 1993). Alteration of the margins of porcelain crowns has been demonstrated as a result of air polishing; therefore, it is advised that the practitioner also proceed with caution when encountering these restorations (Felton et al. 1991; Vermilyea, Prasanna, and Agar 1994). With regard to amalgam and gold restorations, Barnes, Hayes, and Leinfelder (1987) found that a 5-second exposure of these restorations to an air polisher did not produce any appreciable loss of material but did leave the restoration with a dull, matte finish.

TABLE 12–14	
MAINTENANCE OF AIR-POLISHING DEVICES	
TIME INTERVAL	**PROCEDURE**
Start of the day	1. With the system off, unscrew the powder chamber cap (Fig. 12–37). Verify the powder bowl is empty. Turn the unit on for 15 seconds to eliminate residual powder or moisture in the lines. Turn the unit off. 2. Shake powder storage jar to create an even consistency of powder mixture. 3. Pour the powder into the chamber until it reaches the top of the center tube. 4. Secure the cap onto the powder chamber. 5. With the air-polishing nozzle removed, hold the handpiece over a sink to drain. Activate the foot control to flush the water line. 6. Insert an air-polishing nozzle into the handpiece.
End of the day	1. Turn the unit off. 2. Remove the air-polishing nozzle. 3. Clean the air-polishing nozzle with a wire cleaning tool by inserting the wire into the front of the nozzle and moving it back and forth (Fig. 12–38). Remove the wire and use an air syringe to remove any residual powder. 4. Unscrew the powder chamber cap. 5. Remove the powder chamber from the cabinet (Fig. 12–39). Pour the powder into the powder storage jar and secure the lid (Fig. 12–40). 6. Hold the end of the powder chamber *away* from you. Activate the system for 15 seconds to clear the powder chamber. A high-volume evacuator can be used to remove any residual powder from the bowl. 7. Replace the powder chamber into the cabinet. 8. Secure the lid to the powder chamber. 9. Sterilize the air-polishing nozzle and wire-cleaning tool. 10. Clean and disinfect unit in accordance with the equipment procedure supplied with your unit.

FIGURE 12–37

Removal of the powder chamber cap. (Reproduced with permission from Dentsply Preventive Care, York, PA)

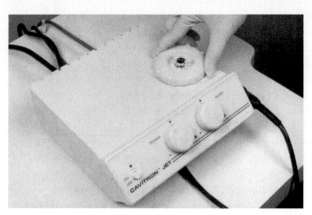

FIGURE 12–38

Use of a wire cleaning tool. (Reproduced with permission from Dentsply Preventive Care, York, PA)

FIGURE 12–39

Removal of the powder chamber from cabinet. (Reproduced with permission from Dentsply Preventive Care, York, PA)

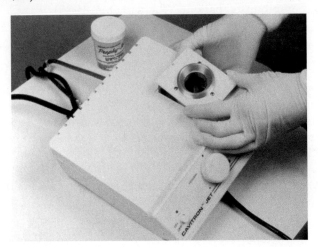

Maintenance

Table 12–14■ and Figs. 12–37■ to 12–40■ highlight the proper maintenance required for an air-polishing device. The major objective of maintenance is to ensure that the powder chamber and the air line are kept free of moisture contamination. If residual moisture is allowed to invade either part of the device, it may lead to device failure.

FIGURE 12–40

Placement of powder in powder storage jar. (Reproduced with permission from Dentsply Preventive Care, York, PA)

Medical conditions

Certain medical conditions (e.g. hypertension renal disease, and resiratory disease) contraindicate the use of an air-polishing device (see Table 12–13■). Since air polishers emit aerosols and use sodium bicarbonate, patients with systemic conditions require prudent consideration by the practitioner to determine if the device can be used safely. In addition, further investigation is required to address concerns raised about the potential for disrupting serum electrolyte levels in certain medically compromised patients (Rawson et al. 1985).

SUMMARY

Clearly, practitioners have several devices from which to choose when attempting to remove extrinsic stains, from the traditional power-driven devices to air-powder polishers, which have expanded applications beyond stain removal. However, regardless of the device used, the final decision to polish teeth should be selective and viewed as a cosmetic procedure only and not therapeutic. Ultimately, the appropriateness of polishing should be determined on the basis of patient's oral conditions, not on conventional practice habits.

KEY POINTS

✣ Update the medical history to avoid polishing when contraindicated.

✣ In the periodontal patient, tooth polishing should be performed only as needed and not as part of routine treatment.

✣ Avoiding exposed root surfaces during the procedure and not having the teeth exposed to the slurry for more than 10 seconds can minimize loss of tooth structure.

✣ High-volume evacuation is the most effective for reducing contamination during air polishing.

REFERENCES

American Dental Hygienists' Association. 1996. Position on polishing procedures. *Education Update* 16(1):2–3.

Atkinson, D. R., C. M. Cobb, and W. J. Killoy. 1984. The effect of an air-powder abrasive system on in vitro root surfaces. *J. Periodontol.* 55:13–18.

Augthun, M., J. Tinschert, and A. Huber. 1998. In vitro studies on the effect of cleaning methods on different implant surfaces. *J. Periodontol.* 69:587–864.

Barnes, C. M. 1991. Management of aerosols with air-polishing delivery systems. *J. Dent. Hyg.* 65(6):280–282.

Barnes, C. M., E. F. Hayes, and K. F. Leinfelder. 1987. Effects of an air-abrasive polishing system on restored surfaces. *Gen. Dent.* (May–June):186–187.

Barnes, C. M., C. M. Russell, L. R. Gerbo, B. R. Wells, and D. W. Barnes. 1990. Effects on an air-powder polishing system on orthodontically bracketed and bonded teeth. *Am. J. Orthod.* 97(1):74–81.

Bergnedal, T., L. Forsgren, S. Kvint, and E. Lowstedt. 1990. Effect of an air-abrasive instrument on soft and hard tissues around osseointegrated implants. *Swed. Dent. J.* 14:219–223.

Berkstein, S., R. L. Reiff, J. F. McKinney, and W. J. Killoy. 1987. Supragingival root surface removal during maintenance procedures utilizing an air-powder abrasive system or hand scaling. *J. Periodontol.* 58:327–330.

Brocklehurst, P. R., R. I. Joshi, and S. E. Northeast. 1992. The effect of air-polishing occlusal surfaces on the penetration of fissures by a sealant. *Int. J. Paediatr. Dent.* 2:157–162.

Brockmann, S. L., R. L. Scott, and J. D. Eick. 1989. Effect of an air-polishing device on tensile bond strength of a dental sealant. *Quintessence Int.* 20(3):211–217.

Brockmann, S. L., R. L. Scott, and J. D. Eick. 1990. A scanning electron microscopic study of the effect of air-polishing on the enamel-sealant surface. *Quintessence Int.* 21(3):201–206.

Brookshire, F. V. G., W. W. Nagy, V. B. Dhuru, G. J. Ziebert, and C. Srinivas. 1997. The qualitative effects of various types of hygiene instrumentation on commercially pure titanium alloy implant abutments: An in vitro and scanning electron microscope study. *J. Prosthet. Dent.* 78(3):286–294.

Brown, D. M. 1995. A scientific foundation for clinical use of air-polishing systems: II. Technique. *J. Pract. Hyg.* (Nov–Dec):14–19.

Brown, D. M., and R. C. Barnhart. 1995. A scientific foundation for clinical use of air-polishing systems: I. A review of the literature. *J. Pract. Hyg.* (May–June):36–40.

Christensen, R. P., and G. J. Christensen. 1986. In vivo effects of polishing on enamel and dentin (Abstract). *J. Dent. Res.* 65:1149.

Clinical Research Associates. 1981. Oral prophylaxis. *Clinical Research Associates Newsletter* 5(10):1–2.

Cooley, R. L., R. M. Lubow, and G. A. Patrissi. 1986. Effect of an air-powder abrasive instrument on composite resin. *J. Am. Dent. Assoc.* 112:362–364.

Dederich, D. N., T. Gulevich, and A. Reid. 1989. The effect of rubber cup versus an air-powder abrasive system on root surfaces. *Probe* 28(3):135–137.

Donnan, M. F., and I. A. Ball. 1988. A double-blind clinical trial to determine the importance of pumice prophylaxis on fissure sealant retention. *Br. Dent. J.* 165(8):283–286.

Eliades, G. C., J. G. Tzoutzas, and G. J. Vougiouklakis. 1991. Surface alterations on dental restorative materials subjected to an air-powder abrasive instrument. *J. Prosthet. Dent.* 65:27–33.

Felton, D. A., S. C. Bayne, B. E. Kanoy, and J. T. White. 1991. Effect of air abrasives on marginal configurations of porcelain-fused-to-metal alloys: An SEM analysis. *J. Prosthet. Dent.* 65:38–43.

Galloway, S. E., and D. H. Pashley. 1987. Rate of removal of root structure by the use of the Prophy-Jet device. *J. Periodontol.* 58:464–469.

Gerbo, L. R., C. M. Barnes, and K. F. Leinfelder. 1993. Applications of the air-powder polisher in clinical orthodontics. *Am. J. Orthod. Dentofac. Orthop.* 103:71–73.

Gilman, R. S., and B. R. Maxey. 1986. Effect of root detoxification on human gingival fibroblasts. *J. Periodontol.* 57:436–440.

Glenwright, H. D., P. J. Knibbs, and D. W. Burdon. 1985. Atmospheric contamination during use of an air-polisher. *Br. Dent. J.* 159:294–297.

Gorfil, C., D. Nordenberg, R. Liberman, and A. Ben-Amar. 1989. Effect of ultrasonic cleaning and air-polishing on the marginal integrity of radicular amalgam and composite resin restorations. *J. Clin. Periodontol.* 16:137–139.

Gutman, M. S. E., V. A. Marker, and J. L. Gutman. 1993. Restoration surface roughness after air-powder polishing. *Am. J. Dent.* 6:99–102.

Gutmann, M. E. 1998. Air-polishing: A comprehensive review of the literature. *J. Dent. Hyg.* 72(3):47–56.

Harrel, S. K. 1998. Advances in air-polishing techniques. *Dent. Connect.* 1(1):1–4, 6–8.

Harrel, S. K., F. Hidalgo-Rivera, and J. B. Barnes. 1997. Reduction of aerosol spatter during air-polishing (Abstract). *OSAP Bull.*

Homiak, A. W., P. A. Cook, and J. DeBoer. 1992. Effect of hygiene instrumentation on titanium abutments: A SEM study. *J. Prosthet. Dent.* 67:364–369.

Horning, G. M., C. M. Cobb, and W. J. Killoy. 1987. Effect of an air-powder abrasive system on root surfaces in periodontal surgery. *J. Clin. Periodontol.* 14(4):213–220.

Hosoya, Y., and J. W. Johnston. 1989. Evaluation of various cleaning and polishing methods on primary enamel. *J. Periodontol.* 13(3):253–269.

Houpt, M., and Z. Shey. 1983. The effectiveness of a fissure sealant after six years. *Pediatr. Dent.* 5(2):104–106.

Huennekens, S. C., S. J. Daniel, and S. C. Bayne. 1991. Effects of air-polishing on the abrasion of occlusal sealants. *Quintessence Int.* 22(7):581–585.

Kee-Nichol, A. 1990. Air-polishing technique and patient selection. *Dent. Hyg. News* 4:6.

Kontturi-Narhi, V., S. Markkanen, and H. Markkanen. 1989. Gingival effects of dental air polishing as evaluated by scanning electron microscopy. *J. Periodontol.* 60:19–22.

Lavigne, C. K., R. K. Nauman, M. M. Munley, and J. B. Suzuki. 1988. In vitro evaluation of air-powder polishing as an adjunct to ultrasonic scaling on periodontally involved root surfaces. *J. Dent. Hyg.* 62(10):504–509.

Lehne, R. K., and A. E. Winston. 1983. Abrasivity of sodium bicarbonate. *Clin. Prev. Dent.* 5(1):17–18.

Liebenberg, W. H., and B. J. Crawford. 1997. Subcutaneous, orbital and mediatinal emphysema secondary to the use of an air-abrasive device. *Quintessence Int.* 28(1):31–38.

Logothetis, D. D., K. B. W. Gross, A. Eberhart, and C. Drisko. 1988. Bacterial airborne contamination with an air-polishing device. *Gen. Dent.* (Nov–Dec):496–499.

McCollum, J. A., R. B. O'Neal, W. A. Brennan, et al. 1992. Effect of titanium implant abutment surface irregularities on plaque accumulation in vivo. *J. Periodontol.* 63:802–805.

Meschenmoser, A., B. D'Hoedt, J. Meyle, G. Elssner, D. Korn, H. Hammerle, and W. Schulte. 1998. Effects of various hygiene procedures on the surface characteristics of titanium abutments. *J. Periodontol.* 3:229–235.

Mishkin, D. J., W. O. Engler, T. Javed, T. D. Darby, R. L. Cobb, and M. A. Coffman. 1986. A clinical comparison of the effect on the gingiva of the Prophy-Jet and the rubber cup and paste techniques. *J. Periodontol.* 57(3):151–154.

Newman, P. S., R. A. Silverwood, and A. E. Dolby. 1985. Effects of an air-abrasive instrument on dental hard tissues, skin and oral mucosa. *Br. Dent. J.* 159:9–12.

Nield, J. S., and G. A. Houseman. 1988. *Fundamentals of dental hygiene.* Philadelphia: Lea & Febiger.

Nunn, P. J. 1997. Selective polishing: Time for a change? *Access* 11(1):38, 40–42.

Orton, G. S. 1987. Clinical use of an air-powder abrasive system. *Dent. Hyg.* 61(11):513–518.

Parham, P. L., C. M. Cobb, A. A. French, J. W. Love, and C. L. Drisko. 1989. Effects of an air-powder abrasive system on plasma-sprayed titanium implant surfaces: An in-vitro evaluation. *J. Oral Implantol.* 15(2):78–86.

Perry, D. A., P. Beemsterboer, and F. A. Carranza. 1990. *Techniques and theory of periodontal instrumentation*, 331. Philadelphia: W. B. Saunders.

Pippin, D. J., W. E. Crooks, B. F. Barker, P. L. Walters, and W. J. Killoy. 1988. Effects of an air-powder abrasive device used during periodontal flap surgery in dogs. *J. Periodontol.* 59:584–588.

Rawson, R. D., B. N. Nelson, B. D. Jewell, and C. C. Jewell. 1985. Alkalosis as a potential complication of air-polishing systems. *Dent. Hyg.* 59:500–503.

Reel, D. C., H. Abrams, S. L. Gardner, and R. J. Mitchell. 1989. Effect of a hydraulic jet prophylaxis system on composites. *J. Prosthet. Dent.* 61:441–445.

Rethman, J. 1997. Polishing angles, cups and pastes. *J. Pract. Hyg.* 6(2):32–35.

Rohleder, P. V., and L. H. Slim. 1985. Alternatives to rubber cup polishing. *Dent. Hyg.* 55:16–20.

Schoen, D. H., and M. C. Dean. 1996. *Contemporary periodontal instrumentation*, 135. Philadelphia: W. B. Saunders.

Scott, L., S. Brockmann, G. Houston, and D. Tira. 1988. Retention of dental sealants following the use of air polishing and traditional cleaning. *Dent. Hyg.* 62:402–406.

Scott, L., and D. Greer. 1987. The effect of an air-polishing device on sealant bond strength. *J. Prosthet. Dent.* 58(3):384–387.

Shultz, P. H., S. L. Brockmann-Bell, J. D. Eick, K. B. W. Gross, R. P. Chappell, and P. Spencer. 1993. Effects of air-powder polishing on the bond strength of orthodontic bracket adhesive systems. *J. Dent. Hyg.* 67(2):74–80.

Steele, P. F. 1975. *Dimensions of dental hygiene*, 2nd ed., 176–177. Philadelphia: Lea & Febiger.

Steele, R. C., A. W. Waltner, and J. W. Bawden. 1982. The effect of tooth cleaning procedures on fluoride uptake in enamel. *Pediatr. Dent.* 4:228–233.

Strand, G. V., and M. Raadal. 1988. Efficiency of cleaning fissures with an air-polishing instrument. *Acta Odontol. Scand.* 46:113–117.

Swan, R. W. 1979. Dimensional changes in a tooth root incident to various polishing and root planing procedures. *Dent. Hyg.* 53:17–19.

Tinanoff, N., S. H. Y. Wei, and F. M. Parkins. 1974. Effect of a pumice prophylaxis on fluoride uptake in tooth enamel. *J. Am. Dent. Assoc.* 88:384–389.

Tolle-Watts, S. L., and E. M. Thomson-Lakey. 1992. Clinical application of the air-polisher. *Pract. Hyg.* (Nov–Dec):27–32.

Vermilyea, S. G., M. K. Prasanna, and J. R. Agar. 1994. Effect of ultrasonic cleaning and air-polishing on porcelain labial margin restorations. *J. Prosthet. Dent.* 71:447–452.

Walsh, M. M., B. Heckman, R. Moreau-Diettinger, and S. A. Buchanan. 1985. Effect of a rubber cup polish after scaling. *Dent. Hyg.* 59(11):494–498.

Waring, M. B., M. L. Horn, L. L. Ames, N. J. Williams, and S. M. Lyne. 1988. Plaque reaccumulation following engine polishing or tooth brushing: A 90-day clinical trial. *Dent. Hyg.* 62:282–285.

Weaks, L. M., N. B. Lescher, C. M. Barnes, and S. V. Holroyd. 1984. Clinical evaluation of the Prophy-Jet as an instrument for routine removal of tooth stain and plaque. *J. Periodontol.* 55:486–488.

White, S. L., and L. A. Hoffman. 1991. A practice survey of hygienists using an air-powder abrasive system: An investigation. *J. Dent. Hyg.* (Nov–Dec):433–437.

Wilkens, E. M. 1989. *Clinical practice of the dental hygienist*, 6th ed., 506–507. Philadelphia: Lea & Febiger.

Wilkens, E. M. 1986. Removal of extrinsic dental stains: Selective polishing. *Can. Dent. Hyg.* 20:59.

Willmann, D. E., B. K. Norling, and W. N. Johnson. 1980. A new prophylaxis instrument: Effect on enamel alterations. *J. Am. Dent. Assoc.* 101:923–925.

Woodall, I. R. 1993. *Comprehensive dental hygiene care*, 4th ed., 648. St. Louis: Mosby–Year Book.

Worrall, S. F., P. J. Knibbs, and H. D. Glenwright. 1987. Methods of reducing bacterial contamination of the atmosphere arising from use of an air-polisher. *Br. Dent. J.* 163:118–119.

SELF-QUIZ

1. In which one of the following medical conditions is air polishing contraindicated during periodontal treatment? (p. 438)

   a. hypertension
   b. bronchitis
   c. viral infections
   d. congestive heart failure

2. Air polishing removes less tooth structure than a curet *because* air polishing uses extremely light pressure on the tooth surface? (pp. 431–432)

   a. Both the statement and the reason are correct and related.
   b. Both the statement and the reason are correct but *not* related.
   c. The statement is correct, but the reason is *not.*
   d. The statement is *not* correct, but the reason is correct.
   e. *Neither* the statement *nor* the reason is correct.

3. Which one of the following precautions can the dental hygienist *best* take to control the aerosols produced by an air polisher? (p. 432)

   a. effective air-conditioning duct system
   b. high-volume evacuation
   c. preprocedural rinse
   d. premedicate with antibiotics

4. Which one of the following steps should be taken to minimize the amount of root structure cementum lost during air polishing? (pp. 433–434)

   a. Apply composite to the tooth before beginning treatment.
   b. Use cold water intermittently to reduce heat buildup.
   c. Expose the tooth to the slurry for no more than 10 seconds.
   d. Rinse with an antimicrobial rinse.

5. Which one of the following effects could air polishing have on porcelain restorations? (p. 435)

   a. scratches the surface
   b. dulls the surface
   c. alteration of margins
   d. creates a porous surface

OCCLUSAL TRAUMA

13

Milton Palat, D.D.S., J.D.

Outline:

Goal:

To educate the dental hygienist about the etiology, identifying features, and therapy of occlusal trauma.

Educational Objectives:

Upon completion of this chapter, the reader should be able to:

Identify and describe two types of occlusal trauma;

Recognize and describe the clinical and radiographic signs of occlusal trauma;

Discuss the interrelationship between occlusal trauma and periodontitis; and

Define the role of the dental hygienist in occlusal therapy.

KEY WORDS

- occlusal trauma
- traumatogenic occlusion
- parafunctional habits
- occlusal therapy
- primary occlusal trauma
- secondary occlusal trauma

*S*oon after the identification of microorganisms as a risk factor for periodontitis, the role of occlusion in periodontal diseases was considered. Although numerous studies using human and animal models have been published on this subject, it still remains a controversial issue.

The Lesion of Occlusal Trauma

Terminology

Occlusal trauma (also termed *trauma from occlusion, periodontal traumatism,* or *occlusal disease*) is defined as injury to the attachment apparatus (bone, periodontal ligament, and cementum) as a consequence of normal or excessive occlusal force(s) applied to a tooth or teeth (American Academy of Periodontology 1992). In addition to periodontal tissue damage, excessive occlusal force also can affect the temporomandibular joint, muscles of mastication, pulp tissue, and integrity of the restoration. Occlusal force is a force (or energy) transmitted to the teeth and their supporting structures by tooth-to-tooth contacts or through food substances or any other intervening material. When the magnitude (size), direction, frequency, and/or duration of these forces exceeds the reparative capacity of the attachment apparatus, the result is occlusal disease. This is determined clinically by signs and symptoms. *Traumatogenic occlusion* is defined as any occlusion that produces forces that directly or indirectly cause injury to the attachment apparatus.

Premature occlusal contact (also called *occlusal interference*) occurs when there are interferences to closure of opposing teeth (Fig. 13–1 ■). That is, a tooth that occludes with an opposing tooth before full closure is achieved in centric occlusion. This premature contact prevents the other teeth in the arch from achieving contact simultaneously. Premature contacts also can occur during lateral movements when the mandible moves from one side to the other. In addition, an extruded (also termed *supererupted*) or a tipped tooth may cause posterior occlusal interferences. Premature contacts should be eliminated if there is evidence of damage to the attachment apparatus or increasing tooth mobility.

Parafunctional habits are activities of the masticatory (chewing) system that are beyond the normal range of function. Chewing and swallowing are normal, whereas grinding and clenching are abnormal or parafunctional activities. Parafunctional activities often occur during sleep or stressful situations. Involuntary or unconscious clenching or grinding of teeth, when the patient is not intentionally chewing or swallowing, is termed *bruxism.* Premature contacts also may predispose to parafunctional habits.

Physiologic occlusion is defined as survival of the dentition despite its deviation from a preconceived hypothetical normal. Most people have some occlusal discrepancies, but in most cases, the dentition has "adapted" to the discrepancies and shows no signs of occlusal trauma. On the other hand, the dentition in a pathologic occlusion generally shows evidence of occlusal disease.

Occlusal therapy is designed to control the forces generated by tooth-to-tooth contact so they are tolerated by the attachment apparatus.

In protrusion (anterior teeth edge to edge), note that the initial interference is on the maxillary incisors, which prevents the right lateral incisor from occluding.

THE ROLE OF OCCLUSAL TRAUMA IN THE INITIATION AND PROGRESSION OF PERIODONTAL DISEASES

Research has concluded that occlusal trauma alone does not cause gingivitis, periodontitis, pocket formation, or gingival recession (Ramfjord and Ash 1981; Svanberg, King, and Gibbs 1995). The gingival unit is independent, having its own blood supply, and is not affected by occlusal trauma (Keller and Cohen 1955). In healthy conditions, the structure and adaptive nature of the attachment apparatus to occlusal forces permit a certain degree of physiologic mobility. *Adaptation* refers to alterations or adjustments that the body develops to accommodate to its environment. However, when occlusal forces are excessive, beyond the capability of the attachment apparatus to repair itself, tissue injury occurs, resulting in occlusal trauma.

A more complex and controversial issue is the interrelationship between periodontal inflammation and trauma from occlusion. Numerous human and animal models were developed to determine the effects of occlusal forces on the progression of periodontitis. It is also debatable whether these factors interfere with wound healing in the treatment of periodontal diseases. The conflicting results of different studies may be due to differences in animal species, the procedures used for producing occlusal trauma, and inherent measurement inaccuracies.

Human studies

Glickman (1963) introduced the concept of codestruction, whereby inflammation and trauma from occlusion are synergistic factors in periodontal destruction. He suggested that while occlusion does not cause gingival inflammation or pocket formation, inflammation of the supporting tissues in the presence of occlusal trauma alters the pathway of inflammation. Subsequently, the inflammatory infiltrate will spread more rapidly through tissue damaged by excessive occlusal forces and move directly into the periodontal ligament space, causing the development of angular bone defects and infrabony pockets. Thus, according to Glickman, inflammation and occlusal trauma become codestructive, whereby the progression of periodontitis is accelerated by the presence of occlusal trauma.

However, other investigators (Shefter and McFall 1984) reported no relationship between occlusal disharmonies and pathoses associated with inflammatory periodontal disease in patients with mild to moderate periodontitis.

Animal studies

In an attempt to reproduce the kind of occlusal trauma that might occur in the human dentition, early studies placed high restorations on teeth to reproduce the jiggling forces caused by premature tooth contacts. Jiggling or reciprocating forces were applied in opposite directions on a tooth at the same time. This prevented the tooth from moving away from the force. Unilateral forces would have allowed the traumatized teeth to migrate away from the occlusal forces. In many studies, tissue inflammation was induced using silk ligatures placed around the teeth near the gingival margin to enhance plaque retention.

Primate Model   Meitner (1975) examined the effects of jiggling forces on marginal periodontitis in squirrel monkeys by forcing wedges into the embrasure between teeth. The wedges were moved every 48 hours, allowing the teeth to be subjected to reciprocating forces every other day. Although this type of trauma is quite different from that caused by premature contacts, there was no accelerated loss of connective tissue attachment.

Polson (1974) also found that there was no difference in loss of connective tissue attachment and bone destruction in periodontally involved teeth of squirrel monkeys subjected to a single episode of trauma.

Beagle Dog Model   The results of several beagle dog studies (Lindhe and Svanberg 1974; Ericsson and Lindhe 1982) showed that when heavy occlusal forces were combined with plaque-induced periodontitis, the rate of clinical attachment loss was accelerated; but this model system also showed that trauma from occlusion does not aggravate gingival inflammation or cause loss of clinical attachment in chronic gingivitis (Ericsson and Lindhe 1977). In the beagle dog, when jiggling forces were applied to a periodontally healthy tooth or a tooth with chronic gingivitis, the tooth became hypermobile.

PATHOGENESIS OF OCCLUSAL TRAUMA

The pathologic features of occlusal trauma are different from those of inflammation. With occlusal trauma, healing of traumatized tissue need not be considered an inflammatory process because no inflammatory/immune cells such as leukocytes, lymphocytes, or plasma cells are present. Thus repair is initiated after the trauma is removed, without the tissue exhibiting the classic signs of inflammation.

The lesion of occlusal trauma in the normal, healthy periodontium usually develops following compression and tension of the periodontal ligament (PDL) fibers and resorption and deposition of bone. Compression of the PDL fibers results in obstruction of blood flow to the fibers, which in turn results in bone resorption. If the destructive process is greater than the repair potential of the periodontal tissue, injury may result. The alveolar bone undergoes osteoclastic resorption in areas of pressure, which results in the widening of the periodontal ligament space (Svanberg, King, and Gibbs 1995). Clinically, increased tooth mobility may result to accommodate for the widened PDL. Regardless of the status of the original attachment apparatus, there will be increasing tooth mobility until the PDL can adapt to the applied force. When adaptation is complete, new lamina dura may be seen radiographically, even though the increased PDL space of hypermobile teeth will remain. When the occlusal trauma is eliminated, bone repair will occur, and a functional width of the PDL will be reestablished. If, however, the trauma continues, excessive widening of the PDL results to accommodate the bone loss. This results in increasing tooth mobility.

The gingival connective tissue attachment is not affected, nor is there apical migration of the junctional epithelium. This same tissue reaction that occurs in a patient with a healthy periodontium also occurs in a patient with a reduced bony support who also has a healthy periodontium.

If the codestructive theory was correct, then the pathway of inflammation would be seen as proceeding not from the gingiva to the bone and finally to the PDL but rather from the gingiva directly into the PDL, inducing the formation of an infrabony pocket with associated vertical bone loss (Glickman and Smulow 1965). Removal of the trauma but not the inflammation does not decrease tooth mobility, and the crestal bone does not repair (Polson, Meitner, and Zander 1976). Kantor, Polson, and Zander (1976) removed both jiggling forces and inflammation, resulting in new bone formation without an increase in alveolar bone height. Collectively, these studies show that occlusal trauma does not initiate gingivitis or periodontitis. Although the importance of the role of dental plaque in inflammatory periodontal diseases is undisputed, the influence of occlusal trauma on the attachment level remains controversial (Hallmon, 1999).

CLASSIFICATION OF OCCLUSAL TRAUMA

Occusal trauma can be can classified as either primary or secondary and either can be localized to a single tooth or generalized, affecting several teeth (Table 13–1■).

Primary occlusal trauma is defined as injury to the supporting structures (PDL, cementum, and bone) caused by excessive occlusal forces (forces greater than experienced during normal chewing function) placed on a tooth or teeth with normal periodontal tissue support (Fig. 13–2■). Examples of causes of primary occlusal trauma include

1. a "high" restoration, where, on biting, the restored tooth creates a premature contact with the opposing tooth;
2. parafunctional habits involving tooth-to-tooth contact such as bruxism, clenching, or object-to-tooth contact such as biting on pencils or nail biting;
3. a malpositioned or maligned tooth, including teeth that are extruded (moved occlusally) or tipped;
4. a periapical (around the apex of the root) abscess or infection causing a tooth to be extruded;
5. physical "blow" to a tooth or teeth;
6. a removable partial denture clasp around an abutment tooth; and
7. orthodontic movement of teeth.

Secondary occlusal trauma occurs when normal (e.g., chewing) or excessive occlusal forces cause injury in a periodontium with reduced bone support (Fig. 13–3■). Bone levels around the tooth are inadequate to support these forces, and

TABLE 13–1

PERIODONTAL OCCLUSAL TRAUMATIC LESIONS

TYPE OF OCCLUSAL TRAUMA	ETIOLOGY	POCKET FORMATION	BONE HEIGHT	MOBILITY	TREATMENT OPTIONS
Primary	Excessive occlusal force(s)	No	Normal height or slight bone loss	Adapted	Selective grinding, appliances, monitoring without treatment
Secondary	Normal or excessive occlusal force(s)	No/Yes Periodontal pockets may be present, but due to periodontal destruction rather than the occlusal trauma	Reduced height (moderate/severe)	Progressive	Splinting if necessary, selective grinding, extraction, orthodontic movement, appliances, monitoring

FIGURE 13–2

Primary occlusal trauma. A tooth with normal periodontal tissues is exposed to excessive occlusal load (arrow). As a result of bone resorption, the periodontal ligament space gradually increases in size on both sides of the teeth as well as in the periapical region.

the tooth is less resistant to occlusal loading. In other words, a tooth in secondary occlusal trauma has insufficient bone support, and normal chewing and swallowing forces are excessive, causing injury to the attachment apparatus. This can occur even when the periodontal tissues are healthy, but there is a reduced bone height. Therefore, the distinguishing feature between primary and secondary occlusal trauma is the amount of bony support surrounding the tooth.

PARAFUNCTIONAL ACTIVITY

Parafunctional activity may result in primary occlusal trauma. This occurs when a tooth is subjected to greater forces over a longer period of time than what nor-

FIGURE 13-3

Secondary occlusal trauma. If a tooth with reduced periodontal tissue support has been exposed to excessive occlusal forces, a widened periodontal ligament space and increased mobility result.

mally occurs in chewing and swallowing. Food chewing is not a cause of primary occlusal trauma because the forces are most likely not long-standing or severe enough to affect the attachment apparatus.

Bruxism usually occurs unconsciously, whether the patient is awake or asleep. Thus many patients are not aware of their habit. When the forces generated during bruxism exceed the adaptive capacity of the periodontium on a regular basis, occlusal trauma is initiated (Caffesse and Fleszar 1992).

Other parafunctional habits such as lip, nail or cheek biting, tongue thrusting, or the placement of foreign objects between the teeth (e.g., pipe clenching and chewing, pencil biting, playing a wind musical instrument, and clenching fingernails or bobby pins) may affect the attachment apparatus. However, these do not appear to occur as frequently as tooth-to-tooth contact habits. A less common cause of primary occlusal trauma is *occupational bruxism,* which occurs in certain stressful occupations (e.g., dental hygienists).

CLINICAL FINDINGS IN OCCLUSAL TRAUMA

TOOTH MOBILITY

The most common sign of occlusal trauma is increasing tooth mobility over a period of time. However, excessive occlusal forces may not always cause tooth hypermobility (Svanberg, King, and Gibbs 1995). Since mobility due to occlusal trauma is an adaptive function, it may not be considered pathologic (resulting in disease). A tooth with excessive occlusal load may adapt to the forces by exhibiting increased but not increasing mobility. However, if there is progressive tooth mobility over a period of several days or weeks, it may then be considered pathologic (Green and Levine 1996). Consequently, for the proper recognition of occlusal disease, tooth mobility has to be assessed on two or more separate occasions (Svanberg, King, and Gibbs 1995).

FIGURE 13–4

A technique for detecting fremitus. The index finger is placed partly on the facial tooth surfaces and the gingiva. Tooth movements can be detected when the patient taps the teeth together and grinds side to side.

A tooth in primary occlusal trauma may show mobility. In this case, the tooth becomes mobile so that it can adapt to the abnormal force placed on it. Thus the mobility of the tooth could be classified as an *adapted mobility* (Tarnow and Fletcher 1986). For example, mobility of a tooth caused by a high restoration will come to a plateau and no longer increase; this is adapted mobility. Tooth mobility in absence of supporting alveolar bone may be characteristic of a parafunctional habit. However, tooth mobility does not occur in all patients who grind and clench their teeth. In some cases tooth wear accommodates for the bruxing habit.

Tooth hypermobility, produced by excessive occlusal forces, does not cause gingival inflammation, worsen the severity of chronic gingivitis, or act as a primary cause for connective tissue attachment loss (Svanberg, King, and Gibbs 1995).

Besides excessive occlusal forces, tooth mobility may result from severe gingival inflammation extending into the connective tissue attachment, the loss of supporting alveolar bone, pregnancy, and orthodontic movement, or may occur following surgical therapy. Tooth mobility will usually decrease by the fourth week after surgery. The cause and progression of the mobility must be determined because treatment options differ.

FREMITUS

Fremitus is the vibrational movement of a tooth under occlusal function. Fremitus is detected by placing the index finger on the gingival-tooth interfaces (Fig. 13–4 ■) of the maxillary teeth and asking the patient to tap the teeth up and down, grind from side to side, and move the jaw into an edge-to-edge (protrusive) occlusion. Centric prematurities are detected by the presence of fremitus.

PAIN

Pain from percussion, pain on biting, and the pain of tooth hypersensitivity are symptoms of primary and secondary occlusal trauma. For example, after receiv-

FIGURE 13–5

A 45-year-old patient with advanced periodontitis. Patient complaints of recently widened spaces, flaring of the maxillary incisors, and extrusion of the maxillary right central incisor are often an indication that the reduced attachment apparatus is reacting to occlusal forces.

ing a restoration, a patient may call to report tooth pain. An evaluation will reveal that the restoration is high, causing pain and mobility on biting or chewing. Once the restoration is reduced in height, the pain and mobility will disappear.

TOOTH MIGRATION

Pathologic tooth migration usually is indicative of moderate to severe periodontitis and secondary occlusal trauma (Towfighi et al. 1997). *Pathologic migration* is defined as a change in tooth position resulting from disruption of the forces that maintain teeth in a normal position (Chasens 1979). Excessive occlusal forces, which include the normal forces of chewing or swallowing applied to teeth, and extensive bone loss, may cause teeth to migrate (Towfighi et al. 1997). Clinically, pathologic tooth migration results in widened spaces between teeth (diastemas), flaring or fanning of anterior teeth, and/or extrusion of teeth (Fig. 13–5 ■). Although it is a common sign of secondary occlusal trauma, pathologic tooth migration may be caused by periodontal surgery or extensive inflammation extending into the PDL.

ATTRITION

Forces generated during bruxism frequently are greater than the adaptive capacity of the periodontium. Consequently, the contoured surface of a tooth may be ground flat, to the point where the dentin may be exposed (Figs. 13–6 ■ and 13–7 ■). This is termed *attrition*. Cracks and pits form on the worn edges and may become plaque traps. Clinical features of attrition include flattened occlusal or incisal surfaces of teeth. The canines and central and lateral incisors most commonly receive the heaviest and earliest lateral wear (Lytle 1990). Exposed dentin may cause a tooth to become sensitive. Wear facets frequently are seen as a flat, shiny worn spots on the side of a cusp of a tooth (Fig. 13–7). The presence of attrition and wear facets does not necessarily indicate occlusal habits. Wear on teeth also may be due to the patient's age or diet. Once a facet has developed, it remains. If a patient has wear facets for many years with no changes, it is probably not an active process.

Anterior view of a 55-year-old woman who was unaware she was a bruxer. Note the generalized heavy wear such that all teeth appear flat and on the same plane.

View of mandibular anterior teeth showing heavy wear through the enamel contributed to by the abrasive quality of the porcelain crown on the maxillary teeth. Note wear facet on the mandibular left canine.

MUSCLE/TEMPOROMANDIBULAR JOINT

Occlusal trauma may cause the muscles that work the jaw, the largest being the temporalis and the masseter, to become chronically sore, resulting in headaches and muscle pain. Pain usually occurs during chewing or on waking in the morning. This type of pain may be emanating from the temporomandibular joint (TMJ). The patient may report muscle spasms in the head, neck, and ear area. Pathology must be ruled out when a patient complains of any type of facial pain, including TMJ pain.

TOOTH STRUCTURE

Tooth fractures and long-term chipping of enamel are additional signs of occlusal trauma related to the magnitude of forces that the teeth endure.

RADIOGRAPHIC FINDINGS IN OCCLUSAL TRAUMA

Along with the clinical examination, radiographs are useful for recognizing the signs of occlusal trauma and/or the signs of adaptation to significant occlusal forces (Caffesse and Fleszar 1992).

Widening of the PDL occurs as an adaptation response to accommodate excessive occlusal loading and also may result in the resorption of alveolar bone. Radiographically, when the PDL space is wider at the coronal third of the root, it is referred to as *crestal funneling*.

Radiographically, a tooth in primary occlusal trauma may or may not show vertical bone loss as a result of widening of the PDL space. However, this should not be confused with bone loss related to periodontitis (Ricchetti 1998; Figs. 13–8■ and 13–9■) because primary occlusal trauma does not show loss of connective tissue attachment, increased probing depth, and related infrabony pockets (Polson and Zander 1983). The presence of angular bony defects is not necessarily a sign of occlusal trauma. If a widened PDL space is present but no tooth mobility exists, occlusal trauma is not necessarily present. The findings may be a functional adaptation to the occlusal forces.

Radiographically, a tooth in secondary occlusal trauma shows reduced bone levels that are inadequate to support the tooth under a normal load without increasing mobility, migration, or fremitus (Ricchetti 1998). Vertical bone loss is accompanied by widening of the PDL. Occasionally, root resorption may occur.

If the codestructive theory were correct, occlusal forces will accelerate the rate of destruction and result in vertical or angular bone defects, in the presence of pre-existing inflammation. However, there is still some questions of whether this occurs.

FIGURE 13–8

A radiograph showing a typical lesion of primary occlusal trauma. Widening of the periodontal ligament space has occurred due to a heavy occlusal force placed on the tooth. Note that there is no alveolar crestal bone loss and no increased probing depths.

FIGURE 13–9

A radiograph showing of a typical lesion of secondary occlusal trauma. The tooth has a reduced bony support and increasing tooth mobility. The tooth has an adverse crown-to-root ratio.

OUTCOMES OF TREATMENT OF OCCLUSAL TRAUMA

The desired outcome of treatment of occlusal trauma is that the patient remain comfortable during chewing and be able to maintain the dentition in a state of health. The dental hygienist can determine if the reversal of signs and symptoms of occlusal trauma has achieved the following outcomes (American Academy of Periodontology 1996). These include:

1. elimination or significant reduction of tooth mobility (the patient should be comfortable when in function);
2. elimination of occlusal prematurities and fremitus;
3. elimination of parafunctional habits;
4. prevention of further tooth migration; and
5. decrease or stability of radiographic changes.

Inadequate resolution of occlusal trauma is identified by

1. increasing tooth mobility;
2. progressive tooth migration;
3. patient continuing to complain of discomfort with pain and tooth mobility;
4. premature contacts remaining;
5. radiographic signs remaining, including widening of the PDL space;
6. parafunctional habits continuing; and
7. TMJ problems remaining or worsening.

OCCLUSAL THERAPY

The objective of occlusal therapy is to control the direction, duration, magnitude, and/or frequency of excessive occlusal forces. Practitioners have different views as to whether occlusal therapy is necessary in the overall periodontal treatment plan.

Table 13–2 ■ lists the most common approaches to treating trauma from occlusion. The key to treatment of occlusal trauma lies in the ability to determine if physiologic or pathologic occlusion exists. Physiologic occlusion does not need to be treated, whereas pathologic occlusion that shows signs and symptoms of occlusal problems requires treatment.

Since primary occlusal trauma is caused by excessive occlusal forces, treatment is aimed at eliminating or reducing the forces. Treatment options include selective grinding, control of habits, orthodontic movement, or monitoring of the condition without treatment.

In contrast to the primary occlusal traumatic lesion, the secondary occlusal traumatic lesion is not reversible, since its cause is loss of bony support around a tooth or teeth. Treatment options for secondary occlusal trauma include splinting, selective grinding, orthodontic movement, extraction, or monitoring of the condition without treatment. Reductions in tooth mobility are limited, because the mobility is due to a reduced periodontal support rather than to excessive occlusal force. Premature contacts on mobile teeth are detected and eliminated by selective grinding.

TABLE 13–2
APPROACHES TO TREATING OCCLUSAL TRAUMA
• Selective grinding
• Control of habits
• Orthodontic tooth movement
• Splinting
• Restorative procedures
• Monitoring without treatment

SELECTIVE GRINDING

Selective grinding is defined as the reshaping of the occlusal or incisal surfaces of teeth to create harmonious contacts between the upper and lower dentition. The goal of selective grinding is to eliminate premature contacts in primary or secondary occlusal trauma. Correction of prematurities should be done in centric occlusion, centric relation, and protrusive and lateral movements so that a traumatic contact of teeth occurs during movements of the mandible (Burgett 1995). Prematurities are detected by the use of wax, articulating paper, or dental floss.

Selective grinding always should be completed after inflammation has been controlled. Once the inflammation is eliminated by periodontal debridement and oral hygiene self-care, the tooth mobility may decrease because the fibers of the connective tissue attachment repair and a tooth with an intact connective tissue attachment has additional rigidity. Once periodontal health is reestablished, the occlusal condition is reevaluated. A decision to perform selective grinding depends on the degree of patient discomfort and function rather than on the assumption that selective grinding is necessary to halt the progression of disease (Gher 1996).

Primary occlusal trauma caused by a high restoration is treated by selective grinding. However, severe discrepancies may be resolved best by replacing the restoration. Selective grinding reshapes the occlusal surfaces of teeth to create harmonious contact relationships between the opposing teeth. This is accomplished with hand instruments or a high-speed handpiece and a bur. Tooth surfaces should be smooth so that patients do not develop secondary occlusal habits by "playing" with a rough surface. Selective grinding also can be performed on teeth in secondary occlusal trauma.

CONTROL OF PARAFUNCTIONAL HABITS

Appliances

If the cause of the occlusal trauma is bruxism, selective grinding usually will not correct the problem; however, counseling the patient may alleviate the psychological component of clenching and grinding. Because such problems are difficult to resolve, a bite plane or Hawley appliance may be fabricated from an orthodontic resin material that disoccludes the posterior teeth. This does not allow the opposing arches to contact and permit the attachment apparatus to heal. The appliance also can be used as an adjunct to selective grinding to stabilize the occlusion and allow the attachment apparatus to rest.

During sleep, a night guard can be worn to control occlusal habits. A night guard serves to protect the teeth from abnormal occlusal wear due to bruxism. Occlusal contacts between the upper and lower teeth are eliminated, thus stabilizing the occlusion and negating the effects of grinding and clenching at night (Chasens 1990). The night guard is made of either hard or soft acrylic, usually covering the occlusal surfaces of all teeth in the maxillary arch (Fig. 13–10■). The night guard is adjusted so that all mandibular teeth make simultaneous contact in centric occlusion.

Exercise

Besides using appliances to alter or control occlusal habits, exercise is important as well, especially if the patient clenches. An exercise to follow includes clenching for 5 seconds, then releasing, and repeating this five times in a row (for a total of 60 seconds). This should be done five times a day for 14 consecutive days. If one day is missed, the exercise must be started again.

ORTHODONTICS

Orthodontic treatment may be indicated in periodontal patients exhibiting drifting, migration, extrusion, or flared anterior teeth. The goal is to move a tooth or teeth into a more functional, less traumatic position.

SPLINTING

Splinting of teeth is considered the treatment of choice for patients who complain of discomfort or if the examination reveals that the mobility interferes with chew-

FIGURE 13–10

A hard acrylic night guard was made for this 35-year-old bruxer. It is used to protect the teeth during the night and help eliminate the habit. Night guards have full occlusal coverage and usually are made for the maxillary arch.

ing (mastication). Although tooth mobility that develops after periodontal surgery usually will subside within a few months, temporary splinting may be necessary to prevent secondary occlusal trauma. Splinting is also done on teeth in primary occlusal trauma if the mobility was caused by avulsion of the tooth or if the patient received a blow to the mouth resulting in loosening of a tooth or teeth.

Splinting permits healing of the attachment apparatus by holding a tooth in a totally fixed position. This allows the PDL to become narrower and the mobility to be reduced (Ricchetti 1998). Instead of one tooth experiencing the brunt of forces, the forces are distributed and spread over several teeth, which are better able to absorb the trauma. If mobility is not increasing over time, it may not be necessary to splint. The attachment apparatus may have adapted to the excessive forces and is in a stage of repair (Chasens 1990). Unfortunately, it is difficult to determine at any given point in time if a patient's attachment apparatus is in a state of repair. That is why monitoring mobility is so important.

Temporary splinting uses wires and composite material, acid etching nylon mesh, or fixed bridges or crowns that are joined or soldered together (Fig. 13–11■). A night guard is considered a type of occlusal splint.

Disadvantages of splinting include compromised aesthetics, reduced plaque-control efficacy, and a changed stable occlusion. Because of these disadvantages, splinting is not done routinely, and if it is selected, it should be considered with the preceding problems in mind.

RESTORATIVE PROCEDURES

To establish a stable posterior occlusion, restorations may be placed if other treatment options, including orthodontics or selective grinding, are not possible. For example, if a patient has anterior teeth and some or all of the posterior teeth on both sides are missing, the anterior teeth may become overloaded. Thus restorations [(e.g., removal partial dentures (RPDs) or crowns)] will restore the posterior occlusion and distribute the load to protect the anterior teeth.

FIGURE 13–11

The fixed prosthesis consists of multiple crowns on the maxillary teeth that have been soldered. This represents a form of permanent splinting.

SUMMARY

Overall, the periodontal response to occlusal trauma can be considered a physiologic adaptation. This adaptation can result in permanently increased tooth mobility if the trauma continues. However, if plaque control is adequate, connective tissue attachment loss should not occur. Removal of the injurious occlusal forces allows the lesion to repair itself, but this may be compromised by the presence of dental plaque. Therefore, maintenance of adequate plaque control is of utmost importance in preventing and reversing the problem. The question of increased periodontal tissue destruction when periodontitis coexists with occlusal trauma remains unresolved.

Occlusal trauma alone does not cause gingivitis, loss of connective tissue attachment, or pocket formation. Unless there is compromised periodontal support, there is little or no damage to the teeth or the attachment apparatus from normal masticatory (chewing) forces. Normal forces are only traumatogenic in secondary occlusal trauma, when the periodontal support is reduced by disease.

The role of the dental hygienist in the identification of occlusal trauma is important for the overall treatment of the patient. Treatment differs depending on the type of occlusal trauma and its etiology. To help distinguish between primary and secondary occlusal trauma, the dental hygienist can use radiographs and present and past dental history. The occlusal forces required to produce occlusal trauma generally are related to the remaining bony support for a given tooth.

KEY POINTS

✢ Occlusal trauma does not initiate gingivitis or periodontitis.

✢ Parafunctional habits may cause occlusal trauma.

✢ The most common clinical sign of occlusal trauma is increasing tooth mobility.

✢ Pathologic tooth migration is usually indicative of moderate to severe periodontitis and secondary occlusal trauma.

✢ Different treatments are available for occlusal trauma.

REFERENCES

American Academy of Periodontology. 1992. *Glossary of periodontal terms,* 3rd ed. Chicago: American Academy of Periodontology.

American Academy of Periodontology. 1996. *Parameters of care.* Chicago: American Academy of Periodontology, Scientific and Educational Affairs Department.

Burgett, F. G. 1995. Trauma from occlusion. *Dent. Clin. North Am.* 39:301–311.

Caffesse, R. G., and T. J. Fleszar. 1992. Occlusal trauma. In *Advances in periodontics,* ed. T. G. Wilson, K. S. Komman, and M. G. Newman, 205–225. Chicago: Quintessence Publishing Co.

Chasens, A. I. 1979. Periodontal disease, pathologic tooth migration and adult orthodontics. *N.Y. J. Dent.* 49:40–43.

Chasens, A. I. 1990. Controversies in occlusion. *Dent. Clin. North Am.* 34:11–123.

Ericsson, I., and J. Lindhe. 1977. Lack of effect of trauma from occlusion on the recurrence of experimental periodontitis. *J. Clin. Periodontol.* 4:115–127.

Ericsson, I., and J. Lindhe. 1982. Effect of long-standing jiggling on experimental marginal periodontitis in the beagle dog. *J. Clin. Periodontol.* 9:497–503.

Gher, M. E. 1996. Nonsurgical pocket therapy: Dental occlusion. *Ann. Periodontol.* 1:567–580.

Glickman, I. 1963. Inflammation and trauma from occlusion: Codestructive factors in chronic periodontal disease. *J. Periodontol.* 34:5–10.

Glickman, I. 1967. Occlusion and the periodontium. *J. Dent. Res.* 46(suppl 53):53.

Glickman, I., and J. B. Smulow. 1965. Effect of excessive occlusal forces upon the pathway of gingival inflammation in humans. *J. Periodontol.* 36:141–147.

Green, M. S., and D. F. Levine. 1996. Occlusion and the periodontium: A review and rationale for treatment. *J. Calif. Dent. Assoc.* 24:19–27.

Hallmon, W. W. 1999. Occlusal trauma: Effect and impact on the periodontium. *Ann. Periodontol.* 4:102–107.

Kantor, J., A. M. Polson, and H. A. Zander. 1976. Alveolar bone regeneration after removal of inflammatory and traumatic factors. *J. Periodontol.* 47:687–695.

Keller, G., and W. Cohen. 1955. India ink perfusions of the vascular plexus of oral tissues. *Oral Surg.* 8:539–542.

Lindhe, J., and G. Svanberg. 1974. Influence of trauma from occlusion on progression of experimental periodontitis in the beagle dog. *J. Clin. Periodontol.* 1:3–14.

Lytle, J. D. 1990. The clinician's index of occlusal disease: Definition, recognition, and management. *Int. J. Periodontic Restorative Dent.* 10:103–123.

Meitner, S. 1975. Codestructive factors of marginal periodontitis and repetitive mechanical injury. *J. Dent. Res.* 54:78–85.

Polson, A. M. 1974. Trauma and progression of marginal periodontitis in squirrel monkeys. II. Codestructive factors of periodontitis and mechanically produced injury. *J. Periodontol. Res.* 9:108–113.

Polson, A. M., and H. A. Zander. 1983. Effect of periodontal trauma upon intrabony pockets. *J. Periodontol.* 54:586–591.

Polson, A. M., S. W. Meitner, and H. A. Zander. 1976. Trauma and progression of marginal periodontitis in squirrel monkeys: IV. Reversibility of bone loss due to trauma alone and trauma superimposed upon periodontitis. *J. Periodontol. Res.* 11:290–298.

Ramfjord, S. P., and M. M. Ash. 1981. Significance of occlusion in the etiology and treatment of early, moderate and advanced periodontitis. *J. Periodontol.* 52:511–517

Ricchetti, P. A. 1998. Treatment of the periodontium affected by occlusal traumatism. In *Periodontal therapy: Clinical approaches and evidence of success,* Vol. 1, ed. M. Nevins and J. T. Mellonig, 132–133. Chicago. Quintessence Publishing Co.

Shefter, G. J., and W. T. McFall. 1984. Occlusal relations and periodontal status in human adults. *J. Periodontol.* 55:368–374.

Svanberg, G. K., G. J. King, and C. H. Gibbs. 1995. Occlusal considerations in periodontology. *Periodontology 2000* 9:106–117.

Tarnow, D. P., and P. Fletcher. 1986. Splinting of periodontally involved teeth: Indications and contraindications. *N.Y. State Dent. J.* (May):24–25.

Towfighi, P. P., M. A. Brunsvold, A. T. Storey, et al. 1997. Pathologic migration of anterior teeth in patients with moderate to severe periodontitis. *J. Periodontol.* 68:967–972.

SELF-QUIZ

1. All the following parts of the periodontium are affected by occlusal trauma *except* one. Which one is the exception? (p. 445)

   a. periodontal ligament

   b. alveolar bone

   c. gingiva

   d. cementum

2. Which one of the following definitions pertains to primary occlusal trauma? (p. 447)

	TYPE OF OCCLUSAL FORCE	BONE SUPPORT
a.	Normal	Adequate
b.	Excessive	Adequate
c.	Normal	Reduced
d.	Excessive	Reduced

3. All the following signs and symptoms are found in occlusal trauma *except* one. Which one is the exception? (pp. 449–453)

   a. tooth mobility

   b. tooth migration

   c. pain on chewing

   d. occlusal erosion

4. Which one of the following radiographic signs is evident in occlusal trauma? (p. 453)

   a. widening of the periodontal ligament space

   b. deposition of acellular cementum

   c. deposition of alveolar bone

   d. receding pulp tissue

5. Occlusal trauma in combination with chronic inflammatory periodontitis *may* result in greater tooth mobility and alveolar bone loss *because* occlusal trauma causes periodontal pocket formation. (pp. 445–447)

   a. Both the statement and the reason are correct and related.

   b. Both the statement and the reason are correct but *not* related.

   c. The statement is correct, but the reason is *not.*

   d. The statement is *not* correct, but the reason is correct.

   e. *Neither* the statement *nor* the reason is correct.

6. Two days after a patient receives an amalgam restoration, he reports back to the office complaining of pain and looseness of the tooth. Which one of the following treatments would be most appropriate? (p. 455)

   a. Replace the amalgam with composite.

   b. Reduce the height of the restoration.

   c. Polish the restoration.

   d. Maintain the restoration as is.

7. Which one of the following factors is the primary cause of secondary occlusal trauma? (pp. 447–448)

   a. tooth with severe bone loss

   b. night and daytime bruxism

   c. tongue thrusting

   d. pipe chewing

8. A patient complains of soreness in the jaw on wakening in the morning. She is having stressful problems at work. She complains that some of her lower teeth are "wearing down." Which one of the following conditions does this patient most likely have? (pp. 444, 449)

   a. fractured jaw
   b. parafunctional habit
   c. severe periodontitis
   d. necrotizing ulcerative gingivitis

9. A patient has returned for a 2-week follow-up visit after periodontal surgery complaining of tooth mobility. There was no mobility before the surgery was done. Which one of the following should be explained to the patient? (p. 450)

   a. Teeth must be splinted immediately.
   b. Mobility will decrease in time.
   c. Additional surgery will be needed.
   d. Systemic antibiotics are indicated.

10. Which one of the following conditions is *best* treated with a night guard? (pp. 455–456)

   a. tooth with severe bone loss
   b. tongue thrusting habit
   c. teeth with severe abrasion
   d. clenching and grinding

PRINCIPLES OF PERIODONTAL SURGERY: GINGIVECTOMY, OSSEOUS RESECTION, AND MUCOGINGIVAL SURGERY

Fadi I. Beydoun, D.D.S., M.S.
Mea A. Weinberg, D.M.D., M.S.D., R.Ph.

Outline:

KEY WORDS

- periodontal surgery
- periodontal diseases
- healing
- gingivectomy
- flap surgery
- mucogingival surgery
- periodontal dressing
- postoperative care

Goal:

To educate the dental hygienist on the basic principles, and postoperative care of periodontal surgical procedures.

Educational Objectives:

Upon completion of this chapter, the reader should be able to:

Discuss the rationale of periodontal surgical therapy;

Describe the indications and contraindications for periodontal surgical therapy;

Compare and contrast the currently accepted surgical treatment modalities;

Counsel patients on postoperative care following periodontal surgery;

Identify and explain the management of postoperative complications; and

Discuss surgical wound healing and how soon after surgery a reevaluation can be performed.

The term *surgery* is a generic word to describe the branch of medical science concerned with the treatment of diseases or injuries by manual or operative means. Periodontal debridement (scaling and root planing) meets this definition, but it is not considered surgery. *Periodontal surgery,* as used in the dental literature, is applied only to surgical procedures used to treat **periodontal diseases** or to modify the morphology of soft tissues and bone.

Different surgical procedures have been proposed to treat gingivitis and periodontitis, as well as to gain access to the underlying root surface and supporting bone. The most common surgical procedures include the gingivectomy, the modified Widman flap, and the apically positioned flap with or without osseous (bone) resection.

OBJECTIVES, INDICATIONS, AND CONTRAINDICATIONS OF PERIODONTAL SURGERY

Over the past several years, root instrumentation techniques and antibiotic periodontal therapy have improved dramatically. Nevertheless, periodontal surgery remains a valid option in many patients. It is imperative for the dental hygienist to have a thorough knowledge of various basic periodontal surgical procedures as well as a clear understanding of the indications and contraindications of these procedures.

The primary objectives of periodontal surgery include the following (Palcanis 1996):

1. Elimination of a pocket results in minimal probing depths, which allows the patient and the dental practitioner access for plaque control.
2. The aim is not necessarily to eliminate the pocket (e.g., in patients with very deep pockets and bone loss) but to gain access to the root and underlying bone to achieve more effective removal of calculus and subgingival bacteria so as to maintain periodontal attachment levels and perhaps even gain "new attachment." *New attachment* is defined as the union of connective tissue with a root surface that has been deprived previously of its original attachment apparatus (American Academy of Periodontology 1992).

3. To regenerate periodontal tissues lost from disease.
4. To arrest disease progression.
5. To create an oral environment that is maintainable by both the patient and the dental team.

After the surgical procedures have been performed, the therapeutic end points of clinical success are measured by (Palcanis 1996) the attainment of stable or improved clinical attachment levels, minimal inflammation (bleeding on probing), and reduced and stable probing depths.

Indications for periodontal surgery include the following:

1. pocket elimination/reduction on teeth with gingival/periodontal pockets;
2. correction of mucogingival defects (e.g., for root coverage, increasing the zone of keratinized/attached gingiva, augmentation of alveolar ridges);
3. establishment of aesthetics;
4. creation of a favorable restorative environment such as lengthening of the clinical crown;
5. placement of dental implants; and
6. incision and drainage of a gingival or periodontal abscess.
7. regeneration of the attachment apparatus that was destroyed as a result of perodontial disease.

Periodontal surgical therapy is contraindicated or at least delayed for the following reasons:

1. systemic diseases that cannot be controlled by medications or otherwise, such as diabetes mellitus, cardiovascular conditions (e.g., hypertension), or in immunodeficiency diseases (e.g., HIV infection) (in these patients, a medical consultation with the patient's physician is warranted);
2. systemic diseases that are associated with excessive bleeding, such as leukemia, hemophilia, and renal (kidney) dialysis (consult with the patient's physician);
3. patients who are noncompliant with plaque control or periodontal maintenance appointments; and
4. concern for cosmetic outcome, especially in anterior areas.
5. treating teeth that have hopeless prognosis

PREOPERATIVE PREPARATION

Preoperative management involving patient preparation for surgery includes removal of soft and hard deposits, reinforcement of oral hygiene self-care, selective occlusal adjustment, and selective adjunctive antimicrobial or antibiotic agents. It is important to complete initial therapy because this may eliminate the need for surgery or at least reduce or eliminate gingival inflammation, which will increase the manageability of the tissues during surgery and allow for better healing. Evaluation for surgery is done at a minimum of 4 to 6 weeks after completion of the initial phase of therapy. At this time, a soft tissue examination will determine the tissue reaction or response to the initial therapy. An evaluation of the patient's oral hygiene status also is made. If there is residual calculus, additional sessions of periodontal debridement may be necessary. A complete periodontal charting is done, including identification and cause of bleeding sites and sites with clinical attachment loss (Carranza 1996).

REQUIREMENTS FOR PERIODONTAL SURGERY

Specific requirements must be met before surgery is performed. Elimination of plaque-retentive restorations should be done before surgery (e.g., overhanging margins of restorations or overcontoured restorations) (Flores-de-Jacoby and Mengel 1995). Any carious lesions should be repaired and hopeless teeth extracted. Risk factors such as smoking have been shown to delay wound healing after surgery (Boström, Linder, and Bergström 1998; Preber and Bergström 1990), and this may need to be addressed with the patient.

TYPES OF PERIODONTAL SURGERY

There are many types of surgical procedures, and selection of the appropriate surgery depends on the pattern of bone loss (e.g., horizontal versus vertical or a combination of both) and the presence of mucogingival involvement. Periodontal surgery usually is done in quadrants or sextants depending on the number of teeth involved and the decision of the surgeon. Most important, the practitioner and the patient should be aware of the limitations of periodontal surgery (Table 14–1 ■).

Lang and Löe (1993) proposed a convenient classification of periodontal surgical procedures. It includes five categories:

1. Procedures for pocket reduction or elimination
2. Procedures for gaining access to root surfaces for debridement (periodontal flap surgery)
3. Procedures for treatment of osseous defects
4. Procedures for correcting mucogingival defects
5. Procedures for regeneration of lost periodontium

HEALING FOLLOWING PERIODONTAL SURGERY

There are four types of **healing** responses of periodontal tissues that can occur after periodontal treatment (Carranza 1996). *Repair* is the healing of periodontal tissues with tissues that do not replicate the original lost periodontium. After periodontal surgery and periodontal debridement, instead of the gingival connective tissue attaching to the tooth, the junctional epithelium re-forms on the root surface by migrating along the root surface, forming a long junctional epithelium attachment. Another example of repair is scar formation, in which the new tissue

TABLE 14–1
LIMITATIONS OF PERIODONTAL SURGERY

- Periodontal surgery does not compensate for the patient's poor plaque control.
- Some adverse effects from surgery include gingival recession, which may compromise aesthetics to some degree.
- It will not routinely produce miraculous and complete regeneration of all lost periodontal tissues.

formed is considered epithelium and connective tissue but does not replicate the original tissue that was lost or damaged. *Reattachment* is the reunion of epithelial or connective tissue to a root surface that was not damaged by periodontal disease. This would occur after an incision or injury. *New attachment* is the union of connective tissue or epithelium with a root surface that was deprived of its original attachment apparatus. This new attachment can include new periodontal ligament, cementum, or bone, but only two of the three tissues. *Regeneration* is the re-formation of the periodontal tissues that were destroyed by periodontal disease with the formation of new cementum, periodontal ligament, and bone. This is the ideal situation and is the goal of various surgical procedures, but it is not always attained and in some cases is not always indicated. Rather, a partial regeneration or new attachment is obtained. Epithelium is the first tissue to move or migrate into the wound area. Epithelium moves very fast, up to 0.5 mm a day. This can interfere with the formation of a new attachment or regeneration.

PROCEDURES FOR POCKET REDUCTION/ELIMINATION

GINGIVECTOMY/GINGIVOPLASTY

Definition **Gingivectomy** is the excision or removal of the soft tissue walls (gingiva) in order to eliminate a pocket. *Gingivoplasty,* on the other hand, refers to surgical reshaping or recontouring of the oral surface of the gingiva without removing any portion of the gingiva that is attached to the tooth.

Indications The main objectives of gingivectomy/gingivoplasty procedures are to reduce or eliminate suprabony periodontal pockets that are associated with a horizontal pattern of bone loss and to eliminate pseudopockets (gingival overgrowth) induced by certain medications, such as phenytoin, cyclosporine, and nifedipine. Enlarged gingiva and interdental papillae seen in mouth breathers also can be treated with these techniques. Frequently, the gingival enlargement will recur, and gingivectomy procedures may have to be repeated. Less frequently, lengthening of the clinical crown can be achieved using gingivectomy.

Contraindications Contraindications for gingivectomy include lack of attached gingiva and the presence of infrabony pockets associated with vertical bone loss.

Technique After the patient receives local anesthesia, the gingivectomy is begun by marking the base of the pockets with a periodontal probe or other instrument. Incisions are made with a surgical blade angled at 45 degrees to the gingiva apical to the base of the pocket (Fig.14–1a,b ■). Incisions are not made into the sulcus, but rather on the outer epithelium, with the blade directed in an occlusal or incisal direction rather than apically. Periodontal debridement is performed followed by gingivoplasty to reestablish a physiologic gingiva. After hemostasis is obtained (bleeding is controlled), the area is dried, and a periodontal dressing is placed. The patient is given postoperative instructions. A sample of postoperative instructions to the patient for any surgical procedure is given in Table 14–2 ■. This includes care of the surgical wound, oral hygiene measures taken during initial healing, and reporting adverse signs and symptoms. The dental hygienist's role in postoperative care is reviewed in Table 14–3 ■. The patient then returns in 1 week for a postoperative visit.

FIGURE 14-1

(a) Clinical picture of a gingivectomy procedure. A 38-year-old patient with pseudopockets (gingival enlargement) due to pheny-toin therapy. The incision is made apical to the bleeding points, which demarcate the base of the pocket. (b) After the incision is made, the tissue is removed, exposing the underlying bleeding connective tissue.

(a)

(b)

TABLE 14-2
POSTOPERATIVE INSTRUCTIONS

Discomfort: Usually minimal discomfort is expected, especially after the anesthesia wears off. If you have been given a prescription, fill it and take the medication as directed. Aspirin should not be used. If discomfort persists, call the office.

Swelling: If swelling occurs, it will peak 48 to 72 hours after the surgery. You may use an ice pack on the outside of your face, 15 minutes on and 15 minutes off, for the next 2 hours. If swelling occurs after the first day, a moistened heated towel may be used on the area. If excessive swelling occurs, call the office.

Bleeding: There may be occasional blood stains in the saliva for the first 4 or 5 hours. This is not unusual; do not be alarmed. If bleeding continues, do not rinse to stop bleeding. Apply firm pressure using a moistened gauze pad or fresh tea bag for 20 minutes, without interruption. Repeat as necessary. If the bleeding does not stop, call the office.

Physical activity: It is recommended that you rest and limit your activities for the rest of the day. Avoid excessive exertion (jogging, swimming, tennis, etc.) for the next week.

Eating: Limit your diet to soft foods on the day of the surgery. Do not drink hot liquids (hot tea, hot coffee, hot soup) for 24 hours following surgery. Do not chew on the area where the surgery was performed. Avoid alcoholic beverages for 1 week following the surgery.

Sutures: If sutures were used, avoid that area. They will be removed approximately 7 to 14 days following surgery.

Dressing: To help minimize irritation, a periodontal dressing may be placed around the surgical area. It will harden within about 2 hours and should not be removed. It is of no concern if a few pieces of the dressing break off. However, if the dressing seems to be loose or has come off, contact the office for instructions.

Smoking: *Do not smoke.* Smoking may negatively affect the healing process, which may result in a poor outcome.

Home care: The most important element required for good healing is meticulous oral hygiene. If a dressing is placed, avoid pressing down on it. Use a soft or ultrasoft toothbrush to *carefully* clean the occlusal surface and the surface of the dressing. If no dressing was placed, *gently* use a soft or ultrasoft toothbrush to cleanse the area. Do not floss the surgical site. Brush and floss the untreated areas as usual. Do not rinse on the day of the surgery. On the second day, use the prescribed mouthrinse as directed.

Medications: In some cases, medications will be prescribed. Use prescribed medications as directed.

	TABLE 14–3	
	SURGICAL CARE PROCEDURES	
SURGICAL PROCEDURE	**POSTOPERATIVE CARE**	**REEVALUATION PROCEDURES**
Gingivectomy	1. Instruct patient not to brush the area where the periodontal dressing is located. 2. At postoperative visit, carefully remove the dressing, irrigate with sterile water or saline and wipe off the white film (this consists of dead epithelial cells). 3. Reapply dressing if needed. 4. Patient may start to brush surgical site gently with a roll technique. Bleeding will occur but will gradually lessen. The patient should continue to brush even if light bleeding is seen.	1. Periodontal probing should not be done until a minimum of 6 weeks after surgery. 2. Final prosthetic restorations should not be completed until 6 weeks or more after surgery. 3. Supragingival scaling can be done after 1 week, but subgingival periodontal debridement should not be performed until 6 weeks after surgery.
Flap surgery	1. Instruct patient not to brush the area where the periodontal dressing is located. 2. At postoperative visit, carefully remove the dressing, irrigate with sterile water or saline and wipe off the white film (this consists of dead epithelial cells). 3. Reapply dressing if needed; patient may start to brush surgical site gently with a roll technique. Bleeding will occur but will gradually lessen. The patient should continue to brush even if bleeding is seen.	1. Periodontal probing should not be done until a minimum of 3 months after surgery. 2. Final prosthetic restorations should not be completed until a minimum of 3 months after surgery. 3. Supragingival scaling can be done after 1 week, but subgingival periodontal debridement should not be performed until 3 months after surgery.
Mucogingival surgery	1. Instruct patient not to brush the area where the periodontal dressing is located. 2. At postoperative visit, carefully remove the dressing, irrigate with sterile water or saline and wipe off the white film (this consists of dead epithelial cells). 3. Reapply dressing if needed; patient may start to brush surgical site gently with a roll technique. Advise the patient not to hit the gums with the toothbrush. The patient discontinue brushing if bleeding is seen and only rinse the area with warm water.	1. Gingival grafts with root coverage would be reevaluated a minimum of 6 months after surgery. 2. Gingival grafts without root coverage can be reevaluated a minimum of 2 months after surgery.

Healing   Epithelialization of the wound surface starts within a few days of surgery. Soft tissue healing is completed within 4 to 5 weeks, although clinically it may appear healed within 2 weeks.

NEW ATTACHMENT PROCEDURES

The objective of new attachment procedures is to remove ulcerated pocket epithelium and the underlying connective tissue in an attempt to obtain a new connective tissue attachment (periodontal ligament fibers) inserting into new cementum.

Subgingival curettage

Indication   The primary indication for subgingival curettage is the presence of shallow pockets with swollen, edematous, and nonfibrotic gingival tissue of adequate width and thickness. This procedure is performed to eliminate or reduce pockets by shrinkage and new attachment, although most healing is by shrinkage and long junctional epithelium. As a definitive treatment, subgingival curettage is not considered to have any benefit, but it is described in this section because some practitioners still use it. Subgingival curettage differs from gingival curettage in that the procedure is performed apical to the junctional epithelium, into the connective tissue, and down to the alveolar crest.

Contraindications   Contraindications to subgingival curettage include the presence of acute infection such as necrotizing ulcerative gingivitis (NUG), medication-induced gingival overgrowth, and periodontitis.

Technique   (Fig. 14–2 ■)   The area is anesthetized with an appropriate local anesthetic. The curet is inserted past the base of the pocket down to the alveolar crest with the cutting edge facing the soft tissue. The tissues attached between the base of the pocket and the alveolar crest are removed. The gingival tissue is then adapted to the tooth surface with finger pressure and is sutured, if necessary. A periodontal dressing is applied, and the patient is instructed to use a mouthrinse (e.g., chlorhexidine gluconate) for 1 week until the postoperative visit. In certain states, the dental hygienist is permitted to perform subgingival curettage. Currently, this procedure is not considered to be a definitive treatment because of the inconsistency of obtaining new attachment. Inadvertent curettage can occur when there is partial debridement of the soft tissue pocket wall during periodontal debridement by the back and lateral edges of the cutting curet.

Healing   Healing of the epithelium is complete by 7 days, and connective tissue maturation occurs by 2 weeks. There is gingival shrinkage and a gain in clinical attachment with a long junctional epithelium.

Excisional new attachment procedure (ENAP)

Yukna and Lawrence (1980) described the ENAP as a means of treating suprabony pockets. In essence, this procedure is subgingival curettage performed with a surgical knife or blade. This procedure has the potential for allowing formation of a

FIGURE 14–2

Subgingival curettage performed using several overlapping horizontal strokes.

new connective tissue attachment (periodontal ligament fibers), in most cases consisting of a long junctional epithelium.

Indications   Indications for ENAP include suprabony pockets (≤5 mm) with adequate width and thickness of gingiva and in anterior areas where aesthetics are a consideration.

Contraindications   Contraindications to ENAP include the presence of an inadequate amount of gingiva and the presence of infrabony pockets.

Technique   The area is anesthetized with an appropriate anesthetic. An incision is made with a surgical blade in the sulcus (this is called a *crevicular incision*) on the buccal and lingual surfaces. The inner part of the periodontal pocket wall (pocket epithelium) is removed. The gingiva is slightly reflected away from the tooth. Periodontal debridement of the exposed root surface is performed, without attempting to remove the connective tissue fibers that are located 1 to 2 mm coronal to the crest of bone. The gingiva is closely adapted to the tooth with interproximal sutures, and the area is covered with a periodontal dressing for 7 to 10 days.

Healing   The pocket epithelium that was removed is replaced with a long junctional epithelium, which forms an attachment or closure to the tooth surface. Healing occurs in approximately 1 month.

Current consensus suggests that subgingival curettage and the other new attachment procedures are ineffective and do not result in new attachment; rather, the attachment or closure is by a long junctional epithelium, which may be capable of being maintained in a stable state over long-term intervals. These procedures are difficult to perform, and in most cases it is impossible to remove all the epithelial lining. Periodontal debridement adequately reduces the inflammation in most cases. The potential for new connective tissue attachment seems to be remote, even though the diseased epithelium is removed.

The modified Widman flap

The modified Widman flap procedure is also considered to be a new attachment surgery. However, because it involves the use of a flap, it is included in the next section on periodontal **flap surgery.**

PERIODONTAL FLAP SURGERY

A *flap* is defined as that loosened portion of the gingiva, alveolar mucosa, and/or periosteum that is separated from the underlying structures except at its base, from which the flap receives its blood supply. Flaps are the most commonly used periodontal surgical procedure. Flap procedures are designed to gain access to the underlying bone and root surface for the purpose of debridement, bone recontouring, or regeneration. Generally, a flap is made by an incision with a surgical blade or knife into the pocket (intracrevicular) or slightly subgingival to the gingival margin (internal bevel incision). The amount of attached gingiva present and the depth of the pockets primarily determine the type of incision made. The flap

FIGURE 14–3

(a) This flap was made to gain access to the underlying root and bone to modify defects in the bone and for root and defect debridement. Since connective tissue remains on the bone, it is called a *split-thickness flap.* (b) Replaced flap-postoperative (Reprinted with permission from James A. Simonds, *Practical Periodontics,* 1991. Continental Education, Santa Rosa, CA)

(a)

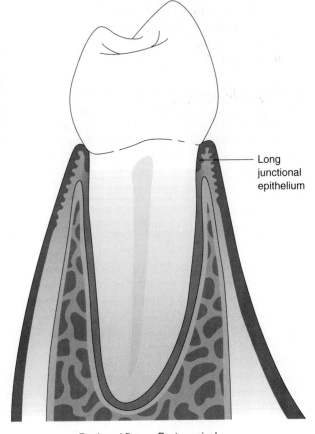

Long junctional epithelium

Replaced flap — Post-surgical

(b)

is then reflected away from the tooth with an instrument called a *periosteal elevator* to expose the underlying tooth and root surface.

Flap classification

Flaps are classified on the basis of tissue components included in the flap and the positioning of the flap at the end of the procedure. In a full-thickness or mucoperiosteal flap, the gingiva, alveolar mucosa, and periosteum are reflected from the root and the underlying bone surfaces (see Fig. 14–3a ■). A partial- or split-thickness flap is a flap in which the periosteum and some connective tissue are left attached to the bone and is not included in the flap. Partial-thickness flaps are used when the bone is thin and exposure to the environment is not desirable, since this would increase the chances of bone resorption. Based on the final positioning of the flap at the end of the surgical procedure, flaps are classified as apically, coronally, and laterally positioned. The most frequently used periodontal flap procedures are the modified Widman flap and apically positioned flap.

Healing following flap surgery

Following traditional flap surgery, the debrided root surface becomes repopulated with epithelial cells that form a long junctional epithelium along the root surface with no new connective tissue attachment (gingival fibers inserting into the cementum). (see Fig. 14–3b ■).

Modified Widman flap

Ramfjord and Nissle (1974) described the modified Widman flap (MWF) as being similar to the ENAP but including a flap for better visualization of the area.

Objective   The specific objective of the modified Widman flap is to gain access to root surfaces for improved periodontal debridement and a reduction in inflammation and pocket depths.

Indications   The procedure is indicated for deep pockets, infrabony pockets, and where aesthetics is important, such as in the anterior region.

MWF procedures, in general, have several advantages over closed subgingival curettage, root planing, and gingivectomy. They facilitate direct visualization and debridement of deep pockets. Widman flap procedures also allow complete removal of pocket epithelium, and since the flaps can be placed in close approximation, healing takes place by primary intention.

Contraindications   The MWF is contraindicated if there are bony defects that need to be recontoured or regenerated.

Technique   After adequate anesthesia is obtained, incisions are made through the crest of the gingiva approximately 1 mm from the margin. This is called an *inverse bevel incision*. This incision is scalloped and extended as far interproximally as possible to preserve the interdental papillae. Gingival tissues are then reflected only far enough to allow the surgeon direct vision of the root surfaces and the crest of bone. After complete debridement of plaque, calculus, and diseased tissue from the root surfaces and bony defects, the flap is readapted to cover the crest of bone. In some cases, bone recontouring is required for better flap adaptation. Interrupted interproximal sutures are then placed, and the surgical area is covered with a periodontal dressing. The patient receives postoperative instructions. The dressing and sutures are removed after 1 week, and the patient is placed on a chlorhexidine mouthrinse.

Apically positioned flap

An apically positioned flap is a full-thickness flap made with an internal bevel incision that is apically positioned at or near the level of the alveolar crest.

Objective   The main objective is to surgically reduce or eliminate deep pockets by apically positioning the gingival complex while retaining the entire width of gingiva.

Indications   This procedure is used to (1) eliminate moderate or deep pockets by positioning the gingival tissue apically, (2) lengthen the clinical crown for restorative/prosthetic procedures, and (3) increase the zone of attached gingiva.

Contraindications   The apically positioned flap is contraindicated for aesthetic reasons, such as in the anterior region, where root exposure would be unaesthetic. This type of surgery is also contraindicated in patients at high risk for root caries. It is also contraindicated in areas of advanced bone loss.

Technique   (Fig. 14–4a,b■)   The apically positioned flap can be used on buccal surfaces of both mandibular and maxillary arches as well as on the mandibular lingual surface. The palatal gingiva cannot be displaced or moved because it is composed entirely of keratinized gingiva without alveolar mucosa, which is what gives the flap its flexibility.

After obtaining adequate local anesthesia, a reverse (internal) bevel incision is made from the gingival margin to the crest of bone. The location of the initial incision in relation to the gingival margin depends on the width and thickness of the attached gingiva, as well as the depth of the pocket. The incision is scalloped interproximally to obtain optimal coverage of alveolar bone when the flaps are sutured. Vertical releasing incisions at the ends of the initial incision may be placed for flexibility and easier positioning of the flap apically. Next, a full-thickness flap is raised, and the incised gingival tissue collar is removed with a curet. Using power-driven scalers and hand instruments, diseased tissue is removed, and periodontal debridement is performed.

If bony defects are present, the bone can be recontoured. Bone recontouring is done with high-speed handpiece and/or hand chisels to establish a harmonious relationship between the gingiva and the bone. The flap is then positioned apically to cover the bone and is sutured. A periodontal dressing can be applied.

Healing   The attachment or closure of the soft tissue to the root surface in the apically positioned flap is by a long junctional epithelium, with no new connective tissue attachment. Complete healing occurs within 30 to 35 days. Postoperative care procedures are reviewed in Table 14–3.

FIGURE 14–4

The apically positioned flap procedure. (a) An inverse bevel incision is made slightly apical to the free gingival margin and the flap is reflected from the alveolar process. (b) The flap is positioned apically and it is sutured. This procedure attempts to help eliminate or reduce the soft tissue pocket depth. (Courtesy of James A. Simonds, D.M.D., *Practical Periodontics,* Copyright 1991. Continental Education. Santa Rosa, CA)

(a)   (b)

PROCEDURES FOR TREATING OSSEOUS DEFECTS

PERIODONTAL FLAP SURGERY WITH OSSEOUS RESECTION

Periodontitis is a disease that involves loss of connective tissue attachment and loss of alveolar bone. This loss creates osseous defects and deformities leading to an uneven gingival architecture, which makes it difficult for the patient and the dental hygienist to maintain a healthy dentition. Osseous surgery is periodontal surgery involving modification of the bone supporting the teeth in order to eliminate pockets and obtain optimal physiologic gingival contours. The elimination or modification of bone defects can be either by resection or recontouring, which is removing bone, or by adding bone, which is termed *periodontal regeneration* (Fig. 14–5a,b,c ■). Periodontal regeneration is discussed in Chapter 15.

Ostectomy and osteoplasty

Ostectomy and osteoplasty are the two types of osseous recontouring during osseous surgery (Fig. 14–6a,b ■). Ostectomy is the removal of supporting bone or bone that is in contact with the root, and osteoplasty is the reshaping or recontouring of nonsupporting bone or bone that is not in contact with the root (e.g., bony ledges) to achieve physiologic contours.

FIGURE 14–5

A periodontal bony defect is treated either by (a) reshaping or recontouring the bone (top diagram) or (b) filling in the defect (bottom diagram) with bone or a bone substitute (regeneration). (c) This three-wall bony defect on the distal surface of the molar (the buccal, lingual, and mesial walls remain) is best treated with a regenerative procedure.

(a)

(b)   (c)

FIGURE 14–6

(a) Ostectomy removes bone attached to the tooth, which is called *supporting bone*. (b) Osteoplasty is the reshaping of the nonsupporting bone.

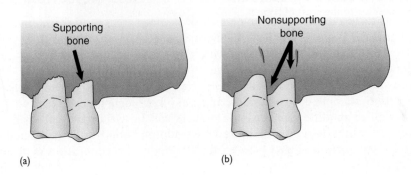

(a)   (b)

Classification of osseous defects

The surgical approach (e.g., resection or regeneration) depends on the pattern of bone loss. The base of a suprabony pocket is coronal to the alveolar crest. The pattern of bone destruction is horizontal, where the bone height is reduced evenly between two adjacent teeth, creating flat interproximal bone. On the other hand, in infrabony pockets, the base is apical to the crest of the alveolar bone. The pattern of bone destruction is vertical (angular), where the bone is "scooped out" along the side of the root. Intraosseous or infrabony defects are classified according to the number of remaining osseous walls and by their predominant morphology: one-, two- and three-wall defects. Most infrabony defects are a combination of 1–2 or 2–3 walled morphology. Most infrabony defects are interproximal, but they can be located on the direct facial or lingual surface. A crater is a specific type of two-wall defect in which the remaining osseous walls are the facial and lingual walls. A hemiseptal defect is a type of one-wall defect in which the remaining wall is usually the facial or lingual. A circumferential defect is a three-wall defect that wraps around the line angle of the tooth to involve the lingual or facial surface. Only by probing, through the soft tissue pocket, but more precisely by surgical entry, can a determination of the type of infrabony defect be made.

Objectives   The objectives of osseous resective surgery are to create optimal physiologic contours that reduce bony ledges or irregular contours in order to permit primary flap closure and to eliminate infrabony pockets by eliminating the bony walls of the defect.

Indications   Indications for osseous resective surgery include the following: (1) to permit optimal flap adaptation by removing bony ledges or exostosis, (2) to eliminate shallow infrabony pockets (1 to 2 mm deep), (3) to open furcations for easier maintenance, and (4) to lengthen crowns for restorative procedures (e.g., crowns).

Contraindications   Osseous resective surgery is contraindicated in the following situations: (1) patients with advanced periodontitis (teeth in these patients already have compromised bone support; additional resection of tooth-supporting

FIGURE 14–7

(a) A horizontal and vertical releasing incision is made on the facial surface. (b) A full-thickness flap is reflected away from the bone. There is a furcation involvement on the first molar. Note the two bony protuberances called *exostoses* (singular: *exostosis*) on the facial surface. A two-wall bony crater exists between the premolar and molar. (c) Osteoplasty removed the exostoses, resulting in a thin, smooth bony surface. Ostectomy removed the bony crater. (d) An apically positioned flap. The flap is moved in an apical position to the crest of bone to eliminate the depth of the pocket.

(a)

(b)

(c)

(d)

structures would be contraindicated), (2) aesthetics (removal of bone in aesthetic areas, especially the anterior maxillary area, will result in an aesthetically unacceptable appearance), (3) isolated deep vertical defects (attempts to reduce or eliminate such defects would result in removing too much supporting bone from the adjacent tooth), and (4) the existence of local anatomic factors, such as the external oblique ridge, maxillary sinus, and flat palate limits achieving the intended results from osseous resection.

Technique (Fig. 14–7a,b,c,d ■) The patient receives local anesthesia. Flap surgery is performed. When the flaps are elevated, the alveolar crest and marginal bone are inspected. If the marginal bone is thick with ledges, osteoplasty is bone with burs on a high-speed handpiece. If infrabony defects are present, ostectomy is performed with burs and hand instruments to flatted the interproximal bone.

A question arises to how much bone should be removed. The answer is enough bone is removed to eliminate or significantly reduce the depth of the defect but not enough to compromise the tooth or adjacent teeth. These procedures will create a harmonious environment for the alveolar process and the overlying gingiva. The apically positioned flap is the technique of choice when pocket elimination is anticipated. If desired, periodontal dressing may be placed over the surgical area. Postoperative instructions are given.

Healing   The soft tissue attachment to the root surface is by a long junctional epithelium. Healing also results in gingival recession with root exposure. Healing is complete by 2 to 3 months.

CROWN LENGTHENING PROCEDURES

Crown lengthening or crown extension is a surgical procedure designed to expose more tooth structure for restorative purposes (e.g., placement of a crown or other restoration). Indications for crown lengthening are as follows: (1) a tooth that is fractured close to the gingival margin and/or alveolar crest and (2) subgingival caries.

Before surgery is performed, the concept of the biologic width must be considered. *Biologic width* is the soft tissue dimension that is occupied by the junctional epithelium and the gingival connective tissue attachment (gingival fibers). The length of the junctional epithelium is 0.97 mm, and the length of the gingival fibers is 1.07 mm, making the dimension of the biologic width approximately 2.04 mm. Thus the biologic width is the soft tissue attachment from the base of the sulcus to the crest of alveolar bone. There must be space available on the root surface to allow for these two attachments. This space is necessary for gingival health. The margin of a crown or other restoration should not be placed within this space, which would create gingival inflammation and could cause damage to the attachment apparatus and bone resorption. Thus, if a tooth is fractured, a radiograph will indicate how close the most coronal part of the remaining tooth structure is to the alveolar bone. Osseous resective surgery may be indicated to create more tooth structure to allow for reestablishment of soft tissue attachments and proper placement of restorative margins (Fig. 14–8a,b,c ■).

Root resection

In patients with substantial furcation involvements (class III or IV) with extensive bone loss around the roots of molar teeth and defective, decayed, or resorbed roots, root resection or hemisection may be indicated (Fig. 14–9a,b ■). *Root resection* or *amputation* is defined as the removal of a root while leaving the crown on a multirooted tooth. Root resection is usually done on maxillary molars. Hemisection is the surgical sectioning and removal of one root and the crown portion and is usually done on mandibular molars that have a furcation involvement with severe bone loss around the root. If a molar is adequately stable with sufficient bony support but with class III or IV furcation involvement, a bisection or bicuspidization procedure can be done. This involves the sectioning or cutting of the molar in half, creating two separate teeth. Endondontics (root canal therapy) must be done before any of these procedures.

FIGURE 14–8

(a) The premolar fractured due to caries. (b) Flap is elevated, and surgical removal of bone was necessary to lengthen the crown so a crown could be placed without impinging on the biologic width. (c) The flap was positioned apically and sutured.

(a)

(b)

(c)

FIGURE 14–9

(Reprinted with permission from James A. Simonds, *Practical Periodontics,* 1991. Continental Education, Santa Rosa, CA.)

Root resection
Pre-surgical defect

(a)

Root resection
Severely affected root removed

(b)

MUCOGINGIVAL SURGICAL PROCEDURES (GINGIVAL PLASTIC SURGERY)

The mucogingival relationship is important in sustaining the health of the gingival attachment. **Mucogingival surgery** is a periodontal surgical procedure used to correct defects in the morphology, position, and/or amount of gingiva.

Indications   Historically, the use of mucogingival surgical procedures was limited to treatment of gingival recession. A certain amount of attached gingiva was considered necessary to maintain gingival health and prevent further recession. However, several studies have shown that periodontal health can be maintained regardless of the width of attached gingiva (Wennström and Lindhe 1983; Salkin et al. 1987). Therefore, gingival augmentation is used in sites with inadequate width and thickness of attached gingiva that exhibit persistent inflammation (bleeding) or progressive recession and sites with inadequate dimensions of gingiva that have subgingival restorations or orthodontics. In sites where crown margins are to be placed subgingivally, recession with exposure of the crown margins may occur when there is inadequate gingival dimensions. Other indications for mucogingival procedures include (1) elimination of frenum and muscle pull at or near the gingival margin, (2) areas in which the base of a periodontal pocket extends to or beyond the mucogingival junction, (3) deepening of the buccal vestibule, (4) aesthetic reasons (e.g., to cover exposed roots), and (5) modifications of edentulous ridges prior to prosthetic reconstruction.

CLASSIFICATION OF GINGIVAL RECESSION

Sullivan and Atkins (1968) classified gingival recession into four categories: (1) shallow-narrow, (2) shallow-wide, (3) deep-narrow, and (4) deep-wide. Miller (1985) expanded this classification (Fig. 14–10 I, II, III, IV■). Miller's classification includes gingival recession not extending to the mucogingival junction and gingival recession extending to the mucogingival junction with bone or soft tissue loss in the interdental area.

TYPES OF SOFT TISSUE GRAFTS

Mucogingival defects are corrected using different types of soft tissue grafts. In addition, guided tissue regeneration procedures also could be used for this purpose.

Pedicle graft or laterally positioned flap

The pedicle graft, as the name implies, is used to move gingiva from an adjacent tooth or edentulous area to a prepared recipient site on another tooth with an inadequate amount of attached gingiva. The pedicle graft is "freed" on three aspects but retains its attachment (blood supply) from its base. This procedure requires sufficient width and thickness of gingiva to be present in the donor site. There should be no underlying bone dehiscence or fenestration. The pedicle graft is best used for single-site recession for root coverage and augmentation (increasing the amount) of attached gingiva.

FIGURE 14–10

P. D. Miller's classification of gingival recession. (Adapted from Miller, P.D., A Classification of Marginal tissue recession. *Int. J. Periodont. Rest. Dent.*, 1985.)

Technique   (Fig. 14–11a,b,c ■)   A V-shaped incision is made around the recipient site, incised tissue is removed, and root planing of the root surface is performed. A full- or split-thickness flap is elevated on the tooth away from the defect and rotated to cover the defect. The flap is sutured, and pressure is applied (this is done with all soft tissue grafts) for about 4 to 5 minutes, ensuring that no blood clot has formed under the graft. A **periodontal dressing** to protect the flap can be placed. If a periodontal dressing is not used, the patient should not brush the area. Postoperative instructions are given to the patient, (Table 14–3) and the patient returns 1 week later. At the 1-week postoperative visit, the sutures and the dressing are removed, and the area either may be left uncovered or may be redressed for an additional week.

Healing   Complete healing occurs in about 1 month.

Double papillae flap

The double papillae flap is a modification of the laterally positioned flap. The papillae from each side of the tooth with the defect are reflected and rotated over the midfacial aspect of the recipient tooth and sutured.

Free gingival soft tissue graft

Unlike a pedicle graft, a free gingival graft (FGG) has a donor site located away from the grafted site. Thus the blood supply is not attached to the graft but depends on the recipient bed. The most common site for donor tissue is the palate, but in many cases, edentulous areas also can be used. Free gingival grafts are more predictable for augmentation of attached gingiva than for root coverage because significant shrinkage of the graft occurs during healing. Thicker free gingival grafts can be used for root coverage because there is less tissue shrinkage.

FIGURE 14–11

(a) Lateral incisor with severe gingival recession with root exposure. (b) A laterally positioned flap was used to move gingiva from the right central incisor to the left central incisor. An anchor suture is around the lateral incisor. (c) Two months of healing shows good root coverage and increased width of attached gingiva.

(a)

(b)

(c)

Technique (Fig. 14–12a,b,c,d ■) After local anesthesia is administered on the palate and the recipient area, split-thickness flaps are reflected at the recipient site. A piece of gingiva about 1 mm thick is obtained from an intraoral area. Although the most common donor site is the hard palate, edentulous areas also can be used. The donor tissue (graft) is placed on the recipient bed, and the graft is sutured in place, making sure that it does not move, since this will interfere with the establishment of a blood supply from the recipient bed and the graft may fail. A periodontal dressing may be applied. Postoperative instructions are given, and the patient returns in 1 week (Table 14–3). Smoking is strictly prohibited because soft tissue grafts are more likely to fail if the patient smokes. A major disadvantage of free gingival grafts is the poor color match between the graft and the existing gingiva.

Healing The graft will swell initially, and then shrinkage occurs. The graft receives blood and nutrients from the underlying connective tissue. Complete healing with keratinization occurs in about 1 month.

FIGURE 14-12

(a) Mandibular central and right lateral incisors have no attached gingiva. (b) A free gingival graft was harvested from the palate and (c) sutured into place at the recipient site. (d) Posttreatment view of the grafted site. Increased width of attached gingiva was achieved. Note that root coverage was not obtained using this type of grafting procedure.

(a)

(b)

(c)

(d)

Subepithelial connective tissue graft

The subepithelial connective tissue graft is the procedure of choice for root coverage of single or multiple teeth. Root coverage in a class II defect is expected to be close to 100%, whereas in a class III defect only partial coverage is expected. The subepithelial connective tissue graft was first described by Langer and Calagna (1982) as having several advantages over the other grafts: (1) there is no open wound on the palate as in a free gingival graft, (2) the graft has a better blood supply coming from both the underlying connective tissue and the overlaying flap, and (3) better aesthetics and tissue and color blend are seen.

Indications   The subepithelial connective tissue graft may be used for both single and multiple adjacent teeth with gingival recession and root exposure.

Technique   (Fig. 14–13a,b,c ■)   After local anesthesia is obtained, a split-thickness flap is raised at the recipient site using a surgical blade. A flap is raised at the donor site on the palate, and connective tissue is harvested while leaving the epithelium from the outside of the flap. This flap is sutured into place. The connective

FIGURE 14–13

(a) Pretreatment view of the mandibular left premolar area. Note the gingival recession and exposed root surfaces. A connective tissue graft was selected to cover the root surfaces. (b) The subepithelial connective tissue graft was harvested from the palate Incisions were made, and the epithelium was reflected. Note the vascular connective tissue underlying the epithelium. (c) The graft was sutured to the recipient site. Part of the connective tissue is visible on the premolars.

(a)   (b)

(c)

tissue is placed on the recipient site and sutured in place. A periodontal dressing may be applied. Postoperative instructions are given to the patient, and the patient returns in 1 week (Table 14–3). At 1 week, the dressing and sutures are removed, and the area is either left uncovered or redressed for another week.

Healing   Healing occurs through a double blood supply. Both the connective tissue from the recipient site and the overlying flap aid in healing of the soft tissue graft. Complete healing occurs in approximately 1 month.

Guided tissue regeneration for root coverage

Guided tissue regeneration (GTR) will be discussed further in the next chapter. Essentially, GTR involves the use of a barrier membrane that is designed to prevent the gingival tissue from establishing contact with the root surface, creating a space for the formation of a new attachment and new bone rather than a long junctional epithelial attachment. This concept was intended originally for the treatment of class

II buccal furcation defects and certain infrabony defects. A newer application is for the treatment of gingival recession and for root coverage (Pini-Prato et al. 1992).

Technique After local anesthesia is obtained, a full-thickness flap is raised at the recipient site. Root planing is completed on the root surface. A barrier membrane is placed over the recession and bone and sutured. The flap is repositioned coronally covering both the membrane and the enamel. If the membrane is resorbable, it is not removed and will resorb in about 6 to 8 weeks after surgery. The flap sutures are removed after 2 to 4 weeks. Patients should not brush the area for at least 6 weeks and are recommended to rinse with chlorhexidine gluconate.

SUTURES

Sutures are used to coapt or closely adapt a flap to a tooth surface until the wound has healed sufficiently to withstand normal functional stresses. Closure of the wound provides good hemostasis and covers exposed bone. Suture material is classified as resorbable or nonresorbable and synthetic or nonsynthetic.

RESORBABLE SUTURES

Surgical gut is a natural material from the intestines of sheep or cows and is resorbable. Surgical gut is not too strong and is hard to handle, getting knotted easily. Chromic gut is plain gut that has been treated with chromic salts, which make it more resistant to absorption. Enzymes in saliva will absorb surgical gut sutures within 7 to 10 days and chromic gut in about 14 days. However, depending upon the patient's saliva, sutures may still be seen up to 2–4 weeks later.

Examples of synthetic resorbable sutures include polyglactin 910 (Vicryl™, Coated Vicryl™, Johnson & Johnson, Somerville, NJ) and poliglecaprone 25 (Monocryl™, Johnson & Johnson). These sutures are easier to handle, the knot will not loosen easily, and they cause less tissue irritation and inflammation than surgical gut.

NONRESORBABLE SUTURES

Silk, a type of nonresorable natural suture, is the most frequently used suture material because of its ease in handling and superior visibility. Examples of nonresorable synthetic sutures include nylon (Ethilon™, Johnson & Johnson, Somerville, NJ), polyester (Ethibond™, Johnson & Johnson, Somerville, NJ), and expanded polytetrafluoroethylene (e-PTFE, Gore-Tex®, W. L. Gore & Associates, Flagstaff, AZ). Silk sutures can elicit tissue inflammation, so they should be removed not later than 10 days after surgery. If sutures need to be left in place for several weeks, e-PTFE sutures are recommended.

NEEDLES

Needle and suture material come in various sizes. Needles also are classified according to their shape and curvature. Needles are available in a 1/4-, 3/8-, 1/2-, and 5/8-in. circle, with 3/8 or 1/2 in. being employed most commonly in periodontal surgery. Suture size is classified numerically. An increase in the number

FIGURE 14–14

An interrupted circumferential (loop) suture.

of zeros indicates a decrease in the diameter of the suture. Thus 4-0 and 3-0 sutures are used most often in periodontal flap surgery. The 6-0 and 5-0 sutures are smaller and are used in more delicate mucogingival surgical procedures (Hutchens 1995).

SUTURING TECHNIQUES

Suturing technique varies among surgeons. Basically, there are different ways to tie the suture. The most common and simplest suture is the interrupted suture which is tied with a square, or surgeon's, knot (Fig. 14–14 ■). After the needle engages the buccal and lingual gingiva, it should be tied on the buccal rather than the lingual so that it is easier to remove and the sutures are in a more protected area. When tying a suture, leave about a 2-mm end. Other types of sutures include continuous sutures, mattress sutures, and sling sutures (Fig. 14–15 ■).

The number of sutures placed should be documented in the chart. When the patient returns for the postoperative visit, count the number of sutures before removing them. This will verify that all sutures were removed.

PERIODONTAL DRESSING

In today's clinical practice, periodontal dressings are of the noneugenol type that does not cause irritation or burning to the tissue or bone. The primary purpose of using a periodontal dressing over a surgical area is for patient comfort. Periodontal dressings also protect the wound area after surgery. Some practitioners prefer not to use a dressing because the dressing creates an anaerobic (nonoxygen) area under itself that favors the growth of pathogenic microorganisms. However, this theory has not been proven.

The most widely used noneugenol dressing is a COE-pak® (GC America, Inc., Alsip, IL). It is supplied in two tubes: the accelerator tube and the base tube. Equal

FIGURE 14–15

Horizontal mattress sutures using 4-0 silk.

FIGURE 14–16

Placement of a periodontal dressing. The packing should not interfere with occlusion or impinge on the gingiva.

amounts of dressing from each tube are mixed for 30 to 45 seconds. In the hard and fast set, the working time is about 5 to 8 minutes; in the regular set, it is 10 to 15 minutes. The material is then formed into a strip. Hemostasis should be achieved before the dressing is applied, and the area should be dried. The end of the facial strip is wrapped around the distal aspect of the last tooth and meets with the lingual strip. Finger pressure is applied interproximally to wedge the dressing into place. A dressing placed on a surgical site should not overextend onto the gingiva, vestibule, or occlusal surfaces (Fig. 14–16 ■). Any excess dressing should be trimmed with a curet.

A light-cured periodontal dressing is available (Barricaid™, Dentsply International, Inc., Milford, DE). It is transparent and is used frequently on anterior areas where aesthetics are a concern. The material is first applied to the area (which does not necessarily have to be completely dry) and then is light-cured.

SURGICAL AND POSTOPERATIVE CARE

The dental hygienist plays an important role in the **postoperative care** of patients.

SURGICAL COMPLICATIONS

Syncope is defined as a temporary loss of consciousness caused by a loss of blood flow to the brain. Patients have been known to faint before, during, or after surgical procedures. If a patient faints, treatment should be stopped and the patient positioned with the head lower than the body. The patient's vital signs, including blood pressure, respiration, and pulse, should be monitored. Oxygen can be administered if necessary. Causes for patient syncope include fear or anxiety about the procedure, the site of blood, or pain.

Immediately after the administration of a local anesthetic containing epinephrine, patients may complain of a fast heart beat or begin to shake or shiver. This is caused by the inadvertent injection of the anesthetic solution into a vein rather than a nerve. Most likely the patient will be fine. To prevent this situation, it is essential to aspirate while injecting.

During periodontal surgery, bleeding will occur because blood vessels are severed and the diseased tissue is vascular. Small blood vessels will be severed or broken when making incisions. However, it is important not to severe certain arteries such as the greater palatine artery in the maxillary palatal area. Once the diseased tissue is removed and the flaps are raised, bleeding should diminish. Excessive bleeding is controlled by finding the source of the bleeding and applying pressure, by administering a vasoconstrictor (e.g., lidocaine 2% with 1:50,000 epinephrine), or by tying the offending artery.

It is important to avoid unnecessary or excessive hemorrhaging or bleeding. The patient's medical history should be evaluated carefully and updated to help avoid these situations. For example, a patient may be taking aspirin every day or even several times a week as a preventive measure for stroke. Aspirin (acetylsalicylic acid) binds to platelets and inhibits the formation of prostaglandins, resulting in a prolonged bleeding time that lasts for approximately 7 days, until new platelets are formed. A similar situation occurs with nonsteroidal anti-inflammatory drugs such as ibuprofen. It is best to consult with such a patient's physician before performing surgery.

POSTOPERATIVE COMPLICATIONS

After periodontal surgery, the patient is given a number of written suggestions and instruction. These instructions must be reviewed carefully with the patient before he or she is allowed to leave the office. An example of postoperative patient instructions is given in Table 14–2. During the first postoperative week, the patient may experience swelling, pain, and sensitivity; these are usually mild and transient. Swelling generally can be controlled by the use of ice packs for the first 2 days. An ice pack should be applied extraorally 20 minutes on and 20 minutes off for the first day. If swelling continues, the patient should switch to warm packs. Swelling can be due to soft tissue inflammation from the surgical procedure or an infection. If swelling continues, advise the patient to return to the office. Pain is usually due to swelling. If there is severe pain, the patient should return to the office. The patient may be given systemic antibiotics and analgesics (pain medication). The dental hygienist should confirm that the patient is taking the appropriate medications as prescribed. The patient should be asked if he or she is taking any over-the-counter medications.

The patient may complain of seeing blood in the mouth for a few hours after the surgery. Most of the time this is residual blood in the saliva probably remaining on the tongue after surgery. If there is frank bleeding coming from the surgical site, the patient should apply pressure to the site and return to the office as soon as possible. Rinsing should not be done because it will prevent a blood clot from forming.

ORAL HYGIENE INSTRUCTIONS

Maintenance of the surgical area is important, and the dental hygienist must instruct the client on proper care (Tables 14–2 and 14–3). Vigorous toothbrushing and flossing should not be done until healing is complete, yet it must be stressed to patients that removal of dental plaque is important for healing. The period of time the patient refrains from toothbrushing varies with each surgeon. While a periodontal dressing is in place, the patient should not brush that area. Rinsing with chlorhexidine gluconate is recommended. After the dressing and sutures are removed, patients are instructed to brush gently with a roll technique. Gradually, as healing occurs, regular brushing can be resumed. After surgery, the interdental papillae are usually absent or blunted, creating large gingival embrasures. Plaque removal in these areas is best accomplished with an interdental brush (single-tuft brush). Also, plaque removal on teeth with Class III/IV furcation involvement is best with a single-tuft brush. If no large interdental spaces develop after surgery, the patient can continue to use dental floss or a small interdental brush.

POSTOPERATIVE VISIT MANAGEMENT

The dental hygienist may be called on to attend to a patient at the first postoperative visit. Table 14–3 describes various reevaluation procedures that may be performed at this visit. At the 7- to 10-day postoperative visit, the dressing and sutures are removed. After the dressing is carefully removed, the number of sutures are counted and compared with the number of documented sutures placed at the time of the surgery. Frequently, parts of or all the periodontal dressing may have come off during the week. When the dressing is removed, care must be taken not to pull the sutures. If the sutures are being pulled by the dressing, cut the interfering sutures before the dressing is further removed. Once the dressing is removed, a white layer can be seen on the tissue surface. This represents dead epithelial cells. A moistened (with water, saline, or chlorhexidine) cotton-tipped applicator is used to carefully cleanse the area. Following suture removal, the area is again thoroughly irrigated with water or saline. Only supragingival debridement should be performed, subgingival debridement should be postponed until complete healing has occurred. The decision to apply another dressing to the area depends on the amount of discomfort the patient is experiencing and the rate of healing.

EFFECTS OF SURGICAL PROCEDURES

As a consequence of surgery, several problems may arise. Patients should be informed about these adverse side effects before surgery. All patients also should sign an informed consent form.

TOOTH MOBILITY

Tooth mobility may increase immediately after surgery and may not return to pre-operative levels for as long as 6 weeks. The patient should be told that this is a normal consequence of surgery. Increased tooth mobility is due to the extension of inflammation into the periodontal ligament and to the surgical manipulation. The occlusion should be checked to verify that there is no occlusal trauma. Any occlusal interferences should be eliminated. Check for fremitus to help determine occlusal interferences.

GINGIVAL RECESSION: DENTINAL HYPERSENSITIVITY AND ROOT CARIES

Gingival recession with longer clinical crowns may occur after surgery. With exposure of the root surface, the patient may experience dentinal hypersensitivity and can develop root caries due to demineralization.

Maintaining adequate plaque control can reduce both the sensitivity and risk for root caries. For immediate hypersensitivity relief, an in-office application of DentinBloc® (Colgate Oral Pharmaceuticals, Canton, MA) is done. Other in-office desensitizing products are available, including chemical agents (oxalates, fluorides), sealants, and bonding agents (see Chapter 10).

It is also helpful for the patient to use at home a dentifrice containing potassium nitrate (Fresh Mint Sensodyne®, Block Drug Corp., Jersey City, NJ; Protect®, John O. Butler Co., Chicago, IL). Unfortunately, the use of dentifrices is controversial, and they may take several weeks to have a positive effect. Once the patient has relief from the hypersensitivity, he or she can start to use the regular dentifrice but should return to the desensitizing dentifrice if the sensitivity returns. An over-the-counter 0.4% stannous fluoride gel (Gel-Kam®, Colgate Oral Pharmaceuticals) that is applied to the toothbrush may reduce dentinal hypersensitivity and prevent demineralization of the exposed root surfaces. A 0.63% stannous fluoride oral rinse (Gel-Kam® Oral Care Rinse, Colgate Oral Pharmaceuticals) is available by prescription for patient use at home. Adverse side effects of stannous fluoride include staining of the dentin and stinging of the soft tissue.

SUMMARY

The range of treatment alternatives for periodontitis is wide. The type of treatment depends on a number of factors, including the patient's level of plaque control, the type of gingival or periodontal pocket, and the type of periodontal defect. Careful assessment and planning of a case are important in the overall surgical treatment.

KEY POINTS

+ Periodontal flap surgery is indicated for increasing access to the underlying root and bone in deeper periodontal pockets.
+ The patient must be able to maintain excellent plaque control before periodontal surgery is performed.

❖ The therapeutic clinical end point of success for surgical pocket therapy is an oral environment that is easily maintainable by the patient and the clinician; there should be minimal inflammation (bleeding) and minimal probing depths.

❖ Cigarette smoking adversely affects the outcome of surgery.

REFERENCES

American Academy of Periodontology. 1992. *Glossary of periodontal terms,* 3rd ed. Chicago: American Academy of Periodontology.

Boström, L., L. E. Linder, and J. Bergström. 1998. Influence of smoking on the outcome of periodontal surgery: A 5-year follow-up. *J. Clin. Periodontol.* 25:194–201.

Carranza, F. A., Jr. 1996. The surgical phase of therapy. In *Clinical periodontology,* ed. F. A. Carranza, Jr., and M. G. Newman, 565–569, 584–587. Philadelphia: W. B. Saunders.

Flores-de-Jacoby, L., and R. Mengel. 1995. Conventional surgical procedures. *Periodontology 2000* 9:38–54.

Hutchens, J. L., Jr. 1995. Periodontal suturing: A review of needles, material, and techniques. *Postgrad. Dent.* 2(4):3–14.

Langer, B., and L. Calagna. 1982. The subepithelial connective tissue graft: A new approach to the enhancement of anterior cosmetics. *Int. J. Periodont. Rest. Dent.* 2:22–23.

Lang, N. P., and H. Löe. 1993. Clinical management of periodontal diseases. *Periodontology 2000* 2:128–139.

Miller, P. D. 1985. A classification of marginal tissue recession. *Int. J. Periodont. Rest. Dent.* 5:15–37.

Palcanis, K. G. 1996. Surgical pocket therapy. *Ann. Periodontol.* 1:589–617.

Preber, H., and J. Berström. 1990. Effect of cigarette smoking on periodontal healing following surgical therapy. *J. Clin. Periodontol.* 17:324–328.

Pini-Prato, G., C. Tinti, G. Vincenzi, et al. 1992. Guided tissue regeneration versus mucogingival surgery in the treatment of human buccal gingival recession. *J. Periodontol.* 63:919–928.

Ramfjord, S. P., and R. R. Nissle. 1974. The modified Widman flap. *J. Periodontol.* 45:601–607.

Salkin, L. M., A. L. Freedman, M. D. Stein, and N. A. Bassiouny. 1987. A longitudinal study of untreated mucogingival defects. *J. Periodontol.* 58:164–166.

Sullivan, H. C., and J. H. Atkins. 1968. Free autogenous gingival grafts: I. Principles of successful grafting. *Periodontics* l6:121–129.

Wennström, J. L., and J. Lindhe. 1983. Role of attached gingiva for maintenance of periodontal health. *J. Clin. Periodontol.* 10:206–221.

Yukna, R. A., and J. L. Lawrence. 1980. Five-year evaluation of the excisional new attachment procedure. *J. Periodontol.* 51:382–385.

SELF-QUIZ

1. Which one of the following prerequisites for periodontal surgery is of primary importance? (p. 465)

   a. meticulous plaque control

   b. placement of interim restorations

   c. low anxiety level

   d. desire to continue treatment

2. Which one of the following healing responses is usually seen after periodontal flap surgery? (p. 473)

   a. new bone, cementum, and periodontal ligament
   b. new bone and cementum
   c. long junctional epithelium
   d. connective tissue attachment

3. Which one of the following surgical procedures is indicated for gingival enlargement in a patient who is taking phenytoin? (p. 467)

   a. mucogingival
   b. gingivectomy
   c. periodontal flap
   d. excisional new attachment

4. When placing sutures, the knot is usually tied on the palatal surface *because* this is a protected area. (p. 486)

   a. Both the statement and the reason are correct and related.
   b. Both the statement and the reason are correct but *not* related.
   c. The statement is correct, but the reason is *not.*
   d. The statement is *not* correct, but the reason is correct.
   e. *Neither* the statement *nor* the reason is correct.

5. After periodontal surgery, which one of the following hygiene aids is *best* recommended to clean exposed furcations? (p. 489)

   a. dental floss
   b. manual toothbrush
   c. powered toothbrush
   d. single-tuft brush

6. Which one of the following surgical procedures is *best* recommended for augmenting the amount of attached gingiva and covering exposed root surfaces before a patient undergoes orthodontic treatment? (p. 483)

   a. gingivectomy
   b. connective tissue graft
   c. modified Widman flap
   d. crown lengthening

7. Which one of the following measures should be advised to a patient who calls the office 2 days after periodontal surgery and states that he or she has bleeding from the surgical site? (pp. 488–489)

   a. rinse with warm salt water
   b. lie down on a couch
   c. remove the packing
   d. apply pressure

8. Which of the following is the primary objective of periodontal flap surgery? (pp. 464–465)

   a. gain access to the bone and root surface
   b. augment the amount of free gingiva
   c. provide easy-to-maintain areas
   d. allow for healing by regeneration

9. A patient has experienced some root sensitivity in the area of flap surgery. Which one of the following recommendations can the dental hygienist make to alleviate the pain? (p. 490)

   a. floss the area
   b. rinse with a nonfluoride mouthrinse
   c. rinse and brush with a baking soda solution
   d. brush with a potassium nitrate dentifrice

10. All the following adverse effects the patient should be informed about before periodontal surgery is performed *except* one. Which one is the exception? (pp. 489–490)

   a. dentinal hypersensitivity
   b. gingival recession
   c. tooth mobility
   d. root caries
   e. open bite

PRINCIPLES OF PERIODONTAL SURGERY: PERIODONTAL REGENERATION

15

Stuart J. Froum, D.D.S.

Outline:

Periodontal Regenerative Surgery
Surgical Procedure
Guided Tissue Regeneration
Regenerative Surgery: Postoperative Care
Root Surface Treatment
Risk Factors for Regenerative Therapy
Biologics and Devices
Summary
Key Points
References
Self-Quiz

Goal:

To educate the dental hygienist on the basic principles of periodontal regeneration.

Educational Objectives:

Upon completion of this chapter, the reader should be able to:

Describe the process of periodontal regeneration, including the type and origin of cells involved in the regenerative process;

Compare and contrast the different clinical procedures used to attain periodontal regeneration; and

Discuss postoperative care after periodontal regenerative surgery.

KEY WORDS

- periodontal therapy
- periodontal regeneration
- bone grafts
- bone substitute materials
- guided tissue regeneration (GTR)
- growth factors

*T*he goals of **periodontal therapy** have long included arresting the disease process, preventing disease recurrence, and providing for the regeneration of periodontium lost as a result of the disease. Over the past three decades, great strides have been made in the field of periodontal regeneration. **Periodontal regeneration** is defined as healing after periodontal surgery that results in the reconstruction of lost tissues, including supporting alveolar bone, cementum, and a functionally oriented periodontal ligament (American Academy of Periodontology 1992). This chapter provides a review of the various regenerative therapies and materials currently in use today (Table 15–1 ■). Future directions in this ever-changing field also will be discussed. Techniques currently in use include open flap debridement, the use of bone grafts and bone substitutes, guided tissue regeneration, combination techniques, and root surface treatment.

PERIODONTAL REGENERATIVE SURGERY

OBJECTIVES

Once inflammation of the gingiva (gingivitis) is resolved with initial therapy (e.g., periodontal debridement and oral hygiene self-care instruction), the periodontitis component still must be treated. Periodontitis is characterized by apical migration of the junctional epithelium resulting in periodontal pocket formation, loss of clinical attachment (connective tissue fibers attached to the tooth surface), and alveolar bone loss. Periodontal regenerative surgery using **bone grafts, bone substitute materials,** and/or barrier membranes and modulators of tissue healing is aimed at regenerating the periodontal attachment apparatus lost due to periodontitis.

The goals of using such bone-replacement materials as bone grafts and bone substitutes in infrabony defects include the following: (1) a reduction in probing depths, (2) a gain in clinical attachment level (this refers to a reduction in probing depth caused by decreased penetration of the probe at the base of the pocket), (3) a filling in of osseous defects, and (4) regeneration of new supporting alveolar bone, new cementum, and a functionally oriented periodontal ligament (Brunsvold and Mellonig 1993; Schallhorn 1977). The latter can only be determined by histologic examination of the healed periodontal tissues.

Regenerative surgery significantly differs from osseous resective procedures, in which the osseous (bony) walls are removed surgically to eliminate the intraosseous component of the defect. Often the morphology of the defect requires

---

TABLE 15–1

PROCEDURES USED TO ENHANCE PERIODONTAL REGENERATION

- Bone and bone substitute grafting to fill the periodontal defect
- Prevention or retardation of junctional epithelial downgrowth:
    Guided tissue regeneration (GTR)
    Acid conditioning of the root surface
- Application of enamel matrix protein derivatives
- Growth factor application to promote specific cell proliferation

the removal of too much bone to obtain complete elimination of the defect (parabolic interdental bone). Periodontal regenerative surgery involves "adding" bone (bone fill) into the intraosseous defect instead of its removal. The type of periodontal defects that respond best to the use of bone grafts include three-wall, two-wall, and combination-type intraosseous defects. This is so because the remaining bony walls contain and hold the bone graft in the defect. Moreover, the additional surrounding bony walls provide more surface area upon which bone can form. Horizontal patterns of bone loss, loss of buccal or lingual plates of bone, and furcation defects cannot be treated predictably with bone graft and bone substitute materials.

The following are different types of regenerative techniques.

OPEN FLAP DEBRIDEMENT

As a surgical technique, open flap debridement, in which a flap is reflected and the roots and pocket area are debrided without the addition of any bone or bone substitute material, has been used primarily as a control for comparison in assessing other treatment modalities (Laurell et al. 1998). In most histologic studies, open flap debridement resulted in repair rather than regeneration of periodontal tissues. A greater recurrence of probing depth has been shown with open flap debridement alone (Smith, Ammons, and van Belle 1980) when compared with traditional osseous resective procedures.

BONE GRAFTS AND BONE SUBSTITUTES

Bone-replacement materials are classified into four categories: autografts, allografts, alloplasts, and xenografts. Bone substitutes can be synthetic (manufactured, not naturally occurring) materials or processed from bone of other species (xenografts). Table 15–2 ■ describes the different types of bone graft materials.

TABLE 15–2	
TYPES OF BONE-REPLACEMENT MATERIALS	
NAME	**FEATURES**
Autografts	Bone harvested from one part of the body and grafted to another part of the same patient's body. The bone can be obtained from an intraoral site such as the maxillary tuberosity area, edentulous area, healing extraction site, or mandibular torus during implant placement or an extraoral site (e.g., iliac crest of the pelvis).
Allografts	Bone material obtained from other individuals of the same species but genetically different. Donors include human cadavers. Allografts are processed under complete sterility and stored in bone banks. The main forms of bone allografts used in clinical practice are demineralized freeze-dried bone (DFDBA) and freeze-dried bone (FDBA).
Alloplasts	A synthetic type of bone substitute. Inert, biologically compatible substances. Synthetic alloplasts include hydroxyapatite, calcium phosphate, bioactive glass, and calcified polymers.
Xenografts	A type of natural bone substitute derived from a genetically different species (e.g., bovine).

Autografts (autogenous grafts)

Autogenous bone is living bone derived directly from the patient's own body and has shown the best potential of any of the bone fill material for periodontal regeneration and bone fill. This bone is often mixed with the patient's blood. However, when a sufficient amount of bone is not available intraorally, or if the patient does not want bone obtained from extraoral sites such as the hip, other materials must be considered. Autogenous bone has long been considered to be the gold standard of grafting materials in terms of stimulating new bone formation.

Allografts (allogeneic grafts)

Allografts such as demineralized freeze-dried bone (DFDBA) obtained from human cadavers have demonstrated bone-forming properties. Bone allografts are obtained from bone banks. The issue of safety (e.g., nontransmission of hepatitis, HIV, and other known diseases) when using allografts has been well established, thus minimizing this factor as a concern (Mellonig, Preuett, and Moyer 1992; Marx and Carlson 1993). Controlled clinical studies have shown greater bone fill in sites treated with DFDBA than in nongrafted controls, with DFDBA reporting a mean bone fill of 2.6 mm (65% defect fill) compared with 1.3 mm (30% defect fill) in nongrafted controls (Mellonig 1984).

Alloplasts (alloplastic grafts)

Alloplastic bone substitutes are manufactured synthetic materials. They are classified as implant material. Alloplasts (implants) are differentiated from *grafts,* which are defined as "any tissue or organ used for implantation or transplantation" (Hallmon et al. 1996). Advantages of alloplasts include no risk of disease transmission as compared with allografts and no additional surgical sites required in the mouth or body to harvest bone (as with autografts). However, alloplasts are not as effective in forming bone as are graft materials. Alloplasts are inert (nonliving) materials acting as a bone "filler" in the defect, and when effective, they act as a scaffold for bone to form around them.

A number of alloplastic materials have been introduced in an attempt to create a readily available material for bone fill of infrabony periodontal defects. Synthetic alloplasts may be divided into ceramic and nonceramic categories. These may be further divided into absorbable and nonabsorbable materials. Absorbable materials will absorb or dissolve (it may take years) and be replaced with new bone, whereas nonabsorbable grafts may never absorb. Ceramic alloplasts are materials that include calcium phosphate such as hydroxyapatite and tricalcium phosphate. The most commonly used ceramic materials are nonporous hydroxyapatite, porous hydroxyapatite, and tricalcium phosphate. Frequently, these materials result in a repair that evidences a long junctional epithelium to the root surface and/or adhesion of connective tissue fibers oriented parallel to the root (Yukna 1993).

Bioactive glass is another type of alloplast. In a recent clinical study of the treatment of infrabony periodontal defects, a bioactive glass (Perioglas, Block Drug, Jersey City, NJ) showed significant clinical superiority in gain of clinical attachment and defect fill compared with sites that were treated with open flap debridement alone (Froum, Weinberg, and Tarnow 1998). Bioactive glass particles contain silicon dioxide, sodium oxide, calcium oxide, and phosphorous pentoxide. Advantages of this material include the ability to bond to both hard and soft tissue (Hench 1988), its cohesiveness (Hench and West 1996), and its ability to inhibit the apical migration of junctional epithelium (Fetner, Martigan, and Low 1994).

While many of these materials serve as scaffolds or fillers that allow bone from the surrounding area to grow over and into them, to date alloplasts have failed to demonstrate human histologic evidence of new cementum and a functionally oriented periodontal ligament. From a clinical standpoint, these materials appear to be biocompatible, nontoxic, nonallergenic, noncarciogenic, and noninflammatory.

Xenografts (xenogeneic grafts)

Heterografts or xenografts are taken from a donor of another species. Bio-Oss® (Osteohealth Co., Shirley, NY) and Osteograf®/N (CeraMed Dental, Lakewood, CO) are types of natural bone mineral obtained from the cow (bovine). This bone is anorganic and deproteinated.

Objectives of bone-replacement materials

Ideally, bone-replacement materials should be able to enhance the formation of new cementum, bone, and periodontal ligament. They should be *osteogenic*. That is, they should cause bone cells, osteoblasts, to migrate and proliferate into the healing surgical site. Bone graft materials (autogenous and allogeneic) may be *osteoinductive* (provide a stimulus for noncommitted stem cells to form bone). These osteoinductive materials induce the transformation of immature cells into bone-producing osteoblasts through growth factors that are found only in living bone (Fox 1997). Autogenous bone is the ideal grafting material because grafted autogenous bone stimulates bone growth by osteoconduction and osteoinduction during surgical healing.

This differs from alloplastic grafts, which when placed into a periodontal defect at best function as an *osteoconductive* material. In these situations, the bone-replacement material acts as a scaffold or framework to allow bone apposition against its surface, with cells originating from the surrounding existing bone. Such osteoconductive materials require the presence of existing bone, and the more bone there is (greater number of bony walls in an intraosseous defect), the greater is the chance of a successful bone fill (Fox 1997). These materials are not osteoinductive and do not produce new bone. The size and shape of the bone-replacement particles influence their osteoconductive capacity. Eventually, the particles of material are either replaced by the bone growing over them or incorporated into the new forming bone.

SURGICAL PROCEDURE

Intracrevicular incisions are made, and a gingival flap is reflected. The root surface and osseous defect are debrided to remove all granulomatous (diseased) tissue. A combination of power-driven and hand instruments is used commonly to ensure that all calculus and plaque as well as altered cementum are removed from the root surface (Brunsvold and Mellonig 1993). The defect is filled and packed with bone or a bone replacement material. The flap is replaced and sutured in an attempt to fully cover the material (Figs. 15–1a,b,c,d ■ and

FIGURE 15–1

(a) A 9-mm intraosseous periodontal defect is present on the mesial aspect of the mandibular incisor. (b) Following reflection of a periodontal flap and defect and root debridement, a demineralized freeze-dried bone allograft (DFDBA) was reconstituted with sterile saline and (c) placed into the defect. (d) The flap is sutured with silk sutures to cover the graft material.

(a)

(b)

(c)

(d)

15–2a,b,c ■). A periodontal dressing may be placed if desired. The patient returns 7 to 14 days later for suture removal, light debridement, and oral hygiene instruction during the first postoperative visit.

GUIDED TISSUE REGENERATION

CELLS INVOLVED IN REGENERATION

The periodontal unit can be divided into five tissue components: the gingival epithelium, the gingival connective tissue, the periodontal ligament (PDL), the supporting alveolar bone, and cementum. In 1976 it was theorized that the type of tissue that predominates in the healing wound after periodontal surgery determines whether the response is either repair (e.g., long junctional epithelial attachment or connective tissue adherence) or regeneration (e.g., new bone, new cementum, and new periodontal ligament) (Melcher 1976).

FIGURE 15–2

(a) A deep crater between the maxillary first and second molars. (b) Probing of the 10-mm-deep defect. (c) After thorough tooth and root debridement, Perioglas® was placed into the defect and the flaps were sutured with silk sutures to cover the graft material.

(a)

(b)

(c)

Epithelium is the fastest growing tissue, migrating at a rate of 0.5 to 1.0 mm per day. A periodontal wound in which unimpeded epithelial migration is allowed to occur results in repair with a long junctional epithelium. This type of healing occurs after open flap debridement and osseous resective surgical procedures. Regeneration does not occur when either gingival (junctional) epithelium or gingival connective tissues (e.g., tissue inside the flap) contact the root surface during healing. In order for regeneration to occur, cells capable of forming new cementum, PDL, and supporting alveolar bone must migrate into the periodontal osseous defect and produce these tissues. It is believed that these cells come from the PDL (osteoblasts, fiberblasts and cementoblasts) and/or alveolar bone remaining around the tooth (Melcher et al. 1987). In order for these cells to migrate into the periodontal defect, apical epithelial migration must be delayed, and the gingival connective tissue from the gingival flap must be excluded. If the flap makes contact with the tooth surface, a long junctional epithelium forms along the root and may prevent the necessary regenerative cells from gaining access to the periodontal defect. This concept lead to the theory of selective cell repopulation or **guided tissue regeneration (GTR)** (Gottlow et al. 1986; Nyman et al. 1982).

Figure 15–3

Schematic illustration of a guided tissue regeneration procedure. (a) The periodontal defect with the junctional epithelium on the root surface. (b) After a flap is raised and the defect debrided, a barrier membrane is placed over the defect to create a space for the defect to heal. The periodontal ligament and bone cells attempt to migrate coronally (arrows) into the defect to produce new cementum, periodontal ligament, and supporting alveolar bone. The flap is then sutured over the membrane covering it. (c) Healing by regeneration. (d) The result of therapy after healing.

(a)　　　　　　　　　　　　　　　(b)

(c)　　　　　　　　　　　　　　　(d)

    This concept has been the basis for clinical techniques using barrier membranes inserted between the gingival flap and the root surface. The membrane maintains a "space" between the tooth and the flap. This procedure is designed to retard apical migration of the junctional epithelium and exclude the gingival connective tissue cells from making contact with the root surface and defect. This then allows cells originating from the PDL space and/or alveolar bone cells to migrate coronally into the defect to form new bone, cementum, and attachment (Fig. 15–3a,b,c,d ■).

SURGICAL PROCEDURE

Barrier membranes have been used in the treatment of Grade II buccal furcation defects in both maxillary and mandibular molars and in two- and three-wall interproximal infrabony periodontal defects. Optimal results are obtained in patients that are healthy nonsmokers who demonstrate adequate oral home care.

Clinically, GTR techniques are performed by making intrasulcular incisions and full-thickness flap reflection. Following debridement of the periodontal defect and the root surface, a membrane barrier is placed on the tooth so as to cover the periodontal bony defect (Fig. 15–4a,b,c,d,e,f ■). The membrane is situated between the inner flap and the tooth and bone. The flap is sutured so that the membrane is fully covered and not exposed to the oral cavity. Frequently, a bone graft is first placed into the periodontal defect to prevent the membrane from collapsing into the defect and to aid in regeneration.

TYPES OF MEMBRANES

Nonabsorbable membranes

Membranes are classified as nonabsorbable or absorbable. Nonabsorbable membranes were the first to be used and studied clinically. Since the body does not absorb (dissolve) a nonabsorbable membrane, it has to be removed. A second surgical procedure therefore is performed a minimum of 6 to 8 weeks later to remove the barrier. The most commonly used nonabsorbable barrier membrane is expanded polytetrafluoroethylene (e-PTFE). An example of an e-PTFE membrane is Gore-Tex® (Gore Associates, Flagstaff, AZ). A similar nonresorbable barrier is TefGen-FD™ (Lifecore Biomedical, Chaska, MN). This barrier is less porous than Gore-Tex®, which may limit the amount of connective tissue ingrowth.

Most studies using nonabsorbable membranes in infrabony defects showed positive results. Over the past two decades, studies of infrabony defects in human beings treated with e-PTFE barriers showed definitive clinical gains in new attachment, with three-wall defects having the greatest improvement (Gottlow et al. 1986). A 12-month study of one-, two-, and three-wall infrabony defects treated with e-PTFE barriers showed a 93% fill of three-wall defects, an 82% fill of two-wall defects, and a 39% fill of one-wall defects (Cortellini, PiniPrato, and Tonetti 1993a, 1993b).

Absorbable membranes

Absorbable membranes appeared half a decade later. These membranes have various compositions. Absorbable membranes offer a distinct advantage over nonabsorbable barriers in that there is no need for a second surgery to retrieve the membrane. The barrier must remain in place a minimum of 3 to 4 weeks (Minabe 1991) for proper wound healing. Several membranes are available commercially (Table 15–3 ■).

The general consensus seems to be that furcation closure in a horizontal dimension is better with absorbable membranes (Garrett 1996). The clinician must choose the appropriate barrier for the appropriate defect. Although nonabsorbable barriers do not have breakdown products that can interfere with tissue healing, the need for a second procedure to remove the membrane is a distinct disadvantage to wound healing.

FIGURE 15–4

(a) A Grade II furcation defect on the buccal aspect of the mandibular first molar probed 10 mm. (b) Sulcular incisions were made, and a mucoperiosteal flap was reflected. (c) After the defect and root were thoroughly debrided, a barrier (Gore-Tex®) was adapted to the tooth and sutured. The flaps were sutured to cover the membrane. (d) Healing after 4 weeks. (e) Approximately 6 weeks later a flap was reflected to remove the membrane. (f) Early healing of site shows a closure of the furca.

(a)

(b)

(c)

(d)

(e)

(f)

TABLE 15–3
ABSORBABLE BARRIER MEMBRANES

MATERIAL	PRODUCT	MANUFACTURER
PLA/PGA (polylactic acid/polyglycolate)	Gore Resolut®	W. L. Gore, Flagstaff, AZ; distributed by Nobel Biocare, Yorba Linda, CA
Polyglycolic acid, polylactic acid, and trimethylene carbonate	Gore OsseoQuest™	W. L. Gore, Flagstaff, AZ; distributed by Nobel Biocare, Yorba Linda, CA
PLA (poly-DL-lactide)	Atrisorb®	Block Drug Corporation, Jersey City, NJ
Collagen	BioMend™ Bio-Gide®	Sulzer Calcitek, Carlsbad, CA; Geistlich, Wohlhusen, Switzerland; distributed by Osteohealth Company, Shirley, NY

The membrane should be covered completely by the flap to prevent bacterial colonization on the outer part of the membrane. This may lead to early infection and poor results. Unfortunately, membrane exposure to the oral cavity occurs with both barrier types. Tissue management when membrane exposure occurs with absorbable barriers may be a problem. Bacteria from the oral cavity may contaminate the exposed membrane by attaching to it. If complete flap closure is not possible, nonabsorbable membranes may be the best choice.

Although GTR using nonabsorbable and absorbable membranes has revolutionized clinical practice, the technique is not as yet predictable for class II, class III and horizontal bone defects. More research in regeneration of furcation and interproximal defects is needed.

REGENERATIVE SURGERY: POSTOPERATIVE CARE

The patient's oral home care is of utmost importance for a desirable outcome. The dental hygienist should give the patient thorough home care instructions. Guidelines for postoperative care are outlined in Table 15–4 ■ (Garret and Bogle 1993; Yukna 1993; Becker and Becker 1993). An antimicrobial mouthrinse such as chlorhexidine gluconate may be prescribed. The patient may be prescribed an antibiotic before and after the surgery to prevent infection. The first postoperative visit is within 7 to 14 days.

Complications can occur during the healing period after GTR surgery. Some complications (Becker and Becker 1993) are outlined in Table 15–5 ■.

ROOT SURFACE TREATMENT

Animal studies have shown that the root surface becomes contaminated by bacteria, bacterial by-products, and endotoxins that will prevent connective tissue attachment and regeneration (Garrett 1977). The classic method of scaling and root planing, while effective in removing endotoxins from the root (Smart et al. 1990)

TABLE 15–4
PERIODONTAL REGENERATIVE SURGERY: POSTOPERATIVE CARE

SURGICAL PROCEDURE	POSTOPERATIVE HOME CARE	IN-OFFICE REEVALUATION PROCEDURES
Bone grafting	If a periodontal dressing is placed, instruct the patient not to brush the area. Instruct the patient to rinse with 0.12% chlorhexidine gluconate twice a day.	At the postoperative visit (7 to 14 days), carefully remove the dressing (cut sutures if embedded in dressing), and wipe off the white film (this consists of dead epithelial cells).
	Following suture removal the patient may start to brush (soft or ultrasoft brush) surgical site gently with a circular technique. Bleeding may occur but will gradually lessen, and the patient should continue to brush.	Reapply dressing if needed (especially if sutures and dressing are removed before 10 days).
	If an antibiotic was prescribed, instruct the patient to continue until all medication is finished.	Periodontal probing should not be done prior to 6 months after surgery.
		Final prosthetic restorations should not be completed until 6 months or more after surgery.
		Initial appointments for professional plaque removal should be every 2 to 3 weeks for the first month, then every month for 4 visits, followed by every 3 months (alternate with visits to the general dentist).
Guided tissue regeneration	A periodontal dressing is usually not placed. Instruct the patient not to floss or brush around the surgical area for 6 weeks after the surgery. However, a soft or ultrasoft toothbrush may be used for coronal brushing of the surgical area.	At the first postoperative visit (1 to 2 weeks), the surgical area is inspected.
	Rinse with 0.12% chlorhexidine gluconate twice a day, and use cotton swabs saturated with chlorhexidine around the surgical area.	The patient should be seen every 2 to 3 weeks for supragingival scaling and tooth polishing with sterile water.
	Instruct the patient to continue to take the prescribed antibiotic until finished.	Between 4 and 6 weeks, the membrane-attached sutures are removed.
		At 6 to 8 weeks, an incision is made to remove the nonabsorbable membrane.
		Periodontal probing should not be done prior to 6 months after surgery.
		Final prosthestic restorations should not be completed prior to 6 months after surgery.

Source: Yukna 1993; Becker and Becker 1993; Garrett and Bogle 1993.

TABLE 15–5
COMPLICATIONS AFTER PERIODONTAL REGENERATIVE SURGERY

COMPLICATION	PROCEDURES TO FOLLOW
Membrane becomes uncovered	Instruct the patient to call the office. Most often the membrane will become exposed within a few weeks after surgery. If there is no infection, instruct patient to keep optimal oral hygiene. Place the patient on an antimicrobial mouthrinse such as chlorhexidine gluconate. Monitor the area. Instruct the patient not to disrupt the membrane.
Gingival recession at the surgical site	If recession occurs, it will usually happen within 1 to 3 weeks after surgery. Since increased plaque accumulation may result, optimal plaque control is stressed.
Pus	If an infection develops, it is most likely at the fourth and fifth postoperative visit. Remove the membrane, and place the patient on an antibiotic. If the patient is already on an antibiotic, change to another antibiotic in a different classification.

in most cases, will not result in new connective tissue attachment but rather a long junctional epithelium. Use of an acid solution such as citric acid or tetracycline HCl has been studied to determine if a new connective tissue attachment results. The proposed purposes of using acidic solutions on contaminated root surfaces are to detoxify the root and expose collagen fibers for a connective tissue attachment. However, a recent review of periodontal regeneration studies with and without the use of citric acid root conditioning showed no clinical advantage to its use (Garrett 1996).

RISK FACTORS FOR REGENERATIVE THERAPY

The same contraindications for any surgical periodontal therapy apply to regenerative therapies. These include any acute or chronic uncontrolled systemic diseases that put the patient at risk (e.g., diabetes mellitus), inadequate plaque control, and smoking (especially more than one pack per day).

BIOLOGICS AND DEVICES

This is a rapidly developing field that has generated few clinical studies thus far. Wound healing is a complex, well-orchestrated sequence of events. In studying the dynamics of cell-to-cell and cell-to-tissue interaction, scientists discovered the presence of growth factors. Attempts have been made to use these factors to enhance would healing (repair and regeneration).

Growth factors are naturally occurring proteins that mediate or regulate cellular events such as cell proliferation. Growth factors are found only in living tissue in cells such as bone, platelets, and macrophages. Bone morphogenic proteins (BMPs) are factors found in bone that help induce new bone formation (Wozney 1995).

There are several problems that have to be addressed before growth factors become part of the clinical periodontal armamentarium. The proper vehicle or delivery system for specific factors has not been identified. There are still questions about the concentration of growth factors when they are used by themselves or in combination with other factors. The variability of growth factor responses locally and systemically is still unknown. However, growth factors may have potential for clinical use in the near future.

Recently, a tissue healing modifier, enamel matrix protein derivative (Emdogain®, BIORA, Inc., Malmö, Sweden; Chicago, IL), has been introduced and used in periodontal regenerative techniques. Early clinical studies have been encouraging in showing improved clinical results and gain in clinical attachment and bone fill in sites treated with Emdogain® versus open flap debridement. Multicenter studies are currently being performed with this material.

Slavkin and Boyde (1975) proposed that enamel-related proteins from Hertwig's epithelial root sheath (HERS), which is the apical extension of the dental organ, are involved in the formation of cementum. In human teeth these enamel proteins are present in areas where cementogenesis (formation of cementum) is initiated.

To prepare Emdogain® to be placed into intraosseous defects, the contents of two vials are mixed together; enamel matrix derivative is mixed with propylene glycol alginate. The gel-like material is syringed onto the root surface, and the flap is sutured (Fig. 15–5a,b■). Newer formulations of this material are available in a premixed, one vial preparation ready for use.

FIGURE 15–5

(a) An 8-mm two-wall intraosseous defect on the mandiular first molar. (b) After flaps are reflected and the root and defect thoroughly debrided, Emdogain was syringed onto the root surface and the flap sutured to cover the material.

(a)

(b)

SUMMARY

Today, the role of periodontics in dentistry focuses not only on stopping the progression of inflammatory periodontal diseases but also on the regeneration of periodontal structures (cementum, PDL, supporting alveolar bone) that were destroyed by disease. Periodontal regenerative therapy uses bone replacement materials and guided tissue regeneration (GTR) techniques. The use of growth factors (e.g., bone morphogenic proteins and tissue modifiers) holds great promise. These factors most likely will be the next addition to periodontal regenerative techniques.

KEY POINTS

- ✤ Periodontal regeneration is defined as healing after periodontal surgery that results in the reproduction of cementum, PDL, and supporting alveolar bone that was lost or destroyed by periodontal diseases.
- ✤ Ideally, after periodontal surgery, healing by regeneration is preferred over repair.
- ✤ Periodontal regenerative techniques include the use of bone grafts, synthetic bone substitutes, guided tissue regeneration (GTR), and a combination of these.
- ✤ Bone-replacement materials may contribute to new bone formation or serve as a filler material for bone formation that starts from the adjacent bone and grows into the defect.
- ✤ GTR is used to delay apical migration of the junctional epithelium and exclude gingival connective tissue (inner flap) from the surgical site. The goal is to allow periodontal regenerative cells to repopulate the wound first.
- ✤ A barrier membrane is placed over the osseous defect and root to create a space for the migration of cells from the PDL and alveolar bone to repopulate the wound.

REFERENCES

American Academy of Periodontology. 1992. *Glossary of periodontal terms,* 3rd ed. Chicago: American Academy of Periodontology.

Becker, W., and B. E. Becker. 1993. Clinical applications of guided tissue regeneration: Surgical considerations. *Periodontology 2000* 1:46–53.

Brunsvold, M. A., and J. T. Mellonig. 1993. Bone grafts and periodontal regeneration. *Periodontology 2000* 1:80–91.

Cortellini, P., G. PiniPrato, and M. S. Tonetti. 1993a. Periodontal regeneration in human intrabony defects: I. Clinical measures. *J. Periodontol.* 64:254–260.

Cortellini, P., G. PiniPrato, and M. S. Tonetti. 1993b. Periodontal regeneration in human intrabony defects: II. Reentry procedures and bone measurements. *J. Periodontol.* 64:261–268.

Fetner, A. E., M. S. Martigan, and S. B. Low. 1994. Periodontal repair using Perioglas® in nonhuman primates: Clinical and histologic observations. *Compend. Contin. Ed. Dent.* 15:932–939.

Fox, J. S. 1997. Bone grafting materials for dental applications: A practical guide. *Compend. Contin. Ed. Dent.* 18:1013–1038.

Froum, S. J., M. A. Weinberg, and D. Tarnow. 1998. Comparison of bioactive glass synthetic bone graft particles and open debridement in the treatment of human periodontal defects: A clinical study. *J. Periodontol.* 69:698–709.

Garrett, S. 1996. Periodontal regeneration around natural teeth. *Ann Periodontol.* 1:621–666.

Garrett, S. 1977. Root planing: A perspective. *J. Periodontol.* 48:553–557.

Garrett, S., and G. Bogle. 1993. Periodontal regeneration: A review of flap management. *Periodontology 2000* 1:100–108.

Gottlow, J., S. Nyman, T. Karrine, and J. Wennström. 1986. New attachment formation in the human periodontium by guided tissue regeneration: Case reports. *J. Clin. Periodontol.* 13:604–616.

Hallmon, W. W., F. A. Carranza, Jr., C. L. Drisko, J. W. Rapley, and P. Robinson. 1996. Surgical therapy. In *Periodontal literature review,* 167–194. Chicago: American Academy of Periodontology.

Hench, L. L. 1988. Bioactive ceramics. *Ann. N.Y. Acad. Sci.* 523:54–71.

Hench, L. L., and J. K. West. 1996. Biological application of bioactive glasses. *Life Chem. Rep.* 13:187–241.

Laurell, L., J. Gottlow, M. Zybetz, and R. Persson. 1998. Treatment of intrabony defects by different surgical procedures: A literature review. *J. Periodontol.* 69:303–313.

Marx, R. E., and E. R. Carlson. 1993. Tissue banking safety: Caveats and precaution for the oral and maxillofacial surgeon. *J. Oral Maxillofac. Surg.* 51:1372–1379.

Melcher, A. H., C. A. G. McCulloch, T. Cheong, E. Nemeth, and A. Shiga. 1987. Cells from bone synthesize cementum-like and bone-like tissues in vitro and may migrate into periodontal ligament in vivo. *J. Periodontol. Res.* 22:246–247.

Melcher, A. H. 1976. On the repair potential of the periodontal tissues. *J. Periodontol.* 47:256–260.

Mellonig, J. T., A. B. Preuett, and M. P. Moyer. 1992. HIV inactivation in a bone allograft. *J. Periodontol.* 63:979–983.

Mellonig, J. T. 1984. Decalcified freeze-dried bone allograft as an implant material in human periodontal defects. *Int. J. Periodont. Restor. Dent.* 4(6):41–55.

Minabe, M. 1991. A critical review of the biologic rationale for guided tissue regeneration. *J. Periodontol.* 62:171–179.

Nyman, S., J. Gottlow, T. Karring, and J. Lindhe. 1982. The regenerative potential of the periodontal ligament: An experimental study in the monkey. *J. Clin. Periodontol.* 9:257–265.

Schallhorn, R. G. 1977. Present status of osseous grafting procedures. *J. Periodontol.* 48:570–576.

Slavkin, H. C., A. Boyde. 1975. Cementum: An epithelial secretory product? *J. Dent. Res.* 53:157 (abstract 409).

Smart, G. J., M. Wilson, E. H. Davies, and J. B. Kieser. 1990. The assessment of ultrasonic root surface debridement by determination of residual endotoxin levels. *J. Clin. Periodontol.* 17:174–178.

Smith, D., W. Ammons, and G. van Belle. 1980. A longitudinal study of periodontal status comparing osseous recontouring with flap curettage: II. Results after 6 months. *J. Periodontol.* 51:367–375.

Wozney, J. M. 1995. The potential role of bone morphogenic proteins in periodontal reconstruction. *J. Periodontol.* 66:506–510.

Yukna, R. 1993. Synthetic bone grafts in periodontics. *Periodontology 2000* 1:93–99.

SELF-QUIZ

1. During periodontal surgery, bone is taken from a mandibular torus and placed into a three-wall periodontal osseous defect. Which one of the following types of bone graft is this? (pp. 497–498)

   a. allograft
   b. autograft
   c. alloplast
   d. xenograft

2. Which one of the following types of cells is required for successful periodontal regeneration? (p. 500)

   a. periodontal ligament
   b. odontoblasts
   c. gingival connective tissue
   d. gingival epithelial

   attachment apparatus

3. Guided tissue regeneration (GTR) focuses on the isolation or exclusion of what type of tissue cells? (p. 501)

   a. junctional epithelial and gingival connective tissue
   b. alveolar bone and sulcular epithelium
   c. connective tissue and alveolar bone
   d. alveolar bone and junctional epithelial

4. Which one of the following types of material is nonabsorbable Gore-Tex® membrane? (p. 505)

   a. polytetrafluoroethylene (e-PTFE)
   b. poly-DL-lactide (PLA)
   c. polylactic acid/polyglycolate (PLA/PGA)
   d. bovine collagen

5. After surgical placement of a barrier membrane around an intraosseous defect, it is important to cover the membrane with the flap because. (p. 505)

   a. brushing the area is easier
   b. bacterial contamination can be prevented

  c. aesthetics are enhanced

  d. tooth mobility is reduced to pretreatment levels

6. Which one of the following defects heals best when treated with bone grafts/bone substitutes? (p. 499)

  a. one wall

  b. two wall

  c. three wall

  d. Class III furcations

  e. horizontal bone loss

7. All the following are objectives of using bone-replacement materials in the treatment of infrabony defects *except* one. Which one is the exception? (p. 499)

  a. reduction in probing depth

  b. reduction of bleeding

  c. gain in clinical attachment

  d. fill of the defect

  e. regeneration of the attachment apparatus

8. Which one of the following materials is a type of allograft? (pp. 497–498)

  a. bone from the patient's chin

  b. demineralized freezed-dried bone

  c. bone from the patient's hip

  d. enamel matrix protein derivatives

  e. bioactive glass particles

9. All the following complications may be seen after placement of barrier membranes *except* one. Which one is the *least* likely? (p. 506)

  a. suppuration

  b. gingival overgrowth

  c. soft tissue recession

  d. membrane exposure

10. All the following postoperative instructions apply to a patient after a regenerative procedure using a barrier membrane *except* one. Which one is the exception? (p. 506)

  a. Floss the surgical area.

  b. Rinse the area frequently with diluted salt water.

  c. Use an antimicrobial mouthrinse.

  d. Use antimicrobial impregnated swabs.

Management of Dental Implants

16

Suzanne K. Farrar, R.D.H., B.S.
Jeanne St. Germain, R.D.H., B.S.
Raymond A. Yukna, D.M.D., M.S.

Outline:

Goals:

To familiarize the dental hygienist with dental implants and the establishment of proper implant evaluation procedures and maintenance.

Educational Objectives:

Upon completion of this chapter, the reader should be able to:

Define the role of the dental hygienist in the management of patients with dental implants;

Explain the various types of dental implants currently in use;

Discuss the general sequence of implant placement, uncovering, and restoration;

Compare the tissues around natural teeth and dental implants;

Discuss the steps in evaluating tissue conditions around dental implants;

Describe proper instrument selection and therapeutic steps for in-office maintenance procedures; and

Recommend appropriate home-care techniques for patients with dental implants.

KEY WORDS

- dental implant
- osseointegration
- perimucosal seal
- peri-implantitis
- nonmetallic materials

513

The Role of the Dental Hygienist

*T*he dental hygienist plays a critical role in implant dentistry, providing valuable information on treatment and maintenance. The dental hygienist should know the type of implant used in his or her dental office. It is usually beneficial to have before and after pictures of patients who have undergone implant procedures in the office to show prospective patients potential end results. Showing prospective patients dental models, descriptive brochures, an actual implant, and/or an instructional video also can be a great help. An intraoral camera can be a very powerful tool to show patients the conditions in their mouths and what happens when teeth are missing, thereby opening a discussion of dental implants.

The **dental implant** serves as an effective vehicle for tooth replacement. Initial acceptance of implants by the dental community was not overwhelming because of their low rate of success. This is no longer the case. More literature is being distributed to laypeople, and they are becoming more aware of implant success rates and the new treatment options that are possible. A potential implant patient must be well educated about the entire procedure, especially the need for follow-up care.

Systemic and Social Factors

Implant therapy may not be an option for patients with certain systemic diseases or adverse risk factors. Systemic diseases such as reduced immune defense (HIV/AIDS) and uncontrolled diabetes mellitus can cause an increased susceptibility to infection and interfere with wound healing. Similarly, social risk factors such as smoking, alcohol intake, drug abuse, and stress have been shown to be associated with an increased frequency of implant problems, including failure (Bain 1996). Consultation with a patient's physician is required if a patient has disturbances of blood coagulation (including anticoagulation therapy), is on long-term steroids, or has a cancer that requires chemotherapy (Belser et al. 1996). An alternate method of replacing missing teeth should be pursued for such patients, such as fixed partial dentures, removable partial dentures, or complete dentures.

Types of Implants

Several types of implants have been used to replace teeth or support prostheses over the centuries. In modern times, a few types have been developed that provide the predictable success rates that clinicians and patients expect (Brånemark et al. 1985; Albrektsson and Sennerby 1991).

The components of a dental implant include the following (Fig. 16–1a ■):

1. The *implant* is the part that is surgically placed into the bone.
2. The *abutment* (or *metal post*) is the part that is attached to the implant and will be fitted with a restoration that can be placed on top of it.
3. The *superstructure* is the prosthetic replacement (e.g., crown or denture) that is either screwed or cemented to the abutment.

FIGURE 16–1

(a) Parts of a dental implant. Osseointegration occurs with direct anchorage of bone to the implant. Diagrammatic (b) and clinical (c) examples of different types of root-form dental implants showing different shapes, surfaces, and coatings.

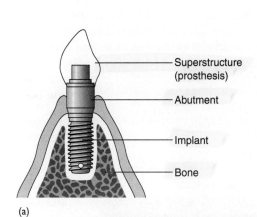

- Superstructure (prosthesis)
- Abutment
- Implant
- Bone

(a)

Core-Vent   Nobelpharma   IMZ   ISIS

ITI Hollow   TPS Screw   Steri-OSS   Integral

FIGURE 1 - Selected Root-Form Implants

(b)

(c)

Implant success and survival rates indicate that the anatomic region of the jaw, the quality of bone, and the length and width of the implant may play important roles in the outcome of treatment (Cochran 1996). Minimal criteria for success should include clinical immobility, absence of persistent and/or irreversible signs and symptoms (e.g., pain, infections), no peri-implant radiolucency, no irreversible mechanical failures (e.g., implant fractures), support and/or retention of functional restoration(s), and lack of progressive bone loss beyond physiologic remodeling. There are four types of implants: endosseous, subperiosteal, transosteal, and endodontic.

ENDOSSEOUS IMPLANTS

Endosseous means "within the bone." Endosseous implants have several different shapes, including blade, cylinder, and screw types, with each manufacturer having its own design. These are the most common implants, and they are placed in edentulous areas of the maxilla or mandible (endosseous). Blade-type implants were popular in the 1960s and 1970s and were associated with a fibrous type of attachment to bone (connective tissue found between the implant and bone). They have been replaced generally by root-form implants, which are associated with a bony attachment called osseointegration (see Fig. 16–1a).

Osseointegration

Osseointegration is a term introduced by Brånemark and coworkers in 1969 to describe the direct contact of a dental implant (inert metal) with bone without any intervening connective tissue. Thus the implant becomes an integral part of the bone and is, in effect, ankylosed, as seen at the light microscopic level (Brånemark et al. 1969). This phenomenon has revolutionized implant dentistry and made it the mainstream form of therapy it is today.

This description has been expanded by the same group of investigators to characterize the long-term success of an osseointegrated implant. Such success requires full occlusal function without pain and, most important, after an initial marginal bone height loss in the first year of 1 to 2 mm at the bone crest, a crestal bone height loss of no more than 0.1 to 0.2 mm per year. Inflammation of the gingiva around the implant neck is acceptable but should not enter the bone or jeopardize long-term implant success rates (Smilth and Zarb 1989).

The implant system that initially showed long-term success was made of machined pure titanium with a screw shape. The titanium surface oxidizes into a thin nonreactive titanium oxide layer to which bone adheres, at least at the light-microscopic level. This type of bone-implant interface is osseointegration. While almost all dental implants today are titanium based (pure titanium or titanium alloy), some are coated, sprayed, or otherwise treated to create a rough surface, thus producing more surface area for the bone to contact or adhere to (Fig. 16–1b, c ■). The coatings used are usually acid-etched and sprayed, a titanium plasma spray, titanium beads, or calcium-phosphate ceramics (hydroxyapatite and others). Some research has shown that the initial bone bonding to hydroxyapatite may be greater and stronger than the bonding to titanium (Weinlander 1991). Endosseous implants are the predominant type (>90%) used in current practice (Fig. 16–2a ■).

SUBPERIOSTEAL IMPLANTS

Subperiosteal means "on top of the bone." Subperiosteal implants are individually designed cast-metal frames that fit intimately over the bone and under the periosteum and gingiva. Resting on the bone for support, the frame may or may not be fixed to the bone. Posts protrude through the gingiva as anchors for the replacement teeth (see Fig. 16–2b ■). Currently, this type of implant is not used frequently except if there is insufficient bone mass for a root-type implant that cannot be corrected with surgery.

FIGURE 16–2

(a) Panoramic radiograph of root-form dental implants in mandible. (b) Panoramic radiograph of supraperiosteal dental implants on mandible.

(a)   (b)

TRANSOSTEAL IMPLANTS

Transosteal means "through the bone." Transosteal implants are mandibular denture anchors placed all the way through the mandible from under the chin into the mouth. They are commonly called *mandibular staple implants.* A curved, flat plate fits under the anterior mandible and usually has five to seven pins. The pins are anchor screws to hold the plate, and the posts are drilled parallel through the mandibular alveolar ridge by means of a jaw-fixation jig with parallel drilling sleeves. This implant has a good success record and is used for very severely resorbed mandibles. However, complications may be more common.

ENDODONTIC IMPLANTS

Endodontic implants are placed "in and through the tooth." They are also called *endodontic stabilizers* because they consist of a long, wide post inserted into the prepared root canal space that purposely extends at least a centimeter beyond the apex. The rationale is that this extension will stabilize the tooth and improve its usefulness as an abutment. However, this type of implant is not used commonly in the United States and has a poor prognosis because of the potential for root fracture, mechanical retention problems, and root resorption.

SURGICAL PROCEDURE

Dental hygienists should be familiar with the basics of dental implant therapy, including the surgical procedures. While dental implant treatment may sound extensive, involved, and painful, most patients receive their dental implants in an outpatient setting and have few postoperative problems such as bleeding, infection, or pain. The general stages of dental implant treatment are outlined in Fig. 16–3 ■.

FIGURE 16–3

Diagram of sequence of dental implant placement using two-stage technique. The body of the implant (fixture) is surgically placed in the bone under the gingiva, allowed to heal for several months, uncovered so that a healing post can be connected to the implant, and the restoration completed.

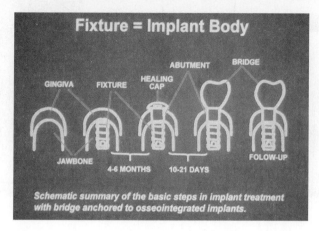

The patient should be aware that several preoperative steps usually are necessary before the actual implant surgery. The restorative dentist (and the surgeon) should do a full workup on the patient. This includes mounted study casts, a wax-up of the planned restoration, fabrication of a radiographic and surgical guide stent, and appropriate pretreatment radiographs such as periapicals, panoramic, and computed or linear tomography for a three-dimensional view of the bone. These steps are needed to ensure accurate planning as to implant number, diameter, length, and location based on the restorative needs of the patient, bone quantity and quality, and anatomic structures.

First-Stage Surgery

Once the patient is made comfortable and the areas of implant placement are anesthetized, the surgical guide stent is positioned and the specific implant locations marked. An incision is made through the crest of the gingiva, and flaps are reflected to expose the bone. A specific sequence of drills/burs is used to create a hole of specific diameter and depth for the implant(s) to be used. The drilling is done at relatively slow speed with copious irrigation to keep the bone cool and minimize trauma to the potential bone-healing cells. The root-form implant is then threaded or gently tapped into position so that its top is flush with the top of the bone. A cover screw is placed on top of the implant to seal the screwhole for cleanliness. The gingiva is then sutured to cover the implant(s) (Fig. 16–4a,b,c,d ■). The implant surgeon may prescribe analgesics and antibiotics as needed. Sutures are left in place for approximately 7 to 14 days. While most patients would like to have a temporary tooth replacement in the implant area immediately, *pressure on top of the implant should be avoided.* A fixed temporary restoration relieved over the implant sites often can be placed in the partially edentulous implant patient.

The implants need to heal undisturbed for 3 to 6 months before second-stage uncovering surgery can be performed. A healing time is usually needed for osseointegration to occur. Osseointegration means the bone fuses tightly and firmly to the implant surface and becomes an integral part of the jaw bone, similar to an

FIGURE 16–4

Clinical case illustrating implant placement. (a) Initial drill hole using surgical guide stent. (b) Test pins placed to verify position and angulation of the planned implants. (c) Two implants placed into properly drilled holes to be level with bone crest. (d) Five-year follow-up radiograph illustrating fixed-bridge design for good oral hygiene and maintenance of bone level.

(a) (b)

(c) (d)

ankylosed tooth. The time period needed for osseointegration varies depending on the bone quality or density and therefore is shortest for the mandibular anterior area, which is composed of dense cortical bone (3 to 4 months), and longest for the maxillary posterior area, which is composed of more fragile cancellous bone (5 to 6 months). However, recent advances in implants surfaces have allowed manufactures to claim implant loading as early as 2 months after placement.

SECOND-STAGE SURGERY

Second-stage or uncovering surgery is performed to expose the top of the implant and replace the cover screw with a temporary healing abutment or post that screws into the implant fixture and protrudes through the gingival tissue into the oral cavity. This surgery is usually performed using local anesthesia. After a small incision is made over the implants, and the cover screw is removed, and the healing abutment is placed. The gingiva is then sutured tightly around the protruding abutment. After 2 to 3 weeks of soft tissue healing, the restoration process continues. Impressions of the implant(s) are taken. Teeth (e.g., crowns) are fabricated to cement or screw onto the implant abutments. A removable replacement tooth also can be attached to the abutment, which allows the patient to remove and clean the tooth. Some implant systems avoid the second-stage surgery with *one-stage implants*. These are implants immediately exposed but not loaded at the time of implantation.

SPECIAL CONSIDERATIONS

While the surgical procedures outlined above are basic and apply to patients with good bone quantity, quality, and form, additional procedures often must be used to build up the bone or gingival tissues to allow proper implant placement and restoration. These extra procedures may include such therapy as bone-replacement grafts, guided tissue regeneration, soft tissue grafts, sinus bone grafts, or combinations of these. These additional procedures may extend the total treatment time until the final restoration can be delivered.

Implant patients and dental office personnel must realize the stages and timeline involved in dental implant therapy. Generally, it takes 9 to 12 months to arrive at the point of delivery of the desired restoration. Longer times are necessary if implant sites require bone grafts or guided tissue (bone) regeneration procedures prior to implant placement. After the final restoration is placed, patients must commit to long-term professional maintenance and optimal oral hygiene self-care.

IMPLANTS VERSUS TEETH

There are obvious differences between implants and teeth in structure and components (Table 16–1 ■). Implants are not prone to caries, endodontic (pulpal) problems, or root sensitivity, as are teeth. However, implants depend on proper restoration and occlusion, good oral hygiene, and regular maintenance, just as teeth do. Having a healthy soft tissue barrier is very important. Superstructures should be designed to help facilitate this. It has been shown that plaque accumulation and excessive occlusal forces are primary causes for implant failures (Meffert, Langer, and Frutz 1992).

TABLE 16–1	
BIOLOGIC ENVIRONMENT	
NATURAL TOOTH	**DENTAL IMPLANT**
Perpendicular connective tissue (PDL) attachment	Parallel connective tissue attachment
Greater blood supply at neck	Less blood supply at neck (scar)
Plaque—less; more confined inflammation	Plaque—greater; more widespread inflammation
Transseptal/supracrestal fibers	No limiting fibers (circular)
Late, slow bone loss	Earlier, faster bone loss
Inflammation not found in bone marrow	Inflammation into bone marrow
May show slight mobility	Any mobility means implant failure

Anatomy

Implant-tissue interface

Natural teeth are surrounded by the periodontium, alveolar and supporting bone, cementum, periodontal ligament, and gingiva. Dental implants are surrounded by peri-implant tissues, including osseointegrated bone surrounding the fixture. There is no periodontal ligament. The abutment, like the crown of a natural tooth, is surrounded by gingiva. After surgery, the gingiva heals around the abutment. During the healing process, a new free gingival margin forms, including a gingival sulcus and free gingival groove.

In natural teeth, the junctional epithelium provides a seal at the base of the sulcus against the invasion of bacterial substances. If the seal is disrupted and/or the gingival fibers are destroyed, the junctional epithelium migrates in an apical direction onto the root surface, forming a periodontal pocket. The evidence supports the fact that a junctional epithelium adheres to implant surfaces and has similar biologic features to the epithelial-tooth interface of a natural tooth. The junctional epithelium, which is referred to as a **perimucosal seal,** separates the inner tissues from the outside environment for both implants and teeth.

On the other hand, the implant–connective tissue interface shows marked differences when compared with teeth. There is a lack of cementum and no connective tissue fibers inserting into the implant surface. Connective tissue fibers subjacent to the epithelium on implants have been shown to be either parallel or circular in orientation to the implant surface, but they do not insert directly into the implant surface. This is sometimes called a *purse-string arrangement,* and it helps to keep the soft tissues tightly adapted to the implant (Listgarten et al. 1991).

Keratinized gingiva

There are conflicting reports concerning the need for keratinized tissue around implants. However, multiple factors may influence the desirability for the presence of keratinized tissue (see Table 16–1).

Blood Supply

Implants have less blood supply near their neck with more of a scar tissue appearance. Lack of a periodontal ligament limits the blood supply to the area to only the periosteal vessels and bone marrow spaces.

Inflammatory Lesion

Dental plaque has been shown to grow faster on titanium than on enamel (Quirynen et al. 1986). When plaque accumulation occurs, it results in more widespread inflammation around implants than the confined nature of the inflammatory lesion seen around teeth (Ericsson et al. 1992; Lekholm 1986). This is due primarily to a lack of limiting attached connective tissue fibers such as the transseptal and supracrestal fiber groups that are present on teeth. Similarly, natural teeth tend to exhibit late slow bone loss, and the inflammation does not usually extend into the bone marrow to any great degree. Infected implants, however, tend to have earlier and more rapid bone loss that extends into the adjacent bone marrow, creating a low-grade osteomyelitis.

SUMMARY

The major difference between implants and teeth, therefore, is the mechanism by which they are attached to the jawbone. Teeth are connected to the bone by means of a connective tissue sling, the periodontal ligament, which is a dynamic, responsive, adjustable attachment mechanism. Implants, by design, become osseointegrated or ankylosed without the cushioning effect of a periodontal ligament. Teeth can move as a result of occlusal or orthodontic forces. Implants do not have any physiologic movement.

BACTERIOLOGY

Neither dental implants nor natural teeth are immune to plaque accumulation. Regular, effective plaque control is imperative for soft tissue health and a good long-term prognosis with both.

Several studies have investigated the amount, rate, and contents of plaque deposits on implants as compared with teeth. Virtually all these studies show that there are no differences in the amount of plaque or the type of bacteria that accumulate on teeth or various implant surfaces. The types of pathogens found on both teeth and implants are similar (Newman and Flemming 1988; Table 16–2 ■). **Peri-implantitis** (inflammation of the tissues around the implant) and marginal bone loss have been associated with the presence of these pathogens in both partially and fully edentulous patients.

For both implants and teeth, smooth surfaces inhibit and roughened surfaces encourage plaque accumulation. Therefore, in-office maintenance procedures should not roughen the surface of implant components (or teeth).

MAINTENANCE PROGRAM

Periodontal maintenance procedures (continuing care) provided by the dental hygienist for implant patients include assessment of the entire oral cavity as well as the implant sites. A thorough assessment of plaque and calculus accumulation, as

TABLE 16–2	
PATHOGENS ASSOCIATED WITH PERI-IMPLANTITIS	
Porphyromonas gingivalis	Fusobacterium nucleatum
Campylobacter recta	Eikenella corrodens
Bacteroides forsythus	Eubacterium species
Prevotella intermedia	Selemonas species
Peptostreptococcus micros	Spirochetes
Actinobacillus actinomycetemcomitans	

well as evaluation of soft and hard tissues, should be a part of the protocol for each maintenance visit. Table 16–3 ■ reviews these assessment procedures.

The goal for maintenance therapy is to continually monitor the stable condition created by active treatment. Recall appointments should take place at 3-month intervals, and the frequency should be increased if that interval is not adequate.

CLINICAL PARAMETERS OF EVALUATION

Soft tissue evaluation

The clinical similarities between the natural dentition and dental implants has led to the use of similar parameters for evaluation of the periodontium and peri-implant tissues. This provides a means of monitoring and observing peri-implant health status and the effectiveness of treatment. Evaluation of the soft tissue surrounding dental implants is very similar to that of natural tooth structure. A basic assessment begins with the color, contour, and consistency (texture) of the surrounding soft tissue. The presence of erythema, edema, and suppuration, which are the traditional signs of inflammation, should be noted. Thorough documentation of the changes in the soft tissue is important because change may signify current disease activity.

Probing Depth Probing depth also can be used to assess the health of peri-implant tissues. However, the use of periodontal probes for evaluation of the peri-implant condition is highly controversial (Brägger 1994). Some clinicians feel that probing depth is not an important clinical parameter in the success of an implant (Smith and Zarb 1989). Concern has been expressed that probing for pockets around an implant may create a pathway for bacteria to attack the peri-implant seal. The probe may carry microorganisms from an infected site and seed a non-infected site. Also, different probing forces allow the probe to penetrate into the

TABLE 16–3
ASSESSMENT OF DENTAL IMPLANTS AND MAINTENANCE PROCEDURES (IN-OFFICE)

1. Review medical history.
2. Head and neck examination, oral cancer screening.
3. Take radiographs every 3 months for first year after implant restoration is placed; then yearly to check for bone loss. Place radiographs in sequential mounts.
4. Remove superstructure if necessary and possible.
5. Clean superstructure.
6. Check tissues for surface inflammation.
7. Check for plaque, and review oral hygiene practices.
8. Record probing depths using a plastic or nylon periodontal probe.*
9. Record bleeding on probing.*
10. Clean implant abutments using special nonmetallic instruments.
11. Irrigate with antimicrobial solution if indicated.
12. Replace superstructure, if removed.
13. Have occlusion checked.
14. Review dental hygiene again with superstructure in place.
15. Reschedule for 3- or 4-month recall depending on evaluation of tissue and oral hygiene.

*Somewhat controversial.

connective tissue/bone region easily because of the lack of a connective tissue attachment. No numerical value has been determined as a "healthy probing depth," as is the case with natural teeth (Rapley 1995). These concepts have not been verified, and thus gentle probing is recommended around implants if the practitioner suspects pathology.

When probing is performed, four measurements around the circumference of the implant should be recorded. As with natural teeth, minimal probing depth (<4 mm) is preferable (Orton, Steele, and Wolinsky 1987; Balshi 1986). Changes in probing depth over a period of time around an implant may be more important as an indicator of disease activity than a single probe depth measurement (Balshi 1986). The use of a plastic or nylon periodontal probe is recommended to prevent scratching of the titanium components. With some abutment and superstructure designs, accurate probing may be difficult because the probe is prevented from reaching the base of the sulcus; thus the probing depth may be underestimated. A more accurate measurement may be obtained by removing the superstructure, which would allow probe insertion parallel to the long axis of the implant. However, more important than the actual probing depth is detecting early changes in the depth of the pocket. Early detection provides an opportunity for therapeutic intervention before irreversible changes have occurred. Probing level has been demonstrated to correlate highly with the marginal bone level (Quirynen et al. 1991; Fig. 16–5a,b,c ■).

Bleeding on Probing   Controversy also can be found in the literature regarding the use of bleeding on probing as a clinical assessment parameter for implants. As with natural teeth, bleeding on probing can be a significant clinical finding. Despite the apparent healthy look of surface tissues and even shallow probing depths, bleeding on probing is an indication that there is underlying disease (Lekholm 1986). Any bleeding site (especially if the same site bleeds from visit to visit) should be inspected closely for the presence of irritants, and appropriate therapy should be instituted. However, some researchers find that bleeding may be related to probing force and wounding of the tissue rather than actual inflammation (Rapley 1995; Esposito et al. 1998) and should not be used as an indicator of healthy or diseased peri-implant tissue.

Keratinized gingiva

The presence of keratinized gingiva adjacent to implants is associated with improved tissue health. As with natural teeth, keratinization improves the strength and stability of the epithelium and promotes long-term implant success. An inadequate zone of keratinized gingiva may lead to increased recession, tissue soreness with toothbrushing or eating, and the ability of metallic components to be seen through mucosal tissues.

HARD TISSUE EVALUATION

Radiographic procedures

Implant bone levels are best determined by regular accurate radiographic evaluations. Panoramic radiographs commonly are taken for baseline data following abutment placement; however, individual periapical or vertical bitewing radiographs should be taken using the paralleling technique with a gridded film (film

FIGURE 16–5

Periodontal probing around implants and tissue health. (a) Plastic probe with pressure-limiting mechanisms showing shallow probing depth. Note health of surface tissue. Also note relative lack of keratinized gingiva. (b) Probing access is easier with superstructure removed. Shallow probing depth and good zone of keratinized gingiva. (c) Inflamed tissue with deeper probing depth and bleeding on probing indicating an unhealthy implant site.

(a)

(b)

(c)

with millimeter markings). Such radiographs are preferable for determining bone height and density. Marginal bone height should be measured both mesially and distally and recorded in relation to a landmark on the implant system. For dental implant success, 0.2 mm or less of bone loss annually along the implant surface is acceptable (Albrektsson et al. 1986). For proper continued evaluation, radiographic examinations are recommended after prosthetic connection, at 6 and 12 months, and subsequently at 1- to 3-year intervals.

MOBILITY

It is recommended that the prosthesis be removed at least once a year to test for implant and abutment mobility. Since the truly osseointegrated implant has no periodontal ligament, there should be zero mobility around stable implants. Mobility of an implant after an appropriate healing period is a sign of implant failure, indicating lack of osseointegraton. Radiographic examinations together with implant mobility tests seem to be the most reliable parameters in the prognostic assessment of osseointegrated implants (Esposito et al. 1998).

Mobility of the superstructure can be evaluated by wedging a curet between the prosthesis and the abutment head or by traditional mobility detection. If the abutment is loose, the screws may need to be examined for possible tightening.

IDENTIFYING THE PROBLEM IMPLANT

While endosseous root-form dental implants are quite successful, with most studies showing greater than 90% long-term success with a variety of systems, some do develop problems. Identification of these problems when they first begin is important for effective management.

CRITERIA FOR SUCCESS

The periodontal criteria for success are similar for dental implants and natural teeth. The basis of success is frequent inspection and debridement. As with natural teeth, shallow and stable probing depths are desirable at each visit. In addition, there should be no bleeding on probing at any evaluation site. An adequate zone of keratinized gingiva may be advantageous to protect the soft tissue interface (Brånemark and Zarb 1985). The main difference in success criteria involves mobility. While unchanging mobility within physiologic limits is acceptable with natural teeth, any implant mobility is unacceptable.

Restoratively, the prosthesis must fit accurately and securely. There should be no trauma from occlusion (excessive occlusal force on the implant), especially in lateral excursions. Moreover, there should be no mobility of the superstructure and especially of the implant itself. Radiographically, no radiolucency should be present around the implant, and less than 0.2 mm of bone loss per year should be present.

Perhaps the most important factor in success is to effect a change in the patient's dental behavior pattern. If this occurs, and the preceding technical aspects are achieved, then a biocompatible interface between the implant and the host tissues can be maintained for a long time. These criteria are summarized in Table 16–4 ■ (Smith and Zarb 1989).

TABLE 16–4
PERIODONTAL CRITERIA FOR SUCCESS WITH DENTAL IMPLANTS

- Frequent inspection and debridement
- Shallow, stable pockets
- No bleeding on probing
- Effective oral hygiene
- Patient ability/accessibility
- Keratinized gingiva
- Accurate, secure fit of parts
- No trauma from occlusion
- No mobility
- Change in dental behavior pattern
- Maintenance of biocompatible interface

OVERLOADING OF IMPLANTS

Mechanical failures of both the implant components and prosthetic superstructures have been associated with occlusal overload and ill-fitting restorative frameworks. Marginal bone loss around implants also has been associated with implant overload.

STAGES OF PERI-IMPLANT DISEASE

Plaque-induced inflammation occurs in a similar fashion around dental implants as around natural teeth. The pathogenesis is very similar for both entities, but there are several differences, as noted earlier in this chapter. Inflammation around implants generally is called *peri-implantitis.*

FIGURE 16–6
(a,b) Radiographic evidence of bone loss around dental implants, indicating peri-implantitis.

(a)   (b)

Peri-implantitis has many of the same clinical manifestations and stages as periodontitis. It can be graded from slight to severe, and its treatment parallels that of the stages of periodontitis (Fig. 16–6a,b ■). Slight problems are treated with improved oral hygiene and nonsurgical local therapy (mouthrinses) (Ciancio et al. 1995). Moderate problems usually require systemic antibiotics (Mombelli and Lang 1992) or flap access surgery. Severe problems require flap surgery for access, with the likelihood of regenerative therapy, including bone-replacement grafts and guided tissue regeneration barriers. The latter has not been shown to be as effective with implants as with natural teeth. The best results in severe cases of peri-implantitis are obtained when the implant can be reburied to recapture the lost osseointegration. Sometimes, the problem is so advanced that the implant must be removed.

INSTRUMENTATION

SUPERSTRUCTURE REMOVAL

On some occasions, the prosthetic superstructure supported by an implant must be removed for better access for maintenance of the implant abutment posts. Some superstructures are removable prostheses anyway, and the patient is familiar with their removal and replacement. Others (increasingly common) are fixed implants (screw-retained or cemented) and must be removed by dental office personnel.

Since the hygienist may be asked to remove a superstructure, he or she must be familiar with the removal and replacement process (Table 16–5 ■). While this may involve the simple unscrewing of a small screw, it is often better left to the dentist, who should know the exact type, length, and diameter of the implant and have the correct instrument and replacement screws for that particular implant system. The prosthetic superstructure should not be removed unless the correct armamentarium is available and the dentist is personally familiar with the implant type used.

TABLE 16–5
REMOVAL AND REPLACEMENT OF SUPERSTRUCTURE

1. Review radiographs and familiarize yourself with the implant location(s).
2. Note location of each implant under superstructure.
3. Have appropriately sized screws and instruments for removal and replacements available.
4. Remove any temporary filling material that may be in the screw hole area.
5. Have small containers, dappen dishes, or envelopes available.
6. Once screws are removed, place in containers labeled as to location.
7. If removing extensive restorations, loosen screws a little at a time. Then return to each screw and loosen fully.
8. Remove superstructure and examine underside for debris.
9. Clean appropriately, keeping the integrity of the interface with the abutments and the screw holes free of debris.
10. Clean around implant abutments (see Table 16–1).
11. Replace superstructure.
12. Using correct screws, screw into place using same sequential technique as was used when removing superstructure.
13. Place temporary filling material over screws if indicated.
14. Check occlusion.

Removing the superstructure generally entails unscrewing it from the abutments. This must be done in a systematic way. For example, a patient may have crowns and bridges from tooth 2 to tooth 15 with six implants under this superstructure. The hygienist should have six containers, small cups or dappen dishes, with markings on them to correspond to the jaw location of the implants. When the screw from implant 2 is removed, it should be placed in the container marked 2. When the screw from implant 6 is removed, it should be placed in the container marked 6, and so on. The hygienist will want to back the screws off a little at a time, alternating among them, much in the way a tire is removed and replaced on a car. Unscrewing one side, for example, implant screws 2, 4, and 6 all the way, and not unscrewing implant screws 11, 13, and 15 may cause the integrity of the implants and superstructure to be compromised. Once the superstructure is removed, better access is available to evaluate the soft tissue and gingiva and provide maintenance therapy to the individual implant. The superstructure itself should be thoroughly inspected and cleaned. The hygienist must be aware that the inside of the screw holes always must be kept free of debris or the screws may not fit, and the superstructure may not seat properly.

When replacing the superstructure, begin with one implant, and slightly tighten the screw. Then move to the next implant, and so on, just like replacing a tire on a car. Once all the screws are in position and slightly tightened, the hygienist can begin to tighten them down fully. Since peri-implant bone loss may result from occlusal overload, always make sure to check the occlusion once the superstructure is in place.

APPROPRIATE INSTRUMENTS FOR IMPLANTS

Deposits that accumulate on supra- and subgingival surfaces of dental implant components should be removed. Normally, calculus on these surfaces is not as tenacious as on natural teeth because the deposits do not penetrate or interlock with the implant surface.

FIGURE 16–7

Several types of nonmetallic scalers and curets for use on dental implant components.

FIGURE 16–8

(a,b) Use of nonmetallic curets.

(a)

(b)

The nature of the surface of implant components must be considered when deciding which instruments to use during office procedures. Most implant components are titanium, a very tough but easily scratchable metal. Stainless steel and carbon steel instruments used directly on an implant can cause marring and scratching of the surface, resulting in roughness, which can increase plaque adherence. Curets made of **nonmetallic materials,** such as plastic, graphite, Teflon®, or nylon, or gold-plated curets are recommended, and these are available from several manufacturers (Figs. 16–7 ■ and 16–8a,b ■). Cleaning around the tissue surface of the prosthesis and implant abutments also can be performed with gauze or tufted floss.

Air-powder abrasive units are effective, but they should not be used directly on implant components for any length of time. The use of ultrasonic and sonic powered scalers with metal tips is also contraindicated with implants. Specific plastic or nylon sleeves placed over the tip are available that allow cleaning of implants without scratching (Fig. 16–9 ■).

FIGURE 16–9

Nylon or plastic sleeve for ultrasonic or sonic instruments to prevent scratching of implant components.

IN-OFFICE IRRIGATION

The purpose of in-office irrigation is to attempt to irrigate to the base of the pocket. Plastic rather than metal irrigation tips or needles should be used when irrigating around implants, and the hygienist should be careful not to become too aggressive in forcing the tip into the pocket. Using an irrigation device with an antimicrobial solution at every maintenance visit is considered to be of some benefit by certain practitioners. Irrigation can be used if pathologic changes are present (Meffert, Langer, and Frutz 1992). However, this information is anecdotal, and *there are not enough controlled clinical studies to support implant irrigation.*

POLISHING COMPOUNDS

Using coarse pumice may compromise implant surface components, so fine or flour of pumice or tin oxide with a rubber cup or point should be used to polish the titanium surfaces (Fig. 16–10 ■).

HOME-CARE PROCEDURES

Diligent home care around tissue-integrated prostheses is imperative for long-term success. Plaque-control procedures must start immediately after uncovering the implants. It is important that the dental hygienist customize a home-care regimen based on the patient's awareness and ability and the type of prosthesis present (Orton, Steele, and Wolinsky 1987).

There are two specific areas of focus for home-care procedures around implants. The first is the portion of the titanium abutment exposed above the soft tissues in the oral cavity, as well as the small portion just below the gingiva. The second area requiring plaque control is the prosthetic component, consisting of the rigid cast framework and tooth replacement materials.

FIGURE 16–10

Polishing implant components with a soft rubber cup and tin oxide.

A multitude of home-care devices exist to assist in mechanical oral hygiene regimes. These devices include various manual (Fig. 16–11a,b,c ■) or powered toothbrushes (Fig. 16–12 ■) and specific interdental aids (Balshi 1986). Soft or ultrasoft manual toothbrushes are the traditional means of plaque removal. However, brush heads come in many different shapes and sizes, and brushes should be prescribed individually depending on the implant type and the patient's abilities. An excellent area-specific soft nylon brush is the single-tufted brush. This brush is for use on individual implants, one implant at a time, and the shaft can be bent for better access.

Various interdental devices are available, including interdental brushes, rubber-tip stimulators, wooden cleaners, and numerous types of dental floss. The brush attachment for interdental brushes is available as a plastic or nylon-coated wire rather than a metal wire to prevent scratching of implant surfaces. Interdental brushes are used only if sufficient interdental embrasure exists. Various floss types, such as tufted floss or floss cords (PostCare™, J. O. Butler, Chicago, IL), along with folded gauze or traditional floss, are effective and safe interproximal plaque-removal aids (Fig. 16–13a,b,c,d ■).

Clinical use of antimicrobials (chemotherapeutic agents) can adjunctively help to inhibit plaque and gingivitis around implants. These agents may be delivered by rinsing or applied topically (via toothbrush, floss, or cotton-tipped applicator). Irrigation can be used if pathologic changes are present (Meffert, Langer, and Frutz 1992). A study conducted by Felo and colleagues (1997) investigated the effects of subgingival irrigation with chlorhexidine gluconate diluted with water on peri-implant gingival health compared with rinsing with chlorhexidine when used as an adjunct to routine peri-implant maintenance. Results suggested that powered subgingival irrigation with chlorhexidine may be better than rinsing in implant maintenance. However, even though the results of this study were favorable toward the use of irrigation at home, patients should not irrigate routinely until more controlled clinical studies can support its use.

The use of chlorhexidine gluconate (Peridex®, Zila Pharmaceuticals, Cincinnati, OH; or PerioGard®, Colgate Oral Pharmaceuticals, Canton, MA) and Listerine® (Warner-Lambert, Morris Plains, NJ) has been shown to be advantageous in the inhibition of bacterial plaque in implant patients (Ciancio et al. 1995).

Some practitioners may recommend home irrigation devices, but patients should be advised to use gentle pressure, ensuring that the irrigant is not forced

FIGURE 16–11

Types of toothbrushes used on implants. (a) Single-tuft brush (also referred to as an *end-tuft brush*). (b) Powered brush used with fixed partial denture superstructure. (c) Powered brush used with overdenture abutments and retention bar.

(a)

(b)

(c)

FIGURE 16–12

Various types of powered brush heads. Many clinicians recommend powered brushes for use around dental implants.

FIGURE 16–13

Oral hygiene aids for interproximal tooth surfaces. (a) Tufted floss used under a fixed denture. (b) Tufted floss used under a fixed bridge. (c) Folded gauze strip can be efficient when access is good. (d) Interdental brush used under a fixed partial denture.

(a)

(b)

(c)

(d)

into the sulcus. Excessive fluid pressure with the tip positioned apically could damage the perimucosal seal. Using either a sideport blunt-tipped canula or a rubber-tip irrigating device is less likely to violate this seal.

While rinsing with antimicrobials has been proven to be beneficial, some rinses do have unwanted side effects, such as staining, altered taste, and increased calculus formation. Awareness of potential side effects may indicate alternative delivery by applying the solution in a site-specific fashion so as to avoid undesirable effects.

SUMMARY

Implant therapy is a rapidly growing part of dental care. With the growing number of implants being placed, the dental team will have an important role in helping attain and preserve the oral health of these patients. Patient education regarding the scope of implant procedures, recommendations for daily home-care regimens, periodic maintenance visits, and regular evaluations are all part of the role of the dental hygienist. The hygienist probably will spend the most time with the patient and can help contribute substantially to the success of dental implant treatment. The dental hygienist has a significant role not only in implant maintenance but also in patient motivation and education. It is important to keep in mind that implant therapy is not for everyone. For this reason, it is crucial that the dental hygienist be educated about implant types, the sequence of therapy, and the social and systemic factors that influence implant success.

KEY POINTS

✦ Controversy exists regarding the use of periodontal probes around healthy implants.
✦ Progressive bone loss is a pathologic sign that can lead to implant failure.
✦ The implant should not be mobile; mobility indicates lack of osseointegration.
✦ Metal (e.g., stainless steel) instruments should never be used on dental implants; use only Teflon®, wood, nylon, gold-plated, graphite, rubber, or plastic instruments.

ACKNOWLEDGMENT

We are indebted to Connie Holland Gandy and Marianne Gabb for assistance with the preparation of this chapter.

REFERENCES

Albrektsson, T., and L. Sennerby. 1991. State of the art in oral implants. *J. Clin. Periodontal.* 16:474–481.

Albrektsson, T., G. Zarb, P. Worthington, and A. R. Eriksson. 1986. The long-term efficacy of currently used dental implants: A review and proposed criteria of success. *Int. J. Oral Maxillofac. Implants* 1:11–25.

Bain, C. A. 1996. Smoking and implant failure: Benefits of a smoking cessation protocol. *Int. J. Oral Maxillofac. Implants* 11:756–759.

Balshi, T. J. 1986. Hygiene maintenance procedures for patients treated with the tissue integrated prosthesis (osseointegration). *Quintessence Int.* 17:95–102.

Belser, U., R. Mericske-Stern, D. Buser, J. P. Bernard, D. Hess, and J. P. Martinet. 1996. Preoperative diagnosis and treatment planning. In *Oral implantology,* ed. A. Schroeder, F. Sutter, D. Buser, and G. Krekeler, 231–255. New York: Thieme Medical.

Brägger, U. 1994. Maintenance, monitoring, therapy of implant failures. In *Proceedings of the 1st European workshop on periodontology,* ed. N. P. Lang and T. Karring. Chicago: Quintessence Books.

Brånemark, P. I., G. Zarb, and T. Albrektson. 1985. *Tissue-integrated prosthesis osseointegration in clinical dentistry.* Chicago: Quintessence Books.

Brånemark, P. I., U. Breine, R. Adell, O. Hansson, J. Lindström, and A. Ohlsson. 1969. Intraosseous anchorage of dental prosthesis. *Scand. J. Plast. Reconstr. Surg.* 3:81–100.

Ciancio, S. G., C. Lauciello, O. Shibly, M. Vitello, and M. Mather. 1995. The effect of an antiseptic mouthrinse on implant maintenance: Plaque and peri-implant gingival tissues. *J. Peridontol.* 66:962–965.

Cochran, D. 1996. Implant therapy I. *Ann. Periodontol.* 1:707–820.

Ericsson, I., N. T. Berglund, C. Marinello, B. Liljenberg, and J. Lindhe. 1992. Long-standing plaque and gingivitis at implants and teeth in the dog. *Clin. Oral Implant Res.* 3:99–103.

Esposito, M., J.-M. Hirsch, U. Lekholm, and P. Thomsen. 1998. Biological factors contributing to failures of osseointegrated oral implants: I. Success criteria and epidemiology. *Eur. J. Oral Sci.* 106:527–551.

Felo, A., O. Shibly, S. G. Ciancio, F. R. Lauciello, and A. Ho. 1997. Effects of subgingival chlorhexidine irrigation of peri-implant maintenance. *Am. J. Dent.* 10:107–110.

Lekholm, M. 1986. Marginal tissue reactions at osseointegrated titanium fixtures. *Int. J. Oral Maxillofac. Implants* 15:53–61.

Listgarten, M. A., N. P. Lang, H. E. Schroeder, and A. Schroeder. 1991. Periodontal tissues and their counterparts around endosseous implants. *Clin. Oral Implant Res.* 2:1–19.

Meffert, R., B. Langer, and M. Frutz. 1992. Dental implants: A review. *J. Periodontol.* 63:859–870.

Mombelli, A., and N. P. Lang. 1992. Antimicrobial treatment of peri-implant infections. *Clin. Oral Implants Res.* 3:162–168.

Newman, M., and T. Flemming. 1988. Periodontal considerations of implants and implant associated microbiota. *J. Dent. Ed.* 52:737–744.

Orton, G. S., D. L. Steele, and L. E. Wolinsky. 1987. The dental professional's role in monitoring and maintenance of tissue-integrated prosthesis. *Int. J. Oral Maxillofac. Implants* 4:305–310.

Quirynen, M., D. van Steenberghe, R. Jacobs, A. Schotte, and P. Darius. 1991. The reliability of pocket probing around screw-type implants. *Clin. Oral Implant Res.* 2:186–192.

Rapley, J. 1995. Dental implants: Maintenance. In *The periodontic syllabus*, 3rd ed., ed P. F. Fedi, Jr. and A. R. Vernino, 183–186. Baltimore: Williams & Wilkins.

Smith, D. E., and G. Zarb. 1989. Criteria for success of osseointegrated endosseous implants. *J. Prosthet. Dent.* 62:567–572.

Smith, D., and G. Zarb. 1989. Criteria for success of osseointegrated endosseous implants. *J. Prosthet. Dent.* 62:567–572.

Smithloff, M., and M. E. Fritz. 1987. The use of blade implants in a selected population on partially edentulous adults: A 15-year report. *J. Periodontol.* 58:589–593.

Weinlander, M. 1991. Bone growth around dental implants. *Dent. Clin. North Am.* 35:585–601.

SELF-QUIZ

1. All the following systemic conditions are contraindications to implant placement *except* one. Which one is the exception? (p. 514)

   a. uncontrolled diabetes mellitus
   b. controlled hypertension
   c. head and neck cancer
   d. AIDS

2. Which one of the following types of dental implants is used most commonly today to support prostheses? (p. 516)

   a. submucosal
   b. subperiosteal
   c. endosseous
   d. transosteal

3. Which one of the following similarities is common between dental implants and natural teeth? (pp. 520–521)

   a. bone interface
   b. microbial flora
   c. connective tissue attachment
   d. probing depths topography

4. Routine periodontal probing around implants is controversial *because* probing may introduce bacteria into the perimucosal seal. (pp. 523–524)

   a. Both the statement and the reason are correct and related.
   b. Both the statement and the reason are correct but *not* related.
   c. The statement is correct, but the reason is *not.*
   d. The statement is *not* correct, but the reason is correct.

5. Which one of the following oral hygiene aids is *best* used for interdental cleaning? (p. 531)

   a. toothbrush
   b. flossing cord
   c. powered toothbrush
   d. interproximal brush with metal core

6. All the following types of instruments are used to clean implant abutments *except* one. Which one is the exception? (pp. 528–529)

   a. Teflon®
   b. stainless steel
   c. gold plate
   d. wood

7. Which one of the following polishing agents can be used for implant abutments? (p. 530)

   a. medium prophy paste
   b. fine pumice
   c. tin oxide
   d. rouge

8. Which one of the following parameters is *most* reliable in the assessment of the prognosis for osseointegrated implants? (pp. 524–525)

   a. color and contour of the gingiva
   b. bleeding on probing and mobility
   c. radiographic changes and mobility
   d. periodontal probing and color of the gingiva

9. Which one of the following signs indicates implant failure? (pp. 525–526)

   a. deep probing depths
   b. edematous tissue
   c. bleeding
   d. mobility

10. Oral irrigation should be used routinely around dental implants *because* there is no periodontal ligament attachment to an implant, allowing for easy access of the irrigant to the implant surface. (pp. 531–532)

    a. Both the statement and the reason are correct and related.

    b. Both the statement and the reason are correct but *not* related.

    c. The statement is correct, but the reason is *not.*

    d. The statement is *not* correct, but the reason is correct.

    e. *Neither* the statement *nor* the reason is correct.

PERIODONTAL MANAGEMENT OF MEDICALLY COMPROMISED PATIENTS

Mea A. Weinberg, D.M.D., M.S.D., R.Ph.

Outline:

Goal:

To educate the dental hygienist in the identification and periodontal management of medically compromised patients.

Educational Objectives:

Upon completion of this chapter, the reader should be able to:

Discuss the different categories of medically compromised patients;

Identify medically compromised patients; and

Describe various dental care considerations for medically compromised patients.

KEY WORDS

- medical risk
- medically compromised
- special care
- universal precautions

*S*ince more people are living longer today than ever before, there is an increased chance of encountering patients with medical conditions that may alter their dental treatment plan and care. Identification of these patients is necessary before treatment commences in order to avoid untoward medical emergencies. Recognition of these patients comes initially from reviewing their health/medical histories. It is the responsibility of every practitioner to identify any patient who may be at a potential **medical risk** and modify his or her care and/or consult with his or her physician. Since it is now recognized that medical conditions can develop as a result of a patient's preexisting periodontal disease, it is prudent to identify such conditions and make sure that they are well controlled. Different categories of **medically compromised** patients or patients with medical conditions that may require **special care** or alterations of the treatment plan will be discussed in this chapter: patients with cardiovascular disorders, endocrine conditions, hormonal conditions, kidney diseases, corticosteroid therapy, chemotherapy/radiotherapy, organ transplant, epilepsy, hepatitis, human immunodeficiency virus (HIV) infection, and tuberculosis.

Cardiovascular Disorders

Cardiovascular or heart disease is one of the more common medical conditions in the United States. Often cardiovascular disease may go undiagnosed. If it is not revealed in the patient's health/medical history, a dental hygienist can recognize certain signs and symptoms to help in the potential identification of patients with the disease.

Hypertension

Hypertension is defined as an elevation of arterial pressure. It is estimated that there are more than 50 million hypertensive people in the United States (Berkow, Fletcher, and Beers 1992). Vital signs, including blood pressure and pulse, should be taken on the initial dental appointment and every subsequent office visit. Blood pressure increases with increasing age from under 110/75 mmHg in children less than 6 years of age to 140/90 mmHg in adults. A long-standing blood pressure of more than 140/90 mmHg in adults is considered abnormal (Little et al. 1997). Most dental clinicians suggest postponing elective dental treatment when the blood pressure exceeds 180/100 mmHg (Perusse, Goulet, and Turcotte 1992). Untreated long-standing hypertension increases the risks for stroke (cerebrovascular accident) and heart attack (myocardial infarction) (Little et al. 1997; Joint National Committee 1993). It is important to control stress and anxiety to avoid elevations in blood pressure. When taking a blood pressure reading, position the patient's arm at chest level. If the blood pressure is elevated, the patient should be referred to a physician; it is not the responsibility of the dentist or dental hygienist to make a diagnosis of hypertension. It is best to avoid any elective dental treatment until the patient seeks medical care. Symptoms the patient may experience include headache, weakness, nosebleeds, and dizziness. Recommendations for dental care of hypertensive patients are reviewed in Table 17–1 ■.

Hypertension can be treated with either diet and/or antihypertensive medications. Nonpharmacologic methods for lowering blood pressure include weight

	TABLE 17–1		
	EVALUATION OF BLOOD PRESSURE IN ADULTS		
SYSTOLIC BLOOD PRESSURE (MMHG)	DIASTOLIC BLOOD PRESSURE (MMHG)	CLASSIFICATION	GUIDELINES
<130	<85	Normal	Proceed with treatment; no special precautions
130–139	85–89	High normal	Proceed with treatment
140–159	90–99	Stage I (mild hypertension)	Proceed with treatment; patient may require conscious sedation and antianxiety drugs; monitor bp and retake within 2 months
160–179	100–109	Stage II (moderate hypertension)	Proceed with treatment; patient may require conscious sedation and antianxiety drugs; refer to a physician.
180–209	110–119	Stage III (severe hypertension)	Delay treatment; refer patient to physician
≥210	≥120	Stage IV (very severe hypertension)	Delay treatment; refer patient to physician

Source: Adapted from Joint National Committee on Detection, Evaluation, and Treatment of High Blood Pressure. 1993. Fifth report. *Arch. Intern. Med.* 153:154–183.

reduction, elimination of smoking, change in dietary habits, and stress reduction (Kaplan 1998).

The dental hygienist should ask the patient if he or she is taking the medication as directed, usually in the morning or at night. Sometimes patients forget to take the medication, or they feel that it is not necessary because they feel "good" today. Some medications can cause orthostatic hypotension. Orthostatic hypotension occurs when blood pressure falls quickly on assuming an upright position. Dizziness and/or syncope (fainting) can result when the patient suddenly sits up after prolonged lying down. To avoid orthostatic hypotension, change the chair position slowly, have the patient sit upright in the dental chair for a few minutes, and then assist the patient in getting out of the chair. Another adverse side effect of antihypertensive drugs is xerostomia. Although not a medical emergency, this is an annoying problem for the patient. It may be necessary to discuss a change in the medication with the patient's physician. Numerous types of over-the-counter synthetic saliva replacements are available.

Anesthesia/anesthetics

Patient care to prevent medical complications involves a stress-free and anxiety-free environment, short appointments, caution in chair positioning, proper medication use, and limited use of vasoconstrictors (e.g., epinephrine) in the local anesthetic. Epinephrine binds to receptors on the heart, causing vasoconstriction, which can increase the force and rate of heart contraction and result in elevated blood pressure. Epinephrine is not contraindicated but must be used with caution. In cardiac patients, the use 0.36 mg of epinephrine is suggested; this corresponds to 2 carpules (1.8 ml) of 2% lidocaine with 1:100,000 epinephrine. Levonordefrin, another, less potent vasoconstrictor found in the local anesthetic mepivacaine, also should be limited to 2 carpules. If a vasoconstrictor such as epinephrine is not used during painful dental procedures, the stress experienced by the patient most likely would cause more elevation in blood pressure and anxiety than use of a limited amount of epinephrine.

Caution should be employed in the use of nitrous oxide to avoid hypoxia ("without oxygen"), which also can elevate blood pressure. If the patient appears to be stressed or fearful of the procedure, treatment should be postponed to a later time.

ANGINA PECTORIS

Angina pectoris is defined as pain or pressure in the chest due to a decrease in oxygen to the heart. Pain can radiate to the left shoulder, left arm, fingers, jaws, and teeth. Angina is usually experienced after exercise, excitement, stress, digestion of a heavy meal, or exposure to cold temperatures. Angina pectoris is classified as stable or unstable. *Stable angina* occurs when chest pain lasts between 3 and 5 minutes. These attacks typically are relieved by rest or nitroglycerin and are provoked by exercise and stress. Usually the patient can predict an attack. Nitroglycerin is a drug that causes vasodilation (dilates blood vessels to reduce the load to the heart). As part of the medical history, the patient should be asked when the last attack occurred. With *unstable angina,* chest pain occurs at rest or after exertion. Such attacks do not respond well to nitroglycerin and usually are very distressing and disabling. These patients should not have dental treatment and should be referred to a physician immediately.

Patients with stable angina may need to be premedicated with antianxiety drugs and/or nitrous oxide. Epinephrine is not contraindicated but should be used with caution. It is better to have profound analgesia than to have the patient release endogenous epinephrine as a result of uncontrolled pain. Cardiac patients generally are given 0.36 mg of epinephrine, which corresponds to 2 carpules (1.8 ml) of 2% lidocaine with 1:100,000 epinephrine.

Patients with angina always should keep their nitroglycerin tablets on the bracket table during dental treatment. If a patient has an angina attack in the dental chair, the dentist should be notified and the following steps should be taken (Rose, Steinberg, and Atlas 1995):

- Stop the procedure.
- Place the patient in a supine position in the dental chair.
- Administer 100% oxygen.
- Administer sublingual nitroglycerin.
- Monitor vital signs.

If after three doses of nitroglycerin, given every 5 minutes, the patient does not respond and pain continues, lasting more than 15 to 20 minutes and accompanied by nausea, vomiting, or syncope, a more serious condition may be occurring. Emergency medical services should be called immediately. Coronary pulmonary resuscitative (CPR) measures may have to be implemented if cardiopulmonary arrest occurs.

MYOCARDIAL INFARCTION

Myocardial infarction (MI) occurs when heart cells are deprived of blood and oxygen, which causes them to lose the ability to contract and soon die. The result is known as a "heart attack." Most heart attack victims have atherosclerosis with occlusion of a coronary vessel due to an atherosclerotic plaque. Symptoms the patient may experience during an MI include deep chest pain radiating to the back, jaw, or left arm. The pain is similar in character to that of angina pectoris but is usually more severe and longer lasting and is relieved little or only temporarily by rest or nitroglycerin (Berkow, Fletcher, and Beers 1992).

Since patients who have had an MI within the last 6 months are more likely to have another MI, it is advised that minimal dental treatment be done within 6 months of an MI and only after a consultation with the patient's physician (Rose, Steinberg, and Atlas 1995). The same management of patients with other cardiovascular conditions as described earlier should be followed with patients who have had an MI.

CEREBROVASCULAR ACCIDENT

Cerebrovascular accident, or stroke, most commonly occurs when the oxygen flow to the brain is disturbed, resulting in neurologic changes. Risk factors for a stroke include smoking, hypertension, diabetes mellitus, advanced age, prior history of stroke, and atherosclerosis. Since recurrences are frequent, no dental treatment should be done (except emergency situations) within 6 months.

Most stroke victims will have some type of memory or speech impairment, paralysis with limited mobility (patient may be in a wheelchair), and impaired emotional status. The patient's appointments should be short, and vital signs should be monitored. The amount of vasoconstrictor (e.g., epinephrine) in the local anesthetic should be minimal; no more than 5 carpules of 1:1,000,000 epinephrine. Oral hygiene self-care may have to be modified, for example, through the use of powered toothbrushes and floss aids. Oral irrigation can be recommended. An antimicrobial mouthrinse such as chlorhexidine gluconate may help in dental plaque control.

Anticoagulation/antiplatelet medications

Patients with prosthetic valves or blood flow disturbances such as stroke are often required to take anticoagulation drugs. Most such patients take warfarin sodium (Coumadin®, DuPont Pharmaceuticals, Wilmington, DE); one tablet taken orally inhibits vitamin K, a natural coagulant (clotting) in the blood. This causes the blood to become "thin," with a resulting increase in flow. Since there is an increased risk of bleeding in these patients, any dental procedures that are likely to cause bleeding, such as an extraction or periodontal surgery, must be discussed with the patient's physician. The physician may decide to discontinue the warfarin for a few days before the surgical procedure but to reinstate it immediately after the procedure. The traditional method for determining the efficacy of anticoagulant therapy is the prothrombin time (PT). After a blood sample is taken from the patient tests are done and the time until a fibrin clot forms, measured in seconds, is reported as the PT.

Because different methods and sources are used to determine the PT it was necessary to standardize the technique. Thus, to resolve the problem of highly variable PTs, the use of the international normalized ratio (INR) or prothrombin time ratio (PTR) has been recommended for monitoring patient's oral anticoagulant therapy. The INR is the ratio of the patient's clotting time to the lab's mean reference value. This recommendation is supported by the American College of Chest Physicians, the National Heart, Lung and Blood Institute and the British Society for Hematology (Nichols and Bowie, 1993).

Thus, INR is a good indicator of bleeding values. The higher the value, the greater are the anticoagulant effects. Nonsurgical or surgical dental procedures can be performed without discontinuation of warfarin if the patient's anticoagulation level (INR) is within the currently recommended therapeutic range and does not exceed 4 (Wahl 2000) and the PTR does not exceed 2.2 (Wahl 2000). If the patient's anticoagulation level exceeds the therapeutic range, the physician may decide to either discontinue the warfarin or reduce the dosage until the level returns to the therapeutic range.

Patients also may be taking aspirin prophylactically, either self-medicated or as prescribed by their physician, to reduce the risk of stroke or a heart attack. Many physicians recommend that aspirin be given prophylactically to patients with cardiovascular conditions at a dose of 81 to 325 mg per day. Platelets (disks found in the blood that are involved in blood clotting) tend to adhere to atherosclerotic plaques in coronary (heart) or cerebral (brain) arteries, increasing the risk of an MI or a stroke. During the medical history, the dental hygienist should ask patients if they are taking aspirin. Aspirin (acetylsalicylic acid), an antiplatelet drug, binds to and inhibits the action of cyclooxygenase, which is an enzyme in platelets that is involved in the formation of thromboxane A_2. Inhibiting the formation of thromboxane A_2 results in inhibition of platelet aggregation, which increases blood flow.

ENDOCRINE DISORDERS

DIABETES MELLITUS

Diabetes mellitus is a syndrome characterized by an absolute or relative lack of insulin. Insulin, a hormone produced by cells in the pancreas, allows sugar (glucose) in the bloodstream to enter all cells of the body and be used as energy. In diabetes, the glucose builds up in the blood instead of moving into the cells. This is termed *hyperglycemia.* Some, but not all, of the excess sugar is carried out of the body (in the urine), and the energy is wasted. Approximately 16 million Americans have diabetes, but only one-third to one-half have been diagnosed. Most of the deaths associated with diabetes are related to its chronic complications. Diabetes is currently the fourth leading cause of death by disease in the United States.

The American Diabetes Association (ADA) has established new guidelines and terms for diabetes mellitus (DM)(American Diabetes Association 1997). Formerly called *insulin-dependent diabetes mellitus* (IDDM), *juvenile-onset diabetes,* or *Type I diabetes,* this form of DM is now called *Type 1 diabetes.* Formerly called *non-insulin-dependent diabetes mellitus* (NIIDM), *adult-onset diabetes,* or *Type II diabetes,* this form of DM is now called *Type 2 diabetes* (American Diabetes Association 1997).

In Type 1 diabetes, the beta cells of the pancreas produce no insulin. Thus insulin must be reintroduced into the blood by injections of insulin. In Type 2 diabetes, the pancreas produces insulin, but the tissues become insulin-insensitive and do not respond to the insulin. This is termed *insulin resistance* and is partly due to obesity and physical inactivity. These patients do not need injections of insulin but require oral medication and changes in diet and exercise levels. Classic signs and symptoms of diabetes include polyuria (excessive urination), polydipsia (excessive thirst), polyphagia (excessive desire for food), and weight loss, which is seen more commonly in Type 1 diabetes but may be seen in Type 2 diabetes. Plasma glucose levels are 200 mg/dl or greater.

When interviewing a diabetic patient, it must be determined if the patient is controlled or uncontrolled. Discuss use of medications and self-testing at home (blood and urine glucose levels). Also inquire about a past history of periodontal disease, including periodontal abscesses. Evidence suggests that DM has an influence on the development of periodontal diseases (Cohen and Rose 1998) not based on microbiologic etiology but rather on host immune responses. Diabetes per se does not cause periodontal disease. It is the altered metabolism of the tissues that lowers resistance to infection and local irritants. Elevated glucose levels decrease leukocyte chemotaxis and phagocytosis. Altered collagen metabolism and microvascular (small blood vessels) changes also may contribute to periodontal disease. The diabetic patient may present with numerous symptoms (Table 17–2■).

The level of metabolic control, duration of disease, types of medications used, and existence and severity of diabetes-related complications influence periodontal treatment care (Mealey 1996). The patient's resistance to infection, wound-healing abilities, and cardiovascular and renal function should be assessed as components of the patient's medical and dental management (Little et al. 1997). Improved wound healing and decreased rates of postoperative infection are associated with good glycemic control.

Frequently, diabetic patients are not well controlled, and there is not enough insulin in their blood. Signs of *hyperglycemia* include decreased blood pressure and acetone breath. Unless treated in time, such patients may lapse into a state of unconsciousness (*diabetic coma*) that can terminate in death. Insulin must be injected, and CPR must be started. Immediate hospitalization is required.

Hypoglycemia occurs when there are low levels of glucose and excessive amounts of insulin in the blood. Signs and symptoms of hypoglycemia, or *insulin shock,* include sweating, nervousness, fainting, and palpitations. Treatment includes the immediate ingestion of sugar (glucose or sucrose). Patients are advised to drink a glass of fruit juice or water with 3 tablespoonfuls of table sugar added or a soft drink and to carry candy or glucose tablets at all times. Hypoglycemia is the most common emergency likely to be encountered in a dental office during treatment of diabetic patients (Mealey 1996). Hypoglycemia in diabetic patients is most likely caused by having taken too much insulin, missing or delaying meals, ingesting alcohol, and undergoing excessive stress (Mealey 1996). If untreated, death can result. Referral to the patient's physician is necessary.

Periodontal management of diabetic patients

The dental practitioner should evaluate the diabetic patient's level of glycemic control, including the ability to maintain optimal glycemic control during and following periodontal appointments. The dental hygienist should discuss with the patient the importance of blood glucose control. Meticulous home oral self-care is an important point to stress with patients. Well-controlled diabetics with good oral hygiene are at lower risk for periodontal diseases and respond better to periodontal therapy. Under good metabolic control, the diabetic patient shows no greater tendency to post-periodontal surgical complications than does the nondiabetic patient (Rose, Steinberg, and Atlas 1995). However, stress reduction is also important in the diabetic patient because stress may increase epinephrine release, which raises glucose levels (Rose, Steinberg, and Atlas 1995).

Treatment modifications include shorter periodontal maintainence visits, control of the environment to minimize stress, prevention of insulin shock or

TABLE 17–2
ORAL SYMPTOMS PRESENTED IN THE DIABETIC PATIENT
• Edematous and deep red color of the gingiva
• Multiple periodontal abscesses
• Lowered resistance to infection
• Poor tissue wound healing
• Dental and root caries
• Dry mouth (xerostomia)
• Burning mouth
• Candidiasis (yeast infection)

diabetic coma, meticulous plaque control, and dietary advice. It is important to make sure that patients have taken their insulin or oral medication as directed, and appointments should be scheduled approximately 1 1/2 hours following insulin administration and breakfast. Shorter, early-morning appointments are advisable. Epinephrine counteracts the hypoglycemic effects of insulin by elevating blood glucose levels; it causes the formation of glucose. Thus it is recommended to use the amount suggested for cardiac patients.

HORMONAL CONDITIONS

Positioning of pregnant patients in the dental chair is critical. Avoiding a supine position (especially during the third trimester) allows better breathing and avoids hypotension (lowering blood pressure) and syncope (fainting) as a result of less uterine pressure on the inferior vena cava. A wedge may be placed under the patient's right side to take the pressure off the inferior vena cava.

Meticulous home oral self-care should be stressed. Appointments should be short, and the patient should be allowed to change position frequently. Supportive periodontal therapy visits can be scheduled throughout the entire pregnancy, but the second trimester is the safest. Lidocaine can be used safely during pregnancy. However, the use of dental radiographs is controversial in pregnant patients (Mealey 1996). The American Dental Association (1989) states that radiographic specifications do not need to be changed because of pregnancy (Mealey 1996; American Dental Association 1989). If antibiotics are necessary, penicillins, clindamycin, cephalosporins, and erythromycins (except the estolate form and clarithromycin) are considered safe; however, consultation with the patient's physician is recommended before any drug is prescribed. All forms of tetracyclines are contraindicated. For pain control, acetaminophen, naproxen, and naproxen sodium are considered safe. Narcotics such as codeine should not be prescribed for a pregnant or nursing patient without consultation with the patient's physician.

KIDNEY DISEASES

The most important function of the kidneys is the production of urine, which is the medium whereby the body eliminates excess water, waste products, salts, etc. In renal failure, the kidneys do not function properly, and the excretion products accumulate in the body. Dialysis is necessary when a patient's kidneys have partly or completely stopped functioning. There are two common methods of dialysis: peritoneal dialysis (no machine is used; the solution is injected into the patient's abdomen) and hemodialysis (a machine acts as an "artificial kidney"). During this "purification" process, blood containing waste products for removal is passed through tubes consisting of thin synthetic membranes immersed in a dialyzing solution. In this way the waste products are removed from the bloodstream. Only patients undergoing hemodialysis need special precautions during dental treatment. On the day of the dialysis, an anticoagulant (a drug that prevent blood clotting) is administered to keep the blood flowing. Thus periodontal treatment should not begin until at least the day after dialysis (24 hours after) to allow for the effects of the anticoagulant to be removed. Of note, hemodialysis patients have a higher incidence of hepatitis (inflammation of the liver).

Bleeding during periodontal treatment is best managed by prevention (Mealey 1996). Coagulation tests [e.g., bleeding time (BT), prothrombin time (PT), and partial prothrombin time (PPT)] should be ordered through the patient's physician. This will help determine the patient's susceptibility to bleeding (hemorrhage). *Bleeding time* is the time it takes for an incision to stop bleeding (this tells about platelet function). *Partial prothrombin time* is the time it takes for blood to clot (this tests for defects in the coagulation pathway).

All dialysis patients should receive initial comprehensive oral examinations with frequent follow-up care. Comprehensive oral hygiene instruction is essential in the overall oral health of such patients (Naugle et al. 1998).

The kidneys are a major route of excretion of many drugs. To avoid drug toxicity (elevated blood levels of a drug), only drugs (e.g., antibiotics or analgesics) that are not eliminated through the kidneys should be used. For example, doxycycline hyclate, minocycline HCl, penicillin V, amoxicllin trihydrate, clindamycin HCl, acetaminophen, and codeine (except if there is liver disease) are safe in patients with kidney disorders. Tetracycline HCl and aspirin should be avoided. Since hypertension is a cause of renal failure, blood pressure should be monitored closely.

SYSTEMIC CORTICOSTEROID THERAPY

Corticosteroids are hormones produced in the body by the adrenal cortex. The principal hormones produced by the adrenal cortex are cortisol (hydrocortisone) and aldosterone. Corticosteroids function primarily to maintain the chemical stability of the body despite changes in the environment; for example, they enable the body to withstand various stresses due to such causes as injury, disease, severe exertion, and mental strain. Steroids also have anti-inflammatory actions (reduce tissue inflammation).

Indications for systemic administration of steroids include asthma, rheumatoid arthritis, inflammatory bowel disease (e.g., ulcerative colitis), and connective tissue/skin disorders (pemphigus, systemic lupus erythematosus). Examples of systemic corticosteroids include prednisone, prednisolone, methyprednisolone, and dexamethasone.

Once systemic corticosteroids are administered, endogenous (within the body) production and secretion are shut down. Thus, when an individual is stressed or excited (e.g., undergoing dental treatment), not enough endogenous corticosteroids are present to allow the body to respond to the stress without leading to adrenal insufficiency. It is necessary to contact the patient's physician (always get approval from the patient to call his or her physician) to discuss this situation. Generally, however, most routine periodontal procedures, including periodontal debridement do not require supplemental steroids (Little et al. 1997). Extractions and surgical procedures may need dosage adjustments.

CHEMOTHERAPY/RADIOTHERAPY

Radiotherapy, or radiation treatment, uses the fact that rapidly growing young tissues, in particular, cancerous tissues, are more sensitive to radiation than mature tissues. The treatment of cancer often requires high radiation doses, which are to some extent also harmful to normal healthy tissue.

Chemotherapy is the application of chemical agents that are not harmful to the patient but which have a specific suppressive or destructive effect on cancer cells. The problem is similar to that of radiotherapy, in that cancer cells are degenerated cells of the human body itself that differ little in character from normal cells. The drawback of cancer treatment with such drugs is that they cannot distinguish cancer cells from healthy cells. Thus they also attack normal healthy tissue in the process of rapid growth, such as the bone narrow, oral mucosa, and intestinal cells.

Such treatments may result in the development of a wide range of oral conditions. There may be a reduction in the volume and character of saliva, resulting in xerostomia. There may be a disruption in the balance of the oral flora, resulting in a greater incidence of infections (Mealey 1996). Patients may develop mucositis (inflammation of the mucous membranes), which is treated on a palliative basis by reducing or eliminating pain and discomfort until the radiation and chemotherapy treatment is completed. Oral candidiasis is the most common fungal infection in these patients. This may be treated with chlorhexidine gluconate rinses. Meticulous oral hygiene self-care is emphasized, as are frequent supportive periodontal treatment visits. Gentle hand instrumentation is recommended; ultrasonic and sonic devices are not recommended. Saliva substitutes and viscous lidocaine are advised for oral discomfort. Consultation with the patient's physician is advisable before periodontal treatment is started.

Organ Transplants

After an organ transplant, patients are given a drug that will help prevent rejection of the new organ. The most commonly prescribed drug is cyclosporine. Patients also may be taking corticosteroids or azathioprine. Cyclosporine is an antibiotic that suppresses the immune system. Frequent adverse effects include renal impairment, hypertension, xerostomia, and gingival enlargement. Cyclosporine has been used in combination with corticosteroids and calcium channel blockers (for hypertension), which also may cause gingival overgrowth. Consult with the patient's physician regarding the use of steroids if periodontal surgery is to be performed; otherwise, no dosage adjustments are required for periodontal debridement.

Meticulous home self-care using a soft-bristled toothbrush and an antimicrobial mouthrinse such as chlorhexidine gluconate is important; however, removal of dental plaque alone does not prevent gingival overgrowth (Seymour and Smith 1991).

Besides organ rejection, infection is another complication after transplant surgery. Therefore, in preparation for such surgery, all questionable and hopeless teeth should be extracted. Routine dental treatment should be avoided during the first 3 months after the transplant surgery until the physician gives clearance (Mealey 1996; Rhodus and Little 1993).

Seizure Disorders

Epilepsy is convulsions (seizures) due to disturbances in electrical activity of the brain. Patients presenting with a seizure disorder should have their condition and level of disease control reviewed. Asking the patient when his or her last seizure occurred may help determine this. Vital signs, including respiratory status, must be taken at every dental appointment. There are numerous types of seizures: grand mal, petit mal (absence), status epilepticus, and myoclonic syndrome. Different drugs are used for specific seizure types. A common adverse side effect of phenytoin is gingival enlargement. Phenytoin adversely interacts with many other drugs, including acetaminophen, alcohol, antidepressants, antacids, aspirin, barbiturates, benzodiazepines, corticosteroids, doxycycline, and metronidazole. A side effect of valproic acid is excessive bleeding and decreased platelet aggregation. Aspirin and nonsteroidal anti-inflammatory drugs (NSAIDs) such as ibuprofen should not be taken with valproic acid.

Blood tests should be performed before dental treatment. Morning appointments are preferred. Meticulous oral hygiene is stressed. If in the event of a seizure, remove objects around the patient, open the airway, and do not restrict patient movement.

LIVER DISEASES

VIRAL HEPATITIS

Hepatitis is inflammation of the liver, usually as a result of a viral infection, but it also can be due to alcohol and drugs. There are at least five forms of infectious or viral hepatitis: hepatitis A, hepatitis B, hepatitis C, hepatitis D, hepatitis E, and hepatitis G. When the liver infection does not resolve after 3 to 6 months, the acute disease becomes chronic active hepatitis.

Hepatitis A is transmitted from person to person by direct contact or through contaminated food or water. Hepatitis A is caused by the hepatitis A virus (HAV), an RNA virus. There is no known chronic carrier state, and HAV plays no role in the production of chronic active hepatitis or liver cirrhosis. There is no evidence that HAV poses an occupational risk to dental personnel as a result of injury or puncture of the skin (Gilllcrist 1999). In 1995, a vaccine became available for immunity against HAV.

Hepatitis B is transmitted from person to person by direct contact of contaminated blood or other body secretions such as saliva. Individuals at risk for hepatitis B include intravenous drug users; persons undergoing tattooing, acupuncture, or body piercing; health care workers; homosexual and bisexual men; patients receiving blood transfusions; and hemodialysis patients. Hepatitis B is caused by the hepatitis B virus (HBV), a DNA virus. Hepatitis B can lead to acute or chronic hepatitis, which causes many of the deaths from chronic liver disease. The presence of HBsAg (hepatitis B surface antigen) in the blood is indicative of ongoing HBV infection. The hepatitis B vaccine is available for prevention.

Hepatitis C is an RNA virus that is transmitted from person to person by direct contact of contaminated blood. Individuals at risk for HCV infection include intravenous drug users, hemodialysis patients, patients undergoing blood transfusions, persons who are sexually active, and health care workers (e.g., undergoing injuries from contaminated sharps) (Little et al. 1997). Onset is usually insidious, with anorexia, vague abdominal discomfort, and nausea and vomiting, progressing to jaundice less frequently than hepatitis B. Hepatitis C may be the most serious of the viral hepatitis infections because of its ability to produce chronic infection. Up to 85% of patients become chronically infected, resulting in liver failure, carcinoma, and cirrhosis (Gillcrist 1999). Immunization against infections with hepatitis C virus is not available.

Routes of transmission of hepatitis D are similar to those of hepatitis B. Hepatitis D is caused by an RNA virus that is found in patients who are carriers of hepatitis B virus. In the United States, infections with HDV most commonly affect persons at high risk of hepatitis B, particularly intravenous drug abusers and persons with hemophilia. Immunization with the hepatitis B vaccine also confers protection against coinfections with HDV-HBV (Gillcrist 1999).

At present, the modes of transmission for hepatitis E virus (HEV) are similar to those for HAV. Hepatitis E is seen more commonly in undeveloped countries with inadequate environmental sanitation and unsafe drinking water, such as India and certain countries in Africa and Asia. Both diseases usually resolve without complications. As with HAV, there is no concern about occupational exposure in health care workers. A vaccine for HEV is not yet available.

Hepatitis G virus (HGV), an RNA virus, was discovered in 1995 (DiBisceglie 1996). The true modes of transmission are not clearly defined, but it is definitely a bloodborne virus. There is no evidence to show that HGV is transmissible by injury or breaking through the skin. Further studies are needed before the cause, clinical features, prevention, and treatment can be established (Gillcrist 1999).

General recommendations

Dental hygienists and dentists should keep up with the latest information regarding viral hepatitis (Gillcrist 1999). All health care workers are advised to have the hepatitis B vaccine, which gives immunity to the virus. Consultation with the patient's physician is needed to determine the status of the patient's hepatitis. It is extremely important to determine whether the patient is a carrier of hepatitis B, C, or D because he or she could be infectious. These carriers of the virus show no symptoms, so the presence of the virus in their blood remains unsuspected. Many times an individual is unaware that he or she has or has had hepatitis. A blood test is needed to determine if the patient is a carrier. If a positive history of hepatitis is reported on the health/medical history, the dental hygienist should further question the patient as to the age of onset of the disease and the possible cause (e.g., food and blood transfusion). If the clinician finds that the information is incomplete, a medical consultation is required. There is no evidence that hepatitis A virus poses an occupational risk to dental personnel as a result of a skin puncture injury (Gillcrist 1999).

If the hepatitis is chronic, active, and ongoing, as determined by the patient's physician, elective periodontal treatment should be postponed. Chronic active liver disease indicates that the virus is actively replicating in the liver. Such patients usually are ill and very weak.

Universal precautions should be used on all patients because many patients and clinicians are unaware of the presence of the disease. Universal precautions is the Occupational Safety and Health Administration's (OSHA's) accepted method of control to protect employees from exposure to all human blood and other potentially infectious materials. The purpose in following specific guidelines is to prevent transmission of the infection. Precautions should be taken in using aerosol-producing instruments, including ultrasonic/sonic scalers, air polishers, and the air-water syringe.

In patients with significant liver damage, there is a possibility for abnormal bleeding (elevated prothrombin time). A medical consultation is necessary to find

TABLE 17–3
DRUGS USED IN DENTISTRY THAT ARE PRIMARILY METABOLIZED BY THE LIVER

Amide local anesthetics
   Lidocaine
   Mepivacaine
   Prilocaine
   Bupivacaine
Nonnarcotic analgesics
   Acetaminophen
   Nonsteroidal anti-inflammatory drugs (NSAIDs), including ibuprofen, naproxen
Narcotic analgesics
   Codeine
Antibiotics
   Tetracycline HCl (doxycycline hyclate and minocycline HCl are eliminated by the kidneys)
   Penicillin V
   Amoxicillin
   Amoxicillin and clavulanic acid
   Metronidazole
   Azithromycin
   Clindaymycin

out the status of the liver function. The liver metabolizes several antibiotics and analgesics to prepare them for final elimination from the body. If these drugs are given to patients with severely impaired liver function, elevated blood levels could occur and could result in drug toxicity. These drugs either should not be given or should be administered in a limited amount (Table 17–3 ■).

HUMAN IMMUNODEFICIENCY VIRUS INFECTION

Acquired immune deficiency syndrome (AIDS) is the end stage of infection with the human immunodeficiency virus (HIV). AIDS is a complex illness that interferes with the body's immune system in a number of ways, particularly that portion responsible for cell-mediated immunity and tumor suppression. Thus the disease attacks the body's immune system, leaving a person vulnerable to otherwise rare life-threatening infections, cancers, and other conditions. The definition of AIDS has changed several times since monitoring began in the early 1980s. Many systems and tissues in the body are affected. HIV can be transmitted from person to person through blood and other bodily secretions. Three basic modes of HIV transmission are (1) sexual contact, (2) blood-to-blood contact, and (3) from mother to child.

HIV is a transmissible retrovirus containing an enzyme called *reverse transcriptase* that converts viral RNA into a proviral DNA copy that becomes integrated into the host cell DNA. HIV preferentially attacks T-lymphocytes, specifically T-helper cells (or CD4+ cells). A person is considered to have AIDS if the CD4 count is less than 200/mm^3. T cells are important to an effective immune response. Because the T-helper cell count in the blood is currently the best indicator of the clinical manifestations of HIV infection, the progress of the chronic infection is now tracked by following the slow decline of patients' CD4+ cells over several years.

HIV infection can range from asymptomatic to full-blown AIDS. HIV affects almost every organ in the body, including the oral cavity. Symptoms associated with HIV infection include fever, fatigue, night sweats, weight loss, dry cough, swollen glands, and diarrhea. These symptoms explain a lot of other medical conditions. The only difference is that in HIV-infected persons, these symptoms are ongoing and do not go away.

The best way to reduce occupational risk of infection with HIV, as well as any other transmissible infectious disease, is to follow universal precautions. Consultation with the patient's physician is necessary before treatment to determine the patient's CD4+ count. Many oral infections are seen in HIV-positive patients. These conditions include hairy leukoplakia (on the lateral boarder of the tongue), linear gingival erythema (distinctive marginal gingival redness), necrotizing ulcerative periodontitis, candidiasis (fungal infection), and Kaposi's sarcoma. Treatment of oral conditions is palliative. Consultation with the patient's physician should be done before prescribing antibiotics, antifungal agents, or pain medications. Meticulous oral hygiene should be stressed. Chlorhexidine gluconate oral rinse can be prescribed to help reduce supragingival plaque accumulation. Lidocaine 2% viscous solution can be prescribed as an analgesic rinse. There seems not to be any contraindications to routine dental treatment for most HIV-positive patients (Mealey 1996). The incidence of postoperative complications following scaling and root planing or tooth extractions is low (Glick et al. 1994), although excessive bleeding, delayed healing, and infections can occur.

TUBERCULOSIS

Tuberculosis (TB) is a chronic, recurring infection most common in the lungs. TB is caused primarily by *Mycobacterium tuberculosis,* which enters the body by inhalation. The presence of HIV infection accelerates the course of TB. Many medications to treat TB are not as effective today as they were in the past. Thus resistance to antituberculosis drugs is a problem with treatment. Also, many individuals infected with TB are not undergoing treatment.

It must be determined if a patient has active TB or if he or she was exposed previously and currently is not active. Often patients with TB remain asymptomatic. A cough is the most common symptom. The cough also may be due to smoking or a cold, but the cough in TB is usually productive (of yellow or green sputum).

If TB is suspected, the patient should be referred to a physician. The tuberculin skin test can be used to help determine if the patient has TB. The skin test is performed by injecting slightly under the skin an extract of the mycobacterium called *purified protein derivative* (PPD). A positive test occurs if the area becomes indurated or hard by 2 days after the inoculation. While this test is not very definitive, it is still a good way to screen individuals for TB. If a patient was exposed previously but did not develop signs and symptoms of TB, the test will be positive. On the other hand, a patient with TB may not have a positive test. If a chest x-ray reveals a scar or cavity in the lung, then the patient is TB-positive.

If the patient has active TB, periodontal treatment should be postponed. If the patient reports a positive PPD test on the health/medical history but no chest x-ray was taken, referral to a physician is necessary. If the patient reports a positive PPD test and a positive x-ray and has not had medical treatment, referral to a physician also is necessary. If the patient reports a positive PPD test and a negative chest x-ray, proceed with periodontal treatment, but follow universal precautions.

Treatment

Isoniazid (INH) is used in adults whose tuberculin skin test converted from negative to positive within the previous 2 years. This is a form of prophylactic (preventive) treatment. Other antimicrobial drugs used in the treatment of TB include rifampin, ethambutol, pyrazinamide, and streptomycin.

Since the disease is transmitted through the air, precautions are necessary in the use of aerosol-producing instruments, including ultrasonic/sonic scalers, air polishers, and the air-water syringe.

Summary

A comprehensive health history is required on every patient. Numerous individuals with acquired diseases present for routine periodontal care and an understanding of these medically compromised states is fundamental for dental practitioners. The student and dental practitioner must be able to recognize these compromised states and prevent complications during periodontal treatment. Additionally, it is important to recognize when to use consultations and referrals to physicians.

Key Points

- Never treat a stranger; review the health/medical history and interview the patient thoroughly to determine if a medical condition requires physician referral or either special precautions or postponement of periodontal treatment.
- Prevention of disease transmission requires an understanding of infection control and modes of disease transmission in the dental office (e.g., power-driven scalers, air-water syringe, and air polisher).

References

American Diabetes Association. 1997. Guidelines: Report of the expert committee on the diagnosis and classification of diabetes mellitus. *Diabetes Care* 20(7):1183–1197.

American Dental Association Council on Dental Materials, Instruments, and Equipment. 1989. Recommendations in radiographic practices: An update. *J. Am. Dent. Assoc.* 118:115–117.

Berkow, R., A. J. Fletcher, and M. H. Beers. 1992. *The Merck manual,* 16th ed., 415. Rahway, NJ: Merck Research Laboratories, Merck & Co.

Cohen, D. W., and L. F. Rose. 1998. The periodontal-medical risk relationship. *Compendium* 19(1):11–24.

DiBisceglie, A. M. 1996. Hepatitis G virus infection: A work in progress. *Ann. Intern. Med.* 125:772–773.

Gillcrist, J. A. 1999. Hepatitis viruses A, B, C, D, E and G: Implications for dental personnel. *J. Am. Dent. Assoc.* 130:509–520.

Glick, M., S. N. Abel, B. C. Muzyka, and M. Delorenzo. 1994. Dental complications after treating patients with AIDS. *J. Am. Dent. Assoc.* 125:296–301.

Joint National Committee on Detection, Evaluation, and Treatment High Blood Pressure. 1993. Fifth report. *Arch. Intern. Med.* 153:154–183.

Kaplan, N. M. 1998. Treatment of hypertension: Insights from the JNC-VI report. *Am. Fam. Physician* 58:1323–1330.

Little, J. W., D. A. Falace, C. S. Miller, and N. L. Rhodus. 1997. *Dental management of the medically compromised patient,* 5th ed., 176–191. St. Louis: Mosby.

Mealey, B. L. 1996. Periodontal implications: Medically compromised patients. *Ann. Periodontol.* 1:256–321.

Naugle, K., M. L. Darby, D. B. Bauman, L. T. Lineberger, and R. Powers. 1998. The oral health status of individuals on renal dialysis. *Ann. Periodontol.* 3:197–205.

Nichols, W. L. & Bowie, E. J. W. 1993. Standardization of the prothrombin time for monitoring orally administered anticoagulant therapy with use of the international normalized ration system. *Mayo Clinical Procedure* 68:897–898.

Perusse, R., J. P. Goulet, and J. Y. Turcotte. 1992. Contraindications to vasoconstrictors in dentistry, part I. *Oral Surg. Oral Med. Oral Pathol.* 74:679–686.

Rhodus, N. L., and J. W. Little. 1993. Dental management of the renal transplant patient. *Compend. Contin. Educ. Dent.* 14:518–532.

Rose, L. F., B. J. Steinberg, and S. L. Atlas. 1995. Periodontal management of the medically compromised patient. *Periodontology 2000* 9:165–175.

Seymour, R. A., and D. G. Smith. 1991. The effect of a plaque control program on the incidence and severity of cyclosporin-induced gingival changes. *J. Clin. Periodontol.* 18:107–110.

Wahl, M. J. 2000. Myths of dental surgery in patients receiving anticoagulant therapy. *J. Am. Dent. Assoc.* 131:77–81.

Self-Quiz

1. Which one of the following procedures should be followed if a 50-year-old patient did not take his medication the morning of the periodontal appointment and has a blood pressure of 180/100 mmHg in the office? (pp. 540–541)

   a. Call the physician immediately.

   b. Give the patient his medication and let him wait in the office.

   c. Notify the emergency medical service (EMS).

   d. Position the patient in a supine position in the dental chair.

   e. Postpone periodontal treatment.

2. A patient is taking an antihypertensive drug called prazosin. After periodontal treatment is completed at an office visit and the patient is ready to be dismissed, which one of the following procedures should be followed? (pp. 540–541)

   a. Have the patient drink orange juice slowly.

   b. Have the patient sit in the dental chair awhile.

   c. Administer more epinephrine.

   d. Administer oxygen.

3. Which one of the following statements is true about use of epinephrine in a cardiac patient? (p. 541)

   a. Use similar amounts as in a noncardiac patient.

   b. Use higher concentrations than in a noncardiac patient.

   c. It is contraindicated.

   d. Use cautiously.

4. Which one of the following time periods should the patient wait after having a heart attack or heart surgery before having periodontal treatment? (p. 543)

   a. 1 month
   b. 3 months
   c. 6 months
   d. 1 year
   e. 2 years

5. Which one of the following medications may be taken prophylactically to prevent a stroke or heart attack? (p. 544)

   a. acetylsalicylic acid
   b. vitamin K
   c. isoniazid
   d. prednisone

6. Which one of the following guidelines have to be followed in a controlled diabetic? (pp. 544–546)

   a. Schedule short, quick appointments.
   b. Antibiotic prophylaxis is required.
   c. Treatment is the same as in a nondiabetic.
   d. Corticosteroid is required before invasive procedures.

7. A patient calls for a periodontal appointment. She has just had hemodialysis at 12:00 P.M. today. When should you make the appointment? (p. 546)

   a. 8 A.M. the next morning
   b. 12:00 P.M. the next day
   c. 6:00 P.M. the next day
   d. 2:00 P.M. the same day

8. A patient has been taking prednisone for arthritis for the last year. Which one of the following precautions needs to be followed for periodontal debridement regarding the drug? (p. 547)

   a. Keep the same dose.
   b. Decrease the dose.
   c. Increase the dose.
   d. Change to a different drug.

9. How soon after a kidney transplant can a patient be seen by a dental hygienist for periodontal debridement? (p. 548)

   a. 2 weeks
   b. 3 weeks
   c. 1 month
   d. 2 months
   e. 3 months

10. Which one of the following medications is used in the prophylaxis of tuberculosis? (pp. 552–553)

     a. rifampin
     • b. isoniazid
     c. prednisone
     d. phenytoin
     e. acetaminophen

PERIODONTAL MAINTENANCE THERAPY

18

Mea A. Weinberg, D.M.D., M.S.D., R.Ph.

Outline:

Goal:

To provide the dental hygienist with an overview of the role periodontal maintenance has in the treatment of inflammatory periodontal diseases.

Educational Objectives:

Upon completion of this chapter, the reader should be able to:

Discuss the objectives of periodontal maintenance;

Describe the components of periodontal maintenance;

Describe the role of the dental hygienist in periodontal maintenance visits;

Discuss the role of the dental hygienist in smoking cessation;

Discuss when retreatment is necessary; and

Explain the factors involved in patient compliance.

KEY WORDS

- periodontal maintenance
- recurrence
- primary prevention
- secondary prevention
- smoking cessation
- retreatment
- patient compliance

*P*eriodontal maintenance also has been referred to as *periodontal recall, supportive periodontal care,* and *continuing care.* All these terms are appropriate, but periodontal maintenance may be a more up-to-date and inclusive term because it is a branch of periodontal therapy.

It is known generally that after periodontal treatment is completed, patients will exhibit a decrease in plaque control and a **recurrence** of gingivitis or periodontitis unless they are enrolled in a regular periodontal maintenance program (Axelsson and Lindhe 1981). Patients must be informed of the need for periodic periodontal maintenance visits throughout their life. Since it cannot be predicted when and if gingivitis will progress into periodontitis, the disease must be monitored, and regular professional removal of dental plaque and calculus must be accomplished.

OBJECTIVES OF PERIODONTAL MAINTENANCE

The primary objectives of periodontal maintenance are (1) to prevent or minimize the recurrence of periodontal diseases by controlling factors known to contribute to the disease process (e.g., dental plaque, calculus) and (2) to preserve the health, comfort, and function of the teeth. Periodontal maintenance is also important for monitoring the overall dental health of the patient and to recognize, identify, and manage other diseases or conditions found within or related to the oral cavity (Wilson 1996a).

INDICATIONS

Periodontal maintenance is indicated for three types of patients: (1) peridontally healthy patients who have never had periodontal disease as a preventive procedure (this type of care is termed **primary prevention** and applies to a large section of the population), (2) patients after active periodontal therapy to prevent or minimize the recurrence and progression of periodontal disease and tooth loss (this type of care is termed **secondary prevention**), and (3) medically compromised patients or patients who maintain poor oral hygiene and are not considered candidates for periodontal surgery.

COMPONENTS OF THE PERIODONTAL MAINTENANCE VISIT

Patient needs at the periodontal maintenance visit vary widely and are modified on an individual basis. Regardless, standard periodontal maintenance procedures include the following steps (American Academy of Peridontology 1991):

1. an update of medical and dental histories;
2. extraoral and intraoral examinations;
3. dental examination and gingival and periodontal assessment;
4. radiographic review;
5. oral hygiene evaluation (amount of plaque, calculus, and stains);
6. review of the patient's plaque-control efficacy; and

7. removal of dental plaque from the supragingival and subgingival areas, root debridement where indicated, teeth polishing, and adjunctive chemotherapy if necessary.

The patient's chart should be reviewed for previous periodontal treatments, including periodontal maintenance care before any current treatment is initiated. Any medications needed before periodontal maintenance, such as antibiotic prophylaxis, can be determined before the patient is seen and acknowledged when the patient arrives at the dental office.

Two aspects emphasized and provided during periodontal maintenance are *monitoring* and *therapy*. The preceding examination steps should be performed on every patient at each periodontal maintenance visit but are subject to the judgment of the dentist and the dental hygienist. The clinical findings obtained at the periodontal maintenance visit should be compared with baseline findings. Baseline values are first established at the initial examination and again following active therapy.

Periodontal maintenance is designed to eliminate or reduce primary and secondary risk factors. The primary risk factor for inflammatory periodontal diseases is dental plaque. Secondary factors include plaque-retentive areas such as calculus and restorations with overhangs or defective margins. The patient removes supragingival dental plaque by toothbrushing and flossing, and the dental hygienist or dentist removes both supragingival and subgingival plaque and calculus by mechanical debridement. The dentist should replace or restore defective or failed restorations. Table 18–1 ■ provides a step-by-step review of the components of an periodontal maintenance visit.

MEDICAL AND DENTAL UPDATE

The patient should be asked if there have been any medication or health changes, including hospitalizations, since the last appointment. Review current medications (prescription and over-the-counter) with the patient. Note any changes in dosage or instructions for use. A medical consultation with the patient's physician may be warranted if new illnesses are recognized or if a previous condition has changed significantly. A chief complaint should be noted, and this should be accompanied by a notation of the degree of comfort or discomfort. The patient and the dentist should sign the amended form.

Counseling of the patient on risk factors that contribute to periodontal diseases, such as cigarette smoking, stress, nutrition, medications (e.g., calcium channel blockers, phyentoin, cyclosporine, oral contraceptives), and systemic diseases (e.g., diabetes mellitus, AIDS), also should be done during the periodontal maintenance visit (Kerry 1995). The patient should be informed about the availability of programs for **smoking cessation** in and outside the office.

Since many patients are on an alternating periodontal maintenance program, seeing both a general dentist and a periodontist, any communication from the last treating office should be reviewed. Any new restorative treatment should be indicated on the chart and evaluated clinically.

EXTRAORAL/INTRAORAL EXAMINATION

An updated examination is performed in the head and neck area and intraoral tissues for the detection of any abnormalities, including enlarged lymph nodes or

TABLE 18–1	
COMPONENTS OF A PERIODONTAL MAINTENANCE VISIT	
EXAMINATION	**REMARKS**
Review and update medical and dental history, take blood pressure, pulse, respiration.	To determine if additional risk factors are responsible for recurrent or progressive periodontal breakdown.

Clinical examination, including
    Extra-intraoral examination
    Plaque evaluation/disclosing
    Evaluating the patient's oral hygiene technique
    Dental charting of caries, restorative care
    Periodontal charting of probing depths, gingival recession, furcation defects, bleeding on probing, exudation, tooth mobility, fremitus
    Implant evaluation: peri-implant tissues, probing depths, bleeding on probing, stability of dental implant (mobility), examination of abutment teeth, occlusal examination
	Changes that should be of concern during a periodontal maintenance visit include sites that have changed from nonbleeding to bleeding, sites that have increased 2 to 3 mm or more in attachment loss or probing depth, and any sites with pus or suppuration.

Radiographic review	Since radiographs only show past activity (e.g., bone loss occurred approximately 6 months ago, not yesterday or today), it is important to correlate the radiographic findings with clinical probing depths and clinical attachment levels.

Treatment options
    Removal of supragingival and subgingival plaque and calculus
    Selective polishing
    Oral hygiene reinstruction
Adjunctive therapy
    Antimicrobial therapy
    Occlusal treatment
    Counseling on control of contributing factors such as smoking cessation, stress reduction, and nutrition
    Restorative and prosthetic care
Reevaluation 2 to 3 weeks after debridement
Scheduling of next periodontal maintenance appointment
	These treatment guidelines depend on the type of periodontal patient. Treatment should not be started unless the data collected are appropriately recorded.

salivary glands and red, white, or pigmented lesions. If any suspicious lesions are found, the dentist should be informed for further examination or treatment.

DENTAL EXAMINATION

The dental examination at the periodontal maintenance visit includes caries assessment as well as documentation of the status of restorations. Restorations should be charted, noting any defective restorations or failures such as fractures or open margins of amalgams, composites, and crowns. The stability of bridges and removable partial dentures also should be noted. Documentation of tooth loss since the last charting should be recorded, including the cause. A good rule to follow is to always count the number of teeth present.

GINGIVAL AND PERIODONTAL ASSESSMENT

Gingival assessment

Initially, a visual examination of the gingival tissues is done to determine the condition of the gingiva. The color, contour, consistency, and surface texture of the gingiva are recorded. Any mucogingival involvement should be noted. If compromised teeth are to receive crowns, augmentation of the attached gingiva may be necessary. If gingival inflammation is found, the location and severity should be noted, as well as etiologic factors (e.g., dental plaque accumulation due to poor oral hygiene self-care, medication-induced, or resulting from a hormonal imbalance).

Periodontal assessment

Next, a periodontal evaluation is performed. This includes recording of probing depths, gingival recession, clinical attachment level, furcation involvement, suppuration (pus), and tooth mobility. The Periodontal Screening and Recording™ (PSR™) system may be used for screening for patients with no history of periodontal disease susceptibility.

Gingival Recession   The position of the gingival tissues on the tooth is defined as the location of the gingival margin in relation to the cementoenamel junction (CEJ). Gingival recession that has progressed since the last appointment must be addressed and treatment options given to the patient. If the recession has remained unchanged, then monitoring is all that is needed. In order to treat gingival recession, the cause must be determined. Etiologic factors include inappropriate toothbrushing technique, attachment loss (disease process), and shrinkage of tissues after initial therapy. Treatment may include educating the patient on proper brushing technique or mucogingival surgery. Common patient complaints concerning gingival include poor aesthetics and tooth pain or hypersensitivity with air or cold application. Any dentinal hypersensitivity can be managed in most patients with desensitizing agents (e.g., potassium nitrate, sodium fluoride, or stannous fluoride).

Disease Stability: Probing Depth and Clinical Attachment Level   Monitoring of probing depths and clinical attachment levels (CALs) currently is the most reliable way to determine periodontal disease stability. It may be time-consuming to determine the CAL, but it is an extremely important measurement. Probing depth recordings should be taken at six sites per tooth. If a patient's periodontal condition has deteriorated rapidly since the last periodontal maintenance visit, systemic disease such as diabetes mellitus, smoking, stress, or use of alcohol must be considered as risk factors.

Measurement of the CAL is made from the CEJ to the apical extent of the tip of the probe. Such measurements are compared with measurements obtained at the last periodontal maintenance visit. *A 2- to 3-mm increase in CAL loss indicates disease progression* (Kornman 1987; Haffajee, Socransky, and Goodson 1983), and more aggressive treatment or **retreatment** may be justified. A patient with a 3-mm probing depth associated with 6 mm of gingival recession, for example, has a 9-mm CAL loss. In such patients, periodontal maintenance must be discontinued and active periodontal therapy started. However, a patient with a 3-mm probing depth without recession has a 3-mm CAL with no attachment loss, and this is not of great concern.

Bleeding on Probing   Probing depths should be interpreted on a patient-by-patient, site-by-site basis. For example, a 5-mm probing depth that does not bleed on probing is viewed differently from a 5-mm probing depth with bleeding on probing and suppuration. Bleeding on probing in deep pockets indicates inflammation within the connective tissue (Armitage 1996), whereas bleeding while stroking the lateral wall of the gingival crevice indicates early gingival inflammation (Van der Weijden et al. 1994). Thus disease stability can be monitored during periodontal maintenance on the basis of bleeding on probing (Lang, Joss, and Tonetti 1996). Bleeding sites in deep pockets seem to have an increased risk for progression of periodontitis (progressive attachment loss) in patients on periodontal maintenance care (Claffey et al. 1990). The absence of bleeding on probing is a better indicator of gingival health than its presence is of periodontal disease (Lang, Joss, and Tonetti 1996). One should chart the sites that bleed on probing (e.g., use a red dot over the site). Thus sites that bleed warrant more attention during the periodontal maintenance visit and may have to be reinstrumented, whereas nonbleeding sites should be left without repeated subgingival instrumentation (Lang, Joss, and Tonetti 1996). Bleeding on probing generally is apparent 10 seconds after probing (Lang, Joss, and Tonetti 1996).

It should be emphasized that the force used while probing (probing force) varies considerably during probing depth measurements, even from tooth to tooth. Therefore, a tooth with healthy periodontium may bleed because "too much" force was used and not because of inflammation. Ideally, a probing force of 0.25 N (25 g) should be used, which clinically represents a "light probing force" (Joss, Adler, and Lang 1994; Lang, Joss, and Tonetti 1996), or probe until slight resistance is felt. A nonmetallic probe should be used to probe around implants.

Furcation Involvement   Furcation involvement for each tooth is noted on the chart. Tooth mobility also should be measured and recorded on the chart as Grade I, II, III, or IV (Carranza and Takei 1996). If there is increasing mobility since the last visit, the cause should be determined and appropriate treatment rendered. The presence of fremitus also should be recorded.

RADIOGRAPHIC REVIEW

Radiographs show past periodontal tissue destruction. It is important to monitor the patient's periodontal status with radiographs and clinical probing. In a periodontal patient with a history of bone loss and periodontal surgery, a full-mouth radiographic series should be taken every few years. Sites that have had bone (osseous) grafting or guided tissue regeneration should be evaluated with radiographs at least 6 months after surgery. In patients without a history of periodontal diseases, a longer interval for radiographs is acceptable. The need for bitewing and periapical radiographs depends on the stage and severity of the disease, risk for caries, and presence of implants. Vertical bitewing views are ideal for periodontal patients because they show more of the alveolar bone than do horizontal bitewings.

ORAL HYGIENE EVALUATION AND PATIENT'S PLAQUE-CONTROL REGIMEN

The next step is to evaluate gross plaque accumulation, determine the quality of oral hygiene self-care procedures, and conduct patient education. A disclosing agent is used for patient education and as a basis for recording a plaque index. Scoring of plaque at a periodontal maintenance appointment may be misleading because patients frequently brush very well just before coming to such an appointment. However, inflammation, if present, will be evident. In any event, monitoring of the plaque level can be used to evaluate the patient's compliance with oral hygiene self-care. The patient's oral hygiene practices are reviewed by asking the patient to brush and use interdental devices while the hygienist watches. The level of patient motivation to perform daily plaque removal must be determined. A patient may understand and show correct technique in the office but may not comply with instructions at home because of lack of interest or time constraints. It is important to recognize such patients and to spend more time explaining to them the importance of performing these tasks.

DENTAL IMPLANTS

Evaluation of a patient with dental implants is essentially the same as that of a patient with natural teeth. However, rather than teeth, the implants and peri-implant tissues are evaluated. If inflammation or disease is detected around an implant, the probing depth should be measured and bleeding and suppuration noted. The stability of the abutment teeth and prosthesis also should be noted by recording mobility. An *abutment* is a tooth or implant used for support and retention of a crown or removable partial denture. The prosthesis is checked for occlusal wear. Any loosened screws should be recorded.

Because there is a correlation between implant failure and bone characteristics, it is essential to take radiographs periodically. Generally, periapical films are indicated at 6-month to 1-year intervals to determine the height of bone around an implant. The accepted standard for a stable endosseous implant 1 year after placement is vertical bone loss less than 0.2 mm per year (American Academy of Periodontology 1989; Albrektsson et al. 1986). Radiographically, an ailing, failing, or failed implant will show varying amounts of alveolar bone loss (Meffert 1992). Mobility will occur with the failed implant.

PERIODONTAL CONDITIONS AND SMOKING

The literature supports the conclusion that smokers, especially cigarette smokers, have increased calculus, greater bone loss, and increased pocket depths but have the same levels of plaque accumulation and the same or less gingival inflammation (American Academy of Periodontology 1996; Haber et al. 1993). It also has been shown that surgical periodontal procedures are less effective for smokers (Bergström, Eliasson, and Preber 1994). The amount and frequency of tobacco use are essential information when evaluating the risk factors associated with smoking (American Academy of Periodontology 1996). Since smoking cessation may decrease the progression of periodontal diseases, it is important that the dental hygienist urge periodontal patients who smoke to stop and perhaps recommend an effective smoking-cessation program. The dental hygienist should perform periodic soft tissue evaluations and recognize any deleterious changes in the periodontium. The dental hygienist can provide assistance in guiding patients to stop smoking, yet he or she needs to realistically assess the effects of this habit on the gingival health and the resulting compromised healing. Education and continued support are beneficial factors influencing the patient's decision to stop smoking.

PRACTICAL STEPS TO SMOKING CESSATION

Smoking-cessation programs can be made available in the dental office. The dental office is a logical place to counsel patients on the effects of smoking on the periodontium and the importance of stopping smoking for improved long-term periodontal health and better results after periodontal treatment. Furthermore, it is important to stress to the patient that smoking cessation also can reduce the risk for other medical diseases such as cancer (Christen, McDonald, and Christen 1991), heart disease, and respiratory disease (e.g., bronchitis). A smoking-cessation program should be a part of comprehensive preventive periodontal care. This includes behavior modification and, if necessary, medications.

The first step in establishing a smoking-cessation program is to get the office organized by selecting a director or coordinator such as the dental hygienist. The role of the director is to become familiar with the National Cancer Institute (NCI) manual and parts of the program, organize records and procedures, assist patients by reviewing self-help material with them, and involve the entire dental office team (Stone and Mattana 1996).

Patients should be reassured that the entire office is going to help them. If a patient shows interest in quitting, then a program can be initiated. If a patient is not interested in quitting, do not force him or her, but rather counsel the patient and give him or her literature to take home. At the next visit ask the patient about smoking cessation again. Once the patient is enrolled in a program (yours or another one), continued maintenance or follow-up visits and communication through phone calls are important.

The role of the dental hygienist includes patient education and counseling in tobacco prevention and cessation. The patient should be informed that smoking influences periodontal conditions such as implant failure (Bain 1996), oral cancer, and periodontal problems such as loss of clinical attachment (Grossi et al. 1994), impaired wound healing (Grossi et al. 1997; Jones and Triplett 1992), halitosis, increased calculus formation, black-brown extrinsic staining, and bone loss (Bergström, Eliasson, and Preber 1991).

A set of guidelines is presented to the patient. Behavior modification should be part of a comprehensive smoking-cessation program. This includes talking to patients about their smoking habits and possibly incorporating hypnosis. Hypnosis has been used for many years in the treatment of habits. Hypnosis is a shift in awareness and not a state of concentration (Weinberg 1986). Hypnosis allows patients to be more susceptible to accepting suggestions, such as quitting smoking. This allows the patient to be in full control of the situation, and responsibility is placed on the patient not to smoke (Weinberg 1986). Patients are put into a situation where they see themselves not smoking anymore. The dentist can perform hypnosis on the patient in the office. The patient is never asleep during this procedure. The patient also can learn self-hypnosis, which can be used anytime and anywhere.

4A smoking-cessation program

The Smoking, Tobacco, and Cancer Program of the National Cancer Institute (1996) recommends guidelines to help patients to stop using tobacco. The 4A Program consists of the following components that are reviewed with the patient during the initial examination and periodically:

"Ask." Inquire whether your patient smokes and, if so, how long he or she has been smoking and how much.

"Advise." Inform the patient of the benefits of quitting and the risks associated with continuing the tobacco habit; strongly suggest that your patient should work toward a goal of complete smoking cessation.

"Assist." Give the patient behavioral self-monitoring techniques and, as appropriate, pharmacologic intervention such as nicotine gum, nicotine patches, or another agent. Encourage the patient to quit smoking. Let the patient set up a quitting date or discuss different therapies.

"Arrange for follow-up." Set up follow-up visits. The patient should return to the office at regular intervals to observe his or her periodontium and to reinforce his or her quitting behavior.

Pharmacologic agents

Acute physical withdrawal symptoms following smoking cessation are not usually long-lasting (seldom more than 1 to 2 weeks), but the success rates of smoking-cessation programs may be augmented by weaning smokers from nicotine gradually through the use of nicotine-replacement therapy. Table 18–2 ■ reviews various types of smoking-cessation methods.

Nicotine-replacement therapy by itself will not result in smoking cessation unless accompanied by counseling and behavior modification. Pharmacologic agents include nicotine gum, transdermal nicotine patches, nasal sprays, and a systemic dosage form. The nicotine-replacement drugs (gum or patches) work by replacing the nicotine that is absorbed in the body while smoking and act as a substitute for the cigarette. The manufacturers of these products claim that they help patients quit while lessening any concomitant nicotine cravings (Stone and Mattana 1996). The efficacy of this method is questionable on a long-term basis. Patient must refrain from smoking while on the gum or patch because nicotine from these products is being introduced into the body. Nicotine therapy should not be used in a patient who continues to smoke. The importance of taking the gum as directed must be stressed to the patient. The gum should be chewed slowly between the cheek and gingiva for about 30 minutes and then thrown away. Currently, the gum is available over-the-counter without a prescription. Nicotine patches are available in different doses that are worn on the skin for variable amounts of time. Indications for use of these products is for the reduction of symptoms associated with smoking cessation, including nicotine craving.

TABLE 18–2
SMOKING-CESSATION METHODS: PHARMACOLOGIC THERAPY

PRODUCT	DIRECTIONS FOR USE	SUPPLIED
Nicotine gum Nicorette® gum (2 mg; 4 mg) (SmithKline Beecham, Pittsburgh PA)	One piece of gum every 1–2 hours for weeks 1–6, every 2–4 hours for weeks 7–9, and every 4–8 hours for weeks 10–12. Do not eat or drink for 15 minutes before chewing a piece of gum.	Over the counter; starter kit has 108 pieces, and refill kits have 48 pieces.
Nicotine transdermal system Nicotrol® patch (McNeil Consumer, Fort Washington, PA)	One patch daily; maximum therapy is 6 weeks.	Over the counter; 15-mg nicotine patch, 7-day supply.
Habitrol® (Novartis Consumer, East Hanover, NJ)	One patch daily; 21 mg/day for 6 weeks, then 14 mg/day for 2 weeks, then 7 mg/day for 2 weeks. Maximum therapy is 3 months.	Over the counter; patch containing 7 mg of nicotine, 14 mg, and 21 mg; 7-day supply.
Nicoderm® CQ (SmithKline Beecham, Pittsburgh, PA)	One patch daily; taper dosage as recommended by manufacturer (21 mg/day for 6 weeks, then 14 mg/day for 2 weeks, then 7 mg/day for 2 weeks). Maximum therapy is 3 months.	Over the counter; 7-mg patch, 14-mg patch, 21-mg patch; 7-day supply in 7-mg dose.
Prostep® (Lederle, Carolina; Puerto Rico)	One patch daily; 22 mg/day for 4–8 weeks, then 11 mg/day for 2–4 weeks. Maximum therapy is 3 months.	Over the counter; box contains 7 patches that deliver 22 or 11 mg/day.
Nicotine Nasal Spray Nicotrol® NS (McNeil Consumer Health Care, Fort Washington, PA)	Start with 2 sprays in each nostril every hour, which may be increased to 80 sprays per day (heavy smokers); maximum therapy is 6 months. Can cause nasal irritation.	Prescription; each spray delivers 0.5 mg nicotine; available in 10-ml bottles.
Nicotine Inhalation System Nicotrol® Inhaler (McNeil Consumer Health Care, Fort Washington, PA)	Reduces craving to smoke. Less nicotine per puff is released with the inhaler than with a cigarette. Best effect is achieved by frequent continuous puffing for about 20 minutes. The recommended treatment is up to 3 months and, if needed, a gradual reduction over the next 6–12 weeks. Total treatment should not exceed 6 months.	Prescription; the inhaler uses nicotine cartridges (10 mg/cartridge) that provide about 20 minutes of active puffing, or approximately 80 deep draws.
Oral Medications Bupropion HCl (Zyban®) Sustained-Release Tablets (Glaxo Wellcome, Research Triangle Park, NC)	Start initial dose while the patient is still smoking to allow for higher blood levels; initial dose is 150 mg/day for 3 days. Maximum daily dose is 300 mg. Should stop smoking within 2 weeks of initiation of drug therapy. Continue drug therapy for 7–12 weeks after the patient stops smoking. Can be used with nicotine transdermal systems (nicotine patches).	Prescription; 150-mg sustained-release tablets.

Bupropion HCl (Zyban® Sustained-Release Tablets, Glaxo Wellcome, Research Triangle Park, NC) is an oral medication prescribed by dentists or physicians to help decrease the withdrawal symptoms and the urge to smoke that accompany smoking cessation. Advantages to this form of therapy are that it is nicotine-free and helps the patient to quit while still smoking. Bupropion is also used to treat depression. Adverse side effects include dry mouth (xerostomia) and insomnia (difficulty sleeping). Both nicotine gum and patches and bupropion should be used in conjunction with behavioral modification therapy.

TREATMENT: RECURRENT PERIODONTAL DISEASE VERSUS A WELL-MAINTAINED PERIDONTIUM

Recurrent periodontal disease occurs when signs and symptoms of disease return after having subsided during active treatment. Clinical signs include bleeding on probing, increasing tooth mobility, continued soft tissue attachment loss (including deep pockets), suppuration from the pocket, and radiographic changes. Recurrent occlusal problems include increasing tooth mobility and fremitus. A good rule to follow may be that when bleeding on probing or the presence of pus is seen 2 to 3 weeks following the periodontal maintenance appointment, then retreatment is plausible (Ramfjord 1987). Another reason for retreatment includes a 2-mm or greater increase in probing depth or attachment loss. Depending on which of these the dental hygienist finds, or combinations thereof, the dentist should examine the patient to determine specific retreatment. This could include periodontal debridement (scaling and root planing), periodontal surgery, antimicrobial agents, occlusal adjustment, splinting, extractions, or a night guard. After the initial therapy is completed, reevaluation should be done. If resolution does not occur after retreatment, then a systemic disease component must be considered.

In a well-maintained patient in whom inflammation is not present (no bleeding on probing) and for whom soft tissue attachment loss or bone loss is minimal, the following treatment is recommended at a periodontal maintenance visit:

1. Point out any areas in the mouth where the patient is having difficulty with plaque control, and correct the patient's technique, if necessary.
2. Deplaquing may be done. In patients with little or no subgingival deposits (usually after active treatment), a deplaquing stroke can be used with a curet or ultrasonic or sonic scaler. The tip of the instrument is "floating" within the gingival sulcus, lightly touching the root surface.
3. Selective tooth polishing can be done. Extrinsic stains may be derived from nicotine, tea, coffee, foods, and chlorhexidine oral rinse.
4. Determine the interval of the next periodontal maintenance visit.

Subgingival instrumentation, including root planing of shallow pockets, has been shown to increase soft tissue attachment loss (Lindhe et al. 1982). Patients with dental implants should be questioned about any difficulty in oral hygiene self-care or discomfort or difficulty in chewing. Plastic periodontal probes, scalers, and curets should be used because stainless steel instruments can scratch the titanium surfaces of implants.

All patients must undergo oral hygiene reinstruction and counseling on control of contributing risk factors such as smoking. Patients should be kept informed of their current periodontal condition and treatment options. Consultation may be required with other dentists who will be providing restorative or prosthetic treatment or who will be involved in the periodontal maintenance program.

CHEMOTHERAPEUTICS

Chemotherapeutic agents may be beneficial in certain patients as an adjunct to standard oral hygiene procedures, but they do not replace brushing and flossing. Since chemotherapeutic agents help to prevent repopulation of potential gram-negative periodontal pathogens between periodontal maintenance appointments, medically compromised patients or those exhibiting poor oral hygiene may benefit from such agents. Since periodontitis is a subgingival malady, rinsing with an agent is ineffective. To target subgingival bacteria, oral irrigation may be helpful between periodontal maintenance visits to prevent repopulation of periodontal pathogens (Jolkovsky et al. 1990). Irrigation with water or a medicament detoxifies and removes unattached dental plaque. Systemic antibiotics are not recommended routinely during periodontal maintenance because of the potential development of bacterial resistance, although antibiotics occasionally may be of some benefit in recurrent and refractory periodontitis cases during periodontal maintenance. Recently approved controlled-release drugs such as chlorhexidine gluconate (PerioChip®, Jerusalem, Israel, Cincinnati, OH) biodegradable film (resorbs without having to be removed), and doxycycline hyclate gel (Atridox®, Block Drug, Jersey City, NJ) may be used in selected recurrent pockets of 5 mm or greater that bleed. Desensitizing agents may be applied at a periodontal maintenance visit to reduce or eliminate dentinal hypersensitivity in patients in whom gingival recession is present.

FREQUENCY OF INTERVALS

Periodontal maintenance intervals are determined on an individual basis according to periodontal disease severity, type of treatment performed, adequacy of oral hygiene self-care, presence of orthodontic and prosthetic appliances, systemic health, and **patient compliance** and cooperation (American Academy of Periodontology 1998). The premise on which a time-interval frame for periodontal maintenance has been based is the repopulation time of periodontal pathogens after the last periodontal debridement. Data suggest that periodontal maintenance intervals of 3 months or less are indicated for continued suppression of potentially pathogenic microorganisms in susceptible patients (American Academy of Periodontology 1998). A 12-month recall interval may be acceptable for patients with limited susceptibility to periodontitis (Rosén et al. 1999). Regardless, the periodontal maintenance interval is determined on a patient-by-patient basis, and the interval may be less or greater than 3 months. Figure 18–1 ■ is a schematic flowchart that reviews suggested time intervals for healthy and periodontal patients. Patients can return 2 to 3 weeks after periodontal debridement for further observations. Any time during a periodontal maintenance program, a patient may temporarily go back into active therapy.

The time required for the periodontal maintenance visit depends on the number of teeth; disease severity; amount of plaque, calculus, and stains; instrumentation access; presence of extensive prosthetic crowns and bridges; orthodontic appliances; depths of pockets; and patient cooperation. Although periodontal maintenance visits usually are scheduled for 45 to 60 minutes, the amount of time should be individualized (American Academy of Periodontology 1998). A suggested schedule is as follows (Caffesse, Mota, and Morrison 1996):

- 15 minutes for the oral/dental examination and oral hygiene evaluation;
- 30 minutes for scaling and selective root planing and fluoride application; and
- 15 minutes for the dentist to evaluate the procedures completed and future needs.

FIGURE 18–1

Schematic illustration describing suggested time intervals for periodontal maintenance.

At the completion of initial therapy (after reevaluation)

↓

PERIODONTAL HEALTH (NO PREVIOUS HISTORY OF PERIODONTAL DISEASES)		GINGIVITIS
Compliant with oral hygiene self-care No extensive restorative or prosthetics No occlusal discrepancies No extensive restorative or prosthetics	No bleeding No periodontally comprised teeth Complaint with oral hygiene self- care hygiene	Generalized or localized bleeding No periodontally compromised teeth Noncomplier or irregular complier
6 months	6 months	3 months or less for the first periodontal maintenance visit; if patient responds to treatment with improvement in oral hygiene then increase interval between visits; if there is no improvement after a few periodontal maintenance visits enroll the patient into active treatment. Risk factors including smoking and systemic diseases (e.g., diabetes mellitus, medications, hormonal imbalance) must be considered.

SLIGHT TO MODERATE PERIODONTITIS (SURGICAL AND NONSURGICAL PATIENTS)	SEVERE PERIODONTITIS (SURGICAL AND NONSURGICAL PATIENTS)
No teeth with less than 50% bone remaining Localized or no bleeding on probing Localized shallow pockets remain A controlled systemic disease that contributes to periodontal destruction Compliers with oral hygiene self-care	If many of the following factors are present: Many periodontally compromised teeth (>50% bone loss) Generalized deep pockets Occlusal problems Systemic disease (uncontrolled or poorly controlled) that predisposes to periodontal destruction (e.g., diabetes mellitus) Extensive restorative and prosthetic appliances Periodontal surgery not performed for medical, psychological, or financial reasons Noncomplier or irregular complier with oral hygiene self-care
6 months to 1 year	3 months or less depending on the number of risk factors present.

GENERAL DENTIST–PERIODONTIST RELATIONSHIP

Periodontal patients should be monitored by both their general dentist and their periodontist, but they should be seen by the periodontist at least once a year for a thorough periodontal evaluation. Periodontal maintenance can be performed alternately by the general dentist and the periodontist.

Gingivitis or mild chronic periodontitis patients can receive total care, including chronic periodontal maintenance, by the general dentist. Moderate chronic periodontitis patients should alternate periodontal maintenance visits between the general dentist and the periodontist once active treatment is completed. Severe chronic periodontitis patients should be seen primarily by a periodontist, with annual appointments with the general dentist for general care. Refractory periodontitis and aggressive periodontitis patients should be seen exclusively by the periodontist for all active periodontal treatment.

PATIENT COMPLIANCE

An essential aspect of periodontal supportive therapy is patient compliance. Most patients do not comply with long-term behavioral changes, especially for conditions that are not life-threatening. Wilson (1996b) identifies three types of compliers: full compliers, irregular compliers, and noncompliers. Periodontal maintenance appointments are essential and important for all groups, but noncompliers have less successful surgical outcomes over time. Better communication may contribute to more successful outcomes. Other methods of improving patient compliance include providing positive reinforcement and attempting to better accommodate patient needs (Wilson 1996b). Furthermore, the severity of the periodontal problem should be stressed because the more threatening a patient perceives a disease, the higher is the compliance.

Wilson et al. (1984) reported that of 100 treated patients who were given the opportunity for periodontal maintenance over an 8-year period in a private periodontal office, 34% never returned to the office for periodontal maintenance, and only 16% completed periodontal maintenance. Becker, Becker, and Berg (1984), in a study of 44 patients who refused to participate in periodontal maintenance, found that in the absence of periodontal maintenance, periodontal surgery was of questionable benefit in maintaining periodontal health.

Some common reasons for patient noncompliance with office visits include the expense, the belief by patients that they no longer require treatment because they no longer have any signs of disease, fear of dental treatment (Mendoza, Newcomb, and Nixon 1991; Wilson 1996b), or lifestyle changes (e.g., job change or move).

Most longitudinal studies have shown that patients who receive therapy maintain their teeth longer than those who do not. A study by Becker, Becker, and Berg (1984) looked at patients in three categories:

1. Patients with untreated moderate to advanced periodontal disease lost an average of 0.33 teeth per year.
2. Patients who had treatment but no periodontal maintenance lost an average of 0.22 teeth per year.
3. Patients who had treatment and periodontal maintenance lost an average of 0.11 teeth per year.

Providing patients with motivational strategies may help to improve compliance. Examples of such approaches include (1) giving patients printed self-care instructions at every periodontal maintenance visit, (2) noting the next periodontal maintenance appointment on the instructions, (3) counseling patients about their condition and the benefit-to-risk ratio of having periodontal maintenance, (4) seeking out patient concerns and responding to them, and (5) sending reminders or calling patients about their next periodontal maintenance visit.

SUMMARY

Professional plaque control, oral hygiene self-care, and periodic periodontal maintenance are and will continue to be the foundation of periodontal therapy. In the majority of patients, periodontal maintenance is started after completion of active periodontal therapy, but it can be used in other phases of treatment. Periodontal maintenance evolved from a dental prophylaxis and now emphasizes treatment of areas with previous attachment loss and areas where clinical signs of inflammation are found (Wilson 1996b). Since the timing interval for periodontal maintenance appointments is not standardized, the decision is empirical, with no real scientific basis. An interval of 3 months between periodontal maintenance visits appears to be an effective schedule to follow, but this may vary according to the clinical judgment of the dentist, the periodontal disease severity of the patient, and clinical findings.

A number of risk factors must be identified and monitored during periodontal maintenance. Increases in bleeding, pockets, and tooth loss will occur in high-risk patients. Clinical decisions during maintenance therapy will be influenced by the presence of risk factors, and better knowledge of these risk factors may lead to improved and more efficient risk-management efforts during periodontal maintenance (Tonetti et al. 1998).

Dental hygienists play an important role not only in the mechanical aspects of periodontal maintenance but also in promoting preventive measures and explaining the importance of periodontal maintenance. Properly motivated patients will stay on a regularly scheduled periodontal maintenance regimen.

KEY POINTS

✢ The desired outcome of periodontal maintenance in patients after active therapy is the maintenance of periodontal health.

✢ Noncompliance with regular periodontal maintenance visits may result in recurrence of progression of disease.

✢ Despite adequate periodontal maintenance and oral hygiene self-care, some patients may show recurrence or progression of disease, and thus active therapy should be reinstated.

REFERENCES

Albrektsson, T., G. Zarb, P. Worthington, and A. R. Eriksson. 1986. The long-term efficacy of currently used dental implants: A review and proposed criteria of success. *Int. J. Oral Maxillofac. Implants* 1:11–25.

American Academy of Periodontology. 1989. Proceedings of the World Workshop in Clinical Periodontics, Consensus report, Discussion section VIII: Implant therapy (VIII-11-18). Chicago: American Academy of Periodontology.

American Academy of Periodontology. 1991. *Current terminology for periodontics and insurance reporting manual,* 6th ed., 22. Chicago: American Academy of Periodontology.

American Academy of Periodontology. 1996. Tobacco use and the periodontal patient. *J. Periodontol.* 67:51–56.

American Academy of Periodontology. 1998. Periodontal maintenance (PM). *J. Periodontol.* 69:502–506.

Armitage, G. C. 1996. Manual periodontal probing in supportive periodontal therapy. *Periodontology 2000* 12:33–39.

Axelsson, P., and J. Lindhe. 1981. The significance of maintenance care in the treatment of periodontal disease. *J. Clin. Periodontol.* 8:281–294.

Bain, C. A. 1996. Smoking and implant failure: Benefits of a smoking cessation protocol. *Int. J. Oral Maxillofac. Implants* 11:756–759.

Becker, W., B. E. Becker, and L. E. Berg. 1984. Periodontal treatment without maintenance. A retrospective study in 44 patients. *J. Periodontol.* 55:505–509.

Bergström, J., S. Eliasson, and H. Preber. 1991. Cigarette smoking and periodontal bone loss. *J. Periodontol.* 62:242–246.

Caffesse, R. G., L. F. Mota, and E. C. Morrison. 1996. The rationale for periodontal therapy. *Periodontology 2000* 9:7–13.

Carranza, F. A., and H. H. Takei. 1996. Treatment of furcation involvement and combined periodontal-endodontic therapy. In *Clinical periodontology,* ed. F. A. Carranza and M. G. Newman, 640. Philadelphia: W. B. Saunders.

Christen, A. G., J. L. McDonald, and J. A. Christen. 1991. *The impact of tobacco use and cessation on nonmalignant and precancerous oral and dental diseases and conditions.* Indianapolis: Indiana University School of Dentistry.

Claffey, N., K. Nylund, R. Kiger, S. Garrett, and J. Egelberg. 1990. Diagnostic predictability of scores of plaque, bleeding, suppuration and probing depth for probing attachment loss. 3 1/2 years of observation following initial periodontal therapy. *J. Clin. Periodontol.* 17:108–114.

Grossi, S. G., J. J. Zambon, A. W. Ho, et al. 1994. Assessment of risk for periodontal disease: I. Risk indicators for attachment loss. *J. Periodontol.* 65:260–267.

Grossi, S. G., J. Zambon, E. E. Machtei, et al. 1997. Effects of smoking and smoking cessation on healing after mechanical periodontal therapy. *J. Am. Dent. Assoc.* 128:599–607.

Haber, J., J. Wattles, M. Crowby, R. Mandell, K. Joshipura, and R. L. Kent. 1993. Evidence for cigarette smoking as a major risk factor for periodontitis. *J. Periodontol.* 64:16–23.

Haffajee, A. D., S. S. Socransky, and J. M. Goodson. 1983. Comparison of different data analyses for detecting changes in attachment level. *J. Clin. Periodontol.* 10:298–310.

Jolkovsky, D. L., M. Y. Waki, M. G. Newman, et al. 1990. Clinical and microbiological effects of subgingival and gingival marginal irrigation with chlorhexidine gluconate. *J. Periodontol.* 61:663–669.

Jones, J. K., and R. G. Triplett. 1992. The relationship of cigarette smoking to impaired intraoral wound healing: A review of evidence and implications for patient care. *J. Oral Maxillofac. Surg.* 50:237–239.

Joss, A., R. Adler, and N. P. Lang. 1994. Bleeding on probing. A parameter for monitoring periodontal conditions in clinical practice. *J. Clin. Periodontol.* 21:402–408.

Kerry, G. J. 1995. Supportive periodontal treatment. *Periodontology 2000* 11:176–184.

Kornman, K. S. 1987. Nature of periodontal diseases: Assessment and diagnosis. *J. Periodontol. Res.* 22:192–204.

Lang, N. P., A. Joss, and M. S. Tonetti. 1996. Monitoring disease during supportive periodontal treatment by bleeding on probing. *Periodontology 2000* 12:44–48.

Lindhe, J., S. S. Socransky, A. Nyman Haffajee, and E. Westfelt. 1982. Critical probing depths in periodontal therapy. *J. Clin. Periodontol.* 9:323–336.

Medoza, A., G. Newcomb, and K. Nixon. 1991. Compliance with periodontal maintenance. *J. Periodontol.* 62:731–736.

Meffert, R. M. 1992. How to treat ailing and failing implants. *Implant Dent.* 1:25–33.

National Cancer Institute, U.S. Department of Health and Human Services. 1996. *Tobacco effects in the mouth,* ed. R. E. Mechlenburg, D. Greenspan, D. V. Kleinman, et al. Bethesda, MD: NCI.

Ramfjord, S. P. 1987. Maintenance care for treated periodontitis patients. *J. Clin. Periodontol.* 14:433–437.

Rosén, B., G. Olavi, A. Baderstan, A. Rönström, G. Söderholm, and J. Egelberg. 1999. Effect of different frequencies of preventive maintenance treatment on periodontal conditions. *J. Clin. Periodontol.* 26:225–230.

Stone, C., and D. J. Mattana. 1996. The role of the dental team in helping patients stop using tobacco. *J. Mich. Dent. Assoc.* (Jan):58–66.

Tonetti, M., V. Muller-Campanile, and V. Lang. 1998. Changes in the prevalence of residual pockets and tooth loss in treated periodontal patients during a supportive maintenance care program. *J. Clin. Periodontol.* 25:1008–1016.

Van der Weijden, G. A., M. F. Timmerman, A. Nijbor, E. Reijerse, and U. Van der Velden. 1994. Comparison of different approaches to assess bleeding on probing as indicators of gingivitis. *J. Periodontol.* 21:589–594.

Weinberg, A. 1986. Instructions in hypnosis, unpublished findings.

Wilson, T. G., Jr., M. E. Glover, J. Schoen, C. Baus, and T. Jacobs. 1984. Compliance with maintenance therapy in a private periodontal practice. *J. Periodontol.* 55:468–473.

Wilson, T. G. 1996a. Supportive periodontal treatment introduction: Definition, extent of need, therapeutic objectives, frequency and efficacy. *Periodontology 2000* 12:11–15.

Wilson, T. G. 1996b. Compliance and its role in periodontal therapy. *Periodontology 2000* 12:16–23.

SELF-QUIZ

1. All the following are goals of periodontal maintenance *except* one. Which one is the exception? (p. 558)

   a. Maintain the patient's oral status and function.

   b. Minimize inflammation and bleeding.

   c. Prevent the recurrence of disease.

   d. Make professional referrals for consultation.

2. Which one of the following assessments *best* determines when periodontal disease activity or destruction is occurring? (p. 561)

   a. clinical attachment level measurement

   b. bleeding localized to certain teeth

   c. redness and edema of the gingival tissues

   d. suppuration

3. The absence of bleeding on probing is a better indicator of gingival health than its presence is of periodontal disease *because* bleeding only indicates inflammation. (p. 562)

   a. Both the statement and the reason are correct and related.

   b. Both the statement and the reason are correct but *not* related.

   c. The statement is correct, but the reason is *not*.

   d. The statement is *not* correct, but the reason is correct.

   e. *Neither* the statement *nor* the reason is correct.

4. Which one of the following procedures is appropriate if a nonbleeding site with a probing depth of 5 mm is found during a periodontal maintenance visit? (p. 562)

   a. Perform periodontal debridement.

   b. Immediately refer the patient to a specialist.

   c. Reevaluate the site at the next appointment.

   d. Prescribe systemic antibiotics.

5. All the following risk factors can be controlled during periodontal maintenance therapy *except* one. Which one is the exception? (p. 559)

   a. stress
   b. smoking
   c. interproximal plaque accumulation
   d. genetic susceptibility

6. Which one of the following protocols is *most* appropriate in a patient who shows generalized recurrence of disease at a periodontal maintenance visit? (pp. 556, 569)

   a. Perform periodontal surgery.
   b. Reinstate Phase I therapy.
   c. Insert tetracycline fibers into the sites.
   d. Prescribe a systemic antibiotic in conjunction with periodontal debridement.

7. All the following determine the *most* appropriate time interval for periodontal maintenance visits *except* one. Which one is the exception? (p. 568)

   a. medical condition
   b. level of plaque control
   c. severity of the disease
   d. number of medications taken

8. Which one of the following types of pockets is *most* appropriate for adjunctive controlled-release drug delivery? (p. 568)

   a. nonbleeding, >5 mm
   b. nonbleeding, <5 mm
   c. bleeding, ≥5 mm
   d. bleeding, ≤5 mm

9. All the following techniques the dental hygienist can use to improve patient compliance to periodontal therapy *except* one. Which one is the exception? (p. 570)

   a. Print self-care instructions.
   b. Counsel patients about their condition.
   c. Call the patient every week.
   d. Seek out patient concerns and respond to them.
   e. Send patients reminders about their next visit.

10. All the following components of the 4A Program are introduced during smoking-cessation sessions *except* one. Which one is the exception? (p. 565)

    a. ask
    b. advise
    c. agrees
    d. assist
    e. arrange

CASE STUDY I

Cheryl Westphal, R.D.H., M.S.

1. All the following are etiologic or risk factors associated with this patient's periodontal condition *except* one. Which one is the exception?

   a. smoking
   b. genetics
   c. aphthous ulcer
   d. pathogenic bacteria

2. Which one of the following classifications of periodontal diseases does this patient belong?

   a. plaque-induced gingivitis
   b. drug-influenced gingivitis
   c. chronic periodontitis
   d. aggressive periodontitis
   e. necrotizing periodontal diseases

3. Bleeding is evident after probing the maxillary anterior teeth. Which one of the following *best* explains the presence of the bleeding in this patient?

   a. lateration of the gingival tissue
   b. accumulation of calculus in the periodontal pockets
   c. increased production of gingival collagen in the connective tissue
   d. engorgement of connective tissue capillaries with ulceration of the sulcular epithelium

4. Which one of the following Angle's classification is evident in this patient?

	RIGHT	LEFT
a.	I	I
b.	II	II
c.	II	III
d.	III	II
e.	III	III

5. Which one of the following instruments is *best* used to inspect and measure the amount of interradibular bone loss on the mandibular right first molar?

   a. William's probe
   b. Nabers probe
   c. CH3 explorer
   d. 11/12 explorer
   e. Columbia 13/14 curet

6. Which one of the following radiolucent areas is evident on the mandibular right second molar?

   a. amalgam restoration

   b. composite restoration

   c. dental caries

   d. root caries

   e. gold onlay

7. Which one of the following radiolucent findings is evident around the mesial root of the maxillary right second molar?

   a. subgingival calculus

   b. maxillary sinus

   c. dental caries

   d. bone loss

8. All of the following treatment procedures in this patient should be planned *except* one. Which one is the exception?

   a. prevention of future decay

   b. assessment of pockets for possible surgery

   c. assessment for prosthetic bridges

   d. exposure to panoramic radiograph

   e. possible antibiotics and periodontal debridement

9. Considering the probing depths, which one of the following treatment plans would be most appropriate?

   a. Premedicate and perform supragingival debridement.

   b. Advise use of sanguinarine rinse and perform full mouth periodontal debridement.

   c. Advise use of chlorhexidine rinse and perform quadrant debridement.

   d. Prescribe tetracycline and reevaluate gingival tissues in 2 weeks.

10. Which one of the following tactics should the dental hygienist take when debriding the mandibular right lateral and central incisors?

   a. Do not debride because the teeth may exfoliate.

   b. Splint the teeth first before debridement procedures are started.

   c. Debride carefully to avoid pain.

   d. Perform supragingival debridement and wait 2 weeks.

Case Study I

MEDICAL HISTORY: This 25 year old male patient denies allergies. The patient has a history of aphthous ulcers, otherwise there is a noncontributory health history. The patient uses Orabase®–HCA (hydrocortisone acetate).

DENTAL HISTORY: Patient has not had previous periodontal treatment. He says he brushes once a day and does not floss. Periodically, for the past 2 months he has experienced spontaneous bleeding.

SOCIAL HISTORY: The patient does not have a full time job. He is a 10 pack/years smoker and does not want to stop.

CHIEF COMPLAINT: "My gums bleed, and spaces are between my teeth."

PERIODONTAL EXAMINATION

PATIENT'S NAME:_____ DATE:_____

Oral Examination

Poor oral hygiene

1. Generalized bleeding on probing
2. Generalized supra/subgingival plaque and calculus
3. Tooth mobility

Class I mobility: teeth #'s 2,4,6,7,8,9, 11,13,14,15,17,18,20,21,23,26,28,29,30,31

Class II mobility: teeth #'s 1,5,10,12,24, 25

R

L

Right side

Left side

R

L

R   L

CASE STUDY II

1. Which one of the following pretreatment procedures should be followed in this patient?

    a. Medicate with 2 g amoxicillin 1 hour before treatment.
    b. Medicate with 1 g clindamycin 1 hour before treatment.
    c. Increase dosage of predisone 2 hours before treatment.
    d. Decrease dosage of predisone to one-half the original dosage.
    e. Increase dosage of atenolol to 100 mg/day.

2. Which one of the following should be avoided in this patient?

    a. use of epinephrine containing local anesthetic
    b. salivary substitutes for xerostomia
    c. stressful situations
    d. systemic antibiotics

3. Which one of the following factors is responsible for the patient's chief complaint?

    a. congenitally long clinical crown
    b. subgingival calculus
    c. primary occlusal trauma
    d. secondary occlusal trauma

4. To which one of the following classifications of periodontal diseases does this patient belong?

    a. chronic, periodontitis
    b. drug-induced gingivitis
    c. aggressive periodontitis
    d. periodontitis associated with systemic disease

5. Which one of the following is the most likely cause of the radiolucency at the junction of the mesial and distal root of the maxillary right second molar?

    a. periapical abscess
    b. periodontal abscess
    c. root caries
    d. furcation involvement
    e. maxillary sinus

6. Which one of the following teeth exhibits a mucogingival involvement or deformity?

    a. maxillary left central incisor
    b. maxillary left second premolar
    c. mandibular right central incisor
    d. mandibular right canine

7. Which one of the following oral hygiene aids is *best* for the proximal surface between the mandibular right central and lateral incisors?

    a. interdental brush

    b. tufted floss

    c. extra soft toothbrush

    d. toothpick-in-holder

8. Which one of the following factors is most likely the cause of the bone loss seen on the maxillary right first molar?

    a. occlusal trauma and subgingival bacteria

    b. bacteria and host response

    c. subgingival calculus

    d. periodontal abscess formation

9. Which one of the following instruments *best* accomplishes plaque and calculus removal on the mesial aspect of the mandibular left second molar?

    a. Gracey 1/2 curet

    b. Gracey 15/16 curet

    c. Gracey 13/14 curet

    d. Columbia 2R/2L curet

    e. Columbia 13/14 curet

10. Which of the following risk factors is associated with this patient's periodental disease?

    a. osteoartritis

    b. dental plaque

    c. heart murmer

    d. hypertension

Case Study II

MEDICAL HISTORY: This 55 year old female patient was diagnosed with osteoarthritis 1 year ago and hypertension last month. Both conditions are controlled with medication. She is taking Prednisone 10 mg per day and Atenolol (Tenormin®) 50 mg per day. She also has a functional heart murmur.

DENTAL HISTORY: The patient brushes twice a day with a soft-bristle toothbrush and flosses occasionally.

SOCIAL HISTORY: The patient is married with two adult children. She has accepted her medical conditions, but at times feels stressed and depressed. She does not smoke.

CHIEF COMPLAINT: "My upper right front tooth is loose and my mouth is dry."

PERIODONTAL EXAMINATION

PATIENT'S NAME:_____   DATE:_____

KEY TO CHARTING

Missing Tooth	-	Draw horizontal line through crown of missing teeth
AL, Attachment Level	-	CEJ to bottom of pocket
PD, Pocket Depth	-	Gingival margin to bottom of pocket
Plaque	-	+ or -
SUP	-	Suppuration or exudate, + or -
Overhang	-	⌐ or ⌐ for mandible; ⌐ or ⌐ for maxilla

Deficient Contacts	-	Draw 2 vertical lines and record space in mm
Endodontics	-	Draw vertical line through root if treated; draw circle at apex if lesion; indicate vitality response at apex
Muscle Attachment	-	∨ for max.; ∧ for mand.
Calculus	-	+ or -
Micro	-	Site for microbiologic sampling

BOP	-	Bleeding on probing, + or -
Migration	-	Drifting, tipping or extruding - indicate an arrow in direction of movement
Mobility	-	Record I, II, or III on facial aspect of crown
Furcation	-	Place I in furca if incipient; II if partial; III if complete

Oral Examination

Fair oral hygiene

1. Moderate supra/subgingival plaque
2. Localized bleeding on probing
3. Class I mobility #'s 4, 5, 25
   Class II mobility #'s 2, 3, 8

R   L

Right side

Left side

R   L

R   L

R   L

R   L

R   L

R   L

R   L

R   L

R

L

R

L

APPENDICES

Section IV

PREVENTION OF INFECTIVE ENDOCARDITIS

Denise Estafan, D.D.S., M.S.

*A*lthough its incidence is rare, *infective endocarditis* (IE) is a critical and potentially lethal condition. The older term, *subacute bacterial endocarditis* (SBE), is no longer used because IE can be caused by microorganisms other than bacteria. The risk of IE associated with dental procedures makes it an important condition for the dental hygienist to be aware of. Equally important is the need for the hygienist to be thoroughly familiar with its causes and prevention. With proper knowledge of what conditions to recognize, which procedures present a risk, and how to pretreat patients at risk, the chances of a dental procedure resulting in IE may be drastically reduced.

Endocarditis most often is the result of an infection of the valves of the heart. The heart valves are made of avascular tissue. In a healthy heart, the cusps of each valve are washed as blood passes over them with each heartbeat. In certain conditions, however, when one of the valves is functioning abnormally, the individual may be susceptible to infection. The avascular nature of the valve tissue enables foreign microorganisms to colonize and literally hide from the immune system. Once bacteria have colonized the valve(s), they continue to proliferate unbeknown to the immune system, and in time, they begin to affect the function of the valve(s). The valve affected most often by infection, be it congenital or acquired, is the mitral valve or bicuspid valve on the left side of the heart. Some medical conditions create a higher risk of IE than others. The conditions and associated risks of IE listed in Table A–1 ■ are based on the potential of an infection resulting in endocarditis. High-risk patients are those patients considered to have the greatest risk of developing severe endocardial infections, often associated with morbidity and mortality. Moderate-risk patients are at a significantly lower risk for endocardial infections yet still must be monitored closely preoperatively for signs of infection. Patients should receive antibiotic coverage if the procedure to be done may cause bleeding. Antibiotic prophylaxis for certain dental procedures is recommended for patients in the high- and moderate-risk categories. The negligible-risk category has been designated to include conditions that do not predispose patients to endocardial infections.

A bacteremia may be caused by many different dental procedures, but it is important to take into account all conditions that may give rise to bacteria in the bloodstream. In addition to toothbrushing, chewing, or flossing, bacteremia has been associated with poor oral hygiene and periodontal or periapical infections. The incidence and magnitude of bacteremia are directly proportional to the degree of oral inflammation and infection. It is therefore essential for patients at risk for endocarditis to establish and maintain the best possible oral health in order to reduce the risk of bacteremia. The best oral health is maintained through regular professional care, as well as routine home care. Table A–2 ■ represents the dental

TABLE A–1
CARDIAC CONDITIONS AND ASSOCIATED RISK OF ENDOCARDITIS

HIGH-RISK CATEGORY	MODERATE-RISK CATEGORY	NEGLIGIBLE RISK
Prosthetic cardiac valves	Other cardiac malformations (other than those in the right column)	Isolated secundum atrial septal defect
Previous bacterial endocarditis	Acquired valvar dysfunction (e.g., rheumatic heart disease)	Surgical repair of atrial septal defect
Complex cyanotic congenital heart disease	Hypertrophic cardiac myopathy	Previous coronary artery bypass surgery
Surgically constructed systemic pulmonary shunts	Mitral valve prolapse with valvular regurgitation and/or thickened leaflets	Mitral valve prolapse without valvular regurgitation
		Innocent (functional) heart murmurs
		Previous Kawasaki's disease without valve dysfunction
		Previous rheumatic fever without valve dysfunction
		Cardiac pacemakers and implanted defibrillators

Source: Adapted from Dajani et al. (1997).

TABLE A–2
ANTIBIOTIC PROPHYLAXIS RECOMMENDATIONS FOR DENTAL PROCEDURES

HIGHER INCIDENCE	LOWER INCIDENCE
Dental extractions	Restorative dentistry (operative and prosthodontic)
Periodontal procedures: surgery, scaling and root planing, probing and recall maintenance	Local anesthetic injections (all except intraligamentary)
Implant placement and reimplantation of avulsed teeth	Placement of rubber dams
Root canal instrumentation when beyond apex (endodontics)	Postoperative suture removal
Subgingival placement of antibiotic fibers or strips	Placement of removable prosthodontic/ orthodontic appliances
Placement of orthodontic bands (not brackets)	Taking oral impressions or radiographs
Intraligamentary local anesthesia injection	Fluoride treatment
Prophylactic cleaning of teeth and implants	

procedures for which prophylaxis is recommended and those for which it is not recommended.

The recommendations listed in Table A–2 are guidelines and not a substitute for clinical judgment. If it is suspected that a patient will bleed during any dental procedures, it is advisable to premedicate the patient. Patients who have not been premedicated and those who are currently taking antibiotics for other reasons will

TABLE A–3		
PROPHYLACTIC ANTIBIOTIC REGIMENS FOR ORAL AND DENTAL PROCEDURES		
SITUATION	**DRUG**	**REGIMEN**
Standard general prophylaxis	Amoxicillin	Adults: 2.0 g orally 1 h before dental procedure Children: 50 mg/kg orally 1 h before procedure
Unable to take oral medication	Ampicillin	Adults: 2.0 g intramusculory (IM) or intravenously (IV) Children: 50 mg/kg IM or IV within 30 min before procedure
Allergic to penicillin	Clindamycin or Azithromycin or clarithromycin or Cephalexin or cefadroxil*	Adults: 600 mg; children: 20 mg/kg orally 1 h before procedure Adults: 500 mg; children: 15 mg/kg orally 1 h before procedure Adults: 2.0 g; Children: 50 mg/kg orally 1 h before procedure
Allergic to pencillin and unable to take oral medications	Clindamycin or Cefazolin*	Adults: 600 mg; children: 20 mg/kg IV within 30 min before procedure Adults: 1.0 g; children: 25 mg/kg IM or IV within 30 min before procedure

*Cephalosporins should not be used in patients with immediate-type hypersensitivity reaction (urticaria, angioedema, or anaphylaxis) to penicillins.

be discussed later in more detail. It is important to note that it is not acceptable to premedicate every patient, since prolonged use or misuse of antibiotics can lead to drug resistance. Furthermore, although it can significantly reduce the risk, antibiotic prophylaxis does not *eliminate* the risk of endocarditis. Clinical judgment is always necessary to evaluate each patient's risk, and close attention should be paid to the patient when risk is suspected.

Table A–3 ■ indicates recommended prophylactic antibiotic regimens for oral and dental procedures. The regimens are most effective when given around the time of dental treatment in doses that allow for adequate levels of the drug in the serum before, during, and after the procedure. In order to reduce the development of antibiotic resistance and maintain minimum serum levels for prophylaxis, the regimens are designed to give the patient adequate serum levels of the drug no longer than necessary.

The bacteria most commonly associated with endocarditis following dental and oral procedures is *Streptococcus viridans* (α-hemolytic streptococci). Amoxicillin remains the most recommended antibiotic for endocarditis prophylaxis. Agents such as ampicillin and penicillin V have an equal antimicrobial effect against these α-hemolytic streptococci, but amoxicillin is better absorbed in the gastrointestinal tract and provides higher, more sustained serum levels than the other penicillins.

Until 1994, the recommended pretreatment dose of amoxicillin for antibiotic prophylaxis was 3.0 g. However, a recent study has indicated that 2.0 g is sufficient to reach adequate serum levels for several hours (Dajani et al. 1997). Previously, it was recommended that a second dose be given postoperatively. Currently, it has been demonstrated that not only will the initial dose of amoxicillin remain above the minimal serum level for long enough following the procedure, but also the inhibitory effect of the drug is sufficient to eliminate the need for a postoperative dose.

Erythromycin, which was approved originally as an effective prophylactic agent for endocarditis in cases of penicillin allergy, is no longer among the recommended agents. Erythromycin can cause severe gastrointestinal upset, and certain formulations (e.g., erythromycin ethylsuccinate) have complicated pharmacokinetics. Instead, second-generation erythromycins, azithromycin, or clarithromycin can be used because they have better absorption and produce much less gastrointestinal upset.

Periodically, patients will present to the dental office for a routine visit during a course of antibiotic therapy with a drug used for endocarditis prophylaxis. Patients receiving antibiotics for other reasons at the time of a routine dental visit who are considered at risk for endocarditis have specific recommendations. Rather than increasing the dose of the drug currently being used, it is advisable to select an agent from a different class of antibiotic. Remember, if you have to choose another antibiotic, it must have the same bactericidal or bacteriostatic activity as the antibiotic taken for prophylaxis. For instance, if the patient is taking tetracycline (a bacteriostatic drug), he or she cannot take amoxicillin (a bactericidal antibiotic) but can take clindamycin, azithromycin, or clarithromycin, which are all bacteriostatic. If possible, the dental procedure is best postponed until at least 9 (Leviner et al. 1987) to 14 days (Simmons et al. 1986) after completion of the antibiotic. This will allow the normal oral flora to reestablish (Dajani et al. 1997).

Since repeated use of antibiotics can lead to the emergence of antibiotic-resistant microorganisms in the oral cavity, it is recommended that there be an interval of at least 7 days between dental appointments.

Generally, patients with mitral valve prolapse do not require antibiotic coverage unless they have a heart murmur or regurgitation associated with the mitral valve prolapse. If at the time of the dental appointment the presence or absence of regurgitation has not been determined, it is best to premedicate the patient with antibiotics and then refer the patient to a physician (Ciancio 1997).

Specific cardiac surgical procedures have varied implications in terms of risk for endocarditis (Steckelberg and Wilson 1993). As the volume and frequency of successful coronary artery bypass graft surgery increase, so does the likelihood of seeing more of these patients in the dental office. There is no evidence to suggest that this type of surgery introduces risk for bypass surgery (see Table A–1). In the case of prosthetic valve` placement, the risk of postoperative endocarditis increases. There is no evidence to suggest that heart transplant patients are at an increased level of risk for endocarditis, but such patients are subject to an increased likelihood of valve dysfunction and are often treated as moderate-risk patients. Whenever possible, patients who plan to have any cardiac surgery should have a carefully executed dental treatment plan in order to complete any dental work necessary before the cardiac procedure. This may decrease the chance of late postoperative endocarditis.

According to the Council on Scientific Affairs, there is no need to premedicate patients with prosthetic joints except for high-risk patients. High-risk or medically compromised patients with prosthetic joints include immunocompromised/immunosuppressed patients (those with rheumatoid arthritis or systemic lupus erythematosus) or patients with disease-, drug-, or radiation-induced immuno-

TABLE A–4
SUGGESTED ANTIBIOTIC PROPHYLAXIS REGIMENS IN PATIENTS AT POTENTIAL INCREASED RISK OF HEMATOGENOUS TOTAL JOINT INFECTION

SITUATION	DRUG	REGIMEN
Standard general prophylaxis	Cephalexin or amoxicillin	2 g orally 1 h before dental procedure
Patients unable to take oral medications	Cefazolin *or* Ampicillin	1 g IM or IV 1 h before procedure 2 g IM or IV 1 h before procedure
Allergic to penicillin	Clindamycin	600 mg orally 1 h before procedure
Allergic to penicillin and unable to take oral medications	Clindamycin	600 mg IV 1 h before procedure

suppression. Other high-risk patients include those with insulin-dependent (Type I) diabetes mellitus, patients during the first 2 years following joint placement, patients with previous prosthetic joint interfaces, and patients with evidence of malnourishment or hemophilia. Table A–4 ■ lists recommendations for antibiotic prophylaxis in these patients.

REFERENCES

Ciancio, S. 1997. Bacterial endocarditis prophylaxis guideline changed. *Biol. Ther. Dent.* 13(2):9–10.

Dajani, A. S., K. A. Taubert, and W. Wilson, et al. 1997. Prevention of bacterial endocarditis: Recommendations by the American Heart Association. *JAMA* 277:1794–1801.

Leviner, E., A. A. Tzukert, R. Benoliel, O. Baram, and M. V. Sela. 1987. Development of resistant oral viridans streptococci after administration of prophylactic antibiotics: Time management in the dental treatment of patients susceptible to infective endocarditis. *Oral Surg. Oral Med. Oral Pathol.* 64:417–420.

Simmons, N. A., R. A. Cawson, C. A. Clark, et al. 1986. Prophylaxis of infective endocarditis (letter). *Lancet* 1:1267.

Steckelberg, J. M., and W. R. Wilson. 1993. Risk factors for infective endocarditis. *Infect. Dis. Clin. North Am.* 7:9–19.

PERIODONTAL INFORMATION RESOURCES

Mea A. Weinberg, D.M.D., M.S.D., R.Ph.

A great number of scientific and clinical resources on periodontology are available from organizations and various journals. This information should be used for continuing education so that the dental hygienist can keep up with current clinical studies and product availability. The Internet provides an excellent opportunity for dental professionals and patients to obtain information related to all aspects of dental hygiene.

ORGANIZATIONS

The *American Academy of Periodontology* (Chicago, IL) publishes patient education brochures, practice management resources, journals, and clinical publications. The website for the American Academy of Periodontology (AAP, Chicago, IL) is *www.perio.org*.

The following materials are available:

1. Patient education brochures
2. Practice management resources
   - "Designing Effective Practice Marketing Materials"
   - "Sample Periodontal Office Forms"
   - "Informed Consent for Surgical Periodontics"
3. Study club kits (binders containing slides, lecture script, consensus reports, article reprints, references)
   - "Epidemiology and Diagnosis of Periodontal Diseases"
   - "The Role of Pharmacotherapeutics in Periodontal Diseases"
   - "Periodic Reevaluation and Supportive Periodontal Therapy"
4. Clinical publications
   - *Journal of Periodontology* (monthly publication); also available on CD-ROM
5. *Annals of Periodontology*
   - *Annals of Periodontology (1996 World Workshop in Periodontics)*, Vol. 1
   - *Annals of Periodontology (1996 Joint Symposium on Clinical Trial Design and Analysis in Periodontics)*, Vol. 2
   - *Annals of Periodontology, (1997): New Directions in Periodontal Medicine*, Vol. 3.
   - *Annals of Periodontology, (1999): 1999 International Workshop for a Classification of Periodontal Diseases and Conditions*, Vol. 4.
6. *Periodontal Literature Reviews: A Summary of Current Knowledge* (1996)

7. *Periodontal Disease Management* (1993)
   - *Glossary of Periodontal Terms,* 4th ed. (2000)
   - *In-Service Exams* (questions given to postgraduate students)
8. Audiotapes from past annual meetings. (www.mobiltape.com or 1-800-369-5718).
9. Guidelines
   - *Guidelines for Periodontal Therapy* (1997)
   - *Guidelines for the Use of Conscious Sedation in Periodontics* (1994)
   - *Position Statement and Guidelines for Soft Tissue Management Programs* (1996)
10. Parameters of care
    - Various papers on the parameters of care of periodontal diseases (2000)
11. Position papers (some position papers are listed below)
    - "The Role of Controlled Drug Delivery for Periodontitis" (1999)
    - "Tobacco Use and the Periodontal Patient" (1999)
    - "The Pathogenesis of Periodontal Diseases" (1999)
    - "Periodontal Disease as a Potential Risk Factor for Systemic Diseases" (1998)
    - "Diabetes and Periodontal Diseases" (1999)
    - "Treatment of Gingivitis and Periodontitis" (1997)
    - "Epidemiology of Periodontal Diseases" (1996)
12. Product and procedure statements
    - "Use of Dental Lasers for Excisional New Attachment Procedure (ENAP)"
    - "Periostast® Systemically Delivered Collagenase Inhibitor of Doxycycline Hyclate" (1998)

Other associations include:

The *American Dental Hygiene Association* (ADHA). The website is www.adha.org.

The *American Dental Association* (ADA). The Web site is www.ada.org.

JOURNALS/BULLETINS

1. *Journal of Periodontology* (American Academy of Periodontology, Chicago, IL; website: www.perio.org).
2. *Journal of Dental Hygiene* (American Dental Hygiene Association, Chicago, IL; website: www.adha.org).
3. *Practical Periodontics and Aesthetic Dentistry* (Montage Media Corp., Mahwah, NJ; 800-899-5350).
4. *Journal of Practical Hygiene* (Montage Media Corp., Mahwah, NJ; 800-899-5350).
5. *Periodontology 2000* (Musksgaard, Copenhagen; e-mail: *fsub@mail.munksgaard.dk*).
6. *Journal of Clinical Periodontology* (Munksgaard, Copenhagen; e-mail: *fsub@mail.munksgaard.dk*).
7. *Journal of Periodontal Research* (Munksgaard, Copenhagen; e-mail: *fsub@mail.munksgaard.dk*).
8. *Perio Reports* (www.PerioReports.com)—research articles are reviewed; (Compendium of Current Research).

9. *International Journal of Oral and Maxillofacial Implants* (Quintessence Publishers, Carol Stream, IL; e-mail: *quintpub@aol.com;* website: www.quintpub.com).

10. *Clinical Oral Implants Research* (Munksgaard International Publishers, ltd., Malden, MA;. e-mail: *fsub@mail.munksgaard.dk;* website: www.munksgaard.dk).

OTHER INTERNET WEBSITES

1. www.dentalcare.com (Procter & Gamble)
2. www.colgate.com (Colgate Oral Pharmaceutical)
3. http://jeffline.tju.edu/DHNet (National Center for Dental Hygiene Research)
4. www.oralhealth.org (Oral Health Letter)

READING THE LITERATURE

Trisha E. O'Hehir, R.D.H., B.S.

ARTICLE CLASSIFICATION

- Clinical trial (in vivo)
- Laboratory study (in vitro)
- Combination studies—part clinical, part laboratory
- Case studies—reports of individual patients and their outcomes
- Epidemiology—incidence and/or prevalence of disease in a population
- Informational
- Review

Research articles include several distinct sections. Each section provides valuable information. These sections do not have to be read in the order they are printed. It depends on what information is being requested. The following is a brief summary of each section.

ABSTRACT

- Brief overview of the entire article
- Hypothesis being tested
- Number of subjects involved
- Methods used
- Results

The last sentence of an abstract often provides the essence of the project. The last sentence is where reading of a research article should begin.

INTRODUCTION

- Lays the groundwork for the project
- Historical information on the subject area
- Past research studies are sited in this area
- Author or authors have to make a case for their project
- Controversies in the area based on previously published work
- Statement of the hypothesis

Most often, a null hypothesis is stated, which says that if the researchers do what they propose, no changes will be seen. The goal of the researchers is to then disprove the null hypothesis. Approaching the hypothesis from the other direction requires stating that the drug, tool, or therapy to be tested will have a specific effect on the test subject, which necessitates quantifying the expected result. Guessing at the outcome before the study begins can be quite difficult. Therefore, disproving a null hypothesis allows for a positive result without the need to estimate the outcome at the start.

Some researchers state their purpose rather than formulating a hypothesis. The following is an example of stating a purpose:

> Thus, this study compares the amount of aerosol produced by a traditional ultrasonic scaler insert and that produced by a new focused style insert. In addition, the effect of using an aerosol reduction device with both types of inserts is evaluated. [Rivera–Hidalgo F, Barnes J, Harrrel S. Aerosol and splatter production by focused spray and standard ultrasonic inserts. *J. Periodontol.* 1999; 70:473–477].

Here is the same statement of purpose restated as a hypothesis:

> The hypothesis to be tested is that no difference is aerosol spray is expected comparing traditional and focused-style ultrasonic inserts, used either alone or with an aerosol reduction device.

> The goal of the researchers remains the same—to determine if there is a difference, thus disproving the null hypothesis.

METHODS AND MATERIALS

This section is often divided into subsections, providing some of the following information:

- *Study population.* Collection of people, items, or observations to be studied
- *People:*
  - *Number of subjects.* Setting a desired outcome in statistical terms allows the statistician to calculate exactly how many subjects are needed.
  - *Random sample.* All subjects of a given population have an equal chance of being selected (e.g., picking names out of a hat or using a table of random numbers to select subjects).
  - *Convenience population.* Sample does not represent the population at large (e.g., dental or dental hygiene students).
  - *Volunteers or paid participants*
  - *Subject solicitation.* Clinic patients, newspaper ads, etc.
  - *Demographics.* Age, gender, general health, oral health, dental history
- *Location of the study.* University, clinical practice, community, etc.
- *Study design:*
  - Timeline of events, including length of the study
  - Indices used and any modifications
  - Description of drugs, tools, or techniques to be tested
  - Who the examiners were and their preparation for the study
  - Characteristics of the clinical study design:
    - (a) *Case control.* Subjects with a certain condition are selected and compared with controls (e.g., subjects without the condition). For example, a group of subjects with oral cancer is compared with a control group without oral cancer for smoking habits over the previous 5 years.

(b) *Crossover.* Each subject receives two or more treatments at different times, and end points are observed after each treatment.

(c) *Cross-sectional.* End points are observed at one given point in time.

(d) *Longitudinal.* End points are observed more than once over a period of time.

(e) *Observational.* Subjects or objects of interest (e.g., teeth) are observed in their natural state with no intervention by researchers.

(f) *Prospective.* Study subjects selected based on a certain treatment or exposure and observed for a specific outcome over a period of time (e.g., subjects selected based on smoking habits and observed for cancer development over a 5-year period).

(g) *Retrospective.* Study subjects are selected based on a certain outcome, and then data are gathered on previous exposure (e.g., subjects selected based on the presence of oral cancer and studied as to smoking habits during the previous 5 years).

(h) *Parallel group.* Experimental groups do not experience the same treatment or products (e.g., a control group and a test group).

(i) *Randomized.* Subjects or objects of interest (e.g., teeth) are assigned to different treatments or interventions randomly.

(j) *Split-mouth.* Each subject receives two or more treatments at different sites within the mouth, and outcomes are observed at a given point in time.

- *Details of laboratory tests:*
  - How specimens are collected
  - How they are stored
  - How the tests are run
  - What equipment is used
  - Who does the testing
- *Statistical analysis.* Selection of mathematical techniques used to assist in the understanding and interpretation of data for the purpose of decision making.
- *Descriptive statistics.* Methods to simply describe data in a numerical way, such as frequency of a given parameter.
- *Inferential statistics.* Methods used to infer something about a population from a sample of observations from that population.

RESULTS

- Factual presentation of the study data
- Statistics

Opinions or conclusion are left for the next section.

DISCUSSION

- Limitations of the study
- Confirmation of earlier findings

- Integration of study findings with previously published data
- Unanswered questions
- New questions raised by the findings
- Interesting side findings that do not relate to this hypothesis
- Subjective opinions of the patients who participated
- Suggestions for future studies
- Conclusions that can be drawn from this study
- Significance of these findings, both statistical and clinical

Statistical significance might be better stated as "statistical difference," since the difference actually may not be clinically significant.

WOMEN'S HEALTH ISSUES IN PERIODONTICS

Robert S. Schoor, D.D.S.

As we enter another century, science is reporting important links between periodontal infection and systemic illnesses. In the last decade, 1990 to the present, early but advancing evidence demonstrated relationships between periodontal diseases and preterm low-birth-weight status, diabetes mellitus, cardiovascular disease, stroke, osteoporosis, and respiratory diseases (Cohen 1998). While ongoing research will present a clearer understanding of the pathophysiology of systemic illness from periodontal sources in the future, enough evidence exists now to prepare a model for the pathogenesis of certain systemic diseases. In this appendix, existing science in these interrelationships will be discussed, together with other intraoral conditions that have an impact on systemic health generally and on *women's health* specifically. This appendix would not be complete without a discussion of *gender differences in responses to periodontal diseases.*

In 1996, Offenbacher et al. published data citing periodontal infection as a possible risk factor for preterm low-birth-weight (PLBW) children. Maternal periodontal infection was studied to determine whether prevalence of periodontitis might be associated with preterm low-birth-weight status. One-hundred and twenty-four pregnant or postpartum mothers were examined for periodontitis at the University of North Carolina. Mothers with a defined preterm low-birth-weight delivery demonstrated that periodontal disease was a "statistically significant risk factor for PLBW." PLBW status is defined as a birth weight of less than 2500 g and/or a gestational age of less than 37 weeks at delivery or premature rupture of membranes. "PLBW cases had significantly worse periodontal disease than respective normal birth weight (NBW) controls." PLBW is a major health problem because it occurs in 1 in 10 deliveries and results in infant mortality, long-term morbidity, and 5 million neonatal intensive care unit hospital stays per year. The emotional, social, and financial burdens on families are extraordinary (Dasanayake 1998). Confirmatory research will mandate early periodontal diagnosis and dental treatment before and during pregnancy. This information will require obstetrical awareness and collaboration with dental professionals.

The mechanism by which this link occurs appears to be through infection and the known risk infection poses for PLBW. According to Offenbacher and coworkers (1996), the increased production of prostaglandin (PGE_2) secreted by the mother, in response to anaerobic periodontal infection, correlates with increases in PGE_2 in the gingival crevicular fluid (GCF) and in the amniotic sac. This twofold elevation in PGE_2 was observed in PLBW compared with normal-birth-weight mothers (Hill 1998).

The hormonal variations that occur during puberty, menstruation, pregnancy, contraceptive use, and menopause have affected GCF flow, one method of assessing periodontal alterations. Higher levels of gonadotropin (follicle-stimulating hormone, or FSH), estrogen, progesterone, and human chorionic somatomammotropin (HCS) have been associated with magnified responses to bacterial plaque. Increased presence of *Porphyromonas gingivalis* and *Prevotella intermedia* has been reported, and their presence is associated with observed increases in gingival bleeding over nonpregnant women (Folkers 1992).

Immunoproteins (IgM) to specific oral microorganisms have been isolated from amniotic fluid, indicating fetal exposure to putative periodontal pathogens in utero. For an engaging overview of existing data and research initiatives in pregnancy outcomes, the reader is urged to read C. Champagne et al., Periodontal medicine: Emerging concepts in pregnancy outcomes. *J. Int. Acad. Periodontol.* 2000; 2:1–8.

Diabetes mellitus is a significant risk factor for periodontal diseases (Aldridge et al. 1995). The periodontal literature is replete with studies demonstrating the impact of uncontrolled diabetes mellitus on periodontal disease progression, response to treatment, tooth loss, and morbidity (Schmidt et al. 1996; Katz et al. 1991). Epidemiologic studies on Type 1 (requires insulin) and Type 2 diabetic (non-insulin-dependent) patients indicate that although persons on optimal control are at equal risk for developing periodontal disease, too few diabetics are optimally controlled, and maintaining strict control is difficult in the long term. There is emerging evidence that untreated periodontal diseases can affect diabetic control, as measured by glycosylating hemoglobin, and intervening periodontal therapy can reduce the challenge of oral infection with diabetic improvement. Grossi, Genco, and Skrepcinski (1998) showed treated periodontitis patients with reduced glycosylates in the blood, as one measure of diabetic control. Women with a family history of Type 2 diabetes or diagnosed as prediabetic may be at higher risk for gestational diabetes. Close periodontal supervision would seem prudent and early intervention vital.

Osteoporosis and its relationship to periodontal disease is under investigation. A number of studies show a correlation between dental bone mass and total bone mass, total bone mass and number of remaining teeth, and tooth loss by periodontal disease as a risk factor for osteoporosis. A study by Jeffcoat (1998) related systemic osteoporosis to oral bone loss, and Kribbs (1990) and Nitta and coworkers (1997) discussed the impact of periodontal health on osteoporosis in postmenopausal women. In the latter study, 12 edentulous postmenopausal women were compared with 14 periodontally healthy postmenopausal women. "The edentulous patients had less bone mineral density of the lumbar spine and less occlusal force." Preliminary evidence suggests that supplementation with biphosphonates, such as alendrolate (Fosamax®, Merck & Co., West Point, PA), may be helpful in stabilizing dental supporting bone because it helps improve total bone mineralization. Calibrating dental radiographs as a diagnostic tool for systemic osteoporosis may help in early detection of both oral and systemic bone loss (Jeffcoat 1998; Hausmann 1990).

Cardiovascular disease has been the number-one killer of men in the United States. In the last decade, preventive measures have helped reduce the incidence and prevalence of this disease in men; however, women, largely spared the morbidity and mortality risk in the past, are at increased risk now as lifestyles are changing prior to menopause and susceptibility is heightened through reduced hormonal protection during menopause (Mattila et al. 1993). Surprising preliminary evidence is implicating periodontal diseases as an independent risk factor for coronary artery disease, myocardial infarction, and stroke (Beck et al. 1996).

Beck and coworkers reviewed bacterial burden from infections, linking inflammation to onset of coronary heart disease. They discussed hyperinflammation, ulceration of the intimal vascular lining, athromata formation, and thromboembolic episodes in patients challenged by bacterial endotoxins. Kinane (1998) considers tobacco use a strong risk factor for cardiovascular disease, as well as a strong risk factor for periodontal disease. Increased tobacco use among women has increased their risk for both diseases and has reduced levels of estrogen in menopausal women, an additional comfounder. It still needs to be determined if reducing periodontal infection will reduce the incidence of cardiovascular disease and stroke.

Studies of the elderly in institutional settings implicate periodontal pathogens as the etiology for certain pulmonary infections. Higher levels of bacterial plaque and lowered immune resistance to plaque antigens in older individuals have been associated with bacterial pneumonia and bronchitis in an analysis of 3854 individuals by Scannapieco and Mylotte (1996), in Buffalo, New York, and by Hayes and coworkers (1998) in Boston. Hayes and coworkers (1998) studied 1312 men in a VA hospital setting for pulmonary function, citing periodontal status as an independent risk factor. Women live longer, they outnumber men 3 to 2, and they will require more effective plaque-control maintenance in these geriatric environments (United States Census 1992).

There is a dramatic difference in orofacial pain and associated myalgias between men and women (Wardrop et al. 1989). Women present with orofacial pain 20 times more frequently than men. Women also present more frequently with tempormandibular joint disorder (TMJD); intermittent, variable low-grade pulpal and periodontal discomfort (Marbach and Varoscak 1980); and altered tongue sensations, which are difficult to manage effectively in a dental office. The clinician may see a higher incidence of depression, higher use patterns of medications, and higher compromised functional status in women (Gorsky, Silverman, and Chin 1987). Vesiculobullous disorders are higher in women, and recurrent apthous ulcers are more problematic in their frequency, severity, and discomfort (Nisengard 1996).

There are gender differences in response to periodontal diseases. Many of the aggressive periodontal diseases show a higher incidence in women. In adults, there may be a heightened response to plaque with generalized inflammatory enlargements and localized inflammatory tumors in women during pregnancy and contraceptive use.

The literature supports a more directed approach to therapy in women, with far more concern for definitive history taking and more rigid preventive maintenance. The clinician must understand these gender differences and institute comprehensive therapy that includes medical consultation (if necessary), reinforced oral hygiene instruction, antibacterial rinses, periodontal debridement, bacterial culturing as indicated for refractory patients, and more frequent recall scheduling. Postmenopausal women may respond dramatically with proper medical supervision inclusive of estrogen-replacement therapy and calcium supplementation and monitoring of systemic osteoporosis improvements in women taking biphosphonates. The clinician is cautioned against the use of antibiotics in women on contraceptives, since interaction reduces the effectiveness of birth-control medication (Barnett 1985).

In summary, the mouth is portal to the body, and pathosis intraorally cannot be separated from illnesses elsewhere. "Most oral problems are complex diseases, their impact on systemic health in women altered by a multitude of factors, multiple genes and gene susceptibility factors interacting with behavioral and environmental variables" (Redford 1997).

The uncovering of the human genome will illuminate intergender and intragender differences predisposing individuals to local and systemic diseases. The impact of oral problems on systemic health of women must be recognized and treated appropriately.

ACKNOWLEDGMENT

I want to acknowledge Dr. Susan Karabin, clinical associate professor, Columbia University, for her invaluable assistance in preparing this chapter.

REFERENCES

Aldridge, J. P., V. Lester, T. L. P. Watts, A. Collins, G. Viberti, and R. F. Wilson. 1995. Single-blind studies of the effects of improved periodontal health on metabolic control in type 1 diabetes mellitus. *J. Clin. Periodontol.* 22:271–275.

Barnett, M. L. 1985. Inhibition of oral contraceptive effectiveness by concurrent antibiotic administration: A review. *J. Periodontol.* 56:18–20.

Beck, J. J., R. Garcia, G. Heiss, P. S. Vokonas, and S. Offenbacher. 1996. Periodontal disease and cardiovascular disease. *J. Periodontol.* 67:1123–1137.

Cohen, W. 1998. The periodontal-medical risk relationship. *Compendium Suppl.* 199(1)11–24.

Dasanayake, A. P. 1998. Periodontal disease as a risk factor in pregnancy. *Ann. Periodontol.* 3:206–212.

Folkers, S. 1992. Periodontal disease in the life stages of women. *Compend. Educ. Dent.* 13(10):852–856.

Grossi, S. G., R. Genco, and F. B. Skrepcinski. 1997. Treatment of periodontal disease in diabetics reduces glycated hemoglobin. *J. Periodontol.* 68:713–719.

Gorsky, M., S. Silverman, Jr., and H. Chin. 1987. Burning mouth syndrome: A review of 98 cases. *J. Oral Med.* 42:7–9.

Hausmann, E. 1990. A contemporary perspective on techniques for the clinical assessment of alveolar bone. *J. Periodontol.* 61:149–146.

Hayes, C., D. Sparrow, M. Cohen, P. S. Vokonas, and R. I. Garcia. 1998. The association between alveolar bone loss and pulmonary function: The VA dental longitudinal study. *Ann. Periodontol.* 3:257–261.

Hill, G. B. 1998. Preterm birth: Associations with genital and oral microflora. *Ann. Periodontol.* 3:222–232.

Jeffcoat, M. K. 1998. Osteoporosis: A possible modifying factor in oral bone loss. *Ann. Periodontol.* 3:312–321.

Katz, P. P., M. R. Wirthlin, S. M. Szpunar, et al. 1991. Epidemiology and prevention of periodontal disease in individuals with diabetes. *Diabetes Care* 14:375–385.

Kinane, D. F. 1998. Periodontal diseases' contributions to cardiovascular disease: An overview of potential mechanisms. *Ann. Periodontol.* 3:142–150.

Kribbs, P. J. 1990. Comparison of mandibular bone in normal and osteoporotic women. *J. Prosthet. Dent.* 63:218–222.

Marbach, J. J., and J. Varoscak. 1980. Treatment of tempormandibular joint and facial pains: A critical review. *N.Y. State Dent. J.* 46:181–188.

Mattila, K., M. Nieminen, V. Vaitonen, et al. 1993. Association between dental health and acute myocardial infarction. *Br. Med. J.* 298:779–782.

Nisengard, R. 1996. Periodontal implications: Mucocutaneous disorders. *Ann. Periodontol.* 1:401–438.

Nitta, H., K. Bando, M. Matsubara, et al. 1997. Impact of periodontal health on osteoporosis in postmenopausal women. Presented at Sunstar–Chapel Hill, Chapel Hill, NC, March 24–25.

Offenbacher, S., B. Katz, G. Fertik, et al. 1996. Periodontal infection as a possible risk factor for preterm low birth weight. *J. Periodontol.* 67:1103–1113.

Redford, M. 1997. Oral Health Working Group: Research on Women's Health for the 21st Century.

Scannapieco, F. A., and J. M. Mylotte. 1996. Relationships between periodontal disease and bacterial pneumonia. *J. Periodontol.* 67:1114–1122.

Schmidt, A. M., E. Weidman, E. Lalla, et al. 1996. Advanced glycation end products (AGEs) induce oxidant stress in the gingiva: A potential mechanism overlying accelerated periodontal disease associated with diabetes. *J. Periodont. Res.* 31:508–515.

United States Census. 1992. Washington: U.S. Department of Commerce, Bureau of the Census.

Wardrop, R. W., J. Hailes, H. Burger, and P. C. Reade. 1989. Oral discomfort at menopause. *Oral Surg. Oral Med. Oral Pathol.* 67:535–540.

NEW CLASSIFICATION SYSTEM OF PERIODONTAL DISEASES AND CONDITIONS

*A*t the 1989 World Workshop in Clinical Periodiontics (American Academy of Periodontology 1989) a classification system was developed that had been used up to 1999. In 1999 the American Academy of Periodontology decided to develop a new classification system that would not overlap in disease categories, add in a classification for gingival diseases (plaque-induced and non-plaque induced), give clearer classification criteria and would not emphasis age as a deciding factor in the classification (Armitage 1999).

A complete outline of the new classification of periodontal diseases (inflammatory and noninflammatory conditions) is reviewed in Figure A5–1.

A section on gingival diseases was added (IA). This includes plaque-induced gingivitis as well as non-plaque-induced diseases (IB). Additionally, gingival diseases can be modified by systemic factors such as diabetes mellitus.

Some other changes included replacing the term adult periodontitis with chronic periodontitis. The Academy decided that adults, as well as adolescents could develop periodontitis and "adult" was too restrictive.

The term, early onset periodontitis was replaced with aggressive periodontitis. Again, the age-dependent nature of the patient was a factor in changing the terms. The older term "early onset periodontitis" included prepubertal periodontitis, juvenile periodontitis (localized (LJP) and generalized), and rapidly progressive periodontitis. Localized juvenile periodontitis is now termed localized aggressive periodontitis and generalized juvenile periodontitis in now referred to as generalized juvenile periodontitis. Prepubertal periodontitis with complicating systemic involvement is now included under the heading of *periodontitis as a manifestation of systemic diseases* (IV). If there are no modifying system conditions it is referred to as chronic periodontitis or aggressive periodontitis.

Refractory periodontitis will no longer have a separate disease classification because any periodontal case can be considered refractory.

It was undecided if necrotizing ulcerative gingivitis (NUG) and necrotizing ulcerative periodontitis (NUP) were considered part of a single disease process or separate diseases. Never the less, the Academy decided to put the two diseases together in a section called *necrotizing ulcerative diseases.*

New classifications were added including *periodontal abscesses* (VI), *periodontitis associated with endodontic lesions* (VII), developmental or acquired deformities and conditions (VIIIA), *mucogingival deformities and conditions* (VIIIB, C) and *occlusal trauma* (VIIID).

REFERENCES

American Academy of Periodontology. 1989. *Proceedings of the World Workshop in Clinical Periodontics*, I/23–I/24. Chicago: American Academy of Periodontology.

Armitage GC. Development of a Classification System for Periodontal Diseases and Conditions. *Ann Periodontal* 1999; 4:1–6.

CLASSIFICATION OF PERIODONTAL DISEASES AND CONDITIONS.

I.   Gingival diseases
    A. Dental plaque–induced gingival diseases*
        1. Gingivitis associated with dental plaque only
            a. Without other local contributing factors
            b. With local contributing factors (see VIIIA)
        2. Gingival diseases modified by systemic factors
            a. Associated with the endocrine system
                (1) Puberty-associated gingivitis
                (2) Menstrual cycle–associated gingivitis
                (3) Pregnancy-associated
                    (a) Gingivitis
                    (b) Pyogenic granuloma
                (4) Diabetes mellitus–associated gingivitis
            b. Associated with blood dyscrasias
                (1) Leukemia-associated gingivitis
                (2) Other
        3. Gingival diseases modified by medications
            a. Drug-influenced gingival diseases
                (1) Drug-influenced gingival enlargements
                (2) Drug-influenced gingivitis
                    (a) Oral contraceptive–associated gingivitis
                    (b) Other
        4. Gingival diseases modified by malnutrition
            a. Ascorbic acid–deficiency gingivitis
            b. Other
    B. Non-plaque-induced gingival lesions
        1. Gingival diseases of specific bacterial origin
            a. Neisseria gonorrhea–associated lesions
            b. Treponema pallidum–associated lesions
            c. Streptococcal species–associated lesions
            d. Other
        2. Gingival diseases of viral origin
            a. Herpesvirus infections
                (1) Primary herpetic gingivostomatitis
                (2) Recurrent oral herpes
                (3) Varicella-zoster infections
            b. Other
        3. Gingival diseases of fungal origin
            a. Candida species infections
                (1) Generalized gingival candidiasis
            b. Linear gingival erythema
            c. Histoplasmosis
            d. Other
        4. Gingival lesions of genetic origin
            a. Hereditary gingival fibromatosis
            b. Other
        5. Gingival manifestations of systemic conditions
            a. Mucocutaneous disorders
                (1) Lichen planus
                (2) Pemphigoid
                (3) Pemphigus vulgaris
                (4) Erythema multiforme
                (5) Lupus erythematosus
                (6) Drug-induced
                (7) Other
            b. Allergic reactions
                (1) Dental restorative materials
                    (a) Mercury
                    (b) Nickel
                    (c) Acrylic
                    (d) Other
                (2) Reactions attributable to
                    (a) Toothpastes/dentifrices
                    (b) Mouthrinses/mouthwashes
                    (c) Chewing gum additives
                    (d) Foods and additives
                (3) Other
        6. Traumatic lesions (factitious, iatrogenic, accidental)
            a. Chemical injury
            b. Physical injury
            c. Thermal injury
        7. Foreign-body reactions
        8. Not otherwise specified

II. Chronic periodontitis†
    A. Localized
    B. Generalized

III. Aggressive periodontitis†
    A. Localized
    B. Generalized

IV. Periodontitis as a manifestation of systemic diseases
    A. Associated with hematologic disorders
        1. Acquired neutropenia
        2. Leukemias
        3. Other
    B. Associated with genetic disorders
        1. Familial and cyclic neutropenia
        2. Down syndrome
        3. Leukocyte adhesion deficiency syndromes
        4. Papillon-Lefèvre syndrome
        5. Chediak-Higashi syndrome
        6. Histiocytosis syndromes
        7. Glycogen storage disease
        8. Infantile genetic agranulocytosis
        9. Cohen syndrome
        10. Ehlers-Danlos syndrome (types IV and VIII AD)
        11. Hypophosphatasia
        12. Other
    C. Not otherwise specified (NOS)

V.   Necrotizing periodontal diseases
    A. Necrotizing ulcerative gingivitis (NUG)
    B. Necrotizing ulcerative periodontitis (NUP)

VI. Abscesses of the periodontium
    A. Gingival abscess
    B. Periodontal abscess
    C. Pericoronal abscess

VII. Periodontitis associated with endodontic lesions
    A. Combined periodontal-endodontic lesions

VIII. Developmental or acquired deformities and conditions
    A. Localized tooth-related factors that modify or predispose
        to plaque-induced gingival diseases/periodontitis
        1. Tooth anatomic factors
        2. Dental restorations/appliances
        3. Root fractures
        4. Cervical root resorption and cemental tears
    B. Mucogingival deformities and conditions around teeth
        1. Gingival/soft tissue recession
            a. Facial or lingual surfaces
            b. Interproximal (papillary)
        2. Lack of keratinized gingiva
        3. Decreased vestibular depth
        4. Aberrant frenum/muscle position
        5. Gingival excess
            a. Pseudopocket
            b. Inconsistent gingival margin
            c. Excessive gingival display
            d. Gingival enlargement (see IA3 and IB4)
        6. Abnormal color
    C. Mucogingival deformities and conditions on edentulous ridges
        1. Vertical and/or horizontal ridge deficiency
        2. Lack of gingiva/keratinized tissue
        3. Gingival/soft tissue enlargement
        4. Aberrant frenum/muscle position
        5. Decreased vestibular depth
        6. Abnormal color
    D. Occlusal trauma
        1. Primary occlusal trauma
        2. Secondary occlusal trauma

*Can occur on a periodontium with no attachment loss or on a periodontium with attachment loss that is not progressing.
†Can be further classified on the basis of extent and severity. As a general guide, extent can be characterized as localized ≤ 30% of sites involved and generalized ≥ 30% of sites involved. Severity can be characterized on the basis of the amount of clinical attachment loss (CAL) as follows: slight = 1–2 mm CAL; moderate = 3–4 mm CAL; and severe ≥ 5 mm CAL.
Source: Armitage GC. Development of a Classification System for Periodontal Diseases and Conditions. Ann Periodontal 1999; 4:1–6.

A

Abrasion   Wearing away of a structure, such as a gingiva or the teeth, through an abnormal mechanical process. Examples would be gingiva or tooth abrasions due to incorrect brushing.

Abscess, periodontal (also called *lateral periodontal abscess*)   Localized accumulation of pus in periodontal tissues formed by the disintegration of tissue.

Abutment (tooth)   A tooth or implant used for support and retention of a crown or removable partial denture.

Accretions   Accumulation on the teeth of foreign materials, such as dental plaque, materia alba, and calculus.

Acellular   Without cells.

Acellular cementum   Cementum that does not contain cementocytes.

Aerobic   Utilizing and dependent on oxygen.

Air polishing   A controlled stream of sodium bicarbonate used to remove extrinsic tooth stains and dental plaque.

Allograft   See Graft, osseous.

Alloplastic   See Graft, osseous.

Alveolar bone   See Bone, alveolar.

Alveolar crest   The most coronal part of the interproximal bone.

Alveolar mucosa   See Mucosa, alveolar.

Alveolar process   Compact and cancellous bone that surrounds and supports the roots of the teeth.

Anaerobic   Non-oxygen utilizing. Oxygen is toxic to these organisms.

Angle's classification of malocclusion   A classification of different types of malocclusion based on the relationship of the anteroposterior relationship of the dental arches.

  Class I (neutroocclusion)   The mesiobuccal cusp of the maxillary first permanent molar occludes in the buccal groove of the mandibular first molar. Crowding has to be present.

Class II (distoocclusion)   The mesiobuccal cusp of the maxillary first permanent molar is mesial to the mandibular first molar; the mandibular dental arch is posterior to the maxillary arch.

Cl II, division 1   Labioversion of the maxillary incisors.

Cl II, division 2   Linguoversion of the maxillary central incisors.

Class III (mesioocclusion)   The mesiobuccal cusp of the maxillary first permanent molar is distal to the mandibular first molar; the mandibular dental arch is anterior to the maxillary arch.

Ankylosis   Fusion of the tooth with the alveolar bone without an intervening periodontal ligament.

Antibiotic   A soluble substance produced by microorganisms that has the capacity to inhibit the growth of or to kill other organisms.

Antibiotic prophylaxis   See Prophylaxis.

Antibodies   Serum proteins synthesized and released by plasma cells. Antibodies bind to and neutralize bacterial toxins.

Antigen   A foreign substance (e.g., bacteria, bacterial toxins, and byproducts) that elicits the formation of antibodies.

Antimicrobials   Chemical agents that inhibit the growth of or kill a microorganism. The terms *antimicrobial* and *anti-infective* are used interchangeably.

Antiseptic   An antimicrobial applied to the skin surface or oral mucosa that inhibits the growth and development of microorganisms.

Apical   Refers to the apical or anatomic end of the root of a tooth.

Attachment apparatus   Comprises the cementum, periodontal ligament, and alveolar and supporting bone.

Attachment level   See Clinical attachment level (CAL).

Attachment loss, connective tissue (also referred to as *clinical attachment loss*)   A pathologic process whereby the gingival collagen fibers become detached from the root surfaces with the concomitant apical migration of the apical aspect of the junctional epithelium along the root surface.

Attrition   The wearing away of tooth structure by tooth-to-tooth normal or abnormal function.

Autograft   See Graft, osseous.

Autoimmune disease   Disease caused by the immunologic response against components of the body's own tissues.

Avascular   Lacking in blood supply (e.g., tooth enamel, gingival epithelium, cementum).

Bacteremia   Presence of bacteria in the bloodstream.

Bactericidal   The ability of a drug or agent to kill bacteria.

Bacteriostatic   Inhibiting the growth of bacteria.

Bifurcation   The anatomic area where roots of a two-rooted tooth separate.

Biodegradable   Resorbable.

Biofilm, plaque   Matrix-enclosed bacterial populations adherent to each other and/or to surfaces or interfaces.

Biologic width   The length of the gingival connective tissue (1.07 mm) and the junctional epithelium (0.97 mm).

Bone   A hard type of connective tissue that contains collagen fibers, calcium phosphate, and hydroxyapatite.

Alveolar bone (also called *alveolar bone proper*)   Compact bone that lines the tooth socket (alveolus).

Bundle bone   Alveolar bone with insertion of Sharpey's fibers.

Cancellous bone   Bone that is spongy with trabeculae, located between the cortical plates and alveolar bone proper. It makes up the majority of a bone.

Compact bone   Bone that is hard and dense.

Cortical (plate) bone   Compact bone found on the facial and lingual aspects of the alveolar process.

Supporting bone   Surrounds and supports the alveolar bone proper. Is composed on the compact cortical plates of bone and cancellous trabecular bone.

Bone loss

Horizontal bone loss   An equal amount of bone loss between two teeth. The entire alveolar process is destroyed.

Vertical bone loss (also called *angular bone loss*)   Bone destruction that does not occur of the entire thickness of the alveolar process. Bone loss affects only a portion of bone surrounding the affected tooth. Examples include one-, two-, and three-wall bony defects. See Periodontal bony defect.

Bone resorption   Bone loss.

Broad-spectrum (antibiotic)   Antibiotic that affects a wide range of bacteria, including both gramnegative and gram-positive microorganisms.

Bruxism   The involuntary and unconscious grinding or clenching of teeth. It is usually triggered by emotional stress, anxiety, or occlusal irregularities and usually results in abnormal wear patterns on the teeth.

Bundle bone   See Bone, bundle.

C

Calculus   Calcified microbial plaque. It is not viable (living bacteria) and thus is a local contributing risk factor for periodontal diseases. Bacteria embed into the porous surface.

Cancellous bone   See Bone, cancellous.

Cementocytes   Cementoblasts from the periodontal ligament that lie close to the root and become surrounded by forming cementum.

Cementoenamel junction The area at which the enamel and cementum are united at the cervical region of the tooth.

Cementum Thin, calcified layer of connective tissue that covers the root of teeth.

Centric occlusion See Occlusion, centric.

Centric relation The most posterior or retruded position of the mandible to the maxilla from which lateral movements of the jaw can be made.

Chemotaxis The process by which cells (PMNs, macrophages) are attracted toward an inflamed area, often by certain substances, including bacterial products, proteins, and interleukins.

Chemotherapeutics The prevention or treatment of a disease by chemical agents.

Cleft, gingival A vertical-shaped slit extending from and into the gingival margin, usually due to the start of pocket formation or improper flossing.

Clinical Pertaining to the signs, symptoms, and course of a condition or disease as observed by a clinician.

Clinical attachment level (CAL) Distance measured from the cementoenamel junction to the location of the tip of the periodontal probe at the most coronal level of the attached periodontal tissues (junctional epithelium). More reliable marker for disease progression than probing depth measurements.

Clinical attachment loss See Attachment loss, connective tissue.

Col A valleylike depression of the interdental gingiva that connects the facial and lingual papillae. It is just below the contact area of the tooth.

Collagen The most abundant protein of skin, bone, and other connective tissues.

Collagen fibers See Fibers, collagen.

Collagenases Belongs to a family of enzymes called matrix metalloproteinases which are responsible for the normal turnover of connective tissue and destruction of host (body's) tissue (collagen). Produced and secreted by bacteria and host cells including PMNs and fibroblasts. Collagenase produced and secreted by PMNs is responsible for the host tissue destruction. Collagenase produced and secreted by fibroblasts is responsible for the normal remodeling and turnover of collagen.

Community periodontal index of treatment needs (CPITN) An index used in population studies of periodontal disease designed by the World Health Organization to assess periodontal treatment needs.

Compact bone See Bone, compact.

Complement A sequence of serum proteins that, when activated, attempt to destroy a foreign substance.

Compliance The patient's ability to adhere to the appointment schedule and oral home self-care instructions given by the dental hygienist or dentist.

Computed tomography (CT) Digitized tomography that results in an enhanced image that is much easier to read than a plane (conventional) tomogram. It measures the amount of energy transmission through an object. It produces a cross-sectional image of a slice of tissue (e.g., bone). Many slices are made of a given edentulous site.

Continuing care See Periodontal maintenance.

Contributing factor Does not initiate the disease process or act independently as an etiologic agent. Helps to allow a condition to become established and/or progress.

Coronal Toward the crown of a tooth.

Cortical bone See Bone, cortical.

Crater Interdental depressions in the gingiva or bone.

Crestal Of or pertaining to the crest or most coronal portion of the alveolar bone.

Curets

   Area-specific curets (also called *Gracey curets*) Designed to be used on specific tooth surfaces of different teeth. Their design includes one cutting edge per end with a rounded back and toe.

   Universal curets Designed to be used on the mesial and distal surfaces of teeth without changing the instrument. Their design includes two cutting edges per end with a rounded back and toe.

Curettage, gingival Removal of the ulcerated soft tissue pocket wall.

Cytokines Proteins produced and secreted by host cells including macrophages and lymphocytes. These proteins signal and modify the behavior or actions of these cells and other cells. Examples are the interleukins, such as interleukin-1 (IL-1), which is responsible for bone destruction.

Cytoxic The ability to kill cells, including human cells.

Debridement The removal of inflamed, devitalized, or contaminated tissue or foreign material from or adjacent to a lesion.

Dental implant An artificial (usually titanium metal) post that substitutes for a tooth root and to which a prosthesis is attached.

Dental plaque Accumulations of bacteria and other microorganisms on tooth surfaces in the area of the sulcus or pocket. Referred to as plaque biofilm.

Dentifrice A powder, paste, or gel used in conjunction with a toothbrush to aid in the removal of plaque, materia alba, and stain from teeth.

Dentinal hypersensitivity The short, exaggerated, painful response elicited when exposed dentin is subjected to certain thermal, mechanical, or chemical stimuli.

Dentogingival junction (unit) Composed of two parts, the gingival connective tissue attachment and the junctional epithelium.

Deplaquing The removal of subgingival dental plaque after the completion of periodontal debridement. It is performed at the reevaluation/supportive periodontal therapy appointments.

Desensitization Reducing or eliminating dentin sensitivity.

Diagnosis

Dental diagnosis Refers to the identification and naming of a disease.

Dental hygiene diagnosis Identifies certain problems or the patient's response to the disease process that can be treated by a dental hygienist.

Diastema A space between two adjacent teeth in the same dental arch.

Digital imaging X-ray images that use a sensor to transmit the image directly to a computer via a cable link. X-ray image appears on a monitor and can be manipulated electronically to change contrast, orientation, resolution, and size of the image.

Disease A process characterized usually by at least two of these criteria: a recognized etiologic agent (or agents), an identifiable group of signs and symptoms, and consistent anatomic alterations.

Disease activity See Periodontal disease activity.

Disease severity See Periodontal disease severity.

Drifting Tooth migration as a result of loss of proximal contact of adjacent teeth in a healthy periodontium.

Edema An abnormal swelling caused by an accumulation of fluid in a tissue or part.

Edentulous Without teeth.

Embrasure The spaces that widen out from the proximal contact area. Each interdental space has four embrasures: facial embrasure, lingual embrasure, an occlusal or incisal embrasure, and a gingival embrasure. An open gingival embrasure is seen frequently in patients with periodontal disease.

Endosseous implant See Implant, endosseous.

Endotoxins Lipooligosaccharide (lipid) complexes formed by gram-negative bacteria. When the bacteria die and break apart (lysis), the endotoxin is released from the cell wall of the bacteria and is capable of having a toxic or harmful effect on the host tissue.

Enzyme A protein substance formed by living cells that acts to speed up metabolic processes or chemical reaction.

Epidemiology The study of the distribution and determinants of illnesses and their associated factors in the human population.

Epithelial ridges Ridgelike projections of epithelium into the underlying lamina propria.

Epithelium (oral) The tissue that lines the intraoral surfaces. It extends into the gingival crevice and adheres to the tooth at the base of the gingival crevice.

Erosion Chemical wearing away of a structure, such as a tooth.

Erythema (erythematous) Redness of the mucous membranes due to inflammation.

Extent The number or percent of diseased teeth or sites in an individual.

Extrusion (extrude) Overruption of a tooth from its normal occlusal position in the dental arch.

Exudate A fluid substance formed within tissues as a result of inflammation. It consists of polymorphonuclear leukocytes, degenerated tissues, dead cells, bacteria, and tissue fluid.

F

Facial   Pertaining to the face. The facial surfaces of the teeth are called *buccal* and *labial.*

Fibers   A filament or thread. In periodontics, the term usually refers to collagenous or connective tissue fibers.

Collagen fibers   White fibers composed of collagen. Found within connective tissue of the gingiva and periodontal ligament arranged in bundles or haphazardly distributed. Characterized by its hydroxyproline and hydroxylysine content.

Gingival fibers (also called *gingival connective tissue* or *supracrestal fiber apparatus*)   Fibers composed primarily of collagen that radiate from the cementum or bone into the lamina propria. Includes alveogingival, circular, dentogingival, dentoperiosteal, and transseptal.

Principal fibers   Collagen fibers of the periodontal ligament. Includes alveolar crest, apical, horizontal, interradicular, and oblique.

Fibroblast   A cell found within connective tissue that synthesizes collagen and ground substance of connective tissue.

Fibrotic   Tissue that is in a state of repair; tissue is hard and not resilient or spongy.

Filtration   The use of absorbers for the selective reduction in intensity of radiation of certain wavelengths from a primary x-ray beam.

Flap   A part of tissue (gingiva) separated from the underlying tissues except at its base.

Fluorosis, dental   Enamel hypoplasia due to the ingestion of water containing excessive amounts of fluoride.

Food impaction   The forceful wedging of food into the interproximal space by chewing pressure or tongue or cheek pressure.

Free gingival graft   See Graft.

Fremitus   Vibrational movement of the tooth under occlusal function.

Frenum   A narrow band of alveolar mucosa radiates from a fixed part to a movable part and limits movement of that part. Example: Frenum runs from the gingiva to the lip, cheek, or under the tongue.

Frequency   The number of times per second the insert tip moves back and forth during one cycle.

Furcation (also called *furca*)   Anatomic area on multirooted teeth where the root base divides.

Furcation involvement (invasion)   Pathologic loss of bone in the furcation of a multirooted tooth.

G

Genetic   Inheritance or transmission of a disease or condition from a parent to a child.

Gingiva   A part of the masticatory mucosa that is attached to the teeth and alveolar process.

Attached gingiva   The portion of the gingiva that is firm, dense, and tightly bound down to the underlying periosteum, tooth, and bone.

Free (marginal) gingiva   The portion of the gingiva that is unattached and forms the wall of the gingival crevice in health. It is continuous with the attached gingiva.

Gingival crevice   A shallow opening between the free gingiva and the enamel or cementum. In gingival health it is called the *gingival sulcus* and in disease a *pocket.*

Gingival crevicular fluid   Fluid originating in the gingival connective tissue that seeps through the sulcular and junctional epithelium. Flow increases in the presence of inflammation.

Gingival pocket (pseudopocket)   See Pocket, gingival.

Gingival recession   Apical migration of the marginal gingiva resulting in exposure of the root surface to the oral environment.

Gingival sulcus   Space between the tooth and the marginal gingiva in gingival health. If bleeding is present, it is not a sulcus but a pocket.

Gingivitis   Inflammation of the gingiva without involvement of the underlying bone or periodontal attachment. The following are gingival diseases listed in the new classification of periodontal diseases (American Academy of Periodontology 1999):

Plaque-associated gingivitis   Gingivitis caused by dental plaque alone.

Drug-influenced gingivitis Gingivitis or gingival enlargement caused by drugs (e.g., Ca channel blockers, phenytoin, cyclosporine and oral contraceptives).

Pregnancy-associated gingivitis Hormonally influenced inflammation and enlargement of the gingiva during pregnancy.

Puberty-associated gingivitis Hormonally influenced inflammation of the gingiva during puberty.

Graft, osseous

Allograft Bone taken from other human beings (cadavers) other than the patient. Bone is bought from tissue banks.

Alloplast Synthetic or natural bone substitutes.

Autograft Tissue such as bone (osseous material) taken from the patient's mouth or extraoral area such as the hip.

Graft, soft tissue

Connective tissue graft Connective tissue (donor) taken from underneath the epithelium and placed in a prepared recipient bed for the purposes of root coverage and increasing the amount of attached gingiva.

Free gingival graft Gingiva taken from an area in the patient's mouth, usually the palate (donor), and placed in a prepared recipient bed primarily to increase the amount of attached gingiva.

Grinding See Bruxism.

Hemostasis Control of and stopping bleeding.

Histopathogenesis (histopathology) Pathologic (disease) changes within the periodontal structures at a microscopic level.

Host Referring to the body or self.

Host cells Cells normally present in the body [e.g., polymorphonuclear leukocytes (PMNs) macrophages, fibroblasts].

Host-derived enzymes Enzymes produced and secreted by cells in the human body such as neutrophils (PMNs) or fibroblasts.

Hypertropy Increase in bulk of a part or organ not due to tumor formation.

Iatrogenic Caused by dental or medical treatment; abnormal condition induced by a clinician.

Immune response Mechanisms used by the body as protection against environmental agents that are foreign to the body.

Immune system Components include the lymph nodes, thymus, spleen, and bone marrow.

Immunity The organism's (or body's) capacity for successfully resisting the actions of harmful foreign substances or pathogenic (disease-producing) microorganisms such as bacteria or viruses.

Immunodeficiency A deficiency in the immune system caused by an upset in the number of lymphocytes.

Implant, endosseous Dental implant placed within bone.

Incidence The rate of new occurrence of the disease in a population over a given period of time.

Indices (singular: *index*) A screening tool designed to quantify and simplify the disease assessment in population surveys. Examples include plaque, debris, calculus, and periodontal destruction.

Infection Pathogenic invasion of the body and the body's response to these organisms.

Infective endocarditis Inflammation of the inner lining of the heart caused by a microbial infection.

Inflammation Protective response elicited by injury or destruction of tissues that attempts to destroy or wall off the injurious agent and tissue. It is also the cellular and vascular tissue reaction that occurs when tissue is injured.

Inflammatory cells Cells involved in the inflammatory response of tissues to injury or infection (e.g., PMNs, macrophages, mast cells).

Inflammatory periodontal diseases A group of inflammatory diseases of the periodontium including gingivitis and periodontitis.

Infrabony defect See Periodontal bony defects.

Interdental Between two adjacent teeth.

Interdental septum That part of the alveolar process extending between adjacent teeth.

Interproximal Pertaining to the area between two adjacent teeth. See Interdental.

Interradicular That part of the alveolar process between the roots of a multirooted tooth (e.g., molars, premolar).

Keratin A protein that is the main component of keratinized epithelium synthesized by keratinmocytes.

Keratinocyte A cell found in the epithelium (a type of epithelial cell) that forms keratin.

Lamina dura A layer of compact bone forming the wall of a tooth alveolus (alveolar bone). In a radiograph, it appears as a thin radiopaque line separated from the tooth by the radiolucent image of the periodontal ligament space.

Lamina propria The gingival connective tissue layer under the epithelium.

Lymphadenopathy Lymph nodes that are abnormal in size, consistency, or number.

Lymph nodes Small, round, or oval organs containing lymphocytes. Found in groups or chains in certain regions, often associated with large blood vessels.

Lymphocyte A type of white blood cell involved in the immune response. There are two types of lymphocytes: T cells and B cells.

Macrophage A large tissue cell responsible for removing damaged tissue, cells, and bacteria through phagocytosis. Increase in number in chronic inflammation.

Malocclusion Deviation from the acceptable relationship of opposing teeth. See Angle's classification of malocclusion.

Marginal Pertaining to the margin or edge.

Marginal ridge A ridge or elevation of enamel that is on the border of the occlusal surface of a tooth.

Mast cell A large tissue cell that releases inflammatory substances or mediators when damaged.

Masticatory (mastication) The process of chewing food.

Microflora Bacteria living in a part of the body (e.g., the mouth, intestines, nose).

Migration, pathologic The movement of a tooth out of its natural position, usually as a result of advanced periodontal disease.

Mobility, tooth The degree of looseness of a tooth beyond physiologic movement. Tooth movement away from its normal position in a buccal/lingual or apical direction when slight pressure is applied.

Mucogingival involvement (defect) A discrepancy in the relationship between the gingival margin and the mucogingival junction. Usually there is minimal to no attached gingiva.

Mucogingival junction Demarcation between the attached gingiva and alveolar mucosa.

Mucosa A mucous membrane.

Alveolar mucosa Mucosa covering part of the alveolar process and continuing into the vestibule and floor of the mouth. It is movable and loosely attached to the underlying periostium.

Masticatory mucosa Mucosa of the gingiva and hard palate.

Murmur A sound produced within the heart at one of its orifices.

National Health and Nutrition Examination Survey (NHANES I) A national survey of adults from 1960 to 1962.

National Health and Nutrition Examination Survey (NHANES III) This is the seventh in a series, beginning in 1960, of national examination surveys of the U.S. population conducted by the National Center for Health Statistics in collaboration with the National Institute for Dental Research (NIDR). The survey was designed to collect data representative of the total U.S. civilian, noninstitutionalized population age 12 months and older.

National Institute of Dental Research (NIDR) Survey A national survey of employed adults between

18 and 64 years of age conducted by the National Institute of Dental Research. It was named the National Survey of Oral Health of U.S. Adults 1985–1986. More than 15,000 people were examined, representing over 100 million working adults in the United States.

Necrotizing periodontal diseases   Formerly known as *acute necrotizing ulcerative gingivitis* (ANUG). Since *acute* is a clinical descriptive term, it should not be used as a diagnostic classification. Thus the correct term is *necrotizing ulcerative gingivitis*. In the new classification, NUG a type of necrotizing periodontal disease. It is an inflammation of the gingiva characterized by necrosis of the gingival margin and interdental papillae. Included in this classification is necrotizing ulcerative periodontitis (NUP), which is characterized by necrosis of gingival tissues, periodontal ligament and alveolar bone.

Neutrophil   See Polymorphonuclear leukocyte.

O

Objective   Based on facts; not affected by personal feelings.

Obligate   Able to survive only in a specific environment (e.g., an obligate anaerobe is only able to live in a nonoxygen environment).

Occlusal adjustment (also called *selective grinding* or *occlusal equilibration*)   Reshaping the occlusal or incisal surfaces of teeth by grinding to create harmonious contact relationships between the upper and lower teeth.

Occlusal trauma   Injury to the attachment apparatus as a result of excessive occlusal forces.

  Primary occlusal trauma   Excessive occlusal forces placed on a healthy periodontium that produces changes in the periodontal tissues. Examples include placement of a "high" restoration and orthodontic movement of teeth.

  Secondary occlusal trauma   Normal forces of mastication on a periodontium with bone loss (periodontitis) produces changes in the periodontal tissues.

Occlusion   Contact of opposing teeth (maxillary and mandibular teeth).

  Centric occlusion   Maximum intercuspation of maxillary and mandibular teeth.

Open bite   Anterior or posterior teeth do not occlude with the opposing teeth.

Oral hygiene self-care   Removal of dental plaque with brushes, dental floss, and other oral aids.

Oral prophylaxis   See Prophylaxis.

Osseointegration (osteointegration)   The biologic phenomenon by which bone grows up to and contacts the surface of implants, thereby anchoring them to the jaw bone.

Osseous   Referring to bone.

Ostectomy   Surgical removal of support bone.

Osteoblast   A cell that forms bone.

Osteoclast   A cell that resorbs bone.

Osteoplasty   Surgical reshaping or removal of nonsupporting bone.

Overbite   Vertical overlap of the upper incisor teeth over the lower incisor teeth.

Overjet   Horizontal projection of the upper teeth beyond the lower teeth.

P

Panoramic film   A type of conventional radiograph showing the entire area of the mandible and maxilla.

Papillary   Pertaining to the interdental papillae.

Parafunctional habit   A habit characterized by abnormal function (e.g., bruxism, pencil chewing, nail biting).

Passive eruption   Physiologic process with recession of the gingiva from the enamel apically toward the cementoenamel junction.

Pathogenic   Disease-producing.

Pathologic mobility   Horizontal or vertical displacement of a tooth beyond its physiologic movement.

Periapical film   A type of conventional radiograph that shows the entire tooth, including the area around the root apex.

Periapical pathology   Disease occurring around the apex of a tooth.

Pericoronitis (also termed *pericoronal abscess*)   Inflammation of the operculum or tissue flap over a partially erupted tooth, especially a third molar.

Peri-implant   Around a dental implant.

Peri-implantitis   Inflammation of the gingival tissues around an implant.

Periodontal   Occurring around a tooth.

Periodontal bony defects   A deviation from the normal form or contour of bone due to periodontal disease.

> **Infrabony defect**   A general term to describe any periodontal bony defect associated with vertical (angular) bone loss. These defects are named according to the number of bony walls remaining in the interproximal area which surround the pocket (e.g., one-wall, two-wall, and three-wall).

> **Crater (interproximal crater)**   A two-wall infrabony defect (facial and lingual bony walls remain).

> **Hemiseptum defect**   The remaining interdental bone septum where the mesial or distal part has been destroyed, with one bony wall remaining (half of a septum).

> **Intrabony defect**   A type of three-wall defect with three bony walls remaining. The defect may or may not be totally lined by cortical bone and may have cancellous bone behind. Not all three-wall defects are intrabony.

Periodontal debridement   The removal of a foreign material (e.g., plaque, calculus) or dead tissue from the crown, root surface, pocket space, pocket wall, and bone surface.

Periodontal disease activity (PDA)   The ongoing loss of connective tissue attachment and bone at a particular point in time (e.g., at the clinical examination appointment). It is difficult to determine disease activity. A 2- to 3-mm change in clinical attachment level must occur before a site can be labeled disease-active.

Periodontal disease severity   The total periodontal destruction and healing that occur prior to the clinical examination. Disease severity is determined after the periodontal assessment (visual, periodontal probing, radiographs) is completed. Severity can be classified as mild, moderate, or severe.

Periodontal ligament (fibers)   See Principal fibers.

Periodontal maintenance   Also referred to as *recare,* or *continuing care.* An extension of periodontal therapy. Procedures performed at selected intervals to assist the periodontal patient in maintaining oral health.

Periodontal pathogen   Bacteria that cause periodontal disease.

Periodontal pocket   See Pocket, periodontal.

Periodontal probing   Measures the location where physical resistance of the probe is met by the junctional epithelial attachment to the tooth.

Periodontics   The specialty of dentistry dealing with the prevention, diagnosis, and treatment of diseases of the tissues that surround the teeth.

Periodontist   A dental practitioner who practices periodontics.

Periodontitis   Inflammation of the supporting tissues of teeth where there is connective tissue attachment loss and alveolar and supporting bone loss. The following is classification system developed by The American Academy of Periodontology (1999):

> **Chronic periodontitis**   Formerly known as *adult periodontitis.* A form of periodontitis that usually is prevalent in adults but can occur in children and adolescents (formerly known as *prepubertal periodontitis*). The amount of periodontal destruction is consistent with the presence of local factors. Bone resorption usually progresses slowly.

> **Aggressive periodontitis**   Formerly known as *early-onset periodontitis* (e.g., juvenile periodontitis, prepubertal periodontitis, and rapidly progressive periodontitis). Except for the presence of periodontitis, patients are otherwise clinically healthy. There is rapid attachment loss and bone destruction. Patients have defects in host defense. Includes prepubesent children who have periodontal destruction without any modifying systemic conditions. The following specific features are identified:

>> **Localized aggressive periodontitis**   Formerly known as *localized juvenile periodontitis* (LJP). Circumpubertal onset. Primarily affects the first permanent incisors and first molars. Attachment loss may progress at a rate three to five times faster than chronic periodontitis. These patients are characterized by a lack of clinical signs of inflammation, harbor *Actinobacillus actinomycetecomitans* in their microflora, and display an altered immune response.

Generalized aggressive periodontitis Formerly known as *generalized juvenile periodontitis*. Usually affects persons under 30 years of age, but patients may be older. Generalized interproximal attachment loss affecting at least three permanent teeth other than first molars and incisors.

Necrotizing periodontal diseases Replaces *necrotizing ulcerative gingivitis* (NUG) and *necrotizing ulcerative periodontitis* (NUP). A form of periodontitis seen in the HIV/AIDS patient. (See necrotized periodontal diseases)

Refractory periodontitis Patients who do not respond to conventional periodontal therapy treatment. It is not considered a single disease entity because it can occur in all forms of periodontitis.

Periodontium Comprises the periodontal tissues that support and surround the teeth, including the gingiva, cementum, periodontal ligament, and alveolar and supporting bone.

Periodontology The scientific study of the periodontal structures in health and disease.

Periosteum Connective tissue covering the outer surface of bone.

Phagocytosis The process of destroying bacteria by devouring and digesting them by phagocytic cells such as polymorphonuclear leukocytes and macrophages.

Pharmacokinetics What the body does to a drug (e.g., absorption, distribution, metabolism, and elimination).

Phase-contrast microscopy A method of using a microscope through which the shape, size, and mobility of bacteria can be viewed.

Phenytoin An anticonvulsant drug that can cause gingival enlargement.

Pocket

Pocket, Gingival A deepening of the gingival crevice due to the coronal migration of the gingival margin without apical migration of the junctional epithelium, (loss of attachment) and bone loss. Examples: drug influenced gingival enlargement, inflammation of the gingiva. Also called a *pseudopocket*.

Pocket, periodontal A pathologic deepening of the gingival sulcus characterized by apical migration of the junctional epithelium and alveolar bone loss. Two types of periodontal pockets: suprabony and infrabony.

Suprabony pocket A periodontal pocket that extends coronal to the alveolar crest or into a suprabony defect with a horizontal pattern of bone loss. The base of the pocket is coronal to the crest of alveolar bone.

Infrabony pocket A periodontal pocket that extends apical to the adjacent alveolar crest or into an infrabony defect (a defect with a vertical pattern of bone loss). There is apical migration of the junctional epithelium and bone loss; the base of the pocket is apical to the crest of alveolar bone.

Polishing The removal of acquired pellicle, bacterial plaque, and stain from the external tooth surface through mechanical means and an abrasive agent.

Polymorponuclear leukocyte (PMN) The major mobile phagocytic white blood cell involved in engulfing, killing, and digesting microorganisms. The first cell to migrate to the acute inflammatory site. Impairment in their function is related to the pathogenesis of aggressive periodontitis.

Prevalence The proportion of individuals in a population having periodontal disease or the number of individuals expected to have periodontal disease in a specific time.

Primary occlusal trauma See Occlusal trauma, primary.

Principal fibers The connective tissue that surrounds the root surface of the tooth and attaches it to the alveolar bone.

Probing See Periodontal probing.

Probing depth The distance from the soft tissue (gingiva or alveolar mucosa) margin to the tip of the periodontal probe. The health of the attachment apparatus can affect the measurement.

Prognosis A prediction or forecast of the course and outcome of a disease.

Prophylaxis Prevention of disease.

Antibiotic prophylaxis Antibiotic coverage necessary before invasive dental procedures that cause bleeding to prevent a bacteremia that ultimately could cause infective endocarditis or serious infections.

Oral prophylaxis The removal of plaque, calculus, and stains from the exposed and unexposed surfaces of the teeth by scaling and polishing as a preventive measure for the control of local irritational factors.

Proximal Surface of a tooth next to another tooth.

Pseudocleft Slit or fissure of the gingiva associated with severe gingival inflammation or certain medications causing the papillae to enlarge and approach each other and not due to pocket formation.

Pseudopocket See Pocket, gingival or Pocket, pseudo.

Pus See Suppuration.

Radicular Pertaining to the root.

Recession See Gingival recession.

Recurrent Signs of disease return.

Regeneration, periodontal Formation of new alveolar and supporting bone, cementum, and periodontal ligament on a previously diseased root surface.

    Guided tissue regeneration Periodontal procedures performed in an attempt at regeneration. Barrier techniques are used with materials that exclude the junctional epithelium from the wound site in an attempt to allow periodontal ligament cells to populate the wound site.

Resistance, antibiotic An antimicrobial agent no longer is effective in killing or inhibiting growth of microorganisms.

Rete pegs See Epithelial ridges.

Rheumatic heart disease A disease of the heart resulting from rheumatic fever, chiefly manifested by abnormalities of the valves.

Risk factors Characteristics that have been shown to directly cause periodontal disease (e.g., dental plaque, diabetes mellitus, tobacco smoking).

Risk indicators Behavioral and socioeconomic characteristics that are associated with periodontal diseases but are not considered to cause the disease (e.g., aging).

Root planing A treatment procedure designed to remove cementum or surface dentin that is rough, impregnated with calculus, or contaminated with toxins or microorganisms.

Scaler A periodontal instrument that is designed to scale primarily supragingival tooth surfaces.

    Sonic scalers Produces mechanical vibrations by means of air pressure rather than electrical energy. The operating frequency is between 3000 and 8000 cycles per second.

    Ultrasonics Devices operating at frequencies between 18,000 and 50,000 cycles per second. They use electrical energy to produce mechanical vibrations that will remove calculus.

        Magnetostrictive ultrasonics A type of ultrasonic instrument. Produces mechanical movement using a low-voltage magnetic signal. The operating frequency is between 18,000 and 45,000 cycles per second. The handpiece contains coils that activate the interchangeable inserts, causing them to vibrate. The working ends can be used on all sides, providing better adaptation to the tooth surfaces.

        Piezoelectric ultrasonics A type of ultrasonic instrument. Produces mechanical movement using a high-voltage magnetic signal. The operating frequency is between 25,000 and 50,000 cycles per second. Only two sides of the working end are adapted to the tooth surface.

Scaling The removal of dental plaque, calculus, and stains from the crown and root surfaces.

Screening A single examination to separate periodontally healthy from diseased patients and to determine the patient's dental needs. It does not make a specific dental hygiene diagnosis or tell the type of treatment to be given. It simply requires probing depth measurements and conventional radiographs.

Secondary occlusal trauma See Occlusal trauma, secondary.

Selective grinding See Occlusal adjustment.

Severity Degree of disease involvement, quantifying the amount of attachment loss or probing depth. May be expressed as mild or slight, moderate, and severe.

Sign Any abnormality indicative of disease, discoverable by the clinician at the evaluation of a patient.

Sonics See Scaler, sonic.

Stem cells   Cells from which all the blood cells "stem" or come.

Stippling   The "orange peel" appearance (depressions) on the attached gingiva. Stippling is not present on the free gingiva.

Subgingival (submarginal)   Beneath the gingiva or gingival margin; into the crevice.

Subjective   As described in an individual's words or opinions rather than facts.

Substantivity   Ability of a substance to absorb or bind to a surface such as the tooth root, tissues, bacterial plaque, or enamel and slowly released over time in its active form.

Sulcus   See Gingival sulcus.

Supporting bone   See Bone, supporting.

Suppuration   The formation of pus. An inflammatory or purulent exudate formed within the tissues. It consists of neutrophils, bacteria, degenerated and liquefied cells, and tissue fluids that form within the tissues in disease and escape through the ulcerated pocket epithelium into the oral cavity.

Supragingival   Coronal (above) to the free gingival margin.

Surface texture   The tactile quality of a material or tissue; the arrangement of parts of the tissue as it affects the appearance or feel of the surface.

Surgery   The act and art of treating injuries or disease by manual operations.

> **Mucogingival surgery**   Periodontal surgery involving the soft tissue (gingival) aspects such as root coverage or increasing the height and width of the alveolar ridge.

> **Osseous surgery**   Periodontal surgery involving the addition or resection (removal) of bone.

Symptom   A departure from the normal in function, appearance, or sensation experienced by a patient. A subjective sign.

Syndrome   The aggregate of signs and symptoms associated with any morbid process and constituting together the picture of the disease.

Systemic   Affecting or pertaining to the whole body.

T

Temporomandibular joint   The connecting sliding hinge mechanism between the mandible (lower jaw) and the base of the skull (temporal bone).

Therapeutic levels (of a drug)   Concentration of a drug in body fluids that causes a pharmacologic effect.

Toxins   Substances that are harmful to the body (e.g., endotoxin).

Trifurcation   Anatomic area where roots diverge in a three-rooted tooth.

U

Ultrasonics   See Scaler, ultrasonic.

V

Vascular   Refers to blood.

W

Wear facet   A flattened, highly polished worn spot on the occlusal or incisal surface of a tooth (usually seen on the side of a cusp). It may be a clinical sign of attrition.

World Health Organization   A specialized agency of the United Nations with primary responsibility for international health matters and public health.

X

Xerostomia   Dryness of the mouth due to inadequate salivary secretion as a result of aging, salivary gland conditions, or medications.

Chapter 1

1. c
2. c
3. c
4. c
5. b
6. c
7. a
8. a
9. d
10. d

Chapter 2

1. c
2. c
3. c
4. b
5. a
6. c
7. d
8. d
9. a
10. a

Chapter 3

1. d
2. a
3. b
4. a
5. c
6. c
7. c
8. a
9. b
10. e

Chapter 4

1. d
2. a
3. c
4. a
5. d
6. d
7. c
8. b
9. c
10. b

Chapter 5

1. b
2. b
3. c
4. b
5. c
6. a
7. c
8. a
9. b
10. a

Case I

1. e
2. d
3. d
4. b
5. a
6. d
7. d
8. b
9. b
10. a

Chapter 6I

1. b
2. c
3. a
4. d
5. b

Chapter 6II

1. a
2. e
3. c
4. a
5. d

Chapter 6IIIA

1. b
2. a
3. c
4. d
5. b

Chapter 6IIIB

1. a
2. b
3. d
4. c
5. e

Chapter 6IIIC

1. d
2. a
3. a
4. c
5. e

CHAPTER 6IIID

1. b
2. b
3. a
4. c
5. c

CHAPTER 7

1. a
2. c
3. d
4. c
5. c
6. b
7. a
8. c
9. a
10. c

CHAPTER 8

1. c
2. d
3. b
4. d
5. b
6. b
7. c
8. b
9. c
10. c

CASE II

1. c
2. a

3. d
4. d
5. c
6. c
7. b
8. b
9. a
10. c

CHAPTER 9

1. a
2. c
3. b
4. e
5. a
6. c
7. a
8. b
9. a
10. a

CHAPTER 10

1. c
2. b
3. c
4. d
5. c
6. a
7. b
8. e
9. c
10. a

CHAPTER 11

1. d
2. d

3. c
4. c
5. c
6. a
7. a
8. c
9. b
10. c

CHAPTER 12I

1. c
2. d
3. c
4. d
5. a

CHAPTER 12II

1. a
2. c
3. a
4. b
5. d

CHAPTER 12III

1. a
2. c
3. b
4. c
5. c

CHAPTER 13

1. c
2. a
3. d
4. a
5. c
6. b
7. a
8. b
9. b
10. d

CHAPTER 14

1. a
2. c
3. b
4. e
5. d
6. b
7. d
8. a
9. d
10. e

CHAPTER 15

1. b
2. a
3. a
4. a
5. b
6. c
7. b

8. b
9. b
10. a

CHAPTER 16

1. b
2. c
3. b
4. a
5. b
6. b
7. c
8. c
9. d
10. e

CHAPTER 17

1. e
2. b
3. d
4. c
5. a
6. c
7. b
8. a
9. e
10. b

CHAPTER 18

1. d
2. a
3. a
4. c

5. d
6. b
7. d
8. c
9. c
10. c

CASE INTER-PRETATION III
CASE STUDY I

1. c
2. d
3. d
4. b
5. b
6. c
7. d
8. d
9. c
10. c

CASE STUDY II

1. a
2. c
3. d
4. a
5. d
6. c
7. a
8. b
9. b
10. b